UCH TEXTBOOK OF PSYCHIATRY

UCH Textbook of Psychiatry
an integrated approach

edited by

Heinz Wolff
Anthony Bateman
David Sturgeon

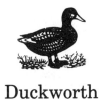

Duckworth

First published in 1990 by
Gerald Duckworth & Co. Ltd.
The Old Piano Factory
43 Gloucester Crescent, London NW1

British Library Cataloguing in Publication Data

UCH textbook of psychiatry.
1. Medicine. Psychiatry
I. Wolff, Heinz   II. Bateman, Anthony
III. Sturgeon, David
616.89

ISBN 0-7156-2289-7 pbk

I MA

W

Photoset in North Wales by
Derek Doyle & Associates, Mold, Clwyd.
Printed in Great Britain by
Redwood Press Ltd, Melksham, Wiltshire

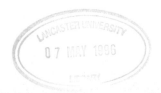

Contents

Part V. Pregnancy, the Puerperium and Gynaecological Disorders

Part VI. Psychiatry and Medicine

Part VII. Child Psychiatry

Part VIII. Treatment Methods

Part IX. Psychiatric Services

Part X. Forensic Psychiatry

To Our Students
who taught us how to teach

Preface

This new comprehensive textbook covers all areas of psychiatry and emphasises an integrated approach, giving equal consideration to the descriptive, biological, psychological, including psychodynamic, and social aspects of the subject. We believe that exclusive emphasis on one or other of these approaches diminishes understanding and impoverishes treatment.

To understand the contribution of personal experience to psychiatric illness it is essential to be familiar with the details of childhood development and the life cycle. Such psychological understanding needs to be integrated with an up-to-date knowledge of biological factors, especially those that affect the brain and mental function in health and illness. These aspects are therefore considered throughout the book. We have paid special attention to the close relationship between psychiatry and medicine, and this is reflected in the chapters on psychosomatic disorders and the practice of liaison psychiatry. At the same time the increasing emphasis on treatment within the community is discussed in the chapters on social and community psychiatry and general practice.

This book replaces *UCH Handbook of Psychiatry* (1975 and 1984) which developed out of the original *UCH Notes on Psychiatry*, first published in 1970. These earlier books were edited and largely written by the late Roger Tredgold and one of the present editors, Heinz Wolff.

In this new book we, as editors, have written many of the chapters ourselves, but our colleagues at University College Hospital and elsewhere have contributed chapters on areas of their special expertise. To maintain a uniform approach we have made changes and additions in several of these chapters, and we are grateful to all the contributors for their friendly collaboration. The ultimate responsibility for the views expressed rests with the editors. Throughout we have used 'he' and 'him' where appropriate to avoid the cumbersome 'he or she' and 'him or her'; no sexual discrimination is intended. The book should serve as a text for medical students, psychiatric trainees, general practitioners and other mental health professionals.

We are particularly saddened by the sudden and premature death of Dr Derek Ricks, author of the chapters on Mental Handicap and Infantile Autism. His work and teaching at UCH will be greatly missed.

We are grateful to the following friends, students and colleagues for their valuable comments and advice: Dr Camilla Bosanquet, Dr Peter Christian, Miss Penelope Crick, Dr Gwen Douglas, Dr Jessie Earle, Dr Peter Hobson, Dr Matthew Hodes, the late Professor John Humphrey, Dr

Morris Katz, Dr Channi Kumar, Mrs Eglé Laufer, Professor Alwyn Lishman, Dr John Paulley, Dr Jean Pigott, Mr Alex Pym, Dr Jeremy Rashbass, Mr Guy Rooney, Dr Bill Smith, Mrs Susan Stuart-Smith, Dr Adrian Sutton, Professor Chris Thompson and Professor Otto Wolff.

We are also grateful to Mr G.R. Peacock, librarian in charge of the University College Clinical Sciences Library, for his help in tracing publications of scientific and historical interest, and to Evelyn Bateman, Jill Bennet, Charlotte Bennie, Kathleen Luckey, Bettine Schneer and Lara Shahabi, who carried most of the secretarial burden between them. Last but not least we thank our publishers for their patience and help in the preparation of this book for press.

Roger Tredgold died shortly before *UCH Handbook* was published. We feel sure that he would have given every support and encouragement to this new venture.

Department of Psychological Medicine   H.W., A.B., D.S.
University College Hospital, WC1

Sadly, Heinz Wolff died shortly before this book was published. In many ways, through the chapters he wrote and his editing, it is very much his book. We hope that it will serve as a fitting tribute to his inspiration and enthusiasm as a teacher of psychological medicine.

A.B., D.S.

Contributors

The chapters written by the contributors are listed below their name and position. Department of Psychiatry, UCMSM = the Department of Psychiatry within the Faculty of Clinical Sciences, University College and Middlesex School of Medicine, University College London. UCH = University College Hospital; UCL = University College London.

Bernard Adams: Consultant Psychiatrist, Department of Psychological Medicine, UCH. Honorary Senior Clinical Lecturer, Department of Psychiatry, UCMSM.
    18. Affective Disorders; 22. Acute and Chronic Organic Mental Reactions; 23. Organic Psychiatric Disorders (with H. Wolff); 48. Psychopharmacology and the Placebo Response; 49. Psychotropic Drugs.

Anthony Bateman: Consultant Psychotherapist, Friern Hospital, and Honorary Consultant Psychotherapist, Tavistock Clinic, London. Psychoanalyst.
    6. Symptom Formation; 10. Interviewing; 11. History Taking; 14. Unusual Situations and Difficult Patients; 16. The Psychoneuroses; 19. Suicide and Acts of Self-Harm; 26. Personality Disorders; 27. Borderline States; 28. Psychosexual Problems; 29. Homosexuality; 40. Disorders of Childhood (with H. Caplan); 51. Psychosurgery; 54. Psychiatric Emergencies; 62. The Mental Health Act 1983.

Joan Bruggen: Psychiatric Social Worker, Department of Psychological Medicine, UCH.
    57. The Hospital Social Worker.

Patrick Campbell: Consultant Psychiatrist, Friern Hospital and Department of Psychological Medicine, UCH. Honorary Senior Lecturer, Department of Psychiatry, UCMSM.
    24. Psychiatric Aspects of Epilepsy; 53. Psychiatric Rehabilitation; 56. Hospital and Community Services.

Harold Caplan: Consultant Child and Adolescent Psychiatrist, Department of Child and Adolescent Psychiatry, UCH. Psychoanalyst. Honorary Senior Clinical Lecturer, Department of Psychiatry, UCMSM.
    40. Disorders of Childhood (with A. Bateman).

Morris Fraser: Consultant in Psychogeriatrics, Department of Psychological Medicine, UCH. Honorary Senior Clinical Lecturer, Department of Psychiatry, UCMSM.

3. Cerebral Structure and Function in Relation to Psychiatry; 25. Psychiatric Illness in Old Age; 50. Electroconvulsive Therapy.

Jeremy Holmes: Consultant Psychiatrist, North Devon District Hospital, Barnstaple, Devon. Formerly Consultant Psychiatrist, Department of Psychological Medicine, UCH.

8. Adolescence and the Life Cycle (with H. Wolff); 45. Marital and Family Therapy.

Sally Hopson: Head of Mental Health and Mental Handicap Occupational Therapy Services, Harringey, London. Formerly Head Occupational Therapist, Inpatient Psychiatric Services, UCH.

60. The Occupational Therapist.

Philip Joseph: Senior Registrar in Forensic Psychiatry, Maudsley Hospital. Barrister at Law. Formerly Lecturer, Department of Psychiatry, UCMSM.

30. Alcoholism; 31. Drug Dependence; 32. Arson.

Julian Leff: Professor of Social and Cultural Psychiatry, Institute of Psychiatry, London. Honorary Research Fellow, Department of Psychiatry, UCMSM.

4. Social and Transcultural Psychiatry; 15. Classification and Epidemiology.

James Mackeith: Consultant Forensic Psychiatrist, Maudsley and Bethlem Royal Hospitals. Formerly Honorary Senior Lecturer, Department of Mental Health, Faculty of Clinical Sciences, UCL.

61. Psychiatry and the Law

George Resek: Consultant Psychiatrist. Formerly Lecturer, Department of Mental Health, Faculty of Clinical Sciences, UCL, and Honorary Senior Registrar, Department of Psychological Medicine, UCH.

46. Behaviour Therapy.

Derek Ricks: Consultant in Paediatric Mental Handicap, Sub-Department of Paediatric Handicap, Department of Paediatrics, UCH. Honorary Research Fellow, Department of Phonetics and Linguistics, UCL.

41. Mental Handicap; 42. Infantile Autism.

Rachel Rosser: Professor of Psychiatry, Department of Psychiatry, UCMSM.

1. A Brief History of Psychiatry.

James Seegolam: Formerly Senior Nurse, Mental Health Unit, UCH.
58. The Psychiatric Nurse (with D. Sturgeon).

Peter Shoenberg: Consultant Psychotherapist, Department of Psychological Medicine, UCH. Honorary Senior Clinical Lecturer, Department of Psychiatry, UCMSM.
35. Menstrual Disorders (with H. Wolff); 36. Gynaecological Surgery (with H. Wolff); 38. Psychosomatic Aspects of Individual Disorders (with H. Wolff).

Valerie Sinason: Senior Child Psychotherapist, Child and Family Department and Day Unit, Tavistock Clinic, London.
43. Child Sexual Abuse.

David Sturgeon: Consultant Psychiatrist, Department of Psychological Medicine, UCH. Honorary Senior Clinical Lecturer, Department of Psychiatry, UCMSM.
12. The Mental State; 13. Formulation; 17. Disasters and the Post-Traumatic Stress Disorder (with H. Wolff); 20. Schizophrenia; 21. Paranoid States; 32. Pathological Gambling; 58. The Psychiatric Nurse (with J. Seegolam); 59. The Clinical Psychologist.

Heinz Wolff: Honorary Consulting Psychotherapist, UCH and Maudsley Hospital. Honorary Senior Clinical Lecturer, Department of Psychiatry, UCMSM. Formerly Honorary Director, Department of Mental Health, Faculty of Clinical Sciences, UCL and Head, Department of Psychological Medicine, UCH.
2. Psychological, Social and Biological Approaches; 5. Psychodynamic Concepts; 7. Personality Development in Childhood; 8. Adolescence and the Life Cycle (with J. Holmes); 9. Bereavement, Death and Dying; 17. Disasters and the Post-Traumatic Stress Disorder (with D. Sturgeon); 23. Organic Psychiatric Disorders (with B. Adams); 32. Shoplifting; 33. Pregnancy and the Puerperium; 34. Termination of Pregnancy; 35. Menstrual Disorders (with P. Shoenberg); 36. Gynaecological Surgery (with P. Shoenberg); 37. Psychosomatic Medicine and the Psychosomatic Approach; 38. Psychosomatic Aspects of Individual Disorders (with P. Shoenberg); 39. Liaison Psychiatry; 44. Psychotherapy; 47. Outcome of Psychotherapy and Behaviour Therapy; 52. Social Therapy; 55. The General Practitioner. Postscript: Psychiatry and Medical Education.

Acknowledgments

The editors are grateful to the following for permission to reproduce material in this book:

Blackwell Scientific Publications Ltd for Tables 22.1 and 22.2, taken from W.A. Lishman, *Organic Psychiatry*, 2nd ed. (1987). Cambridge University Press for Figure 20.2, taken from J. Leff, L. Kuipers, R. Berkowitz, C.E. Vaughn and D.A. Sturgeon, 'Life events, relatives' expressed emotion and maintenance neuroleptics in schizophrenic relapse', *Psychological Medicine* 13 (1983). The Royal College of Psychiatrists for Figure 20.1, adapted from C.E. Vaughn and J.P. Leff, 'The influence of family and social factors on the course of psychiatric illness', *British Journal of Psychiatry* 129 (1976). Chatto & Windus and The Hogarth Press for the extracts from *Virginia Woolf: a biography* by Quentin Bell (1972) and *Cider with Rosie* by Laurie Lee (1959). Faber & Faber Ltd for the extract from *A Grief Observed* by C.S. Lewis (1961). Hamish Hamilton Ltd for the extract from *In the Springtime of the Year* by Susan Hill (1974).

All information about the use and dosage of drugs recommended in this textbook has been carefully checked. However the possibility that mistakes may have been overlooked cannot be excluded. Readers are therefore advised to check the information against relevant and up to date pharmaceutical literature.

Part I
History and Basic Principles

1

A Brief History of Psychiatry

Are people who report unusual subjective experiences or exhibit deviant behaviour inferior, special in some way, or ill? If they are ill, how should their states be described and classified? What are the causes of mental illness? How far should sufferers take responsibility for their state? Should they be treated separately from the rest of society? To what extent can treatments be based on the same principles as treatments of physical illness? What is the importance of intuitive judgment in psychiatric practice? What are the rights of the mentally ill? Is psychiatry a valid academic discipline and if so, what is the relationship between academic psychiatry and clinical practice? These are some of the issues facing modern psychiatry, but their origins can be traced to the beginning of civilisation.

THE ANCIENT WORLD

Archaeological evidence dating back to the beginning of the third millennium BC shows that medicine in Egypt combined specialised physical treatment methods with magical or religious rites and incantations. Healing practices were originally performed by priests, and Imhotep, the originator of Egyptian medicine, was deified after his death and became the Egyptian God of Healing.

It is not clear how far the early Egyptians understood the function of the brain. The Edwin Smith papyrus (2000 BC) advises against operating on the brain. Evidence from mummies shows, for example, cranial injuries in people with paralysis, and suggests that the importance of the brain, which was removed during mummification, may have been recognised.

The role of what might now be called a psychosomatic approach seems to have been appreciated. Temple sleep was used as a treatment at Thebes in Egypt; the faithful would be treated by means of dreams, sometimes drug-induced. The Egyptians knew a great deal about the uses and abuses of drugs which affected the mind. They imported opiates from China and India and other drugs from Crete. The Ebers papyrus, in addition to describing surgical procedures, describes tranquillisers and plants containing scopolamine, as well as a variety of stimulating, relaxing, hallucinogenic and analgesic extracts from plants containing hyoscyamine and atropine. It is not clear, however, to what extent the treatment of the mentally ill differed from that of the physically ill.

In Mesopotamia mind-influencing drugs, including belladonna, were in common use. However, here the balance between the irrational possession theory of illness and the rational disease theory was tipped towards magical explanation and treatments.

In China, medicine was initially practised by priests and witch healers, but later on medicines were also prescribed. Of these the best known is ginseng, which was used for psychosexual disorders, fatigue and neuro-endocrine disorders. The crucial element in the maintenance of health was the world spirit, Tao, with its contrasting components within the human body, Yin and Yang. Health depended on the proper balance between these two opposing forces. Institutions were set up for the treatment of the insane during the Chou dynasty (1027-221 BC). Ancestor-worship prevented the dissection of human bodies, and notions of anatomy and physiology were primitive. Surgery was almost unknown. It was first practised in the third century AD by Hua To, using narcotic analgesia rather than acupuncture. He offered brain surgery to a prince for a neuropsychiatric condition manifest by headaches and paranoid ideas. However, just as the operation was about to start, the prince became terrified and suspicious and accused the surgeon of plotting to murder him on behalf of an enemy. The surgeon was executed and his writings destroyed, so it is hardly surprising that psychosurgery failed to become popular.

Although there has been speculation about contact between the cultures of China and Central and South America, it seems that the latter were wrestling with the problem of the nature of mental illness in relative isolation.

Clay figures from several separate cultures in Western Mexico indicate the origins of syphilis there, whence it travelled to Europe with the returning Spanish invaders and became an important cause of insanity. Aztec art shows that illness was seen as a punishment for sin. For example, epilepsy is depicted as being inflicted by offended deities who had then to be placated with human sacrifice. Philip II of Spain (1527-1598) commissioned Dr Francisco Hernandez to compile a work on the New World in which he identified 1,200 drugs and other treatments used by the Aztecs. Here again there seems to have been tension between healers who were priests and soothsayers and those who were genuine physicians. There was specialisation to the same degree as in ancient Egypt, and powerful drugs were used. In Peru, cocaine was used as a recreational drug as early as 500 BC. Special to Peru are the Mochican figures which depict the results of cerebrovascular disease and evocatively portray the emotional impact of endocrine, neurological and other illnesses. Peruvian mummies reveal that skull trepanning was a common treatment amongst the Mochicans, with a survival rate perhaps as high as 95 per cent. The reasons for surgery are not clear, but it may sometimes have been carried out to release evil spirits from the insane. The Mochican skulls are as yet our best examples of primitive neurosurgery, but there have been similar finds at stone age sites elsewhere, including Northern Europe.

Another isolated culture was that of the Indus empire in India, which reached its zenith at the beginning of the second millennium BC and was eliminated by Aryans some 500 years later. The invading culture produced the Hindu Vedas. Neuralgia, headache, epilepsy and insanity are all described in the Vedas and attributed to sin or possession. Treatment was mainly by spells and exorcism, but in the Atharga Veda, the Rig Veda (1500 BC) and the Ayur Veda (700 BC) there are passages about specific surgical and medicinal treatments with drugs, indicating the basis of a rational system of medicine. Knowledge of the Ayur Veda has been passed on to us through the writings of the Indian physician Susruta who practised and taught medicine and surgery in Benares, probably during the first or fourth century AD. The Ayur Veda was especially concerned with medical and surgical practice. Its fourth part was called the Bhutavidya and dealt with mental disease and its treatment by the 'restoration of the faculties from a disorganised state, induced by demonical possession'. Susruta himself identified aspects of the personality – intellectual, social, spiritual, moral and emotional – which might contribute to the development of mental diseases.

Like the Hindus, the followers of the Buddha sought relief from suffering by means of asceticism. The Buddhist doctrine of a life of good works overcame the harsh caste system for a time in the fifth century BC. Indian kings built the first hospitals in which there was special concern with good clinical practice. We cannot be sure whether these were open to the mentally ill, but there is a record of an exclusively psychiatric hospital in Manchu in 1000 AD.

An important and peculiarly Indian contribution to psychosomatic medicine was the practice of Yoga, which is recorded as early as the third millennium BC. By relaxation, concentration and meditation, the mind could be freed from the influence of the external world, reducing appetite and sensitivity to pain, and lowering heart and respiration rates. These practices have influenced modern physicians and led to experiments with suggestion and hypnosis that were the antecedents of twentieth-century dynamic psychiatry (see Chapter 5).

Indian culture later became permeated by Greek ideas on medicine. Greek medical practice was highly developed by the time Alexander invaded India (326 BC) and Babylon, where he died in 323 BC at the age of 32. At that time the view that mental illness was due to organic disease of the brain was consistent with Greek theories. Alcmaeon of Croton (fifth century BC) thought that the brain, not the heart or liver as hitherto believed, was the seat of mental life. Plato (427-347 BC) supported this, whereas Aristotle (384-322 BC) claimed that intelligence was located in the heart and that the brain was only a temperature-regulating gland. Hippocrates, who practised medicine in the fourth century BC until his death in 377 BC and had studied medical practice in Egypt, argued that both normal temperament and madness arose from the functioning of the brain. Madness was due to the impact of such bodily humours as blood, phlegm and bile on the brain. Hence the term melancholia, which he thought was caused by the influence of black bile. Greek scholars, including Herophilus and Erasistratus of the Alexandrian School in the third century BC, developed these more scientific concepts further on the basis of dissections. For example, Erasistratus of Chios argued that, since the gyri of the brain were more developed in humans than in animals, these were the location of intellectual ability.

It is customary to distinguish these later scientific concepts from the earlier religious explanations and healing practices used in the Aesclepieia. However, it seems that the two approaches – one seeking specific organic causes and treatments and the other attending to the well-being of the whole person – were at first seen as complementary, but that this insight was later forgotten. The Aesclepieia, named after Aesclepios (Aesculapius), the Greek God of Healing, were small temples built in pleasant rural parts of Greece – for example at Epidauros and on the island of Kos – Turkey and some parts of Northern Europe. They had a wide range of facilities, including temples and theatres. Treatment was by 'temple incubation', dream interpretation and tranquillisation with the sound of running water and music. Patients were also encouraged to watch Greek drama in the theatres where the staff would gauge their state of health from their ability to respond appropriately to Greek comedy, drama and tragedy.

The town of Pergamon has an important Aesclepion; it was also the home of the scientist Galen (AD 129-199) who advanced the organic approach to psychiatry. Galen considered that it was the solid part of the brain and the ventricular system which were important in determining mental function. He pioneered the concept of cerebral localisation. Imagination was said to be located in the fore-brain, thought in the mid-brain, and memory in the hind-brain. He described the corpus callosum but took the retrograde steps of ignoring the actual convolutions and insisting that there were only seven cranial nerves.

The Romans inherited Greek ideas, but, despite the enlightenment of Galen, their practice was derived mainly from astrology, religion and primitive superstition. The medical school at Alexandria declined in Roman times, dissections were forbidden, and medicine became a despised occupation practised by slaves and immigrants. None the less the Romans made important contributions to mental health legislation. Their laws distinguished between insanity, mental defect, and disorders due to strong passions, and made provisions for property, marriage and criminal responsibility of the mentally ill.

Roman culture came into contact with the Judaic tradition, and that in turn with early Islamic thinking. The Old Testament viewed insanity as a punishment for sin: 'The Lord shall smite thee with madness ...' (Deuteronomy 28:28), and death might legitimately occur by stoning

(Leviticus 20:27). However, when an evil spirit caused King Saul to be depressed, he was cured by the music of David: 'And it came to pass when the evil spirit from God was upon Saul that David took an harp and played with his hand: so, Saul was refreshed, and was well, and the evil spirit departed from him' (I Samuel 16:23). The concept of possession by devils continued into the New Testament, as described in the miracle of the casting of the devils into swine (Matthew 8:31; Mark 5:12).

By contrast the Talmud did not regard mental illness as a consequence of possession and stated that during periods of insanity the sufferer was not responsible for his actions. It identified different types of mental abnormality, including organic state, psychosis, confusion and mental defect.

In the early Islamic period the mad were distinguished from defectives and from people with disorder of judgment or temperament. The causes of madness were classified as congenital, passionate, bilious and satanic. It appears that Jewish and Islamic attitudes towards madness were in advance of those of Christian culture until the fifteenth century.

THE DARK AGES AND MEDIEVAL EUROPE

The Romans laid the foundation for attitudes to mental illness in Europe. There is scant evidence about attitudes to mental illness in the Dark Ages. The Anglo-Saxons seem to have believed that mental illness was due to possession by demons; they used herbal medicines, ceremony and sometimes violence to drive them out. In Britain monastic hospitals were established by missionaries, for example at St Albans (794) and York (937). After the Norman conquest, there was some revival of interest in Galen's neuro-anatomical and humoral approach and for a while the insane seem to have been regarded as ill in the same way as those with physical symptoms. Almshouses and hospitals such as those of St John at Ghent (founded 1191) and St Mary of Bethlehem at Bishopsgate in the City of London (founded 1247), later called Bethlem or Bedlam, provided for the acutely ill of any kind. Hospitals throughout Europe were run by priests and monks. During the Inquisition physical and mental abnormality were considered to be the work of the devil and evidence of witchcraft. The mentally ill were therefore often tortured or beaten, and some were burnt at the stake as witches. Others were treated with exorcism.

ISLAM

The European Renaissance was preceded by conceptual advances in the Islamic world. Moslem scholars learned Greek philosophy from the Syrians, and in Persia they had access to Sanskrit texts on mathematics and astronomy. Prominent Islamic medical scholars also took an interest in philosophy and psychology. Averroes, born in 1120 in Cordoba in Spain, though not a Greek scholar, doubtless benefited from the new college of translators at nearby Toledo. His works, commenting on Aristotle and arguing for the impersonal immortality of the intellect, were translated and had a wide impact on academics at the Sorbonne and on the Franciscans. In the twelfth and thirteenth centuries Jews lived in harmony with the Moors of Spain, absorbing and transmitting their intellectual culture. With the dawn of Islamic orthodoxy, Aristotelian Moslem scholars, fearing persecution, fled from Spain to take refuge with Jews in Provence, providing yet another means of disseminating ideas and medical knowledge to Western Europe.

Psychiatric hospitals made their appearance against this flourishing intellectual background; the first was built in the mid-ninth century at Cairo. The first sufitic house was opened near Baghdad soon after, offering psychological and social interventions for emotional and psychosomatic problems in a setting without physical restraint. Such establishments spread throughout the Ottoman empire in the thirteenth to fifteenth centuries. In Damascus in 1154, a mental hospital opened which later became the first Turkish medical school. Treatments included medication, especially opium, and music therapy. Music therapy was also used in hospitals in Cairo, Aleppo and Constantinople, and at Edirne, where a hospital with a medical school was designed exclusively for psychiatric use with acoustics adjusted for music therapy. These hospitals provided the inspiration for similar developments in Western Europe. A psychiatric hospital was founded by a priest in Valencia in 1409. In London, the Bethlem Hospital began to specialise exclusively in psychiatry in the fifteenth century. With the dissolution of the monasteries at the time of the Reformation, hospitals in England passed from monks to physicians. The City of London became the custodian of Bethlem in 1547, but the hospital's district commitment diminished and by the end of the sixteenth century four of its twenty-one patients came from outside London.

THE RENAISSANCE

The spread of the principle of freedom of ideas at the beginning of the Renaissance led to a questioning of the possession theory of mental illness and a renewed search for evidence of natural causes. The origins of the Renaissance are complex, but it is clear that the exchange of ideas and translation during the Crusades, the movement of Greek scholars following the fall of Constantinople in 1453 and the invention of printing in 1451, were some of the many causes of the growing intellectual ferment. This led to prolonged tension between mediaeval magical and religious beliefs and the new rationalism.

The archetypal Renaissance man, Leonardo da Vinci (1452-1519), based his paintings and anatomical drawings on detailed empirical knowledge acquired from dissection. This led to accurate drawings of, for example, the blood vessels of the head. The revival of human dissection had begun at the University of Bologna in 1156. The first Professor of

Anatomy, Mandino de Luzzi, thought that the choroid plexus controlled the flow of psychic spirit within the cerebral ventricles. The fourth and seventh volumes of Versalius' *De Humani Corporis Fabrica* (1543) covered respectively the nervous system and the brain, the latter dissected in horizontal slices. However, misconceptions about the vascular system of the brain were not corrected until the English physician Thomas Willis (1621-1675) published *Cerebri Anatome* in 1664, where he also described the circle of Willis. This book was illustrated by Sir Christopher Wren, a member of a group of scientists who met to form the Royal Society in 1660.

The growing body of empirical data came to the attention of theoreticians. Paracelsus (1493-1541) emphasised that mental disorders were the consequence of natural diseases. Francis Bacon (1561-1626) anticipated the dawn of a scientific society and was a pioneer of inductive method. He taught the important doctrine of 'double truth', maintaining that it was possible to support two complementary but contrasting theories derived respectively from reason and revelation. Such a doctrine had been favoured by Averroes, but it was condemned by both the Church and Islam. The 'double truth' doctrine was also apparent in *The Anatomy of Melancholy* (1621) by Robert Burton (1577-1640). It was a fresh way of expressing the creative tension between reason and intuition, both of which are essential to psychosomatic medicine and to a comprehensive style of psychiatric practice today.

René Descartes (1596-1650) introduced the dual concept of body and mind which has remained controversial ever since. His central theme was the primacy of consciousness. He separated reality into two 'substances', one underlying all forms of matter and the other underlying all forms of mind. He expected to explain everything except God and the soul by mechanical and mathematical laws, derived by reason. Cartesian dualism therefore denied the unity of mind and body, but it encouraged systematic scrutiny of the mind itself and thus prepared the way for modern psychiatry, and for the psychosomatic approach (see Chapter 37) which emphasises and studies the interaction between mind and body.

Mental illness also became the subject of legislation. In Britain the Poor Law Act of 1601 brought together and changed previous legislation and formalised common law practice. Following the mediaeval practice of providing refuge for some mentally ill in institutions and general hospitals, and the early Renaissance introduction of specialised psychiatric hospitals, this was the first experiment in formally legislated community care. Before this, the rich usually looked after their own mentally ill relatives within the family or in private institutions or madhouses, but there were few provisions for the poor. The Poor Law Act specified that each parish should take responsibility for the old and the sick, including idiots and lunatics, and provide work for the poor. The first statute law requiring the confinement of vagrants, including the dangerously insane, was the Vagrancy Act of 1714. Magistrates could commit vagrants to gaol or to 'houses of correction' known as 'Bridewells' where the insane were often mixed with criminals and treated as such. Furthermore, the insane were often kept in degrading conditions; at Bethlem hospital, which moved from Bishopsgate to Moorfield in 1676, the inmates were chained and put on display to visitors.

THE MODERN ERA

The consequences of this legislation and other developments in psychiatric practice are disputed. Some historians view the eighteenth century as a period of shameful psychiatric practice. Foucault (1971), for example, refers to it as 'The Age of the Great Confinement', arguing that all over Europe the mad and the eccentric continued to be shut away in institutions. However, for Britain at least, the figures do not support this. During the seventeenth and eighteenth centuries, only the rich arranged private psychiatric care, either by fostering or in small private hospitals which were extremely variable in their standards. It was not until the second half of the nineteenth century that the proportion of mad people confined to institutions climbed rapidly. The legality of physical restraint, straitjackets, beating and other degrading treatments such as confinement in rotating chairs or in cold baths, has also been misinterpreted as no more than a sign of contemptible cruelty. It seems likely, however, that these methods were really believed to be the only effective treatments available. They were used to treat George III (1738-1820) who, during his periods of remission from psychosis, had considerable power over the lives of his physicians!

An alternative view is that psychiatry reached a peak in the eighteenth century with influence at court and in the medical scientific world. In 1751 St Luke's Hospital opened in the City of London, aiming to provide a more humane alternative to Bethlem, and to increase knowledge in psychiatry by teaching, recruitment to the subject and research. Medical students were taught on its wards from 1753. Its first superintendent, Dr William Battie (1703-1776) was a Fellow of the Royal Society and the only psychiatrist to become President of the Royal College of Physicians. Battie brought together the concepts of humane care and rigorous classification of psychiatric disorders. His *Treatise on Madness* (1758) argued that mental illnesses could and should be differentiated and that some would be found to have specific organic causes. The book was consulted by Dr Francis Willis, who looked after George III during his last illness, an atypical psychosis, probably manic-depressive (Leigh 1979), but attributed to porphyria by Macalpine and Hunter (1969). However, Battie's views were not universally accepted, and John Monro (1715-1791), superintendent at Bethlem, asserted that madness was a single indivisible entity.

Humane care became the trend by the end of the eighteenth century. In France it was pioneered by Philippe Pinel (1745-1826), who removed the chains of patients at the Bicêtre and the Salpêtrière in Paris. In Britain, the leading role is attributed to William Tuke (1732-1822), a Quaker who in 1792 established the Retreat at York for mentally ill members of the Society of Friends. Another Quaker leader, born in Philadelphia, was Dr Benjamin Rush (1745-1813) who studied medicine in Edinburgh and was influenced by Pinel. He later became physician at the Pennsylvania Hospital in America where he developed a special interest in psychiatric patients and had a strong influence on the practice of psychiatry in the USA.

Despite the growth of humanitarian treatment, voluntary admission to mental hospitals did not become possible in England until the 1930s, although it had been introduced in Scotland at the end of the nineteenth century (see p. 689). Mental hospitals were however established in great numbers during the early nineteenth century, and legislation provided counties first with the option of building asylums and then, in 1845, with the obligation to do so. These asylums were originally intended to be small hospitals caring for some 100 patients in the centres of towns. Later they became vast overcrowded institutions, largely self-supporting and remote from city centres. They provided protection and care but often at the cost of social stigma and institutionalisation.

The segregation of severely disturbed psychiatric patients in asylums led to a change in the relationship between psychiatry and the rest of medicine; to the separation of the treatment of neurotic conditions from the mainstream of psychiatry, which concerned itself with psychoses and other severe mental disturbances; to closer interaction between neurology and psychiatry; and to problems and delays in the development of university departments of psychiatry. The divisions in the services for the mentally ill were reflected in entirely different conceptual approaches. The tension between the rational and the mystical approach to mental illness, which had been maintained for so long in many different cultures, was undermined. Descriptive psychiatry, rooted in the rational tradition, emerged as the dominant approach to diagnosing the psychotic illnesses observed by psychiatrists working in mental hospitals. Dynamic psychiatry provided a way of understanding and treating the neurotic difficulties which presented to physicians and neurologists. Although both approaches were applicable to the full range of psychotic and neurotic conditions, they were often regarded as mutually exclusive rather than complementary.

Descriptive psychiatry

Descriptive psychiatry was pioneered in France, but in the mid-nineteenth century the leadership passed to Germany. Pinel (1745-1826) and his pupil Jean-Etienne Dominique Esquirol (1772-1840) conceived of psychiatry as a branch of medicine and emphasised objective observation and classification of the symptoms of the inmates of lunatic asylums. Pinel, an admirer of Hippocrates, divided insanity into mania, melancholy, dementia and idiocy.

At the Royal Hospital of Charenton, the French psychiatrist Antoine

Bayle in 1826 reported a collection of case histories of patients with intellectual impairment, grandiose delusions and paralysis and showed that at post-mortem their brains showed evidence of chronic arachnoiditis. A history of syphilis was obtained in some of these patients and this was suspected to be the cause of the inflammation and hence of general paralysis of the insane. It was however not until 1913 that Noguchi and Moore demonstrated the treponema pallidum in the brain. Bayle's crucial discovery in 1826 provided a stimulus to descriptive psychiatry, for it was hoped that accurate classifications of mental diseases would reveal specific organic causes, a hope that continues to inspire biological research today. Another contributor to early biological psychiatry was Benedict Augustin Morel (1809-1873) who was born in Vienna but studied and practised medicine in Paris. He first studied goitrous cretinism and subsequently argued that all mental abnormalities reflected central nervous system degeneration although their specific manifestations were the consequence of cultural, environmental and hereditary factors. He is best known for his invention of the term 'démence précoce' (dementia praecox) which he applied to young mentally ill people who did not recover and eventually appeared to be demented (see p. 227).

The early neuropsychiatrists such as Carl Wernicke (1848-1905) contributed to a change in German psychiatric thinking from speculation to observation and experiment. Wernicke was especially interested in cerebral localisation and aphasia. A similar development occurred in Russia where Korsakoff (1854-1900) created a diagnostic system while he was Director of the Psychiatric Teaching Hospital, founded in Moscow in 1888. In 1889 he described the psychosis due to chronic alcoholism, since known as Korsakoff's psychosis.

Emil Kraepelin (1855-1926), one of the greatest German psychiatrists, was appointed at the age of 30 to a Chair at Dorpat in Russia but then moved to Heidelberg and subsequently to Munich. Kraepelin made painstaking summaries of every one of the 1,000 annual admissions to the hospital in Munich and spent his university vacations trying to group these so as to derive classifications which he modified in the light of the French and German literature. In his early work he was concerned with classifying mental states, but later he placed more emphasis on the course of the illness. His *Compendium of Psychiatry*, first published in 1883, later retitled *Textbook of Psychiatry*, passed through eight major revisions (8th ed. Kraepelin 1909-15). He eventually distinguished between dementia praecox – later called schizophrenia by Eugen Bleuler in 1911 – and manic-depressive psychosis. The concept of dementia praecox was never generally accepted in France, and psychiatrists there retain an idiosyncratic classification (Pichot 1984). However, Kraepelin's classification had an enormous impact on British psychiatry, for Munich served as a model for the Maudsley Hospital and the Institute of Psychiatry in London.

The German philosopher Karl Jaspers (1883-1969) gave descriptive psychiatry a philosophical basis in phenomenology. He moved from law to medicine and then to philosophy, spending only five years in psychiatry. The first edition of his influential *General Psychopathology* was published when he was 30 in 1913, but he continued to update it for the next 40 years. Jaspers (1923) distinguished between the subjective phenomena of morbid mental life and the objective manifestations and symptoms of the phenomena which he termed 'objective psychopathology'. He was concerned not so much with the content and meaning of the experiences patients reported, which were the concern of dynamic psychiatry, but with the form they took. For example, it was more important to identify whether a reported idea was an obsession or a delusion, than to know the precise content of the idea.

In Britain descriptive psychiatry was slower to develop after its early lead at St Luke's but eventually became dominated by the European descriptive approach. John Conolly (1794-1866), the first Professor of Medicine at University College, intended that his medical students, to whom he lectured in psychiatry, should walk the wards of asylums. However, after two years he resigned and later achieved prominence as Superintendent of Hanwell Asylum. In 1830 he insisted on the abolition of physical restraint, still widely practised at that time. This aided the development of a more humane attitude in the treatment of the insane, and encouraged a more medical, descriptive approach (Conolly 1856).

Henry Maudsley (1835-1918), a University College graduate, made an important contribution to descriptive psychiatry with his *Physiology and Pathology of the Mind* (1867), which drew on the descriptive classification of Esquirol. His approach was almost entirely descriptive and organic, and he suggested that mental illness might be cured by a treatment which induced convulsions; he even looked forward to the discovery of the molecular basis of mental disorder.

One of Maudsley's pupils, Frederick Mott (1853-1926), visited Kraepelin's Clinic and Research Institute at Munich and wrote a proposal for a similar University Psychiatric Hospital in England. Maudsley provided the funds, and it fell to Mott, because of his interest in neurological anatomy and physiology, to develop the laboratories at the Maudsley Hospital in London and to Edward Mapother, another University College graduate, to shape the clinical departments. Mapother brought with him ideas which he had developed at Longrove Hospital, an asylum where the highest standards of care were provided. He was strongly influenced by a tour of European centres in 1922 and worked to establish the tradition of descriptive psychiatry at the Maudsley, which became the leading postgraduate teaching hospital in Britain and later merged with the Bethlem Hospital.

Another psychiatrist at Longrove Hospital was Bernard Hart, also a University College graduate. He was particularly interested in psychological aspects of psychiatry and was a Founder Member of the London Psychoanalytical Society. In 1912 he published *The Psychology of Insanity* and in 1913 became the first consultant psychiatrist in the

Outpatient Department of Psychological Medicine at University College Hospital, London.

The development of academic psychiatry and the establishment of University Chairs of psychiatry in Europe and in Britain were also strongly influenced by the development of descriptive psychiatry.

The first French Chair of psychiatry was created within the Faculty of Medicine in Paris in 1877. Eventually, after much debate, Benjamin Ball, who came from a neurological and university background, was appointed. The other candidate was Valentin Magnan (1835-1916), who had a distinguished background in mental hospital psychiatry. This struggle between university psychiatry, rooted in general medicine and neurology, and mental hospital psychiatry, took place throughout Europe. The appointment of Theodor Meynert (1833-1892), a neuroanatomist, to the Chair of psychiatry in Vienna at about the same time provoked a similar debate. In both instances there was resistance, after the appointment of university men, to the establishment of teaching clinics within mental hospitals. In German-speaking countries no fewer than twenty-one Chairs of psychiatry were created between 1804 and 1880, and a further eight before the First World War. They were predominantly occupied by neuropsychiatrists with a special interest in neuroanatomy. The multiplicity of Chairs in Germany reflects the emphasis placed on higher education and research, and the lack of political centralisation, for it seems that here scientific advances in psychiatry followed, rather than preceded, the investment by the universities.

The first Chair of psychiatry in an undergraduate medical school in Britain was established in Durham in 1910, followed by Leeds in 1912. In London, it was not until 1961 that the first Chair in an undergraduate school was established at the Middlesex Hospital, with which the St Luke's Foundation had merged in 1948.

Dynamic psychiatry

While the historical development of descriptive psychiatry led to better diagnosis and classification of psychiatric illnesses and to a better understanding of their aetiology in biological, mainly anatomical and pathological terms, less attention was being paid to the study of the psychological aspects of mental disease. This section describes how the development of psychological methods of treatment from mesmerism through hypnosis to psychoanalysis and related methods of psychotherapy has led to the concepts of dynamic psychiatry. Dynamic psychiatry complements descriptive and biological psychiatry. It is concerned with the way in which psychological understanding can contribute to the diagnosis, aetiology and treatment of some psychiatric disorders, especially the psychoneuroses, personality disorders and some psychosomatic conditions (see p. 23).

Primitive methods of healing and the early explanations of mental illness in terms of possession by evil spirits are sometimes seen as precursors of dynamic psychiatry. However these primitive views and treatment methods were based on religious and supernatural concepts and not on psychological understanding of the patient's experience, as is the case in dynamic psychiatry.

The origins of modern dynamic psychiatry can be traced to the work of Franz Anton Mesmer (1734-1815) at the end of the eighteenth century. Working first in Vienna and then in Paris, he introduced *animal magnetism* as a form of treatment for such disorders as convulsions and paralysis. He brought about these cures with the help of so-called magnets, with which he touched his subjects. He found that he could thereby also induce convulsions and states of trance in normal subjects. Interest in this treatment spread from Paris to London, where its chief exponent was the flamboyant John Elliotson (1791-1868), Professor of medicine at University College. In 1838 Dr Wakley, editor of the *Lancet*, conducted what might now be called a single blind placebo-controlled trial of 'magnetic' treatment, using as subjects two patients under the care of John Elliotson at University College Hospital. Wakley secretly replaced a nickel rod Elliotson was using, claiming that it had 'magnetic' powers, by a 'non-magnetic' rod made of lead. The experiment demonstrated that changes in the mental state could be induced just as well by 'non-magnetic' means. The outcome was that Professor Elliotson was discredited and forced by the Medical Committee to resign (*University College Hospital Magazine* 1951). Regrettably, the extra-ordinary observation that subjects who believe in the effectiveness of a treatment, whatever its properties, can develop abnormal mental states, lose their symptoms or perform strange feats of strength, attracted no interest, and it was many years before the existence of such unconscious phenomena and the placebo effect were recognised and studied (see p. 599).

Thereafter mesmerism was gradually replaced in France and in England by what soon became known as *hypnotism*. The Manchester surgeon James Braid (1795-1860) first introduced the term. In France there was a growing interest in hysteria and other neuroses. August Ambroise Liebeault (1823-1904) and Hippolyte Bernheim (1840-1919), working in Nancy, used hypnosis for the treatment of hysterical symptoms. Pierre Janet (1859-1947) who had a great influence on the early development of dynamic psychiatry, especially in France, studied hysterical phenomena in detail. Independently of Freud, he recognised the importance of unconscious mental phenomena in the origin of hysteria and other psychological disorders; he also used suggestion and hypnosis in their treatment. The famous Parisian neurologist Jean Martin Charcot (1825-1893) published a paper in 1882 describing the effect of hypnotism on hysterical illness, especially hysterical convulsions known as 'grande hystérie'. Later Charcot became interested in hysterical paralyses and amnesia and distinguished these from organic conditions due to neurological lesions.

An important turning point in the development of dynamic psychiatry occurred when Sigmund Freud (1856-1939) came to study with Charcot at the Salpêtrière for four months in 1885. Freud was at that time working as a neurologist and neuropathological research worker in Vienna. Having come across patients with hysterical symptoms, he wished to see how Charcot treated such patients with hypnosis, and as a result became interested in what they talked about while in an hypnotic trance. After his return to Vienna he replaced the technique of hypnosis with the technique of listening to the patient's free associations, and applied this not only to patients with hysteria but also to other neuroses. He thus embarked on his major achievement, the study of unconscious mental phenomena, their role in the aetiology of the neuroses, and the development of psychoanalysis as a treatment method (see p. 558). He and his colleague Joseph Breuer (1842-1925) published their early findings in *Studies on Hysteria* (Breuer and Freud 1895). Freud also distinguished between anxiety, phobic and obsessional neuroses.

Freud's work is usually divided into three phases (Sandler *et al.* 1973). During the first phase, which ended in 1897, he recognised the importance of repressed memories, unconscious mental processes, and conflict, resistance and defence. The second period, which ended in 1923, included the recognition of the importance of fantasy and the distinction between the Unconscious, Preconscious and Conscious – the so-called topographical model of the mind. In the third and final period he introduced the concepts of the id, ego and superego – the so-called structural model of the mind. His theories were based on his observations of the experiences reported by patients, at first during hypnosis and subsequently during psychoanalysis. They were mainly concerned with the patient's inner or subjective experience, or 'psychic reality', in contrast with physical or external reality. Freud shed light on the origin not only of neurotic symptoms but also of such everyday experiences as dreams, forgetting and slips of the tongue ('Freudian slips').

Following his early publications *The Interpretation of Dreams* (1900) and *The Psychopathology of Everyday Life* (1901), Freud began to develop his theories of the dynamic unconscious and instinctual drives. He recognised the influence of early childhood development, including infantile sexuality, on normal and abnormal personality development. He published *Three Essays on the Theory of Sexuality* in 1905 and wrote many papers on psychoanalytic technique. He gradually developed a 'metapsychology', a term which he first used in 1896 to denote a set of theoretical viewpoints on psychoanalytic phenomena. The concept of the id, ego and superego appeared in *The Ego and the Id* in 1923. In 1926 his last major psychopathological work, *Inhibitions, Symptoms and Anxiety*, was published. He continued to publish many more observations and summaries of previous work until his death in 1939.

The psychoanalytical movement began in 1902 when Freud started regular Wednesday meetings for his colleagues and pupils. In 1908 the 'Meeting for Freudian Psychology' in Salzburg attracted participants from six countries, and International Congresses were held regularly thereafter. The International Psychoanalytic Association, incorporating local societies, was established in 1910. The British Psychoanalytical Society was founded in 1913 by Ernest Jones, a University College Hospital graduate. He first met Freud in 1908, remained his strong supporter throughout his life, and published a biography of him (Jones 1964).

Freud's insistence on unquestioning commitment to his ideas from his colleagues resulted in many schisms within the psychoanalytic movement, including the departure of Alfred Adler in 1911 and of Carl Gustav Jung in 1913. Adler (1870-1937) adopted a more social and interpersonal approach to understanding and changing a person's lifestyle. Modern psychosomatic medicine, group and family approaches were influenced by his work. Jung (1875-1961), working in Zürich, split from the Freudian group in 1913, after several years of close collaboration (The Freud/Jung letters 1974). Jung's own work began with his experience of schizophrenic patients, and he introduced the concept of archetypal images and of the collective unconscious (see p. 42). He and his successors were more interested than Freudian analysts in working with older patients, and he insisted that the analyst must himself be analysed. His concepts are discussed further on p. 562.

For a time the descriptive and dynamic approaches were brought together by Professor Eugen Bleuler (1857-1939), Director of the Burghölzli Clinic in Zürich. Bleuler claimed to apply Freudian and Jungian ideas to the descriptive work done by Kraepelin on dementia praecox. He coined the term 'schizophrenia', arguing that the dissociation of psychic functions was an important characteristic of the disorder (Bleuler 1911). He first distinguished, albeit in vague terms, between primary symptoms originating from the pathological process and secondary symptoms which were a manifestation of the disturbed psyche.

Within mainstream psychoanalysis much was learned from the development of psychoanalytic work, including play therapy with children. This was developed further by Anna Freud (1895-1982) who moved with her father to London in 1938 and founded the Hampstead Child Therapy Clinic. She also studied children in the Blitz and during the evacuation from London, and demonstrated the consequences of family disruption and separation from the mother. Her best known work is *The Ego and the Mechanisms of Defence* (1936).

Melanie Klein (1882-1960), a psychoanalyst who had arrived in London from Germany in 1926, had early on become interested in the psychoanalysis of children using play therapy. She emphasised the importance of the earliest experiences of the infant, and her work also helped in the understanding of psychotic states. She defined two constellations in psychic development, the earlier and more primitive paranoid-schizoid position and the later depressive position (see p. 70). Her work had a profound influence on psychoanalysis, especially in Britain, where separate Kleinian and Freudian schools within the British Psycho-analytical Society continue to the present day.

Psychoanalytic theory and practice have undergone many further changes in the last fifty years. Among these the development of object relations theory (see p. 64) under the influence of Balint, Fairbairn, Klein, Winnicott and Bowlby, is particularly important. These concepts and the practice of psychoanalysis today are described in Chapter 44.

Behaviourism

Psychoanalysis emphasised the continuity between normal and abnormal psychic functioning and profoundly influenced people's views of themselves, of society and of the arts. Behaviourism offered an alternative, empirically-based approach to neuroses which was also applicable to normal behaviour and affected patterns of child-rearing and education.

Ivan Petrovich Pavlov (1849-1936) did research on animal behaviour at the Imperial Military Institute in St Petersburg. He showed that simple sensory stimuli, such as the sound of a bell, paired with physiological stimuli, could induce 'conditioned reflexes', such as an increase in salivation in dogs. Conflicting stimuli could produce states in animals which resembled neurotic behaviour in man. Pavlov was a physiologist but not a psychiatrist. The psychiatrist Vladimir Bekhterev (1857-1927) at the same Institute did similar work with more direct clinical relevance.

Clinical behaviourism was pioneered by John B. Watson (1878-1938) at the Phipps Clinic attached to the John Hopkins Hospital in Baltimore. Watson published his findings on behaviourism in 1919 and 1925, and Skinner (1938; 1953) distinguished between operant conditioning and classical Pavlovian conditioning. Behaviour therapy, which arose out of these developments, is described in Chapter 46.

Although behaviourism was introduced at the Phipps Clinic, its Director Adolf Meyer (1866-1950) who had a background in anatomy and pathology, encouraged a pluralistic approach to psychiatry, integrating a person-oriented with a biological approach. As a result he became a leading figure in American psychiatry.

Biological psychiatry and physical treatment

Dynamic psychiatry and behaviourism both offer a method of assessment and treatment. By contrast, descriptive psychiatry provides a diagnostic system which might prove useful in selecting treatments, but is not in itself helpful to the patient. The hope is that the underlying aetiology for different categories will be identified and specific treatments found, but progress in this direction has been limited. None the less, biological psychiatry draws almost exclusively on the descriptive approach. Interest in biological psychiatry was further stimulated by the encephalitis epidemic which started in 1916. This resulted in extrapyramidal signs, sleep disorders, mood disturbances, delusional states and, where it affected children, personality disorders and behaviour problems. In adults Parkinsonism was one of its sequelae (see p. 289) and has received a great deal of attention from biological psychiatry.

New methods of clinical investigation were invented. In 1929 the electroencephalogram was introduced by Berger. It immediately came into widespread use and was the subject of a great deal of research during the next forty years.

W.B. Cannon's work on *Bodily Changes in Pain, Hunger, Fear and Rage* (1929) was done in the Harvard Physiological Laboratory and first published in 1915. At Cornell, a team led by Harold G. Wolff (1950) worked on the body's response to stress and the role of the sympathetic nervous system. Their work led to great advances in the field of psychosomatic medicine. The first modern research on psychiatric genetics was published by Rüdin (1916) in *On Heredity and the Origin of Dementia Praecox* from the Department of Genetics in Munich.

Important advances were also made in biological treatment methods, offering fresh hope to people who had hitherto suffered chronically or permanently. Wagner-Jauregg demonstrated in 1917 that deliberate induction of malaria was beneficial in general paralysis of the insane and received the Nobel Prize for this discovery. The use of penicillin for treating general paralysis was demonstrated in 1943 and an important cause of long-term admission to mental hospital was thus eliminated. Continuous narcosis was introduced in 1922, and insulin coma treatment for schizophrenia was reported in 1933 but abandoned later. Convulsive treatments were introduced soon after and chemical induction was soon replaced by electrical treatments as demonstrated by Cerletti in 1937 (see pp. 617-18). Prefrontal leucotomy, which was for some years a common treatment for chronic depression, was introduced by Egas Moniz in 1936. Major advances in the treatment of the affective disorders and schizophrenia have resulted from the discovery of psychotropic drugs, especially the antidepressants and major tranquillisers, such as chlorpromazine, since the 1950s (see Chapter 49).

Psychiatry since 1945

Two World Wars have had a dramatic effect on the development of psychiatry. Trench warfare in the First World War brought its toll of conversion hysteria and neurotic disorders, bringing psychiatry into the limelight. Massive social changes followed. The Second World War brought civilian injuries but, contrary to expectations, fewer psychiatric casualties.

Jewish psychiatrists and psychoanalysts fled from Europe. Whereas Freud and his daughter Anna settled in London in 1938, one year before he died, the majority of psychoanalysts emigrated to America. There, in a favourable economic climate, psychoanalysis flourished and became the dominant school in American psychiatry. This movement was accompanied by an increase in the importance of clinical psychologists and an enormous increase in their numbers.

Meanwhile, in Europe and in Britain descriptive and biological psychiatry and the new pharmacological treatment methods flourished. In the late 1960s, disillusioned with the exaggerated claims of psychoanalysts and impressed by the greater diagnostic precision of European psychiatrists, American psychiatrists began to move back towards the descriptive model and a more medical and biological emphasis.

Throughout the Western world the demand for medical care of all kinds increased and exceeded supply. Psychiatric patients continued to occupy a large proportion of hospital beds. In Britain, the National Health Service provided a new setting. When it was set up in 1948 there was a desperate shortage of staff of all disciplines, especially psychiatrists at consultant level. Other resources were also short, and the nineteenth-century asylums were in poor condition. Gradual replacement of the mental hospitals by district general hospitals and local facilities for crisis intervention, rehabilitation, psychotherapy and support were planned, but there was and still is continuing concern about insufficient community care to replace the old asylums (see Chapter 56). Developments in neuroradiology and neurochemistry added momentum to the move back to the general hospital.

The new methods of investigation and treatment were applied to an ageing population and psychogeriatrics became an important sub-speciality. Psychosomatic medicine gained increasing attention and led to the introduction of liaison psychiatry. Drug and alcohol dependency reached epidemic proportions, requiring services of a new type.

High costs and short supplies led to the definition of priorities. Funds, whether from the NHS in Britain or from insurance companies in other countries, had to be allocated in the best possible way. The time had come to apply scientific methods to evaluating the effectiveness of the full range of treatments, from ECT and pharmacological treatments on the one hand, to the various forms of psychotherapy and different patterns of service delivery on the other. Over the past 20 years, an impressive amount of information has been gathered about the relative effectiveness of different treatments, separately or in combination, but much work remains to be done. There is reason to hope that greater integration of the descriptive, biological, social, behavioural and psychodynamic aspects of psychiatry will lead to further progress in the understanding, diagnosis and treatment of the wide range of psychiatric disorders.

FURTHER READING

Bynum, W.F. (1983). 'Psychiatry in its historical context' in *Handbook of Psychiatry*, vol. 1 (Shepherd, M. and Zangwill, O.L., eds). CUP, Cambridge.

Ellenberger, H.F. (1970). *The Discovery of the Unconscious: the history and evolution of dynamic psychiatry*. Allen Lane, The Penguin Press, London.

Gay, P. (1988). *Freud: a life of our time*. Dent & Sons, London and Melbourne.

Hunter, R. and Macalpine, I. (1963). *Three Hundred Years of Psychiatry, 1535-1860*. OUP, Oxford.

Lader, M. and Allderidge, P. (no date). *The SK&F History of British Psychiatry: 1700 to the present.* Smith Kline & French Laboratories Ltd., Welwyn Garden City.

Thompson, C. (ed.) (1987). *The Origins of Modern Psychiatry.* John Wiley, Chichester.

Zilboorg, G. (1941). *A History of Medical Psychology.* Norton & Co., New York.

2

Psychological, Social and Biological Approaches

In many respects the practice of psychiatry is similar to the practice of the rest of medicine. Both are concerned with the care of patients suffering from symptoms or clearly defined illnesses, with the causation, diagnosis and treatment of these illnesses and, whenever possible, with their prevention. One essential difference, however, is that in psychiatry we are mainly dealing with mental symptoms and abnormal behaviour, while in other branches of medicine we are concerned mainly with physical symptoms. This is not to say that the psychological and social aspects can be ignored in general medicine, or the physical aspects in psychiatry. On the contrary, all branches of clinical medicine, psychiatry included, are concerned with the whole person in relation to his environment, i.e. with the biological, psychological and social factors involved in the origin, course and treatment of mental and physical disorders.

As psychiatry is especially concerned with mental function in health and illness it tends to attract students and doctors with a major interest in people, their personal experience, their inter-personal and social relationships and their behaviour. For the same reason it has much to contribute to the understanding of the psychological and social aspects of other branches of medicine, including general practice. This will be considered further in the chapters concerned with the work of the general practitioner (Chapter 55) and with the psychosomatic aspects of medicine and medical-psychiatric liaison work (Chapters 37 to 39).

It is helpful to distinguish between three main approaches to psychiatric illness, namely the psychological (including the psycho-dynamic), the social, and the biological (sometimes called the organic approach). It must be stressed, however, that these are not alternatives; all three must be taken into account in understanding and helping patients with psychiatric problems or disorders. The relative importance of each approach depends on the particular disorder, the patient's personality, life experience and social or cultural environment. In psychiatry a multi-factorial approach to the aetiology of the various conditions and to the understanding of the course of the disorder is often essential. This is why psychiatrists need to combine their knowledge of the psychological, social and biological aspects, even though the degree to which individual psychiatrists may be interested in one or other of these is bound to vary.

THE PSYCHOLOGICAL APPROACH

This will be considered first because psychiatric disorders usually present with psychological symptoms. It is essential to gain as much information about a psychiatric patient's subjective experience, including his thoughts, feelings and fantasies, as about any objectively observable psychological phenomena he presents. These include cognitive processes, intelligence, memory, attitudes and behaviour.

There has been a tendency for psychologists to concentrate on the scientific study of objective and observable behaviour, and to pay less attention to or even ignore the individual's subjective experience. This exclusive emphasis on observable behaviour stems partly from John B. Watson's attempt to explain all mental phenomena in purely behavioural terms (Watson 1925). The view that behaviour alone is the proper field of psychological study ignores the important role of subjective experience, which by the very nature of psychology and psychiatry should constitute a central topic of psychological enquiry. An attempt on the part of some psychologists to solve this problem by broadening the use of the term 'behaviour' so as to include all such intra-psychic processes as feelings, thoughts, desires and fantasies as well as behaviour itself, is unhelpful, especially in clinical psychiatry. Nowadays many psychologists contribute a great deal to clinical psychiatry and research by paying attention to both subjective and objective psychological phenomena (see Chapter 59).

The psychodynamic approach

The study of subjective experience and intrapsychic processes has become the special concern of what is known as the psychodynamic approach. This will be considered further in Chapters 5 and 44. In essence, it is concerned with conscious and unconscious mental processes and their influence on interpersonal processes and behaviour. The psychodynamic approach emphasises especially the influence of personality development on mental health and illness (see Chapters 7 and 8). It stresses the importance of the relationship between patient and therapist, especially of transference and counter-transference phenomena in interview and treatment situations (see p. 560). Although the psychodynamic approach has its origin in and hence has much in common with psychoanalysis (see p. 558), it is not confined to any one school or theoretical model.

In clinical practice the psychodynamic approach is particularly relevant to the aetiology, understanding and treatment of personality disorders, some psychosexual problems, the psychoneuroses and borderline states and some psychosomatic symptoms or disorders. It has much less to contribute to the treatment of organic psychiatric disorders. Its place in the functional psychoses, schizophrenia and manic-depressive psychosis is controversial. In treatment the psychodynamic approach makes use of the various forms of insight-directed psychotherapy: psychoanalysis, analytical psychotherapy, and some forms of group, marital and family therapy. It also helps the medical and non-medical staff looking after psychiatric patients to understand the interaction between themselves and their patients and thereby to create and maintain as therapeutic an environment for them as possible.

THE SOCIAL APPROACH

It is now clearly established that stressful situations in the patient's family or social environment play an important role in the causation and course of many psychiatric disorders (Paykel 1978) (see p. 39). These *life events* include bereavements, other losses and separations, physical illness and disability, family tension, marital disharmony, stress at work, retirement, unemployment and so on. They influence especially the onset and course of such common disorders as depression, schizophrenia, the psychoneuroses and some psychosomatic conditions. It is important to recognise that life events will affect people differently, according to the exact meaning the event has for each individual, and that this is in part determined by the individual's personality make-up and past experience. Taking bereavement as an example, an insecure woman whose husband suddenly dies will experience his death as a severe and almost unbearable loss if they have been married for many years and she has been very close to and dependent on him; another stronger and more self-reliant woman who has been unhappily married to an alcoholic and unfaithful husband may experience her husband's death as a relief and an opportunity to make a new beginning. The meaning and significance of what is happening to an individual thus needs to be understood in the context of his present social relationships, as well as his past experience and personality. Cultural and religious factors also influence the way an individual copes with life events.

In treatment the social approach directs attention to the need to improve the patient's social environment, the provision of support in the community by community nurses and social workers, day hospital care, occupational therapy and rehabilitation.

THE BIOLOGICAL APPROACH

This, sometimes also called the *organic approach*, is concerned with the physical basis of mental disease, either disorders of the brain itself or cerebral dysfunction secondary to disorders elsewhere in the body.

Many psychiatric disorders are of organic origin (see Chapters 22 and 23). The brain may be affected by genetic abnormalities, e.g. Down's syndrome and Huntington's chorea; by infection, e.g. general paralysis of the insane (general paresis) due to tertiary syphilis; by degenerative disorders, e.g. senile or presenile dementia; by trauma, e.g. dementia due to brain injury; or by neoplasms, e.g. frontal lobe tumours or secondary deposits. Cerebral function may also be disturbed secondarily by disease elsewhere, e.g. in myxoedema madness due to hypothyroidism, organic confusional states due to electrolyte disturbances, hypo- or hyperglycaemia, toxaemia and high fever in systemic infections, and renal or hepatic failure.

Rapid progress is being made in research on the genetic and biochemical factors in the aetiology of the so-called functional psychoses, i.e. manic-depressive psychosis and schizophrenia. Abnormalities in monoamine transmission in the former (see p. 195) and dopamine transmission in the latter (see p. 238) have been found to play an important role. These developments have increased our knowledge of the biological factors and brain mechanisms involved, but this does not mean that psychological and social factors are unimportant. All three play their part. In some conditions, e.g. reactive depression, life events such as losses are of major aetiological importance, while better understanding of the biochemical abnormalities in the brain throws light on the cerebral mechanisms involved in the disorder. In endogenous depression, on the other hand, genetic and biochemical factors may be of major aetiological significance, while life events and psychodynamic aspects may be precipitant or maintaining rather than causative factors.

In treatment, the biological approach is concerned with the use of psychotropic and other drugs, and the use of electroconvulsive therapy (ECT). Great advances have been made since the Second World War in the discovery and use of psychotropic drugs (see Chapter 49) to control the manifestations of major psychiatric disorders, especially the psychoses.

THE MIND-BRAIN RELATIONSHIP

Consideration of the psychological, social and biological aspects of psychiatry would be incomplete without referring to the controversial issue of the mind-body or mind-brain relationship.

Ever since Descartes (1596-1650) introduced the concept of what is now called mind-body dualism, it has been the subject of philosophical controversy. He considered the mind to be non-material, akin to or the same as the soul, and hence fundamentally different from the body, which is material. This dualistic concept made it difficult to conceive how the non-material mind or soul could have an effect on the material body and vice versa. Since then several alternative philosophical views have been put forward. These include the belief that all mental phenomena, such as conscious self-awareness, feelings, thoughts and wishes, are ultimately reducible to or identical with cerebral processes; these views are referred to as reductionism and the identity theory respectively. Neither makes the necessary distinction between the cerebral mechanisms responsible for psychological experience and the individual's experience itself. It is, of course, accepted nowadays that all mental processes depend on the functions of the brain. But experiences like feeling happy, sad or angry, falling in love, enjoying music and art, or the excitement of making a scientific discovery, are not the same as the electro-physiological processes in the brain. The latter provide the necessary physical mechanisms for the existence of such experiences, but subjective experiences cannot be described or communicated to others in the language of cerebral physiology. Human experience can only be communicated in a language that is meaningful to oneself and others.

Another view is that mental phenomena like self-awareness are mere side-effects or 'epiphenomena' of the neurophysiological processes in the brain. They are thought to have no influence on decision-making or behaviour, which are supposed to be the direct and predictable outcome of cerebral function. This viewpoint, called epiphenomenalism, denies that mental activities like thoughts, feelings and wishes have any influence on what we do. These and other philosophical theories have been critically discussed by Popper in Part 1 of *The Self and Its Brain* (Popper and Eccles 1977).

The present position

Modern psychophysiological research has taken us some way towards formulating a more realistic answer to these questions. First, the mind is no longer confused with the soul, which is a religious concept. Secondly, it is now recognised that 'the mind' is in fact neither a thing nor a substance but a word used to describe the totality of human mental functions, including conscious self-awareness, subjective experience, thoughts, feelings, desire and so on. Thirdly, and this is of special importance, modern biology has recognised the fact that there are different levels of biological organisation, each with its own structure and function. At each higher level of organisation processes take place which cannot take place at lower levels; what happens at the higher level is therefore not necessarily reducible to lower-level processes. In ascending order this is the case when one considers the levels of sub-atomic particles, atoms, molecules, enzymes, cells, organs and man as a whole living organism. This idea is often expressed by saying that 'the whole is greater than the sum of its parts'.

These biological concepts can equally be applied to the level of the brain and the next higher level of psychological or mental function, 'the mind'. Cerebral functions or neuronal activity provide the mechanisms necessary for mental life and subjective experience, but the latter cannot be reduced to the cerebral processes which take place at the next lower level of biological organisation (D. Hill 1970, 1981; J. Hill 1982; Wolff 1983). Many further advances are bound to be made in our knowledge of the relation between cerebral and psychological functions, but this does not mean that the distinction between these two levels of organisation can be ignored or denied.

Another consequence of the recognition that psychological and cerebral processes take place at different levels of biological organisation is that, by what is called 'downward causation', psychological processes can influence cerebral function. Downward causation applies to all successive levels of organisation. Thus, the behaviour of the whole organism or person influences the function of his component organs – if a person starts to run fast this will produce an increase in his heart and respiratory rates. Similarly, the experience of feeling frightened will influence cerebral activity and this in turn produces changes in physiological activity in various parts of the body. There is thus constant interaction between cerebral and psychological processes; for example, if fear occurs in response to being threatened by another person, it is through the organs of perception and consequent changes in cerebral activity that the experience of being threatened and feeling afraid arises; the fear in turn affects cerebral function which increases the activity of the autonomic nervous system. The concept of mind-brain dualism, if by this is meant that the mind is altogether different in nature from the brain, like a soul or a 'ghost in the machine', is no longer acceptable, but interaction between the two levels of organisation, the cerebral and the psychological, is crucial to our understanding of the mind-brain relationship.

CAUSATION IN PSYCHIATRY

It is helpful to bear in mind the interaction between cerebral and psychological processes, and the biological, psychological and social aspects of mental illness when considering the problem of causation in psychiatry.

Some psychiatric disorders, mainly those of organic origin, are due to a clearly identifiable physical cause, e.g. mental subnormality due to phenylketonuria, a biochemical abnormality of genetic origin. The majority, however, are multifactorial in origin, biological, psychological and social factors all playing a part. It is often difficult to decide what aetiological role the different factors play. In schizophrenia, for example, life events may precipitate the onset of a schizophrenic episode in someone with a genetic predisposition, and social factors may prolong the illness. In practice it is useful to distinguish between *predisposing, precipitating* and *maintaining factors*.

Predisposing or *vulnerability factors* include genetic factors and constitutional factors in the individual's personality. The latter are often the result of emotional deprivation in childhood, e.g. separation from or death of the mother, or a seriously disturbed parental background. Such deprivations have been shown to predispose to the development of a depressive illness. The role of *precipitating factors* such as life events has already been described.

Maintaining or *perpetuating factors* are those that maintain or prolong the illness. For example, an hysterical conversion symptom like hysterical paralysis may be maintained by the attention the patient gets from those who are looking after him, so-called secondary gain (see p. 175). Here the perpetuating factor is itself the result of the illness but then serves to prolong it. In a schizophrenic patient the illness may relapse or be prolonged if he lives in an emotionally highly charged family atmosphere; in that case the perpetuating factor is not due to the illness but may have a profound effect on its course. Once the patient is helped to live away from his family, e.g. in a community home, the relapse rate may be reduced (see p. 251).

There is often a complex interaction between predisposing, precipitating and maintaining factors so that no one single or major cause of the disorder can be readily identified. Sometimes research clarifies the issue in a particular disorder, e.g. by identifying a chromosomal abnormality, as has recently been demonstrated in some families with manic-depressive psychosis (see p. 194), or as happened in the case of hysteria when the role of repression and unconscious conflict was recognised by Freud (see p. 175).

Another difficulty of historical origin has arisen from the distinction made by the German psychiatrist and philosopher Karl Jaspers (1883-1969) in his book on *General Psychopathology* (Jaspers 1923). He distinguished between what he called *meaningful* and *causal connections*. Meaningful connections are arrived at by 'understanding' the individual's subjective, psychological experience through empathy, but Jaspers considered that meaningful connections had no causal significance. Causal connections, by contrast, were arrived at through regular observation of observable events, as in the natural sciences, and these connections had causal significance which could be used to explain the origin of a mental disorder in general, independent of the individual's experience. He thus related 'understanding' to individually meaningful connections, and 'explaining' to general causal connections. Moreover, he considered that only somatic events in the brain could be regarded as causal. This distinction has perpetuated the view that only physical processes in the brain can act as causes, not the meaningful experiences of an individual.

Bolton (1984) and J. Hill (1982) have re-examined Jaspers' concepts in the light of up-to-date knowledge of the mind-brain relationship. As has been pointed out earlier, the dualistic approach which considered psychological and cerebral processes as entirely separate has been replaced by the biological concept of two levels of organisation, the cerebral and the psychological. The psychological phenomena have a cerebral basis, and psychological and cerebral processes constantly interact with and influence each other.

In particular, Bolton and Hill have drawn attention to the distinction between *reasons* and *causes*. To give one example, let us consider the effect of a bereavement. The loss of a close and loved one will make the person left behind feel sad and tearful. Here the loss is the reason for the sadness, but there are many intermediate cerebral mechanisms involved in this process. They include the cerebral processes of perception and those underlying the knowledge that the other person will not return, changes in neurotransmitter levels at synapses linked with affective changes, and the nervous impulses leading to stimulation of the lachrymal glands, to mention only a few. These are the physical causes or mechanisms involved. Both the *reason* for sadness and crying, i.e. the bereavement, and the *physical mechanisms* involved in the process thus have *causal* significance.

In other words, it can now be readily accepted that both meaningful connections or reasons and cerebral mechanisms, or a combination of both, can play a causal role in the origin of psychiatric illness. Biological, social and psychological factors, including subjective experience, can all contribute to the causation of the illness.

It is, however, important to note that while known physical causes in terms of abnormal cerebral structure or function may give rise to fairly specific mental abnormalities, social and psychological causes are often non-specific. For example, stressful life events may precipitate the onset or relapse of a variety of illness, e.g. a depressive illness, schizophrenia, a psychosomatic disorder like ulcerative colitis, or a psychoneurotic illness like hysteria or an anxiety state. Similarly, such predisposing causes as emotional deprivation in childhood may be involved in the causation of various disorders, including depressive illnesses, personality disorders and antisocial behaviour. Some authors are still reluctant to use the term causal for predisposing, precipitating or perpetuating factors because this might suggest that the particular factor invariably causes the same mental disorder and by itself is responsible for it. This is not in fact implied. The various factors are causal in the sense that in different disorders and in individual patients they can all, to a greater or lesser degree, have a causal effect and contribute to the development and course of the disorder. This fits in with the view that many mental disorders are multifactorial in origin.

FURTHER READING

Bolton, D. (1984). 'Philosophy and psychiatry' in *The Scientific Principles of Psychopathology* (McGuffin *et al.*, eds). Academic Press, London.

Hill, D. (1970). 'On the contributions of psychoanalysis to psychiatry: mechanism and meaning'. *Brit. J. Psychiat.* 117, 609-615.

Hill, D. (1981). 'Mechanisms of the mind: a psychiatrist's perspective'. *Brit. J. Med. Psychol.* 54, 1-13.

Jaspers, K. (1923). *General Psychopathology*, English translation by J. Hoenig and M.W. Hamilton (1963). Manchester University Press, Manchester.

3

Cerebral Structure and Function in Relation to Psychiatry

Psychiatric disorders are usually categorised as either 'organic' or 'functional'. Organic disorders arise from identifiable structural or biochemical change either in the brain or elsewhere. The most common example of a chronic disorder originating in the brain substance is dementia, where there is primary brain-cell degeneration. Disorders originating from change outside the brain, e.g. severe chest infection, often cause acute confusion and are therefore sometimes grouped together as the 'acute confusional states'. However, disorders of the brain itself can also cause acute confusional states, e.g. a cerebrovascular accident or encephalitis. The terminology is discussed on p. 262.

Functional psychiatric disorders are those for which there is no such identifiable organic cause; common examples are depression and schizophrenia. There are theories about underlying biochemical change, each with some evidence to support it, but there are no physical tests for depression or schizophrenia.

This subdivision is to some extent artificial. An organism interacts continuously with its environment, so psychiatric illness is rarely determined purely by internal physical change (as in the case of organic mental illness), or purely by external events (as in some cases of functional illness). However, in most instances an aetiology of one type or another is predominant (see also Chapter 2).

ORGANIC PSYCHIATRIC DISORDERS

Acute confusional states
(acute organic psychiatric reactions)

Brain cells are highly vulnerable to any form of interference with their nutrition, so that disorders in this category are exceedingly hazardous in their liability to cause permanent brain damage. The possibility of extracerebral disease should normally be considered first when any acute psychiatric symptoms of organic origin are being investigated.

Impairment of brain function due to extracerebral disease occurs, broadly speaking, as the result of (a) intoxication, e.g. alcohol or metabolic disorders like renal or liver failure, (b) deprivation, e.g. hypoxia or vitamin deficiency, (c) trauma, e.g. head injury, or (d) infection, e.g. septicaemia. The various extra- and intracerebral causes of acute confusional states are listed in Table 22.1 (pp. 263) under the heading of acute organic reactions. As a set of general principles, diagnosis is made on the following:

(1) The history. The main pointers are that the pattern of onset is likely to have been fairly acute and the state of confusion is likely to fluctuate; there may be associated features indicative of extracerebral disease, e.g. cough, chest pain, dysuria.

(2) Thorough physical examination and screening.

(3) Possible specific patterns of mental disturbance. For example, in chest infections or alcohol withdrawal there may be visual hallucinations, and in hypothyroidism there are commonly paranoid ideas or auditory hallucinations. Some vitamin deficiencies may cause a relatively isolated memory loss.

The individual acute and chronic organic psychiatric disorders are described in Chapter 23.

Primary brain disease with regional affiliations

Most primary brain disorders present with symptoms that have so-called *regional affiliations*, i.e. the psychiatric symptoms are strongly determined by the site of the lesion. This applies whether there is an isolated lesion, resulting in a few characteristic symptoms, or a diffuse disorder, giving rise to a wide range of deficits. The regional affiliations of such symptoms have major diagnostic importance; a psychiatrist can sometimes make an accurate diagnosis on the basis of 'localising signs' discovered on mental state examination, just as a neurological examination may indicate the site of the lesion responsible for a neurological disorder.

The following sections deal with the various brain areas in which disorder leads to typical psychiatric symptoms.

The frontal lobes

Two frontal lobe functions are of particular importance in psychiatry. First, the frontal lobe is the seat of the 'higher' intellectual functions and can be said generally to govern personality and most of the ways in which the individual makes a finely-judged emotional response to his environment. Anterior frontal integrity is necessary for the maintenance of the 'learned' behaviours which, acquired from infancy onwards, gradually assert themselves over behaviour that is more 'primitive'. Therefore, most of the symptoms that arise from anterior frontal lobe disorder can be classified as *release phenomena*. Emotional control is diminished, giving rise to lability; the emotions are shallow, and the individual is easily moved to laughter, rage or tears. ('Sham rage' can be induced in animals by partial frontal lobe ablation.) Self-care deteriorates; there is personality change with general coarsening of behaviour, disinhibition and a return to infantile patterns of self-gratification. This is called the *frontal lobe syndrome*. If there is severe frontal damage there may be 'primitive' reflexes, e.g. a grasp reflex or an extensor plantar response. A patient with advanced dementia will sometimes exhibit the *sucking reflex* of babyhood: if a finger is brought towards his lips he will purse them as if to suck.

In the posterior part of the frontal lobe, Broca's area in the dominant hemisphere governs language. Disorder of language, or *dysphasia*, is a significant and easily elicited marker of frontal lobe disease. At an early stage there is some degree of expressive dysphasia, beginning with difficulty in naming fairly complex objects (the buckle or winder of a watch, perhaps), then extending to simpler objects; in advanced disease language may degenerate to a meaningless babble. Receptive language function is often relatively preserved, and one should always remember that even a person who is apparently severely confused can often understand more than he can express.

The frontal lobe is especially sensitive to the effect of drugs or alcohol, which are of course taken largely in order to inhibit the frontal 'censor'. Tranquillisers work similarly, although they do not exert their effect directly on the cells of the frontal cortex. Release of frontal control is more likely brought about by their effect on ascending impulses from subcortical nuclei; the nerve endings which bind tranquillisers are largely situated in the brain stem.

The mechanism of frontal release is also utilised therapeutically in the now rare operation of leucotomy, whereby some of the thalamo-frontal tracts are divided in order to relieve intolerable anxiety or depression (see p. 619). The procedure has been almost totally replaced by the use of tranquillisers and antidepressants.

The parietal lobes

The parietal lobes co-ordinate fine movements and complex sensory input. Disorder is thus commonly evident either as *dyspraxia* or *agnosia* (the prefixes 'a-' and 'dys-' are used virtually interchangeably to denote disorder). A severely dyspraxic patient will be unable to perform even simple tasks, such as washing and dressing; early dyspraxia can best be tested clinically by means of simple drawing tests. One of the most sensitive of these is to ask the patient to draw a clock-face, including all the figures, or to copy a simple geometrical drawing (see p. 127). A patient with agnosia is unable to recognise the nature and use of objects, e.g. a pen or a pair of scissors. Tests are less easy to perform since naming ability can be affected by dysphasia; the most effective tests are those that determine whether an object is correctly used. Patients with parietal lobe disorder may also show a failure of right-left orientation and two-point discrimination.

The temporal lobes

Each temporal lobe consists of an outer neocortical division and an older medial portion, made up mainly of the hippocampus and hippocampal gyrus on the inferomedial margins of the temporal lobes. This hippocampal formation processes incoming information and acts as a short-term memory (STM) store. It can only retain a string of eight to ten items, however; items then have to be passed on to the long-term memory (LTM) storage sites. These are principally in the temporal lobes, but the encoding of memory is highly complex and the mechanisms and storage areas involved have not yet been clearly identified. The amnesic syndrome due to bilateral lesions of the hippocampal formation is described below. The primary defect in chronic organic brain disease, especially dementia, is probably an inability to transfer information from STM to LTM stores. The latter stores information about both recent and more remote events. A highly sensitive test of recent memory is that of 'delayed recall', in which the patient is given a fictional name and address and is asked to repeat it after a brief distractor task, such as repeating digits forwards and backwards. If recent memory is impaired the name and address will usually have been 'lost' while the new information was being processed. Asking a patient to repeat numbers backwards and forwards (digit span test) is of limited value as this is a test for immediate memory, which may be intact even in advanced organic brain disease, and of concentration.

Failure to lay down new information in organic brain disease means that memory for recent events is impaired to a much greater degree than that for more remote events. Defects in recent memory can also be elicited by testing a patient's orientation for time, place and person; or he can be asked about recent personal events. Further details of memory testing are described on p. 126.

If lesions of the dominant temporal lobe affect the posterior superior portion various forms of dysphasia may develop. Long-standing temporal lobe epilepsy may cause severe personality change or the development of a psychotic disorder indistinguishable from schizophrenia (see p. 317). The often highly organised nature of the aura of *temporal lobe epilepsy* may be mistaken for a psychogenic symptom, especially if, as is quite common, the aura is not followed by a fit (see p. 314). Temporal lobe epilepsy is at times associated with violent aggressive behaviour. It has been claimed that lesions affecting the amygdaloid nucleus in the temporal lobe may be responsible for such behaviour, and attempts have been made to treat violent and aggressive patients by stereotactic removal of the amygdaloid nucleus. However, the results of such operations are variable and the functions of the amygdala are still uncertain.

Amnesic syndromes of organic origin

The role of the hippocampal formation in the temporal lobes in laying down recent memory has already been referred to. Bilateral lesions of the *hippocampal formation* give rise to a characteristic amnesic syndrome. Immediate recall remains unimpaired so that the patient can immediately repeat a name or a few digits but these will have been forgotten after a few seconds. There is a severe defect of recent memory so that new learning becomes impossible but long-term or remote memory is better preserved.

An almost identical amnesic syndrome can arise as the result of lesions in the *hypothalamic-diencephalic system*; this includes the posterior hypothalamus, the grey matter around the third ventricle and the mamillary bodies. This amnesic syndrome is the central feature of *Korsakoff's psychosis* and is due to thiamine deficiency, usually due to alcoholism. Unlike the amnesic syndrome due to lesions of the hippocampal formation, it may be accompanied by confabulation. After recovery there is a retrograde amnesia for events during and preceding the illness. The condition is described further in Chapter 30 (see p. 381).

Differential diagnosis

It is essential to distinguish organic from functional memory loss due to, say, *hysterical amnesia* or *depression*. When the amnesia is due to repression and dissociation as in hysterical amnesia (see p. 176) it usually covers a circumscribed period of days or weeks in the recent past, or the memory loss may be so global that the patient may even have forgotten his own name and identity. At the same time there may be variations and inconsistencies in his account. It may later emerge, perhaps from information obtained from relatives, that the patient's amnesia covered a period of severe stress.

In depressive illness an apparent loss of memory, sometimes called *pseudodementia*, may result from lack of concentration or psychomotor retardation, but in such cases other evidence of depression should help to distinguish it from organic memory loss. It will also tend to lack the selective impairment of recent memory that is so characteristic of organic memory loss.

FUNCTIONAL PSYCHIATRIC DISORDERS

In the functional psychiatric disorders, such as the affective disorders and schizophrenia, there is no known structural disorder in the brain or any known systemic disease outside the brain which is responsible for the disorder. Biological research into the functional psychiatric disorders has therefore concentrated largely on possible biochemical causes, especially neurotransmitter abnormalities in the central nervous system.

The evidence for neurotransmitter abnormalities is indirect; for example, it may be inferred from the effect of drugs, from measurement of urine or CSF metabolites, or from observations in animals. Occasionally an increase or decrease of neurotransmitter substances may be found at post-mortem examination in parts of the brain.

The following brief account describes the biochemical abnormalities that are thought to be involved in some of the symptoms of functional disorders.

Anxiety states

The biochemical changes that occur in the central nervous system in anxiety states are not clearly understood. Certain drugs such as the benzodiazepines which reduce anxiety bind to specific receptors in the CNS and thereby enhance the inhibitory synaptic actions of the neurotransmitter *gamma aminobutyric acid* (GABA) (see p. 602). These receptors are found especially in the septo-hippocampal part of the limbic system, and also in the spinal cord. The GABAergic system appears to inhibit anxiety and arousal; the benzodiazepines by increasing the effects of GABA therefore have both anxiolytic and anticonvulsant effects. Decreased activity of the GABAergic system therefore may be one of the cerebral mechanisms operative in anxiety states.

In the same way as research on opiate pharmacology led to the discovery of endogenous opioid peptides, the endorphins and enkephalins, research has been directed towards the discovery of endogenous anxiolytics in the central nervous system, but so far without success.

Depressive illnesses

These are associated with reduced activity of *monoamine transmitters* in the central nervous system, specifically noradrenaline and 5-hydroxytryptamine (5-HT). Evidence has emerged haphazardly and biochemical theories of depression have mainly originated from the fact that certain drugs have been found, more or less by good fortune, to treat depression effectively. These are almost all drugs which enhance monoamine transmission. The corollary is also true: drugs which deplete monoamines, e.g. reserpine, can cause depression. The monoamine hypothesis (see p. 195) and the pharmacological action of antidepressant drugs will be considered in more detail in Chapters 18 and 49.

Schizophrenia

The most favoured biochemical theory is the *dopamine hypothesis*, i.e. that dopamine overactivity is responsible for the acute symptoms of schizophrenia. This may be due to either excessive dopamine production or oversensitivity of the postsynaptic dopamine receptors. Evidence rests largely on the observation that the drugs which are most effective in schizophrenia block dopamine receptors. There is also somewhat weak post-mortem evidence; in some brains of schizophrenic patients a slight dopamine increase in the caudate nucleus has been demonstrated. The likelihood is that dopamine overactivity is responsible for only some of the symptoms of schizophrenia, namely the so-called positive symptoms such as delusions, hallucinations and excitement. These symptoms as a group are more susceptible to drug management, in contrast to the negative symptoms such as emotional flattening and loss of volition. The dopamine hypothesis in schizophrenia will be considered further on p. 238.

It will be seen that words like 'probably' have to be used to qualify almost everything written about the biochemistry of functional psychiatric disorders. Almost all modern treatments came into use simply because they worked; theories, right or wrong, followed much later. Even now, the living human brain is virtually impossible to observe directly, and the advanced diagnostic tools available, e.g. CT scanning or EEG, are insensitive when it comes to the detection of subtle biochemical changes. Techniques such as magnetic resonance imaging (MRI), previously called nuclear magnetic resonance scanning (NMR), are more responsive to biochemical activity but are still unlikely to be helpful in the diagnosis of affective disorders or schizophrenia. Indirect tests, such as the measurement of amine metabolites in the cerebrospinal fluid or urine have proved equally disappointing; it is probable that no clinician of the near future will have diagnostic tests for functional psychiatric disorders that are more sensitive than the evidence of his own eyes and ears.

FURTHER READING

Baddeley, A. (1983). *Your Memory: a user's guide*. Penguin Books, Harmondsworth.

Fraser, M. (1987). *Dementia: its nature and management*. John Wiley, Chichester.

Green, A.R., and Costain, D.W. (1981). *Pharmacology and Biochemistry of Psychiatric Disorders*. John Wiley, Chichester.

Kopelman, M.D., (1987). 'Amnesia: organic and psychogenic'. *Brit. J. Psychiat.* 150, 428-442.

Lishman, W.A. (1987). *Organic Psychiatry: the psychological consequences of cerebral disorder*, 2nd ed. Blackwell, Oxford.

Scientific American Book (1979). *The Brain*. W.H. Freeman, Oxford and New York.

Shaw, D.M., Kellam, A.M.P., and Mottram, R.F. (1982). *Brain Sciences in Psychiatry*. Butterworth Scientific, London.

4

Social and Transcultural Psychiatry

Man is one of the most social of all animals. He is born into a social group, brought up in it and continues to live in it. Apart from unusually solitary individuals, people develop bonds with relatives, friends and workmates. In addition, they relate on a wider scale to a culture and to a nation. An extensive body of scientific work has been built up concerning the effect of the social environment on the origin and course of psychiatric disorders.

SOCIAL PSYCHIATRY

Distribution of psychiatric illness

Some of the earliest work employed epidemiological techniques (see p. 151). At the end of the last century, Durkheim (1897), a French sociologist, studied the geographical distribution of suicides in France. He discovered that they were concentrated in cities, and also found that individuals were at greater risk if they did not marry or have children. To explain these findings, he developed the concept of *anomie*, by which he meant absence of social bonds. He postulated that social relationships protect people against suicide, and that the lifestyle imposed by cities disrupts social networks and makes people more vulnerable to suicide (see p. 216). His findings have been replicated many times over the years, and his concept of anomie has had a seminal influence. It has even entered public consciousness in the generalised form that industrialisation and urbanisation drive people mad (see, for example Chaplin's film 'Modern Times'). However, Durkheim's proposition is weakened by such a generality, for which there is very little evidence. On the other hand, his ideas have been profitably extended to psychiatric conditions other than suicide.

In the 1930s, Faris and Dunham (1939) charted the distribution of psychiatric illnesses in the city of Chicago. They found that patients admitted for the first time with schizophrenia were concentrated in the central districts of the city, which were characterised by a deteriorating physical and social environment and a high proportion of single-person households. In a later study of the city of Bristol, Hare (1956) confirmed the concentration of schizophrenia in the central districts, and demonstrated a significant association with the proportion of single-person households. These observations do not necessarily prove that the isolation of deteriorating urban environments leads to schizophrenia. An alternative explanation is that individuals who will later develop schizophrenia leave their families and migrate to the centre of cities, where they choose to live on their own. This possibility was explored in a study by Dunham (1965), carried out in Detroit 25 years after his original work in Chicago. He selected two contrasting areas, a desirable outer suburb and an inner-city district, and calculated the first admission rates for schizophrenia. As anticipated, the rate for the inner-city area was three times the rate for the suburb. Dunham then divided the patients into migrants, who had lived in the district for less than five years, and those with more than five years' residence. The rates for the geographically stable patients were almost identical for the two districts, showing that the excess in the inner-city area was entirely due to individuals who had migrated there within five years of the onset of their first episode of schizophrenia.

This geographical drift of pre-schizophrenic individuals is mirrored by social drift. In Western countries, patients with a first schizophrenic illness are always found to be over-represented in the lowest social classes. Interestingly, the reverse seems to be true in non-Western countries. When the fathers of Western schizophrenic patients were studied, it was found that their social class distribution was no different from that of the general population. Hence the patients must have drifted down the social scale before the onset of their first schizophrenic episode. The social and geographical drift of pre-schizophrenic individuals strongly suggests that the illness affects aspects of their relationship with others and their capacity to function in society long before the appearance of the characteristic symptoms (Goldberg and Morrison 1963).

Family influences on schizophrenia

Studies of family influences on schizophrenia illustrate the problems of interpreting associations between social and clinical factors, in particular the difficulty of determining what is cause and effect from what is observed without any interference, so-called 'naturalistic data'. One approach to this problem is to conduct an experiment, attempting to alter the social factor(s) considered to be exerting an influence, and looking for concomitant changes in clinical factors. Such an approach has been adopted as part of a body of work on the effects of social factors on the course of schizophrenia.

This work began in the 1950s, at a time when cogent criticisms had been levelled at psychiatric institutions, and had led to a change in the attitudes of staff (Goffman 1961). There was a move away from custodial care and towards resettlement of patients in the community. A follow-up study of a group of schizophrenic patients discharged from psychiatric hospitals revealed that those who went to live with relatives were more likely to be readmitted than those living alone (Brown *et al.* 1958). This suggested that some aspect of the relationship between patients and their relatives might be exerting a deleterious influence on the course of their illness. Brown and Rutter (1966) developed a technique of measuring relatives' emotional attitudes towards patients, based on an interview with the relatives. On the basis of the relatives' response to questions, they were categorised as high or low on an index of *expressed emotion* (EE). The commonest reason for assigning a relative to a high EE category was excessive criticism of the patient or emotional over-involvement with the patient. High EE attitudes in relatives were found to be associated with a worse outcome from the patients' schizophrenic illness.

This finding could be viewed as evidence for an effect of the emotional relationship between relative and patient on the course of schizophrenia. An alternative, and equally plausible, explanation is that some quality in the patient both provokes the relative to become critical or over-involved and leads to a worse prognosis. A powerful way to distinguish between these alternatives is to conduct the kind of experiment referred to above. In this instance it involved therapeutic intervention with high EE families, with the aim of ameliorating critical and over-involved attitudes. Several trials have been conducted and have shown that if the family atmosphere can be altered in the desired direction, the outcome for patients is substantially improved (Leff *et al.* 1985; Hogarty *et al.* 1986). Hence there is good evidence that relatives' emotional attitudes do indeed exert an influence on the course of schizophrenia. These findings are discussed more fully in Chapter 20 (see p. 250).

It should be noted that these findings do not constitute proof of a role for relatives' emotional attitudes in the aetiology of schizophrenia. That issue can only be investigated directly when it is possible to identify individuals who will later develop schizophrenia. Otherwise, it is a matter of attempting to reconstruct retrospectively the family atmosphere before the patient fell ill, a dubious endeavour.

High EE attitudes are by no means confined to the relatives of schizophrenic patients. The spouses of depressed patients have been found to be as critical of their partners as the spouses of schizophrenic patients. Furthermore, the degree of relatives' criticism predicts relapse of depression, albeit at a lower threshold than is the case for schizophrenia. Over-involved attitudes have been identified in the parents of anorexic girls, mentally subnormal individuals, and children with diabetes. It is clear that these emotional attitudes are non-specific stress factors, which may operate across a wide range of psychiatric and physical disorders.

Life events and psychiatric illness

Life events constitute another source of stress in the social environment that has been extensively studied. They are sudden, often unexpected, happenings which necessitate some degree of psychological adjustment on the part of the individual to whom they occur. Major events, such as births, marriages and deaths in the family, occur in everyone's life and clearly exert a significant psychological influence. However, less dramatic happenings, such as starting a new job, or a course of study, or acquiring new neighbours, may also produce important effects. In research on life events it has proved crucial to define carefully the onset of the illness being studied, to determine as accurately as possible the timing of events, and to distinguish between *independent* and *dependent life events*. Events defined as dependent are those that might conceivably be brought about by the individual's illness, e.g. giving up his job because he is depressed. The exclusion of these from consideration lessens the likelihood of circular reasoning about cause and effect.

Independent life events have been shown to play a part in the origin of episodes of psychiatric and physical illnesses. They cluster in the three weeks before bouts of schizophrenia (Brown and Birley 1968), and during the three months preceding episodes of depression (Leff and Vaughn 1980). They have also been identified as precipitating manic illnesses. Several studies have suggested that the events preceding depression have a particular quality, in representing losses of one kind or another to the individual concerned. Death and separation are obvious examples, but the loss of health involved in a serious illness, or the loss of self-esteem in failing to gain an expected promotion, can also be included in the category of loss events. Furthermore, for loss events to bring about depression, certain vulnerability factors have also to be present. These include the loss of one's mother by death or separation before the age of 11 (Brown and Harris 1978), and for women the lack of a job, the presence of three or more children under the age of 15, and the absence of an intimate relationship with another person, usually a spouse. Other work has confirmed that a poor marital relationship renders people more liable to develop depression in response to a life event.

There are also particular examples of the role of social support in buffering individuals against stress. For both schizophrenia and depression, relatives with warm and supportive attitudes can help patients adjust to life events and hence prevent a worsening of their condition. Whether social support confers a similar advantage on patients with other types of illness is currently under study, but it is evident that Durkheim's ideas about the importance of social bonds for a healthy existence continue to stimulate research.

In addition to the psychiatric conditions mentioned, life events have been studied in relation to a number of physical illnesses. They have been shown to cluster in the three weeks before a myocardial infarction (Connolly 1976) and also are connected with abdominal pain mimicking appendicitis (Creed 1981). When patients who were found at operation to have a normal appendix were compared with those with an inflamed appendix, the former had experienced an excess of life events in the preceding three weeks. These findings emphasise the non-specific nature of the stress occasioned by life events, and suggest a close parallel with relatives' EE. Each represents an aspect of environmental stress, the one short-lived, the other enduring, which can be measured accurately and which has been incorporated in a large number of studies. Both have proved to be influential in a wide variety of conditions, psychiatric and physical. They appear to explain in many instances why individuals fall ill, but they do not determine the nature of the illness. It seems likely that this is shaped by factors within the individual, either inherited or developmental.

The therapeutic environment

One social environment that has been extensively studied is that of the psychiatric hospital. Sociologists such as Goffman (1961) and Etzioni (1961) described psychiatric institutions in terms of their power structure, and saw patients as occupying the lowest rung of the ladder. They identified the ways in which patients were deprived of their individuality and treated as objects. The classical study of hospital environments by Wing and Brown (1970) demonstrated that the more custodial the care, the more time patients spend doing nothing, and the worse certain aspects of their symptoms were. These studies have been influential in fuelling the movement for community care, and have led to major changes in the pattern of psychiatric services (see also p. 621). Over the last few decades, the evaluation of psychiatric services has grown into a major area of social psychiatry. The work is difficult because it is rarely possible to conduct controlled experiments, and the great majority of studies have to be naturalistic, with all the problems of interpretation that involves. Furthermore, some of the key issues, such as the nature of the social environment in a community facility and the quality of life for an individual, pose considerable measurement problems. Despite its scientific limitations and the methodological hurdles, this type of evaluative work is of great importance as it can influence the process of planning services at a local or national level.

Prevention in psychiatry

Studies of the incidence of diseases can lead to the identification of aetiological factors, and hence to the institution of measures for primary prevention. Unfortunately, there is only a handful of conditions in psychiatry for which the aetiology is sufficiently well understood to implement primary prevention. Huntington's chorea (see p. 280) and Down's syndrome (see p. 525) are two examples of inherited conditions for which genetic counselling is an appropriate measure. Secondary prevention concerns the amelioration of the course of an illness once it has appeared, and becomes feasible when the factors that maintain an illness have been identified. The studies of relatives' expressed emotion, described above, have indicated that therapeutic intervention in families can prevent relapse of schizophrenia, at least over a two-year period (Leff *et al.* 1985). Tertiary prevention is aimed at the handicaps that accumulate in the course of chronic relapsing conditions.

Rehabilitation programmes (see Chapter 53) are an integral part of psychiatric treatment. They aim to return patients suffering from schizophrenia and other disabling conditions to as normal a life as possible. Programmes involve training in everyday skills, such as self-care, domestic activities, shopping and work-like activities. The last usually take place in day centres and sheltered workshops. Schizophrenia often impairs a patient's ability to form relationships with other people, and social skills training, either on an individual or a group basis, is employed to remedy the resulting defects (see p. 682).

TRANSCULTURAL PSYCHIATRY

Cultural influences on delusions and hallucinations

Transcultural psychiatry is sometimes seen as a minor branch of psychiatry, dealing with unusual ethnic and cultural groups and exotic conditions. In fact, the concepts central to this discipline provide a basis for understanding psychiatry as a whole. As an example, let us consider the standard definition of a delusion, namely a false belief which cannot be shaken by evidence to the contrary, and *which is inconsistent with the individual's cultural background*. This last proviso is necessary to allow for cultural groups which adhere firmly to beliefs that are irrational and, if not contravened by evidence, are not based on facts. This would apply to all religions, whether established by the state and numbering their believers in millions, or obscure and practised by a handful of adherents. It follows that we are no more entitled to label a belief in the Yoruba god of iron, Ogun, a delusion than a belief in the Holy Trinity. In many non-Western cultures, beliefs in witchcraft flourish and are firmly held by mentally healthy people. When a group emigrates from such a culture to a Western country, the contrast in systems of belief can pose problems for the psychiatrist. Faced with a West Indian client who complains that evil spells have been cast on him, the psychiatrist may well be uncertain whether this belief constitutes a paranoid delusion or not. One approach is to ask a member of the same cultural group whether the client's beliefs are acceptable to him or not. An enquiry of this nature is essential when the psychiatrist is unfamiliar with the client's cultural background. Psychiatrists working in large cities may encounter representatives of many different ethnic and religious sub-groups, and cannot be expected to become conversant with the variety of beliefs involved.

The argument that delusions can only be judged in relation to the client's culture applies equally to hallucinations. In some traditional cultures, hearing voices or seeing visions is taken to be a sign of a special link with the spirit world, which confers an increase of status on the individual. Where attitudes to such phenomena are favourable, individuals are more likely to report them, and possibly to experience them as well. Evidence for this view comes from a population survey of hallucinations conducted in Florida. It was found that ethnicity and religious affiliation were both significantly associated with the likelihood of reporting hallucinations. In particular this was increased in black respondents and members of fundamentalist religious sects. Since the diagnosis of a psychotic condition almost always depends on the presence of delusions and hallucinations, it is incumbent on the clinician to pay careful attention to the client's cultural background, even if he does not obviously belong to an unusual minority group.

Universality of schizophrenia

Two complementary issues are whether psychiatric conditions are universal, i.e. occur in all cultural groups, and whether any culture-bound conditions exist, i.e. illnesses which are peculiar to a single cultural group. The first question was tackled by the World Health Organisation (1973) in a study called the International Pilot Study of Schizophrenia (IPSS), which involved nine centres distributed between developed and developing countries. The psychiatrists taking part were trained in the use of the *present state examination* (PSE) (Wing *et al.* 1974), a standardised clinical assessment schedule. It emerged that psychiatrists in seven of the nine centres used the diagnosis of schizophrenia in a very similar way, and included patients under this rubric whose clinical pictures resembled each other closely. This was not true of the centres in Washington and Moscow, where psychiatrists employed a much broader definition of schizophrenia, including patients who would have been diagnosed as manic or depressed by their colleagues in the other centres. Apart from these two exceptions, the evidence from the IPSS supports the universality of schizophrenia, at least in literate cultures. Similar studies need to be conducted in pre-literate cultures.

Culture-bound conditions

The related question whether culture-bound psychiatric conditions exist appears to merit a positive answer, for conditions such as koro and amok are confined to particular cultural groups and geographical areas. However, a closer look at these states casts doubt on their unique character.

Koro affects people of Chinese ethnicity, occurs in south-east Asia, and can take an epidemic form. The affected individual develops a belief that his penis is shrinking into his abdomen, and that if this is allowed to happen he will die. At first sight, this might appear to be a delusion. However, the sufferer is always able to recruit relatives and friends to aid him in the situation by firmly holding on to his penis, and it is clear that this belief is shared by his cultural group. Rather than being a psychosis confined to a particular ethnic group, it is a hypochondriacal anxiety state, common to mankind, but given an exotic (to us) form by local beliefs.

Amok was first described among Malayan people, but it also occurs in other parts of south-east Asia. The word, in Malay, means 'to engage furiously in battle'. The condition begins with a period of brooding followed by a sudden, unprovoked outburst of wild rage. It causes the affected person to run about attacking, maiming and killing indiscriminately any people and animals who are in his way until he is overpowered or commits suicide. In most instances, so-called culture-bound conditions are found to be familiar entities when allowance is made for their local context.

Traditional healing

Traditional healers are found in every culture, including our own. Their methods range from pharmacological, usually herbal remedies, to psychological and spiritual treatments. It is a mistake to dismiss traditional treatments as irrational because they emerge from explanatory systems that conflict with the Western medical model. For example, the Ayurvedic system, which consists of Indian texts over 2,000 years old, recommends *Rauwolfia* for madness because it was believed to be caused by snakes in the brain, and the plant concerned has snake-like roots. In fact, reserpine, the active agent in *Rauwolfia*, does have some antipsychotic effects.

The psychological treatments employed by traditional healers, such as divination, exorcism and spirit possession, are almost always conducted in group sessions. The patient is treated as an integral part of his family and his wider social circle, who are often involved in the healing rituals. The prescriptions of the healer are usually aimed at strengthening social bonds and regulating the patient's behaviour. Studies of schizophrenia in traditional societies have shown that the social support available has a markedly beneficial effect on the course of the illness. Traditional healers serve not only immigrant groups in Britain but also the indigenous population. Faith healing, spiritualism and herbal remedies continue to flourish, and eastern imports, such as acupuncture and meditation, are attracting increasing numbers of clients. Alternative therapies survive in areas of medicine in which cures are lacking. Unfortunately, this is particularly true of psychiatry, with the result that traditional healers, wherever they operate, treat a high proportion of clients with psychiatric conditions.

All these considerations make it clear that the doctor practising psychiatry cannot afford to ignore patients' cultural values and affiliations in diagnosis, treatment and management.

FURTHER READING

Leff, J. (1988). *Psychiatry Around the Globe*, 2nd ed. Gaskell Books, London.

5

Psychodynamic Concepts

Psychodynamic concepts are concerned with the study of intrapsychic phenomena and subjective experience, and their relation to interpersonal processes and behaviour. Psychodynamic considerations are relevant to both normal and abnormal mental function; in the latter case they are referred to as dynamic psychopathology. In fact there is considerable overlap between the two. Many of the mental processes underlying normal experience and behaviour also play a part in causing such abnormal phenomena as psychoneurotic symptoms, personality disorders, psychosexual problems and difficulties in human relationships.

UNCONSCIOUS MENTAL PROCESSES

Fundamental to the understanding of patients' problems and symptoms is the recognition that mental processes may be either *conscious, preconscious* or *unconscious*. Sigmund Freud (1856-1939) regarded the Unconscious as a distinct part or sub-system of the mind or 'mental apparatus', as he called it. This reflected his wish to apply the mechanistic tradition of the natural sciences, including biology and medicine, prevalent at the time, to the study of human psychology. Nowadays the word unconscious is more often used as an adjective to describe memories, fantasies, wishes, fears or conflicts of which a person is unaware and which he is unable to bring into consciousness unaided. This may be the result of *repression* of impulses, thoughts, memories and feelings which had originally been so painful and unacceptable that they were repressed from consciousness. Some early and primitive unconscious processes like aggressive, destructive or sexual impulses may be innate and at first not accessible to consciousness. Repression may also lead one to forget the name of a person one dislikes, or forget an appointment, or make a slip of the tongue – a 'Freudian slip'. Such mistakes, sometimes referred to as *parapraxes*, were described by Freud (1901) in *The Psychopathology of Everyday Life*. Loss of memory can of course also be due to organic brain disease (see p. 34).

Unconscious material does not enter consciousness except under special circumstances, e.g. in dreams which often contain unconscious material in disguised form (see p. 50). Return of unconscious material into conscious awareness can be aided by suggestion under hypnosis, during abreaction or *catharsis*, i.e. the release of memories and feelings induced by a tranquilliser or a hypnotic, or during free association as in classical psychoanalysis (see p. 559).

By contrast, the term preconscious is used to describe thoughts or memories which are not available to one's awareness at a given moment but which can usually be recalled after a while with some mental effort. This is, of course, a common experience, e.g. of students during an examination. It is best to think of conscious, preconscious and unconscious mental processes as being part of a continuous spectrum rather than representing three different systems of the mind.

Experimental psychology has provided ample confirmation of the importance of unconscious and preconscious mental processes. For example, sensory stimuli can have physiological effects and influence experience and behaviour without reaching conscious awareness. Thus tachistoscopic stimuli, i.e. sensory stimuli presented at such low intensity or for such short duration that the subject remains unaware of the stimulus, can have profound physiological effects and influence such experiences as dreaming, images, attitudes, feelings and behaviour. Dixon (1981) has studied experimentally the psychological and physiological effects of such *subliminal perception* and has described the role of preconscious and unconscious mental processing. He also quotes Popper from Popper and Eccles (1977; p. 431): 'All experience is already interpreted by the nervous system a hundredfold – or a thousandfold – before it becomes conscious experience.'

Freud was not responsible for discovering the unconscious. Writers long before him had been aware of the influence of hidden thoughts and fantasies on human experience. Shakespeare was aware of the importance of our fantasy life in the deeper layers of the mind and of 'things unknown'. In *A Midsummer Night's Dream* Theseus says:

> Lovers and madmen have such seething brains,
> Such shaping fantasies, that apprehend
> More than cool reason ever comprehends.
> The lunatic, the lover, and the poet
> Are of imagination all compact:
> One sees more devils than vast hell can hold,
> That is, the madman: the lover, all as frantic,
> Sees Helen's beauty in a brow of Egypt:
> The poet's eye, in a fine frenzy rolling,
> Doth glance from heaven to earth, from earth to heaven;
> And, as imagination bodies forth
> The forms of things unknown, the poet's pen
> Turns them to shapes, and gives to airy nothing
> A local habitation and a name.

And Antonio at the beginning of *The Merchant of Venice* says:

In sooth, I know not why I am so sad:
It wearies me; you say it wearies you;
But how I caught it, found it, or came by it,
What stuff 'tis made of, whereof it is born,
I am to learn;
And such a want-wit sadness makes of me,
That I have much ado to know myself.

The German philosopher Arthur Schopenhauer (1788-1860) wrote about unconscious forces and resistances which interfere with our wishes and may cause 'madness' to 'break in upon the mind'. And the French psychiatrist Pierre Janet (1859-1947) described the role unconscious ideas play in the origin of hysterical symptoms (Janet 1907, 1920). Ellenberger (1970) has written a detailed history of *The Discovery of the Unconscious*.

Freud, however, was the first to explore and to apply systematically the concept of unconscious mental processes to the understanding of normal mental functioning and behaviour and of psychoneurotic and related symptoms. In these endeavours he was much helped by his early followers and collaborators, among whom Carl Gustav Jung (1875-1961) and Alfred Adler (1870-1937) are most widely known. Each later separated from Freud as a result of various disagreements, both personal and theoretical, and founded a school of his own. Jung, who was of Swiss Protestant origin and especially interested in the religious and spiritual aspects of human experience, contributed a great deal to the study of unconscious processes and introduced the concept of the *collective unconscious* (Jung 1943). He thought this to be innate, common to all mankind, and existing at a deeper layer of the mind than the individual's personal unconscious described by Freud. He based this view on the finding that the beliefs, symbols and mythology of widely different religions and cultures have a great deal in common throughout the ages and in different parts of the world (see p. 562).

INSTINCT THEORY AND OBJECT RELATIONS THEORY

A central psychodynamic concept, based on Freud's early findings, concerns the fundamental influence which infantile and childhood experiences have on personality development and on adult psychological function in mental health and illness. This is now widely accepted and will be considered in detail in Chapter 7. In his initial formulation Freud stressed particularly the role of early instinctual, especially sexual drives (Freud 1905). Only later did he also emphasise the important role of destructive and aggressive impulses in normal development and in the origin of the neuroses and other psychiatric disorders (Freud 1920, 1930).

Since the 1930s psychoanalysts have placed increasing emphasis on the role which the relationship to people, originally the mother, and later others, plays in human development from infancy onwards. The strong emphasis originally placed on instinctual gratification has thus been modified by the recognition that the search for close relationships to people and objects and their internalisation is of at least equal, and probably of greater significance in human psychological functioning and behaviour. *Object-relations theory* (Fairbairn 1952; Guntrip 1961; Kernberg 1977b) has thus largely replaced the earlier instinct theory. Both concepts need to be taken into account and integrated in understanding the functions of the mind or inner world, sometimes referred to as inner reality, and its interaction with the real world outside (Klein 1959). This will be discussed further in Chapter 7 (p. 64).

ID, EGO AND SUPEREGO

Freud (1923) described three parts or structural components of the human personality: the id, ego and superego. These are nowadays best thought of as useful terms to describe certain aspects of psychological functioning, rather than as structural entities.

The term *id* refers to the basic inborn drives like self-preservation and the sexual and aggressive impulses. In as far as they demand immediate gratification they are said to be governed by the *pleasure principle*. Some of these impulses and accompanying wishes and fantasies are conscious but others are unconscious, either because they are repressed or because they are innate and have not yet reached conscious awareness. The term *ego* is used to describe the more rational, reality-orientated and controlling aspects of the personality, again partly conscious and partly unconscious. They are concerned with the need to control the more primitive id impulses and to adapt these to outer reality, in accordance with the demands of the social and cultural environment, the so-called *reality principle*. The term *superego* is used to describe our conscience and ideals; these are derived through internalisation from parental and cultural, especially moral and religious, influences from childhood onwards and therefore vary from person to person and in different cultures. The ego not only has to try to adapt the instinctual demands of the id to outer reality but also has to cope with the conflicting demands of the id and supergo. An over-developed conscience may lead to perfectionism, excessive feelings of guilt, preoccupation with what is the right or wrong thing to do, and hence to indecision and obessionality; it plays an important role in the aetiology of some forms of depression, obsessional neurosis and sexual disorders like impotence or frigidity. Although id, ego and superego are valuable theoretical and clinical concepts it is important not to overlook the fact that the human personality functions as one unit, often referred to as the Self. Self-psychology (Kohut 1977, 1978) is an important aspect of present-day psychodynamic theory and practice, and integration of the personality – or individuation, as Jung called it – is an important aim of all forms of analytical psychotherapy.

CONFLICTS AND DEFENCE MECHANISMS

A number of defence mechanisms have been described which become mobilised when conflicts threaten to disturb a person's psychic equilibrium. Anna Freud (1936), daughter of Sigmund, called these the ego-mechanisms of defence, the implication being that they are functions of the ego. These defence mechanisms and their relation to symptom formation will be discussed below (see Chapter 6), but two particularly important ones will be briefly described here.

Repression has already been referred to. If, for example, a child is faced with a conflict between loving and hating his mother, the conflict can be resolved by repressing all angry and destructive thoughts and feelings so that only feelings of love will be consciously retained.

Splitting, a primitive defence mechanism, serves a similar purpose. Staying with the example of an infant or child in relation to its mother, the child will, in his mind, split the mother into two separate persons, the bad mother whom he hates and the good, idealised mother whom he loves. By thus mentally keeping the good and the bad mother strictly separate, the ambivalent conflict between loving and hating his mother who is in reality one and the same person and a mixture of good and bad, can be avoided. This widespread tendency to see the world in terms of either good or bad, white or black, right or wrong, often persists throughout adult life and profoundly affects our attitude not only to individuals and to ourselves but also to social institutions and political, religious and other organisations. Concepts like heaven and hell, goodies and baddies, or the frequent theme in fairy tales of dangerous witches and beautiful fairies are examples of the same phenomenon.

CONFORMITY VERSUS ORIGINALITY

There has been a tendency in classical psychoanalysis to overemphasise the view that primitive id drives and unconscious mental processes are aspects of the personality that need to be controlled, if not replaced by the more rational, adaptive functions of the ego. So-called *ego psychology*, developed under the influence of Heinz Hartman (1964), an American psychoanalyst, emphasised the need to use rational ego functions in order to adapt and conform to society. Nowadays it is more readily acknowledged that the irrational, unconscious id functions can in fact be the very source of human imaginative thinking, originality and creativity. In the *New Introductory Lectures*, Freud (1933; p. 80) wrote 'where id was, there ego shall be'. Today it would be more appropriate to speak of integrating the more chaotic but potentially creative id functions with the more rational and controlling functions of the ego. In this way the necessary degree of social adaptation can be achieved without giving up one's sense of identity, the ability to stand up for onself, to protest and to be original and creative.

A related issue concerns the distinction made by Freud between *primary* and *secondary process thinking*, the former being characteristic of the id and of unconscious mental phemonena, the latter of the ego and conscious phenomena. Secondary process thinking, as we know it, is rational and follows the ordinary laws of logic, time and space. In primary process thinking, on the other hand, the laws of time and space and the distinction between opposites do not apply; the distinction between past, present and future no longer holds and different events may occur simultaneously in the same location; one symbol may represent a number of different objects, or one object or symbol may have several different and even contradictory meanings. Dreams in particular make use of primary process thinking, and the same applies to some psychotic manifestations.

Nowadays many analysts consider that primary process thinking can be the source of much, if not most, of our imaginative thinking and is essential for adult creativity, not only in literature and the arts but also in the intuitive insights characteristic of original discoveries made by scientists, mathematicians and others. Secondary process thinking is then needed to test, evaluate and give expression to the imaginative insights that have arisen from the chaotic but creative aspects of primary process phenomena. The following discussion of dreams illustrates some aspects of primary process thinking.

DREAMS

When Freud began to use *free association*, i.e. asking patients to say aloud whatever came to mind, he found that by asking them to apply this to their dreams, repressed unconscious material could be brought into consciousness. He therefore called the analysis of dreams 'the royal road to the Unconscious'. In *The Interpretation of Dreams*, first published in 1900, he reported his findings, including the analysis of some of his own dreams, and formulated his psychoanalytic theory of dreams. The following is a brief account of the modern psychoanalytic theory of dreams; it is based on Freud's original views, modified in later years by himself and subsequently by other analysts and psychotherapists in the light of findings in normal people as well as in patients in psychoanalysis or analytical psychotherapy.

It is now widely accepted that dreams have meaning and psychological significance for the dreamer. Many of Freud's original views still hold, but his early theory that dreams express in disguised form unconscious, usually sexual wishes and their fulfilment has been replaced by the recognition that their significance extends to many other areas of human experience. Freud called the content of the dream, as remembered on waking, the *manifest content*; the hidden, unconscious meaning he called the *latent content*. This can be uncovered by asking the patient to tell the therapist what comes to mind when thinking of different parts or aspects of the dream. Events from the previous day often contribute to the content of the dream and are called the *day residue*.

A fundamental feature of dreams is that they follow primary process thinking so that in a dream the ordinary laws of time and space do not apply; one person or object in a dream may have multiple meanings, and the significance of the dream or part of it is frequently expressed in symbolic form. For example, a comfortable house may represent a safe place and may thus stand for a caring and supportive mother. A threatening figure like an animal that attacks and bites may symbolise frightening, bad aspects of mother, father or of other significant persons in the dreamer's life. At the same time the dangerous biting animal may also represent the aggressive intentions of the dreamer himself. The latent content of the dream is converted into the manifest content by means of *symbolisation, condensation* (one image in the dream having several meanings), or by *displacement* when, for example, aggressive or sexual impulses which are actually those of the dreamer himself are attributed to, say, a stranger in the dream. Sometimes, however, the manifest content may reveal directly the meaning of the dream so that free association is not always needed to uncover its significance.

The more recent psychoanalytic view is that dreams can express many different aspects of mental functioning (Rycroft 1979). They may express conscious or unconscious conflicts and problems, both past and present, and attempts at solving such problems, as well as hidden wishes or unacceptable aspects of the personality. When a patient is in psychotherapy or analysis a dream often refers to aspects of his relationship to the therapist, especially feelings experienced in the transference (see below). Dreams may also express creative ideas and may subsequently lead to creative, imaginative work when awake.

The role of *symbolism* in dreams and, for that matter, in many other human mental processes during the waking state, is of central significance, but any one symbol may have different meanings for different people, depending on each individual's past and present experience and cultural background. In this context it should be noted that Jung always stressed the wide significance of symbolism in dreams, including religious and mythological aspects. He put forward the view that dreams not only reveal aspects of the dreamer's personal unconscious but at times more universal meanings, expressed by the appearance of what he called 'archetypal images' in symbolic form (see p. 563).

Lastly, modern neurophysiological findings have made it possible to study the underlying cerebral mechanisms of dreaming in considerable detail. These studies have shown that everyone dreams for about 20 per cent of the night, and that, when woken up during the rapid eye movement periods of sleep (REM sleep), on 80 per cent of occasions one will vividly remember dreaming. The neurophysiological aspects are considered further on p. 305.

TRANSFERENCE AND COUNTER-TRANSFERENCE

These important psychodynamic processes will be dealt with in greater detail in Chapter 44, but they are briefly described here because of the central role they play in modern psychoanalysis and analytical psychotheraphy. Briefly, *transference* is that process by which a patient in psychoanalysis or psychotherapy relives in relation to his therapist feelings and fantasies he once experienced in childhood in relation to other significant people, like his parents.

Counter-transference originally referred to the process by which the analyst experiences feelings towards his patient which he has displaced on to him from significant figures in his own life, but nowadays the term is used instead to describe the analyst's reactions, both feelings and thoughts, experienced while listening to his patient. These reactions often provide him with a clue to what is going on in his patient's unconscious. In this way the counter-transference can serve as an important tool in the course of the analyst's or psychotherapist's work with his patient (Heimann 1950). The use made of the patient's transference and of the analyst's counter-transference is central during psychoanalysis and analytical psychotherapy as practised today (see Chapter 44). These phenomena are often not sufficiently recognised or used in other psychological treatment methods or in psychiatric practice.

FURTHER READING

Brown, J.A.C. (1961). *Freud and the Post-Freudians*. Penguin Books, Harmondsworth.

Fancher, R.E. (1973). *Psychoanalytic Psychology: the development of Freud's thought*. Norton, New York and London.

Freud, S. (1940). *An Outline of Psychoanalysis*, Standard Edition, vol. 23. Hogarth, London.

Guntrip, H. (1971). *'Psychoanalytic Theory, Therapy and the Self*. Maresfield Reprint, Karnac, London.

Jones, E. (1964). *Life and Work of Sigmund Freud*. Penguin Books, Harmondsworth.

Jung, C.G. (1963). *Memories, Dreams, Reflections*. Collins and Routledge & Kegan Paul, London.

Rycroft, C. (1968). *A Critical Dictionary of Psychoanalysis*. Pelican (1973), Penguin Books, Harmondsworth.

Rycroft, C. (1979). *The Innocence of Dreams*. Hogarth, London.

Segal, H. (1979). *Klein*. Fontana/Collins, London.

Storr, A. (1973). *Jung*. Fontana, London.

Sulloway, F.J. (1979). *Freud, Biologist of the Mind: beyond the psychoanalytic legend*. Fontana, London.

Taylor, D. (1984). 'Psychoanalytic contributions to the understanding of psychiatric illness': in *The Scientific Principles of Psychopathology* (McGriffin, P., Shanks, M.F. and Hodgson, R.F., eds). Grune & Stratton, London.

Whyte, L.L. (1962). *The Unconscious before Freud*. Tavistock, London.

6

Symptom Formation and the Mechanisms of Defence

The personality and healthy psychological functioning of an individual is not normally threatened by inner conflicts, thoughts and feelings. This integration of psychological functioning depends partly on the so-called mechanisms of defence. These play an essential part in normal mental functioning and help to shape character and personality; it is their failure or their excessive or inappropriate use that leads to the formation of some psychiatric symptoms.

SYMPTOM FORMATION

It has been pointed out that the term 'ego' describes those aspects of psychological functioning of an individual which act as a mediator and problem solver. As such, the ego has to meet varying demands arising from the id, the super-ego and the external world (see p. 48). The mechanisms of defence are used to meet some of these demands. A psychological crisis occurs when inner conflicts or external circumstances threaten to overwhelm the normal psychological balance of the individual. *Inner conflicts* alone may threaten this balance. For example, a married man with high moral principles may also have strong promiscuous desires; this conflict between his conscience and inner urges may lead to anxiety, guilt and depression. Sometimes *external circumstances*, such as loss of a loved one, the end of a relationship, the failure of a business or a physical illness re-awaken dormant past conflicts; this helps to explain how some external events affect one individual severely but leave others unscathed. For example, a man whose wife had recently had a baby became anxious, sleepless and depressed as he struggled to adapt to the presence of the new-born child whom he loved but also resented. It transpired that the jealousy he had felt at the age of five towards his new-born brother had been re-awakened. This jealousy was being re-experienced in relation to his wife and new-born baby and led to anxiety and depression.

In both these examples the conflict between opposing demands had resulted in anxiety. Anxiety acts as a signal indicating that some form of adaptation must take place. In some cases this can be brought about by realistic action, but in neither of the two cases mentioned is there any obvious realistic solution. If realistic action is not possible or fails, the mechanisms of defence are mobilised. For example, the man caught between his conscience and his promiscuous sexual urges may use the unconscious mechanism of defence called repression to remove his erotic desires from consciousness and be relieved of the conflict. If repression is excessive, however, he may lose his sexual desire altogether and become impotent with his wife. If, on the contrary, repression fails, the conflict will persist and his symptoms of anxiety, guilt and depression will continue to trouble him.

Sometimes the symptoms which arise from a psychological conflict serve as a compromise between opposing psychological forces. The symptoms may even express some aspect of the underlying conflict in symbolic form. If we take the example of the man who became jealous of his new-born baby, the conflict is clear. On the one hand he loved the baby and his wife; on the other he was jealous of the attention his wife was giving to the baby just as he used to be jealous of the attention his mother gave to his new-born brother. As a result he felt himself in danger of shouting at his wife and the baby to express his anger and jealousy. As his fear of loss of self-control became worse he developed hysterical aphonia and his anxiety diminished. The symptom of aphonia now served as a compromise in that it prevented him from expressing his rage by shouting; it also had a symbolic meaning in as much as it symbolised his fear of giving verbal expression to his angry feelings.

MECHANISMS OF DEFENCE

The use of defence mechanisms, their success or their failure and the concepts of compromise formation and symbolic meaning of symptoms are all of considerable help in understanding the development of psychoneurotic symptoms.

The following are some of the important mechanisms of defence (A. Freud 1936). They all take place outside conscious awareness. Each is illustrated with an example to show how they work. The excessive use of certain mechanisms of defence, i.e. splitting and projection, suggests more severe psychopathology. For example, severe splitting, projection and projective identification are common in paranoid states, while rationalisation and intellectualisation play a part in normal adolescence and adult life. Regression is also a commonly used defence against anxiety. It is described elsewhere (see p. 71).

Repression

Repression is the fundamental mechanism of defence. The other defence mechanisms may only come into operation if repression fails to prevent unacceptable wishes entering consciousness. An individual remains unaware of unbearable impulses, feelings, thoughts, images and memories when they are confined to the unconscious by repression. The process occurs automatically and takes place normally throughout life. Repression is characteristic of hysterial conversion (see p. 175) where the repressed impulse may find symbolic expression in the patient's symptoms, as in the patient with aphonia.

In contrast, *suppression* is the volitional exclusion of thoughts and feelings from conscious attention.

A clear example of repression was observed in a patient suffering from depression. During psychotherapy, he burst into tears when talking about the death of his mother years ago. He then became aware that he had 'forgotten' that the cause of her death was an overdose of tablets. Only after having faced the fact that she had killed herself was he able to work through his long-delayed grief reaction and recover from his depression. In this example the painful memory of his mother's suicide had been repressed from consciousness but returned during therapy.

Splitting

This defence mechanism is considered elsewhere (see p. 70). In essence it consists of the good and the bad aspects of others and of oneself being kept strictly separate, i.e. split apart in order to avoid having to cope with ambivalent feelings of love and hatred towards the same person.

Denial

Any individual confronted with a painful external event may deny it has happened. For example, a common human response to personal catastrophe is to say 'it can't be true', 'I refuse to believe it'. Usually reality supervenes rapidly but this is not always the case. Denial is common after a bereavement. For example a woman whose husband has died may keep all his possessions in the house as if he were still alive, sometimes for years. In denial there is thus a cognitive acceptance of the painful event but an emotional rejection of it. This is in contrast to delusional conviction (see p. 122) in which cognitive insight is also lost, so that the woman mentioned above would have believed her husband was still alive.

Displacement

In displacement an emotion or wish is transferred from one person, towards whom it was originally felt, to another person or object. This process is unconscious and allows the emotion to be expressed more freely. For example, a person who feels angry towards his superior may displace his anger on to someone lower in the hierarchy, or he may remain polite at work but smash crockery at home or get angry with his children.

Magical undoing

Magical undoing is seen in the obsessional neuroses. It may also be observed in superstitions and primitive religious ceremonials. In magical undoing an individual attempts to negate a thought, word, gesture or action by making use of the thought or behaviour which has the opposite meaning. For example, a person who believes that aggressive thoughts may result in someone else's death may relieve his anxiety by making himself have loving thoughts about the same person instead, thus undoing the feared effects of his destructive thoughts.

Projection

In projection unacceptable wishes or impulses are attributed to someone else and may then be experienced as being directed back at oneself. For example, someone may repress his own angry feelings towards another person and believe instead that the person is angry with him. Projection causes an individual to misinterpret the environment. In extreme cases this may lead to the formation of paranoid delusions.

Projective identification

This mechanism, first described by Melanie Klein (1946) differs from projection in several respects. In projection unwanted impulses and feelings are attributed to someone else, but in projective identification whole parts of the personality are split off and projected into another person or object who then represents and becomes identified with these split-off parts; attempts are then made to control these parts of the self by asserting control over the other person. The following two examples illustrate this process.

A man who was working as a teacher was put in charge of a form of teenage boys; he soon began to resent any boy who was disobedient, rude or otherwise badly behaved to such an extent that he became frightened before each lesson lest he would be unable to control the class. He hated these pupils and feared that he might lose control and hit one or other of the boys. During psychotherapy it emerged that throughout his own adolescence he had been a 'good boy', obedient, working hard and never causing trouble either at school or at home. He had split off all those destructive and rebellious aspects of himself which, as the result of his upbringing, he considered to be evil, dangerous and unacceptable. By means of projective identification he was now projecting all these unacceptable aspects of himself into his adolescent pupils. They had become identified with his own split-off rebellious parts. In them, he hated these unwanted aspects of himself and he desperately but unsuccessfully tried to control these aspects by wanting to control and punish his pupils. In therapy he soon understood that these pupils represented hated aspects of his own personality. He then added that as a boy he used to collect and play with toy animals like tigers and crocodiles who were dangerous but, as they were toys, he could control and make them do exactly what he wanted, including making them attack and devour other animals and human beings. These toy animals had at that time also become identified with the projected aggressive parts of himself. By projecting all these parts into them he had, however, lost any inner sense of being strong enough to stand up for himself and to fight other boys and, later on, adults who might insult or oppose him.

Projective identification can thus also leave a person feeling deprived of essential aspects of his own personality. Good aspects of the self can also be projected into others.

A young woman who had always tended to regard herself as unattractive, worthless and unlovable became dependent on and envious of a slightly older woman friend whom she regarded as very competent, beautiful and successful in all her relationships with men. During psychotherapy it became clear that she had projected all her own positive qualities which she felt unworthy of, and hence unable to contain inside herself, into this other woman, who thus became identified with all her own assets. This made her feel even less attractive and less worthy of being loved so that she felt impoverished inside herself. She made constant demands on her friend, as only in her presence and with her backing did she feel able to do anything worthwhile. When her friend married and moved away she became depressed because she felt her friend had taken away with her everything good that she no longer contained within herself. In therapy is also emerged that as a child she had for a while owned a beautiful doll who, she felt, unlike herself, was loved by everyone. This doll had, by projective identification, also become identified with all her own good and lovable qualities.

Projective identification and the related process of splitting can thus play an important part in personality development from childhood onwards. When used excessively they can lead to personality disorders and psychiatric symptoms.

Introjection

Introjection is the process by which an individual takes in another person's inherent qualities and makes them part of himself. This process is important during normal development. A baby or child introjects good aspects and experiences from his mother and lays down memories associated with safe, pleasurable feelings. In this way an inner representation of a good mother may be built up, allowing the child later on to separate from his actual mother without suffering excessive anxiety.

A similar process occurs in bereavement. The pain associated with the loss of a loved one is diminished by introjecting various qualities and characteristics of the deceased. This creates the feeling that the loss is not complete and so lessens the psychological suffering.

Identification

Identification is similar to introjection but extends further. An individual not only assimilates an aspect or attribute of another person but is wholly or partially transformed by it. This plays an important part in normal personality development but can also lead to neurotic symptoms. For example, an hysterical personality may develop someone else's symptoms by identification.

Identification can also play a part in depression and mourning. For example, a woman mourning the loss of her grand-daughter appeared to have resolved her grief. However, some months later she developed intractable abdominal pain for which no physical cause was found. Her grand-daughter had died of intestinal volvulus and the patient's symptoms were a result of identification with the symptoms of the dead child. She was helped to recognise this during bereavement counselling and this led to the disappearance of her symptoms.

Identification is an unconscious process. In contrast, *imitation* is a conscious attempt to mimic the behaviour of someone else.

Rationalisation and intellectualisation

Both these defence mechanisms are common in everyday life. Intellectualisation is most prominent during adolescence but may persist throughout adulthood. Many individuals attempt to give explanations for their attitudes, ideas or behaviour which appear logically consistent but, in reality, serve to cover up true motives. This is *rationalisation*. It is often used to justify irrational behaviour to oneself and others. For example, a man who insists on driving the car when his wife is in the car with him may explain his insistence by saying his wife does not like driving, when his real motivation is an attempt to dominate her and prove himself superior.

Intellectualisation differs in that it attempts to keep emotions at bay. For example, someone who is uncertain whether or not to marry his girlfriend may continually and intellectually discuss the relative merits of monogamy and free love rather than allow his personal ambivalent feelings about his girlfriend to emerge. Plausible explanations for emotions, attitudes, ideas or behaviour are not offered.

Sublimation

Unconscious wishes which are unacceptable to the individual or society are diverted into socially acceptable outlets by sublimation. Both society and the individual may benefit from this. For example, excessive aggressive or angry feelings may be diverted into sporting activities, or latent homosexual wishes turned into close male friendships.

Reaction formation

An individual may protect himself from wishes, feelings or ideas which provoke anxiety by adopting diametrically opposed psychological attitudes. This is reaction formation. For example, someone who joins the anti-vivisectionists to oppose cruelty to animals may in fact be sadistic towards his wife and harbour violent fantasies. In that case his decision to join the anti-vivisectionists may, at least in part, be a reaction-formation against his own sadistic wishes.

*

The mechanisms of defence are useful in the understanding of many normal and abnormal psychological phenomena. In addition to having a descriptive value they also have an explanatory value at the level of mental functioning. An individual who uses defence mechanisms inappropriately or excessively will either suffer from psychiatric symptoms or function as a vulnerable personality. As such, certain defence mechanisms are associated with particular personality types. For example, excessive splitting and projective identification occur in borderline personality disorders, while repression, intellectualisation and rationalisation are common in hysterical personality disorders. Consequently some psychiatrists discuss personality in terms of the mechanisms of defence instead of using descriptions of observable behaviour (see Chapter 26).

FURTHER READING

Freud, A. (1936). *The Ego and Mechanisms of Defence*. Hogarth, London.
Freud, S. (1926). *Inhibitions, Symptoms and Anxiety*, Standard Edition, vol. 20. Hogarth, London.
Klein, M. (1946). 'Notes on some schizoid mechanisms' in *The Writings of Melanie Klein*, vol. 3, *Envy and Gratitude and Other Works, 1946-1963*. Hogarth, London (1975).
Sandler, J. (ed.) (1988). *Projection, Identification, Projective Identification*. Karnac, London.

Part II

Personality Development and the Life Cycle

7

Personality Development in Childhood

Each stage of psychological development from infancy onwards influences what happens at all subsequent stages. In order to understand the mental functioning and behaviour of an adult it is essential, therefore, to know as much as possible about his earlier development, starting from the very early period of his relationship as an infant to his mother. These early experiences in infancy, and later as a child and adolescent, are retained in our minds or inner world at a conscious or unconscious level throughout life so that, as it were, the infant and the child are still part of the adult.

From time to time, especially when under stress, not only mentally disturbed patients but also normal people will revert or *regress* to earlier stages of mental functioning and behaviour. For the practice of psychiatry and psychotherapy it is therefore essential to be familiar with normal and abnormal psychological development. Equal attention must be paid to objective facts concerning a person's past experiences and behaviour and to the meaning these experiences have for him, as well as to the fantasies which may have modified and be associated with them. In this way a picture can gradually be built up of the patient's inner world. This contains the so-called mental representations of all those people – mother, father, siblings, etc. – parts of people and other objects which at one time or another have played a significant part in his development. Of course physical factors, especially inherited characteristics and acquired physical vulnerability, also have an important effect on an individual's development, but in this chapter we are concerned with psychological aspects.

The account that follows, though based on some of Freud's formulations early this century, differs from them in many important respects. In *Three Essays on the Theory of Sexuality* (1905) Freud expressed the view, based on clinical observations, that the sexual drive or instinct played a central role in development from infancy through childhood and adolescence into adulthood. In this context he used the term sexual or 'libidinal' in a much wider sense than adult sexuality and included in it all forms of pleasurable bodily sensations, arising from successive *erotogenic zones*. He considered that these started with sensations experienced during sucking, the so-called *oral stage*; leading on to sensations associated with expelling or retaining faeces, the *anal stage*; then moving on to auto-erotic pleasurable sensations, the *phallic or infantile genital stage*, soon followed by the *Oedipal stage*; and ultimately, after puberty, to the ability to experience orgasm associated with real or fantasied contact with other people's genital organs, the *adult genital stage*.

One of the most important advances in our understanding of personality development is the much greater emphasis now placed on the nature of the relationship to mother, father and other significant people or objects, rather than on the gratification of sexual, aggressive or other instinctual desires as such. Freud was always aware of the important role of the person or object required for instinctual gratification, e.g. the mother who feeds or the partner to have sex with, but in modern *object relations theory* (Fairbairn 1952) it is the real or fantasied relationship to people like mother or parts of mother, say her face or breast during feeding, which is central to the understanding of psychic functioning and development. Both are important, but the need for close and reliable relationships is nowadays considered to be of primary importance, while the search for pleasurable, instinctual gratifications is of secondary importance in the development of the personality. Modern object relations theory stresses that throughout children's development important people in their environment, like mother or father, are internalised and form internal *mental representations* or 'internal objects' within the mind. Thereafter there will be constant interplay between the external world and the world within. For example, somebody who has internalised a demanding and punitive conscience (superego) from an authoritarian father may later misinterpret a simple request made by an employer as if it were a critical or authoritarian command.

Progress is also being made through objective observation by psychoanalysts and developmental psychologists of the behaviour of infants in relation to others, especially their mother, at early stages of development. These objective findings are gradually being integrated with psychoanalytic concepts concerned with the development of the infant's and child's inner or subjective experience. Stern (1985) has investigated and discussed these issues and thrown light on the development of the sense of Self and the infant's way of relating to others.

MOTHER-INFANT RELATIONSHIP

Donald Winnicott (1896-1971), a British psychoanalyst and paediatrician, studied the nature of the relationship between mother and baby in depth and has provided much of our understanding of the early phases of development. An American analyst, Margaret Mahler, who carried out systematic observational research on mothers and their babies (Mahler *et al.* 1975), has further provided much information on the early 'symbiotic phase' and the next phase of 'separation-individuation', to be discussed below. Balint (1968) used the term *primary love* to describe the very early relationship of the infant to its mother.

Initially the new-born infant is totally dependent on its mother. Winnicott (1963a) called this the state of *absolute dependence*. As pregnancy progresses the mother becomes increasingly concerned with her baby and when the baby is born she will be in a mental state of what he called *primary maternal preoccupation*. This enables her to recognise and respond appropriately to the infant's early needs to be comfortably held, fed, smiled at, cared for and loved. The infant is, however, not yet sufficiently developed for it to perceive its mother as a separate person. The baby has no sense of 'I' or, to use different terminology, it has not yet developed any ego-boundaries and feels merged or fused with its mother. This is why we speak of a state of *symbiosis* or *fusion* of the baby with its mother, or of the mother-baby unit or dyad, at this early stage of development.

The experience of being held by the mother and fed from breast or bottle, and the pleasurable sensations that accompany sucking, form an important aspect of the infant's relationship to its mother at this stage, but it is the nature of the whole relationship in the context of which these feeding experiences take place which is crucial rather than the process of being fed as such. The wish later in life to return to a state of fusion to some extent survives in everyone but may be particularly strong in an individual whose mother was unable adequately to meet her baby's needs. Such individuals continue to search for a perfect, conflict-free relationship to others, be it in friendship, love affairs, marriage or social relationships; they cannot tolerate the inevitable disillusionments encountered when differences and conflicts have to be accepted in their real lives as opposed to the hoped-for and fantasied perfect or idealised relationship to others which still dominates their inner world. Sometimes states of mystical union, enlightenment or, in religious terms, of being 'at one with God', or moments of inspiration and creativity may provide in sublimated form the longed-for fulfilment of the wish to have such fusion experiences.

It should be noted that present research by developmental psychologists, reviewed by Stern (1985), has thrown doubt on the existence of an early symbiotic phase. Their findings suggest that from birth onwards an emergent sense of self exists, as shown by the infant's reactions to others, and that this progresses to a more fully developed sense of self and others by the age of fifteen months.

If during the phase of absolute dependence the infant has been exposed to a preponderance of bad as opposed to good experiences, in the sense of having felt let down and emotionally 'dropped', these impingements, as Winnicott called them, may have serious consequences later on. These may take the form of being unable to trust others, and of severe anxiety, sometimes called existential or annihilation anxiety, when threatened by a loss or rejection. Outwardly such people may appear to be coping well, but their outer armour or *false self* (Winnicott 1975) often hides an inner sense of extreme vulnerability, emptiness and isolation. Schizoid and borderline personality disorders (see Chapters 26 and 27) can sometimes be traced back to impingements or let-downs during the early phase of dependence.

It is important, however, not to make mothers feel that they should or could be perfect and that they alone are responsible for any future disturbances their children may develop. No mother or father can be a perfect parent and, as Winnicott has pointed out, a mother can at best be 'good enough'. Moreover, no two new-born babies are alike; inborn individual differences, the social and family circumstances, especially the relationship between the parents, and the father's own relationship to the baby and developing child all make important contributions, for better or for worse, to the infant's and child's experiences and development. Winnicott (1965) has stressed particularly the need for parents or parent substitutes to provide a *facilitating environment* to allow the process of maturation to take place. We shall discuss later how psychotherapy may contribute to recovery from the effects of early painful experiences and lead to further growth in years to come.

There is evidence that not only in humans but also in monkeys disturbances in the early mother-infant relationship can have profound effects on future development. Experiments on rhesus monkeys by Harlow (Arling and Harlow 1967; Harlow and Harlow 1969; Suomi and Harlow 1978) have shown that infant monkeys separated at birth from their mothers remain prone to seriously disturbed behaviour. They are unable later on to socialise when introduced as adults to a group of other monkeys. Their sexual behaviour remains impaired, and if a female monkey who has not received mothering herself as an infant later becomes pregnant, if necessary by artificial insemination, she rejects her own offspring and behaves aggressively towards them.

SEPARATION AND INDIVIDUATION

When the infant is about three to six months old his behaviour indicates that he is beginning to recognise more clearly that he and his mother are separate individuals, and his mother is now being responded to in a highly personal and specific manner. Margaret Mahler calls this the beginning of the *separation-individuation phase*, and Winnicott speaks of the stage of relative as opposed to absolute dependence. This gradual process of separation and individuation continues until the child reaches the end of his third year, with many fluctuations as well as individual differences. These depend on the child's genetic endowment, the nature of the earlier infant-mother relationship and the family setting, including the child's relationship to his father and siblings. The child's increasing ability to recognise a greater variety of objects and people, and the development of motor skills which enable him to walk away from his mother to explore the surrounding world and then return to her, all promote the development of a separate sense of self.

Particularly important is the development of the child's *cognitive abilities*; this has been studied in detail by the Swiss psychologist Jean Piaget (1953, 1965). He speaks of an early *sensory-motor stage*, characterised by more or less automatic or reflex sensory and motor responses to the immediate environment; this is followed by the growing ability to recognise particular objects and people and what they represent, the *representational stage*. This leads to the ability to give names to objects and to the beginning of speech, usually during the first year, though there are considerable individual variations. Gradually during succeeding years this concrete form of thinking and intelligence leads to being able to think in more abstract, operational and symbolic terms, an ability which is not fully developed until early adolescence. While Piaget's work was mainly concerned with the development of thought and intelligence, psychoanalysts and child therapists have continued to explore the emotional and intrapsychic development and especially the internal fantasy life of the child. Piaget's contributions to childhood development have been reviewed by Hobson (1985).

An important consequence of having become aware of being a separate person from mother is the experience of *separation anxiety*. When the child is aware of his mother not being there or immediately available, and especially when the child is apart from his mother for longer than he can readily tolerate, he becomes anxious, looks for her and, if she cannot be found soon enough, will become distressed and cry. Such normal separation anxiety starts to show itself from about the age of four to six months, tends to be more marked during the second year and gradually diminishes under favourable circumstances during the third year. If the mother, and soon also the father, are 'good enough' in the sense of not exposing the child to over-long periods of separation, the child will learn that the parent will return and his separation anxiety will remain within tolerable limits.

The child also turns to sucking his fist or thumb to comfort himself when anxious, and many small children get attached to a special soft toy, like a teddy bear, or a rag or blanket which they hold on to, play with and take to bed with them before they can feel safe enough to go to sleep. Winnicott (1953) has called these toys *transitional objects* and has studied the many ways in which children use them to bridge the gap when their mother is absent, to express feelings of love or anger towards them and to endow, say, a teddy bear with special significance and meaning. Some games, such as playing bo-peep or dropping a toy and asking for it to be picked up and given back again and again, also help the child to master separation anxiety.

Children who during the first few years of life have had 'good enough' parenting, who have been spared excessive or traumatic separation experiences and have learnt how to cope with gradually increasing and hence acceptable periods of separation, will enter adult life with what Erikson (1965) has called a sense of *basic trust* and confidence in themselves based on an internal image or *mental representation* of reliable mother and father figures.

If, however, children aged between six months and three to four years are exposed to more prolonged, traumatic periods of separation or emotional deprivation from their mother, this may lead to immediate or short-term disturbance of behaviour; this in turn may be followed by long-term psychopathological sequelae and predispose to psychiatric illness later in life. Bowlby (1969, 1973, 1980) at the Tavistock Clinic in London has done a great deal of research on what he calls *maternal deprivation*. His earlier studies (Bowlby 1951) included observations made on children who were separated from their mothers through hospitalisation; similar findings were obtained from studies of children who were brought up in institutions.

If a child aged between about six months and three years is admitted to hospital and not visited by his mother he will, for the first few days, show marked distress and cry a great deal, the so-called *stage of protest*. If mother does not return he will enter the second *stage of despair* when he cries less but appears listless and miserable, and is prone to outbursts of anger. He then enters the third *stage of detachment*, characterised by apparent calm and disinterest in his parents. When his mother ultimately returns, say after a few weeks, to take him home, he no longer appears to recognise her. This is a very painful experience for the mother and it may take several days, depending on the length of separation and hence the degree of detachment, before the child begins to recognise her again. From then onwards and for varying lengths of time his relation to her is marked by extreme dependency, as shown by anxiously clinging to her, and anger and distress as soon as she shows signs of leaving the room or is absent even for a short while. Children who have experienced prolonged or repeated separation experiences of this kind are likely to remain extremely dependent and insecure whenever their parents leave them, sometimes for years to come; they also tend to suffer from severe home-sickness if, say, they are sent to boarding school later on. Long-term sequelae may include a persistent tendency to neurotic anxiety or depression, sometimes to agoraphobia, and to the development of an insecure, dependent personality, finding it difficult to trust others or to tolerate losses and to be on their own.

As a result of these and similar findings, Bowlby (1979) has formulated the view that during the first few weeks and months of a baby's life the formation of what he called the *affectional bond* between the child and his mother or mother-substitute is of central importance for future development. If such a bond is not established from the start or broken later on, the child's subsequent development will be seriously affected. He also drew attention to the close similarity between *attachment behaviour* and bond formation between parent and offspring in animals, including birds and mammals, as described by ethologists, and bond formation between mother and children in humans.

It is largely as a result of Bowlby's work that so much emphasis is nowadays rightly placed on the need for children to be accompanied by their mothers if they have to be admitted to hospital, or at least for the parents to visit them daily. Similarly if a child has to be taken into an institution, like a residential nursery, every effort must be made to ensure that each child is given as much warm and close maternal care by the same person or mother substitute as possible to avoid the ill effects of prolonged maternal deprivation.

Rutter (1981) has drawn attention to the fact that many factors other than maternal deprivation as such may influence the effects of separation experiences. These include the presence or absence of the father, the relationship between the parents, and whether or not the child, if separated from one or both parents, remains in his own familiar environment with a parent or parent-substitute already known to him, as opposed to being taken away to a strange, affectionless or frightening environment. It has also become clear that failure of intellectual development which may occur in some of these children, is not due to maternal deprivation but the result of insufficient play and stimulation in the institution or foster home where the child is being looked after. These multiple factors may account for the considerable individual differences observed in the response of children to separation experiences, some children being severely affected while others may show little adverse immediate or long-term effects. In spite of this the importance of the relationship of the child to his mother during the early phases cannot be over-estimated. It is during this period that the affectional bond becomes established, and the child learns to tolerate gradually increasing and non-traumatic degrees of separation. Good enough mothering during the symbiotic and separation-individuation phases of development seems essential for healthy personality development, and failure in these respects can lead to serious short-term and long-term disturbance and psychological ill-health.

AMBIVALENCE

Another consequence for the child of recognising his mother as a person separate from himself is that he experiences divided or ambivalent feelings towards her. Feelings of love are directed towards the mother when she satisfies the child's needs and is therefore experienced as a good mother, while feelings of anger or hatred are directed towards her when she frustrates his wishes and is experienced as bad. These two aspects of his mother may initially be kept strictly apart from each other so that the child first experiences and internalises the good and the bad mother as two separate images in his inner world, the good one who is loved and the bad one who is hated. When these two images gradually become recognised as being in fact aspects of one and the same whole person – mother – the child experiences mixed or ambivalent feelings of love and of hatred towards her. As a result the child feels guilty and sad, afraid of having damaged his mother and of no longer being loved by her. He begins to feel concern for her, wants to make reparation and needs to be reassured that she still loves him even though he has felt angry and destructive towards her. Later in life, if conflicts between love and hate become too great, the child or adult may return to the earlier phase of once more splitting the other person, originally his mother, into either all good or all bad so that the anger and destructiveness is no longer felt to be directed towards the person who is loved.

Melanie Klein called the early stage the *paranoid-schizoid position* because the child not only splits his mother into good and bad but also fears being counter-attacked and hated by her in response to his own destructive wishes. She called the subsequent stage of ambivalence the *depressive position* because the child now recognises his mother as a whole person, both loved and hated, so that he experiences feelings of remorse, depression or sadness when he fears he has hurt or destroyed and lost her (Segal 1978, 1979; Klein 1946, 1952).

The terms paranoid-schizoid and depressive position must not be confused with such psychiatric disorders as paranoid schizophrenia or depressive illness. They are normal stages of development, not illnesses. Winnicott (1954) therefore prefers to speak of the child having reached the *stage of concern* to describe the ability to have mixed feelings and concern for another person, originally the mother; this is preceded by or may alternate with periods during which the child experiences persecutory anxiety because he is afraid of being punished and counter-attacked in response to his own destructive feelings. Winnicott also stressed that the stage of concern or the depressive position may not be reached until later in childhood or adult life.

Much of children's play and fantasy life gives expression to these fears and anxieties. Fear of the bogey man, fear of the dark, and later on fear of ghosts or evil spirits, or games in which a doll or teddy bear is torn to pieces and then comforted and made whole again, may serve as examples. It should be added that while this account refers to the child's relation to his mother or mother substitute, the same applies to his relation to his father and other people, although usually at a somewhat later stage of development.

The capacity to tolerate ambivalent feelings and to express concern through making reparation and forgiving other people their failures remains crucial in maintaining lasting and trusting relationships throughout life. Failure to reach the depressive position as a child or adult leads to mistrust, excessive fear of being hurt or hurting others, and hence to an inability to form and maintain close relationships, isolation and withdrawal. These difficulties are particularly prominent in paranoid and schizoid personality disorders (see p. 330), and may interfere with normal mourning after a bereavement (see p. 94).

PSYCHOSEXUAL DEVELOPMENT

The classical psychoanalytic concepts of so-called oral, anal, phallic and Oedipal stages of psychosexual development have already been referred to briefly, but their relation to the above more up-to-date description of personality development requires further clarification. To anticipate the main point, pleasurable physical sensations derived from the mouth, anus and genital organs undoubtedly play an important part in childhood and later sexual development. However, it is the relationship to the person – mother, father and others – in the context of which these physical sensations are first experienced, rather than the physical sensations as such, that determines the influence they have on the development of the personality and on sexual functioning in particular. It is also essential to recognise that to talk of successive stages of psychosexual development is to some extent artificial, as pleasure derived from these different physical functions overlaps and co-exists to a considerable degree, not only in children but also in adults.

The oral stage

The pleasurable experience of sucking and of being fed, be it from the breast or from the bottle, during the symbiotic and early separation-individuation phases is undoubtedly of great significance at the time, as well as for later development. After the child has been weaned, he continues to put his fist or thumb and soon many other objects into his mouth, and oral gratification continues to play an important part throughout adult life, including various forms of adult sexual activity. Under stress both children and adults may *regress* to oral activities; for example, a toddler who has stopped sucking his thumb may start doing so again after the birth of a younger sibling. Adults may start to overeat and put on weight, or start smoking again if they have previously stopped doing so, when they feel lonely after a loss, or during a crisis in their personal life or at work. More serious disorders due to disturbance of oral activity are anorexia nervosa and bulimia, common forms of eating disorders (see p. 440) which occur in adolescents and young adults; and loss of appetite or compulsive overeating are symptoms which frequently accompany a depressive illness.

Oral activity can also be used aggressively and destructively, so-called oral sadism. Infants, when frustrated during a breast-feed, may bite the nipple. Biting may remain a way of expressing anger later in life, and we speak of 'biting remarks' when we refer to angry words used in the course of attacking someone else in arguments or personal quarrels. Biting may also continue to play a significant part in adult sexual behaviour.

The anal stage

During the second year of life when the child has reached a separate sense of Self he is also beginning to gain control of his sphincters and to derive pleasure from expelling or retaining his faeces. As pleasure in defaecation succeeds the earlier pleasure associated with feeding, Freud spoke of the oral stage being followed by the anal stage of libidinal development. It would appear, however, that the concept of an anal stage is too narrow in the context of object relations theory. What seems to be more significant is whether the child is allowed and encouraged by his parents gradually to gain and enjoy mastery of his own function of defaecating or whether excessive parental control is imposed upon the child, in which case a battle for control is likely to ensue.

In fact, the issue of control applies to many functions other than toilet training. These include the growing child's eating habits, his activities and behaviour in general, including such potentially dangerous activities as playing with matches or sharp instruments; and later on his behaviour towards other children and adults, his homework and so on. The growing child develops a will of his own, and while he undoubtedly needs structure, guidance and control, parents or other adults who try to impose their own will upon him to an excessive degree are likely to cause a battle of wills. This can lead to the appearance of character traits like obstinacy and rebelliousness, or, if the child gives in, to the opposite, i.e. fear and submissiveness. Erikson (1965) speaks of a *battle for autonomy* instead of the child developing his autonomy in his own time. It seems more appropriate therefore to speak of the development of a sense of autonomy rather than in the narrower terms of an anal stage.

This does not mean, however, that inappropriate handling of toilet training may not lead to more specific disturbances in childhood and later on. Refusal to defaecate, constipation, soiling, encopresis and the use of faeces to make a mess, are all well known behaviour disturbances in children who rebel against over-strict parental standards and control (see p. 508). Personality traits like obstinacy, obsessional cleanliness and meanness, characteristics of the obsessional personality (see p. 331) are among the later effects, as may be preoccupation with bowel function. It is also important to recognise that anal activity may remain an aspect of normal adult sexuality, while excessive anal stimulation in childhood may predispose to over-emphasis on anal aspects of sexual behaviour.

The infantile genital stage

At some time during the second year and sometimes earlier, the child begins to derive pleasure from contact with his or her own genitals, so-called infantile auto-erotic activity. Freud originally called this the *phallic stage* because he considered that the penis or phallus was the only genital organ children of either sex were aware of. This one-sided masculine attitude to sexual development has since been superseded and the term *infantile genital stage* is more appropriate; it also distinguishes this period in a child's development from the later adult genital stage which commences at puberty. The preceding oral and anal stages described above are often referred to as 'pregenital' stages. Their significance extends well beyond the child's sexual development, influencing, as we have seen, many other aspects of personality development.

During the infantile genital stage boys and girls also begin to show interest and curiosity in each other's genitals. The boy may develop the fantasy that as the girl does not have a penis he might lose his, the beginning of so-called *castration anxiety*. Conversely, the girl may resent the fact that the boy has an organ she lacks, and in families or cultures in which parents seem to favour boys this may lead the girl to behave in a tomboyish fashion and to express envy of boys having a penis.

Parental attitudes have an important influence on the way in which children handle these problems and on the fantasies and beliefs they develop. If parents accept the boy's or girl's auto-erotic play as a normal part of childhood development a healthy basis is laid for the child's attitude to his or her own sexuality in years to come. Disapproval or a threatening and punitive parental attitude on the other hand will lead the child to associate guilt and fear of punishment with sexual activity. Such threats, fortunately rarely heard nowadays, as 'I will cut it off if you touch it again' are bound to increase any castration anxiety the little boy may already have; and if the girl is made to feel similarly guilty when she touches herself she, too, will begin to associate feelings of guilt, anxiety and inadequacy with her developing sexuality. As a result her confidence that she will develop into a woman, capable of sexual enjoyment, of conceiving and of giving birth to healthy children of her own when she gets older may be undermined. Guilt about masturbation, impotence in men and anorgasmia in women, and uncertainties about sexual identity are among the disorders likely to arise as a consequence in adolescence (see p. 83) and adulthood. It is important but often difficult, even today, for parents to respond realistically to the little boy's or girl's questions about the anatomical differences they have observed and to help them appreciate the different biological functions of men and women once they are grown up. The existence of a rich and sometimes totally unrealistic fantasy life in children is often not acknowledged by parents, especially where their sexual fantasies are concerned; the need therefore to listen to children and to respond to them in a realistic and helpful manner cannot be stressed enough.

The Oedipal stage

Closely associated with the infantile genital stage is the period during which the child enters what Freud called the Oedipal situation. According to classical psychoanalytic theory this occurs between the ages of three and five although it may take place earlier. To a greater or lesser extent, at a conscious or unconscious level, unresolved Oedipal problems may persist into adolescence and adult life.

In its widest sense the *Oedipal situation* refers to the recognition by the child that he or she is now involved in a three-person or triangular relationship as opposed to the earlier two-person one. Taking a small boy as an example, he experiences his father as a rival in his relationship to his mother; his wish for an exclusive, close and affectionate relationship to her makes him feel jealous of his father whom he resents and wants to displace. Similarly, a small girl wants to have a close, affectionate relationship to her father and feels jealous and resentful of her mother.

In a more specific sense, following Freud's classic formulation, the Oedipal situation has a sexual significance, the child, boy or girl, desiring sexual closeness to the parent of the opposite sex and wanting to get rid of the rival parent of the same sex. Freud, who first became aware of this conflict in his self-analysis and in the course of psychotherapeutic work with patients, called this the Oedipal conflict following Sophocles' tragedy *Oedipus Rex*. Oedipus, the son due to be born to the king and queen of Thebes, Laius and Jocasta, was said by the Delphic oracle to be destined to kill his father. As soon as he was born, therefore, he was left exposed on a mountain to die, but he was rescued and brought up in Corinth without any knowledge of his real origin. As a young man, on a journey to Thebes, he was involved in a fight and killed a man in a chariot, unaware of the fact that this man was his father Laius. Subsequently he married the widowed Queen Jocasta, again unaware of the fact that she was his real mother and the widow of the man he had killed. When years later he discovered that he had killed his father and married his mother he blinded himself as a self-punishment.

The term Oedipal situation, although applicable in the Greek myth only to the boy, is nowadays used equally to describe the girl's corresponding situation of rivalry with her mother in her search for closeness to her father. Boys and girls, therefore, have to struggle with conscious or unconscious ambivalent feelings towards the parent of the same sex, and with incestuous feelings towards the parent of the opposite sex. Although these conflicts, and especially their sexual content, are usually repressed and therefore no longer accessible to conscious awareness when we grow up, observation of children in the family setting readily reveals the existence of these conflicts in the child's behaviour. In the course of psychotherapy of children and adults these Oedipal problems frequently come to light again. Recognition of the frequent occurrence of child sexual abuse within the family has once more focused attention on these problems in our society (see Chapter 43).

Before discussing the influence of Oedipal conflicts on subsequent sexual development we need to consider how the Oedipal situation is resolved in favourable circumstances. Briefly, children have to accept that their father and mother are married and belong to each other and that the wish for exclusive, including sexual, closeness to the parent of the opposite sex cannot be fulfilled. Instead the boy has to identify with his rival father, whom he also loves, in anticipation of being able to choose his own sexual partner, other than his mother, in years to come; similarly the girl has to identify with her mother in anticipation of finding a sexual partner other than her father when she is grown up. The resolution of the Oedipal situation in either sex therefore depends on successful identification with the parent of the same sex, and on the capacity to tolerate delay and frustration. Such resolution may be only partly achieved in childhood, and Oedipal conflicts almost inevitably return in adolescence when there may be further opportunities for their resolution.

The following are some of the common disturbances of sexual development which may result from unresolved Oedipal problems. A boy who sees his father as an authoritarian and punitive figure may fear being punished by him for his forbidden rivalrous and incestuous wishes. As a result he may as an adult remain guilty and afraid of competing for a woman with other men and lack confidence in his masculinity. More specifically, he may continue to suffer from repressed castration anxiety, i.e. doubts about his manhood and genital potency, a frequent finding in men suffering from impotence. His original fear of punishment for wanting to defeat and displace his father may also find expression in areas other than sexuality. As a result he may feel afraid of success and tend to lose out in competitive situations in his social or professional life. Alternatively, if he has a weak or absent father and a strong, possessive or seductive mother he may identify with her instead, develop feminine characteristics and uncertainty about his sexual identity, possibly becoming homosexual (see p. 372).

Correspondingly, a girl whose unconscious incestuous attachment to her father persists may, as an adult, suffer from anorgasmia out of guilt associated with sexual relationships; or she may repeatedly become attracted to older married men and fail to find a partner who is free to marry her. If instead she identifies with her father she may develop strong masculine tendencies and perhaps become a lesbian. The occurrence of actual incestuous relationships between a girl and her father, as mentioned above, may lead to serious problems in her later sexual development (see Chapter 43).

In summary, Oedipal problems which remain unresolved can cause a variety of sexual and psychoneurotic disorders, but instead of giving them a central place in the understanding of the neuroses, as Freud did originally, in modern psychodynamic understanding Oedipal problems take their place alongside the many other psychopathological considerations outlined earlier; many of these date back to earlier stages of infantile development and emotional deprivation.

THE ROLE OF PLAY

The important role of play in the development of the personality has only been recognised fully since the early 1950s. We mentioned earlier that such games as playing bo-peep or hide-and-seek help the child to master separation anxiety and learn that what is lost is not necessarily lost for ever but can return. However, Winnicott in *Playing and Reality* (1971) pointed out that play has a much wider significance in the child's development and continues to be an essential part of adult living. Through play we learn early in life how to express ourselves in imagination and how to relate to the world around us. 'It is in playing and only in playing that the individual child or adult is able to be creative and to use the whole personality, and it is only in being creative that the individual discovers the self' (Winnicott 1971, p.62).

Already in infancy the child derives pleasure from his mother or father playing with him, perhaps at first by smiling at him and making noises to which he can respond; or throwing him up in the air and catching him. Soon the child begins to invent his own games, sometimes by playing with others, sometimes by playing on his own. Play thus becomes a deeply absorbing activity, and objects like toys, pictures and story books can all be used to stand for or symbolise aspects of real living and of the child's inner fantasy life. For example, a few cushions put on the floor in a row can represent a train and the child, sitting on the cushion in front, can 'drive the train', being fully engaged in the game he has created. Milner (1952) has emphasised the role of symbolism and play in the development of creativity, and has applied this especially to the way in which children and adults learn to draw and paint (Milner 1957). The central role of play in the development of thought and intelligence has also been described by Piaget (1962).

As the child grows older, e.g. when he goes to school, play and learning continue to be closely related, and educational achievements are best promoted by parents and teachers who can make the subject enjoyable and exciting by stimulating the child's curiosity, imagination and sense of discovery. Play also serves a vital role in promoting the child's relationships to other children outside the family, either in organised games at school or, perhaps more importantly, by the imaginative and creative activity of children who invent their own games.

Children who are not given sufficient stimulation and opportunities for play may be held back in their emotional and cognitive development, and the same applies to children who are frightened and inhibited so that they cannot let themselves go in play and in imaginative activity. The consequences of such impairment may extend into adult life.

Personality development does not end with childhood but continues through adolescence into adulthood. These later stages will be considered in Chapter 8.

FURTHER READING

Bowlby, J (1979). *The Making and Breaking of Affectional Bonds*. Tavistock, London.

Erikson, E.H. (1965). *Childhood and Society*. Penguin, Harmondsworth.

Hobson, R.P. (1985). 'Piaget: on the ways of knowing in childhood' in *Child and Adolescent Psychiatry: modern approaches*, 2nd ed. (Rutter. M. and Hersov, L., eds). Blackwell, Oxford.

Mahler, M.S., Pine, F. and Bergman, A. (1975). *The Psychological Birth of the Human Infant: symbiosis and individuation*. Karnac, London.

Mitchell, J. (1986). *The Selected Melanie Klein*. Penguin, Harmondsworth.

Piaget, J. (1953). *The Origin of Intelligence in the Child*. Routledge & Kegan Paul, London.

Rutter, M. (1981). *Maternal Deprivation Reassessed*, 2nd ed. Penguin, Harmondsworth.

Segal, H. (1978). *Introduction to the Work of Melanie Klein*. Hogarth, London.

Segal, H. (1979). *Klein*. Fontana, London.

Stern, D.N. (1985). *The Interpersonal World of the Infant: a view from psychoanalysis and developmental psychology*. Basic Books, New York.

Winnicott, D.W. (1965). *The Maturational Processes and the Facilitating Environment: studies in the theory of emotional development*. Hogarth, London.

Winnicott, D.W. (1971). *Playing and Reality*. Penguin, Harmondsworth.

8

Adolescence and the Life Cycle

Although the basis for an individual's personality is to a large extent laid down during his development from infancy through childhood, important further development takes place during adolescence. This will be considered next, followed by a consideration of the remainder of the life cycle, i.e. adulthood, including middle age and old age. Just as at each of the earlier stages the individual is faced with problems and conflicts characteristic of that particular period, so he will in adult life be confronted with situations and conflicts more or less specific for that period, and the new experiences may lead to further growth in some, to breakdown in others. How a person copes with such problems when they arise will, in part, depend on his development at earlier stages.

ADOLESCENCE

Adolescence is the period of transition from childhood to adulthood. As is the case with all transitions, it is hard to define its precise boundaries. In our society adolescence can be divided into three phases: (1) Early adolescence, which starts around the onset of puberty and lasts until the mid-teens, in which the young person rapidly matures physically but remains emotionally and physically dependent on his parents. This coincides with the formation of strong peer relationships, usually in groups of the same sex. (2) A middle phase, in which pairing becomes apparent, both with the same and with the opposite sex, and in which the adolescent begins to assume a definite identity and sense of who he is and what his hopes and aims are. (3) A phase of late adolescence in which sexuality begins to become established and in which the adolescent explores the balance between intimacy and individuation, grappling with fears of merging on the one hand, and isolation on the other. Social and emotional, and sometimes also financial separation from the parents begins to be achieved rather than merely striven for.

Such an account is inevitably class-, sex- and culture-bound, and adolescence in different societies and historical epochs takes and has taken many different forms. For example, the prolonged adolescence of modern life in Western society reflects the time required to acquire the technical and social skills needed for survival in an industrialised, competitive and often disrupted society. Urban life with its attractions and temptations may be particularly threatening to adolescents. Despite these differences, the tasks of adolescent development are similar in all cultures and involve three main and interconnected themes: the body, identity and independence.

The body

The physical changes in adolescence, including the development of the sexual organs and secondary sexual characteristics, are associated with marked hormonal changes. Androgen and oestrogen production begins to increase from about the age of eight in both boys and girls; this is followed, shortly before puberty, by a further sharp rise of androgens in boys and of oestrogens in girls. The increased sexual drive in adolescence is largely due to the greater production of androgens, and this applies to both sexes. Puberty and adolescence are also accompanied by an increased growth rate. This growth spurt tends to start earlier in girls than in boys, but there are marked individual variations. These physical changes lead to and are accompanied by profound psychological changes in the adolescent's attitude to his body.

Before adolescence a child's bodily powers are limited but in imagination all is possible. Princes and princesses can fall in love, marry and live happily ever after; battles can be won, space explored, and planets reached or destroyed. In reality the child is still dependent on his or her parents, and sexual maturity and other physical achievements have not yet been reached. After puberty the adolescent acquires genital maturity and real potency but loses the sense of unlimited possibilities.

Adolescents must learn to accept the person they are. This includes the body they have got, their sex, size and physical and mental abilities. There is often an intense preoccupation with appearance and change in body image. The adolescent can alter the colour of his hair and determine which latest fashion to assume, but he cannot stop or influence the hormonal changes which are driving him towards adulthood. Changes in the genitals and increasing sexual awareness become associated with masturbation which occurs in almost all males and is common in females. Whether or not an adolescent can accept masturbation and the fantasies associated with it without guilt depends on his attitude to sexuality, which is largely determined by experiences at earlier stages of development, as described in Chapter 7.

For most adolescents bodily changes, like breast development, the appearance of pubic hair and the start of menstruation in girls, and corresponding changes in boys, including wet dreams and the capacity to ejaculate during orgasm, will be welcome signs of growing up. For others, especially those who are unprepared for what is happening to them, and for those who were brought up with fear and guilt about anything sexual, these changes can be deeply disturbing and may lead them to hate their own bodies, a topic to which we shall return shortly.

Identity

A crucial issue for adolescents is the development of a new sense of identity. The process of identity formation has been discussed by Erikson (1965, 1968) who says that identity 'connotes both a persistent sameness within oneself and a persistent sharing of some kind of essential character with others'. Erikson has also described the process of identity formation in a biography of Martin Luther (Erikson 1958). The adolescent has to create a new identity out of the various identifications with parental and other figures carried within himself since childhood, and out of a range of recent models and identifications with different ideals, values, heroes and images. The old identifications and more recent influences do not necessarily have to be given up, but they need to be questioned and modified and choices have to be made in order to achieve a unified sense of identity or sameness of one's own. This process may involve periods of uncertainty and confusion, sometimes referred to as *identity diffusion*. Rebelliousness is an integral part of this struggle, and at times the adolescent may organise himself around a negative identity. Here he defines himself not so much by what he *is* but by what he is *not*, not by what he is *for* but by what he is *against*. At the same time he wants to make relationships outside the family, with peers and social groups, to feel part of a wider society and to belong, but without giving up his growing or hard-won individuality by excessive conformity.

The development of an adolescent's *sexual identity*, in keeping with his biological sex, and a positive attitude to his new body image is a particularly important aspect of the wider process of identity formation. Once genital maturity has been achieved it brings with it the ability to have sexual relationships with another person. At what stage an adolescent has his or her first sexual experience depends on many factors, including family, social, moral and religious influences, and the adolescent's own attitudes, hopes and fears. One important issue is the ability or lack of ability to integrate sexuality with friendship and affection towards the partner. Some adolescents who start a sexual life are capable of doing so early on, and their relationships may be relatively stable, while others have a series of brief relationships, the end of which may cause distress to one or other of the partners. This applies equally to heterosexual and homosexual relationships.

Some adolescents who do not feel ready to start having a sexual relationship may feel isolated and inferior to their peers who may have started to do so, especially if there are strong social pressures to find a sexual partner. Others may experience disturbing conflicts between heterosexual and homosexual wishes. This may lead to anxiety about their future sexual orientation, especially if they do not realise that such sexual conflicts, as well as homosexual experiences, are common in adolescence on the way to heterosexuality.

Choices about sexual orientation and behaviour are not the only decisions that face adolescents. These may include choices of study, future occupation, religious, moral and political convictions, and choices between conformity and rebellion. Those who are not yet ready to make important choices in one or more of these areas may need what Erikson called a *moratorium*. This is a conscious or unconscious postponement of making a decision so that time, sometimes months or years, is available before the person is ready to decide which direction to choose. This is becoming more difficult in modern society, where expectations are often more pressing, and where mass unemployment makes the prospects of finding satisfying work more difficult. Unemployment also casts a shadow over the spontaneity and optimism of many adolescents and young adults. Fear of nuclear war and, in the sexual sphere, of contracting AIDS may also prevent some adolescents from feeling able to enjoy life and to look forward to the future.

Independence

Adolescence is the second of the three great periods of separation-individuation in the human life cycle. The first occurs during the first two years of life, when the infant gradually emerges from a state of symbiosis with his mother to become a separate person in his own right (see p. 66). The second, to be discussed here, is the period of separation of the adolescent from his family. The third occurs towards the end of life when a person begins to detach himself from life, relatives and friends, and prepares himself to die alone.

An adolescent has to detach himself from his parents and family and begin to lead his own life, and probably at a later stage to start a family of his own. The path between insufficient separation from parents with persistent dependence, and excessive detachment with isolation can be a narrow one. The adolescent has to learn to be separate, and yet to be able to relate.

The move from dependence to independence can be helped or hindered by the parents, and it is much influenced by their earlier relationship to their child. Earlier experiences of having had parents who provided a sense of security and non-intrusive intimacy while encouraging the child's growing separateness and initiative will assist the adolescent's move towards independence. Such an experience leaves the adolescent with an inner sense of security and with a model, through identification, of how to relate to others outside the family. It also paves the way for the future adult to relate to his parents as equal adults and friends. If, on the other hand, parents cling excessively to their child, perhaps because they need him for their own satisfaction and security, he will either feel bound to stay with and hence remain dependent on them, or he will rebel excessively in his struggle towards independence. This may lead to total rejection of the parents, and in extreme cases to involvement with drugs or other antisocial behaviour.

The development from dependence to independence inevitably arouses anxiety and conflict in the adolescent, and to a greater or lesser extent also in the parents. Social rituals, sometimes called puberty rites, exist in many societies to mark and facilitate this transition from childhood to adulthood. In our society religious ceremonies like confirmation, or examinations and the public awarding of certificates or degrees have replaced the symbolic, often sexual rites that used to be practised in primitive societies. Eccentricities of dress, sexual initiation and minor antisocial activities practised in groups of teenagers may take the place of more conventional ceremonies.

The large majority of teenagers pass successfully through these stages of adolescence and accompanying emotional turmoil. Some become seriously disturbed and a few develop an adolescent breakdown. These complications will be considered next.

Adolescent disturbance

Adolescents often challenge the established order and cause anxiety among those who are close to them. Adolescents themselves, their parents, teachers, doctors and others are thus often confronted by the question of whether a particular feeling or form of behaviour is 'normal' or not. A vital distinction here is that between *adolescent disturbance* as part of normal adolescent development, and *adolescent breakdown*. If this distinction is not made, a phase of developmental disturbance, likely spontaneously to improve, may wrongly be seen as illness; conversely a deeply confused and mentally ill teenager desperately in need of help may be mistaken for a normal adolescent going through a 'difficult patch'. The fact that adolescents are often very secretive and may not reveal their problems to anyone, least of all their parents, makes it particularly difficult to come to the right decision. The distinction is easier to make in theory than in practice, and sometimes only the passage of time allows a clear picture to emerge.

Normal disturbances in teenagers include minor episodes of depression, anxiety, guilt about masturbation, fears of homosexuality, experimentation with 'soft' drugs like alcohol and cannabis, and minor infringements of the law. All can be an aspect of 'normal' development, though this is not to say that they do not reflect personal, social and family conflicts with which adolescents may need help and guidance from peers, parents, teachers, counsellors or psychotherapists. Provided the teenager is willing to accept help this may prevent a more serious adolescent breakdown.

In adolescent disturbance the teenager usually functions normally in most areas. He continues to mix with peers, goes to school or work, looks after himself and eats normally. In adolescent breakdown there is a serious failure in one or more of these areas.

Adolescent breakdown

A study of fourteen to fifteen-year-old adolescents on the Isle of Wight (Graham and Rutter 1973; Rutter *et al*. 1976a) showed that the one-year prevalence of overt psychiatric disorder in this age group was 10 to 15 per cent. In addition there was a group of adolescents who on interview were found to be severely psychiatrically disturbed but whose parents and teachers were unaware of their disturbance. The total figure of adolescent psychiatric disorder in this study therefore amounted to 21 per cent. Male and female adolescents were about equally affected. The rate of psychiatric disorder among adolescents is greater in inner cities than in rural areas (Rutter *et al*. 1975b).

The various forms of adolescent breakdown will be considered under two main headings: breakdown due to an adolescent identity crisis, and breakdown due to other psychiatric disorders. In practice this distinction is often difficult to make.

Identity crisis

This is the commonest form of adolescent breakdown but is difficult to define. As the name implies, the adolescent feels defeated in his search for an identity of his own and lost in almost all aspects of his existence. Neither child nor adult; torn by the desire to rebel against his parents and to invite their disapproval, and yet wanting to retain their care and protection; unsure of his sexual identity and feeling unable to accept the changes in his body; without any ideas or plans about future work or career; lonely in his isolation and yet afraid of close relationships, he may break down more or less completely. Such a breakdown may take many forms.

Depression, sometimes with suicidal thoughts, is common. Acts of self-harm and suicide also occur; their frequency is discussed below. Anxiety states, panic attacks and confusion may occur in association with depressive features or separately. Psychosomatic or hysterical symptoms and eating disorders may take the place of more overt mental symptoms. Self-hatred and dislike of the sexual body and guilt about sexual fantasies and desires (Laufer and Laufer 1984) may lead to further depression, acts of self-harm or suicide.

Abnormal behaviour may consist of truancy or school refusal (see p. 509), lying in bed all day, almost total withdrawal, or serious involvement with drugs or delinquent behaviour. In adolescent girls the disturbed behaviour may take the form of extreme promiscuity, perhaps leading to repeated unwanted pregnancies. If the adolescent is very disturbed and unable to express himself coherently it may be difficult to differentiate between an identity crisis and schizophrenia. However, delusions and hallucinations do not occur and observation over a period of time may be the only way of reaching a decision.

Other psychiatric disorders

Psychiatric disorders may occur during adolescence without necessarily being caused by an identity crisis or other adolescent problems (Graham and Rutter 1985). The disorder may also be a continuation of a disorder already present in childhood. Adolescent problems, including identity crises, do however often act as precipitating or perpetuating factors and influence the nature and course of the illness. In clinical practice the patient's relation to his parents, teachers and peers and his reaction to his adolescent development should always be taken fully into account when considering the diagnosis and management.

The following are some of the psychiatric disorders seen during adolescence. The reader is referred to the relevant chapters where the conditions are described in detail, independent of the age of the patient affected.

The commonest are the *affective disorders*, depressive illnesses being more common than mania. As in depressive illnesses among other age groups, *suicide* and *acts of self-harm* may occur (Hawton 1986), and the prevalence of suicide increases rapidly during adolescence (Shaffer 1974; Shaffer and Fisher 1981; McClure 1984, 1987). Completed suicide hardly ever occurs before the age of twelve. By the age of fifteen to nineteen the suicide rate has risen to 40 per million population in males and 20 per million in females (Office of Health Economics 1981). The higher rate in male than in female adolescents has been found in all studies. There has also been a marked increase in adolescent suicides over the years from 1941 to 1980.

Acts of self-harm (attempted suicide) also increase rapidly between the ages of fourteen and nineteen (Hawton and Goldacre 1982; Hawton *et al.* 1982). In contrast to completed suicide acts of self-harm are more common in girls than boys.

Suicide and acts of self-harm are often preceded by arguments with a boyfriend or girlfriend, rows with parents, threats of disciplinary action or punishment, and poor relationship with peers. Parental discord and early loss of a parent are among the predisposing factors (Stanley and Barter 1970; Shaffer 1974). As in other age groups, repeated attempts are common after an initial act of self-harm.

Anxiety states are also common in adolescence; obsessive compulsive neurosis and hysteria are seen less often. Adolescents often suffer from social inadequacy, especially in relation to adults, and antisocial or delinquent behaviour may present serious problems. *Eating disorders*, especially anorexia nervosa, have already been referred to (see p. 440).

Schizophrenia is rare in early adolescence, the one year prevalence being less than 1 per 1000 compared with 3.3 per 1000 in adults. It increases in late adolescence and early adulthood.

Children who have organic brain damage and those who are mentally handicapped (see Chapter 41) present many personal, social and educational problems when they reach adolescence.

Treatment in adolescence

A sense of shame and embarrassment almost invariably accompanies adolescent difficulties. This makes it hard for teenagers to admit that anything is wrong. They are trying to be adults and to become independent of their parents, so asking for help from adults feels like failure. Some of them prefer to seek help in walk-in centres without telling their parents or family doctors. For this reason a sensitive, non-intrusive and flexible approach is essential so that the young person feels the doctor, counsellor or psychotherapist can be trusted and is on his side. At the same time adolescents may long for boundaries to be drawn, and parents and doctors must feel able to set firm limits when appropriate.

In some milder cases family therapy (see p. 577) may reduce the adolescent's feelings of being a scapegoat, help restore parental authority and assist the adolescent's move towards independence. More often individual counselling or psychotherapy is the only setting in which a young person can be helped to share his fear of madness, his doubts and confusion, his depression and suicidal thoughts, his fear of or guilt about homosexuality, and other sexual problems.

In severe cases hospital admission is essential. Unfortunately provision for inpatient or day-patient care for adolescents, separate from children or adults, is inadequate in the NHS as there are few adolescent units. The units that do exist may lack the staff that can provide the necessary psychotherapeutic help. Once admitted, the atmosphere of a therapeutic community, including the use of individual and group therapy, occupational therapy and educational facilities can be very effective (see p. 621). Behavioural treatment methods are useful in some cases. Drug therapy may be needed to control severely disturbed behaviour, and will be essential when treating a psychiatric illness like severe depression or schizophrenia in an adolescent.

ADULTHOOD

Two particularly important aspects of adult life will be considered here: marriage, including parenthood, and work.

Marriage

In our society 90 per cent of adults marry. 30 per cent of first marriages and 40 per cent of second marriages end in divorce or separation. The separation rate of couples who marry under the age of twenty is 50 per cent. The increase in marriage rates outstrips the increase in divorce rates as more and more marry more than once. These figures indicate the strength of the forces that lead people to get married and at other times drive them apart.

Marriage also varies greatly in different classes and cultures. In some cultures marriages are arranged by parents, often when the future couple are still children. Authoritarian and traditional attitudes tend to dominate in such families, with strong prohibitions on divorce. If such a family moves into a less traditional society, problems arise as the children, when they grow up, may rebel against their parents, for example by deciding to choose their own marriage partner. Similarly, in some strict or orthodox religious families the parents may object to their son or daughter marrying a member of a different faith, thus causing serious conflicts within the family.

In contrast, modern marriage is more often based on romantic love and the parents have little or no say in their offspring's choice of partner. This kind of marriage is usually associated with a nuclear type of family and easy divorce, unless religious convictions make this difficult.

Another important dimension concerns the role of the two sexes. In some cultures males and females have very different roles, in others their roles are blurred. In our society the traditional distinctions between male and female roles are much less rigid than they used to be. The feminist movement has stressed the equality of men and women, especially in the social field. Women now have greater freedom to follow their own interests or careers, while men may be willing to accept a more domestic role and assume greater responsibility for looking after the children, combining masculine with more maternal functions. These changes have helped some marriages but have brought with them new problems which may lead to difficulties in others.

In some patterns of marriage teamwork is essential and husband and wife are together for long periods, e.g. in farming communities. In other marriages the men are away for long periods, e.g. migrant workers, and the wives have to combine their nurturing female role with the more disciplinarian or authoritarian role traditionally assumed by the husband.

Choice of marriage partner

The choice of one's marital partner is one of the most, if not *the* most, important decisions in a person's life. At a conscious level people tend to marry those with similar backgrounds, education, intelligence and interests as themselves, but it is far more difficult to say what determines why two people fall in love with each other and decide to marry. While sexual attraction plays a major role, unconscious factors are also of great importance.

Taking a woman as an example here, her partner may, by a process of projection, come to represent an idealised version of an internal image of a near perfect man, perhaps based on what, as a child, she had wanted her father to be. In this sense projection of feelings dating back to childhood often plays a central role, similar to what happens in the transference in a psychotherapeutic relationship (see p. 560).

Alternatively, the partner may represent an aspect of the Self which a person feels is lacking in himself: a man who feels unsure of himself and lacking in confidence may find himself attracted to a woman who is more sure of herself, or even somewhat domineering and controlling. This may cause problems later on; for example, when the husband, as he gets older, becomes more confident, he may begin to resent his wife's attempts to control or dominate him.

To take another example, a rather gentle, submissive woman who denies all her aggressive impulses may fall in love with a man with strong, though often partly concealed aggressive tendencies; if, after having married him, his aggressive behaviour becomes more overt she may object and the marriage may become punctuated by quarrels and mixed feelings of love and hatred. How such marital problems can be dealt with will be considered in Chapter 45 (see p. 575).

In other cases, however, the choice of marital partner based on mutual projection may fulfil the needs of both, so that husband and wife continue to complement each other and each learns to accept the strengths and weaknesses, or the acceptable and less acceptable aspects of the other.

Marriage can be divided into a number of phases, each with its own pleasures and pitfalls. Romantic love, with intense mutual concern, sexual excitement and emotional involvement may continue, sometimes lasting a long time. However, powerful feelings of possessiveness accompanied by jealousy may complicate the relationship. Earlier experiences of excessive intimacy and closeness dating back to childhood may be reawakened and lead to a sense of being trapped and to an ambivalent attitude towards the partner. This, in turn, may lead to sexual problems; for example, a couple may have a mutually satisfying sexual relationship before getting married, but afterwards the man may become impotent because he feels he has lost his freedom so that he begins to resent his wife. The marriage may thus be in danger of breaking up. In order to prevent this happening it is essential for the couple to learn how to balance closeness and intimacy with the necessary mutual respect for each other's separateness and individual needs and preferences. Such a balance between closeness and separateness is in fact crucial in all marriages (Skynner 1976; Skynner and Cleese 1983).

As romantic love subsides the relationship may break up unless it is transmuted into conjugal love where companionship, shared interests, mutual care and support and, in many cases, rearing a family, predominate. The ability to maintain conjugal love depends on the level of maturity of the partners and especially on finding a balance between stability and excitement, closeness and separateness, and self-interest and regard for the other person's needs. Perhaps most important of all is the capacity to tolerate and survive mixed feelings towards the partner when faced with inevitable differences and disagreements in the relationship.

Parenthood

If the couple have children the marriage will be punctuated by their arrival, growth and development, and their departure when they leave home. Couples with a young child have to learn to accept the change from a two-person to a three-person relationship, with attendant rivalry; in either or both of them this may reawaken unresolved feelings of jealousy they experienced at the Oedipal stage in their own childhood. For example, the father may feel displaced in his wife's affection when she devotes much of her time to looking after her baby and small children. The arrival of a new baby may also stir up earlier feelings of sibling rivalry experienced in his own childhood.

Mothers may feel overwhelmed by the demands of their baby or small children and become depressed as a result. The psychological aspects and psychiatric complications of pregnancy and the puerperium are discussed in Chapter 33. It is at this stage that the husband's ability to support his wife and take an active part in caring for the children is particularly important. Both partners must accept that they will often have to put their children's needs before their own, while at the same time safeguarding their own privacy and intimacy.

If, as the children get older, the relationship between the parents deteriorates, the father's frustration and search for affection may stir up his incestuous wishes and lead to such damaging and disruptive events as child sexual abuse (see Chapter 43).

As the children reach adolescence they present different challenges to the marriage. Their emergent sexuality may evoke anxieties that one or other parent experienced in their own adolescence. This may prevent the parents from talking to their children about sexuality, or they may become over-anxious about their adolescent children's sexual interests or behaviour. Alternatively, they may envy their son's or daughter's first sexual experience and seek extra-marital affairs themselves. As the children become more independent and question or rebel against parental authority, the couple need to be able to work as a team, set limits when necessary and not permit the adolescent to drive a wedge between them and to undermine their role as parents.

The problems posed by children are usually outweighed by the enjoyment and pride they engender. This does, however, depend on the parents' ability to share their activities and their play. Parents who have since childhood retained their own capacity to play will find it easy to do so, while those who are no longer in touch with the playful child aspects within themselves will find this difficult, at a considerable loss to themselves and their children (see p. 75). The ability to remain playful is helpful not only in bringing up children but also in the relationship between the parents themselves.

Another difficult phase of married life arises when the children leave home. When parents who have devoted themselves mainly or only to looking after and providing for their children are once more alone together they have to re-think their relationship. The mother may, perhaps for the first time, have to find new interests outside the home, and both partners may have to learn new ways of enjoying and sharing life by themselves. Interest in grandchildren and other activities may fill the gap the children have left.

The final phase of marriage involves facing and coping with illness, death and bereavement, and with the prospect of being alone. How couples deal with these painful experiences is often a function of their earlier relationship, their individual development earlier in life, and their present social environment (see Chapter 9).

Marital breakdown

Several factors contribute to marital breakdown.

Developmental factors

The more emotionally immature the partners, the less likely is a marriage to survive. At the same time, immaturity in one or both partners is itself a factor that pushes people towards premature marriage. This creates a repetitive cycle in which people from emotionally deprived backgrounds and unstable homes are themselves likely to be agents of marital breakdown. In others marriage and learning how to resolve marital problems may enhance personal development. Alternatively, if psychological problems remain unresolved they may lead to separation or divorce.

Social factors

Unemployment, poor housing and financial difficulties all put great strains on a marriage and may contribute to marital breakdown. Fagin and Little in their study *Unemployment and Health in Families* (1981) have described the effects of the husband's unemployment on his wife and children and the marital problems this can give rise to. Mattinson (1988) has described similar findings.

Mental illness

Marital difficulty is both a cause and a consequence of mental illness. Men with marital problems may drink excessively; women who are unhappily married often become depressed. Major chronic mental illness, such as schizophrenia or affective disorders, and, indeed, chronic physical illness, can put an intolerable burden on marriage. Mental illness rates in married men are lower than for unmarried men, whereas for women the reverse is true. Being married appears to be a protective factor in men but a vulnerability factor for mental illness in women if the marriage is disturbed and unhappy. In morbid jealousy (see p. 256) the marriage itself becomes the focus of a psychosis in which one partner, usually the husband, develops delusions of his wife's infidelity.

Presentation of marital problems

Doctors should be alert to the possibility of indirect presentation of marital difficulties. Drinking problems, persistent nightshift work, infidelity, unexplained psychosomatic complaints, depression, acts of self-harm and behaviour problems in the children may all be manifestations of marital problems. The presenting patient may cast the doctor in the role of an understanding substitute for the unsatisfactory spouse, but the doctor should resist the temptation to take sides. Concerned neutrality combined with empathic understanding is the best strategy for helping troubled couples, as described in Chapter 45.

Separation, divorce and single parents

Our society, however liberal its ideology, discriminates against the single. Being divorced or separated may put an individual at a financial and social disadvantage which compounds the already low self-esteem and loneliness created by the unhappiness of separation itself. It is not surprising therefore that consultation rates in general practice for the recently separated are higher than for any other social group. Parents bringing up children without a partner, whether previously married or not, are particularly vulnerable, and doctors should be sensitive to their problems and difficulties. Self-help groups such as Gingerbread in the UK exist to support single parents.

Work

Work plays an important role in the life of adults, but its meaning varies from person to person and over time. At its most obvious, to have a job is essential to earn money for oneself and one's family. Ideally a person's occupation should provide a sense of achievement, but in most societies there are many whose work provides little satisfaction and may be experienced as a boring necessity. Only relatively few have the opportunity to choose a job they really like, or to train for a career that provides a sense of enjoyment and creativity. Everyone will at times be anxious about his success or failure at work and about his chances of being promoted or the risk of losing his job.

Other important aspects of work are the sense of belonging to a group of workers and professionals, and the relationships to fellow workers, subordinates and superiors which it provides. Throughout adult life, therefore, either a person's work and occupation will contribute to a sense of security and self-esteem, or problems related to work may be responsible for a sense of failure, both economically and as a person, and contribute to such feelings as anxiety, depression, envy, resentment and isolation.

Unemployment

It is hardly surprising therefore that unemployment, which has become such a serious problem in many countries, is associated with poor mental and physical health, as has been shown in the Black Report on Inequalities in Health (Black *et al.* 1982), and by Warr (1984). Mattinson (1988) has provided a study of the meaning of work to individuals and how losing a job and unemployment can affect both husband and wife, their marital relationship and their family.

Several studies have also shown that suicide and acts of self-harm are considerably more common among the unemployed. In Edinburgh in the years from 1978 to 1982 unemployed men showed a significantly higher incidence of acts of self-harm than men who were employed, and the risk rose significantly with the duration of unemployment. The ratio of acts of self-harm of the unemployed to the employed was 6:1 during the first 5 months of unemployment, 10:1 during the period from 6 to 12 months and 19:1 for those who were unemployed for longer than 12 months (Platt and Kreitman 1984). Similarly, Hawton and Rose (1986) found that in Oxford between 1979 and 1982 the rates for acts of self-harm for unemployed men were 12 to 15 times as great as those for men who were employed.

MIDDLE AGE

There is no agreed age at which a person can be said to enter middle age, although in women the menopause constitutes a biological landmark. It is a period when a person may have to accept some limitations to his physical abilities. Physical ill-health may accelerate this process. Some will have to face the fact that they are reaching the limits of their personal achievements and may feel frustrated and depressed. For many it is a time when achievements and ambitions are consolidated. Yet others may be able to embark on new ventures with even greater responsibilities and enjoyment than in earlier years.

Changes in family life, such as children leaving home, have already been referred to. Sooner or later there may be some falling-off of sexual interest. In many cases, however, an active and enjoyable sex life will last well into middle or even old age, depending more on the nature of the relationship between the partners than on age itself. Women will, however, have to accept that their ability to bear children is coming to an end.

How each individual adjusts to the inevitable changes associated with no longer being young depends on how he has learnt to deal with other losses earlier in life. Those who feel dissatisfied with their earlier achievements and cannot tolerate losses may give up hope and become depressed, while others may accept the challenge of having to create a new and fulfilling life in keeping with their age. Yet others may deny that they are middle-aged and go through a period of behaving as if they were young adults or even adolescents, perhaps leaving their married partners and starting a relationship with a much younger person. They, too, may become depressed and need help when their denial no longer works and they have to face reality.

OLD AGE

About one in six of the population of the UK is sixty-five or over, and somewhat arbitrarily this is the age when people are said to become elderly. This is also the age when most people have to retire.

Nowadays more people are living to the age when the diseases of degeneration, e.g. coronary disease and cerebral arteriosclerosis, may start to affect them. This is also the age when hearing and eyesight may begin to deteriorate. As people get older some mild impairment of memory may develop, but the majority retain their mental abilities. Only about 2 per cent of those aged sixty-five to seventy, and 20 per cent of those over eighty develop moderate or severe degrees of dementia due to Alzheimer's disease (Royal College of Physicians 1981).

Many individuals do, however, become more isolated as they get older. Apart from the effect of physical factors there are several social factors responsible for this. These include the following:

(1) Retirement may lead to the loss of friends and contact with fellow workers, accompanied by a loss of status and belonging. As a result the elderly may have less contact with others and feel lonely and unwanted unless they prepare for their retirement and develop new and stimulating interests.

(2) The longer we live the fewer relations and contemporaries may be alive to keep us company. The death of a husband or wife, or of a son or daughter who provided company and support, may be a devastating blow from which someone may find it difficult to recover; this may be aggravated by any physical disability which makes the elderly person dependent on others. The effects of bereavement are described more fully in Chapter 9.

(3) Financial stress, having to live alone, and no longer being able to go out or look after themselves, may all contribute to the isolation of the elderly.

It is not surprising, therefore, that depression is common in this age group, sometimes combined with dementia or other psychiatric illness. The psychiatric disorders of old age and their treatment are described in Chapter 25.

It must be stressed, however, that there are many elderly people who remain active and enterprising, with plenty of interests and friends, well into their seventies or longer. Much depends on their physical and mental health, social and economic circumstances, and on their personality.

It is important to consider how the more serious consequences of becoming old can be prevented or ameliorated. The need to plan for one's retirement has already been mentioned. In addition doctors, including geriatricians, must do all they can to treat any physical disabilities the person has developed, and the social services play a most important role in providing financial support and assistance in finding suitable housing and accommodation. Day centres for the elderly are particularly useful to counter isolation and to stimulate new interests. Those who live alone and can no longer look after themselves may be helped by meals on wheels and, in general, visits by social workers, community psychiatric nurses or voluntary workers all provide the social contacts which are so essential in preventing social isolation in old age.

FURTHER READING

Black, Sir Douglas *et al.* (1982). *Inequalities in Health. The Black Report* (Townsend, P. and Davidson, N., eds). Penguin, Harmondsworth.

Calarusso, C.A. and Nemiroff, R.A. (1987). 'Clinical implications of adult developmental theory'. *Am. J. Psychiat.* 144, 1263-1270.

Erikson, E.H. (1968). *Identity, Youth and Crisis.* Faber & Faber, London.

Jacques, E. (1965). 'Death and the mid-life crisis'. *Int. J. Psychoanal.* 46, 502-514.

Mattinson, J. (1988). *Work, Love and Marriage: the impact of unemployment.* Duckworth, London.

Skynner, R. and Cleese, J. (1983). *Families and How to Survive Them.* Methuen, London.

9

Bereavement, Death and Dying

BEREAVEMENT

The loss through death of a close and loved relative or friend can be one of the most painful events anyone has to cope with. Few if any of us are spared such an experience and the grief that follows. It takes a long time to get over a serious bereavement, and it is not unusual for sad and painful memories to persist for many years. In clinical practice it is helpful to distinguish between normal and abnormal mourning, or a normal and abnormal grief reaction, but there are many individual variations and the distinction is far from clear-cut and hence often difficult to make.

A bereavement can also be the cause or precipitant factor of a psychiatric, especially a depressive illness (see p. 171), and it often precedes the onset of psychosomatic symptoms and disorders (see p. 438). There is also evidence of an association between the death of a spouse and an increased risk of death, especially in men, from coronary disease or cancer (Parkes *et al.* 1969; Parkes 1986; MacAvoy 1986; Bowling *et al.* 1985). This applies particularly to widowers during the first six months and to widows a year or longer after the bereavement.

Many factors influence a person's reaction to a bereavement. These include his earlier development, the nature of his relationship to the deceased, his personality and psychological vulnerability, age, social and cultural circumstances, religious beliefs, and especially the support he may or may not be getting from relatives or friends. The psychodynamic aspects have been reviewed by Pedder (1982).

Bowlby, in his work on attachment and loss, has frequently drawn attention to the similarity between a child's reaction to separation from its mother, in terms of the stages of protest, despair and detachment (see p. 68), and mourning in adult life. He has summarised his findings in his books on *Attachment and Loss* (Bowlby 1969, 1973, 1980). The comprehensive study of bereavement by Parkes (1972, 1986) in adults has been much influenced by Bowlby's concepts. Much earlier Freud (1917) had drawn attention to the relation between mourning and melancholia, pointing out that melancholia, now called depression, more often followed a bereavement if there had been a preponderance of negative feelings in the relationship to the deceased, as opposed to normal mourning when positive feelings had predominated (see also p. 196).

Melanie Klein's concept of the depressive position during personality development (see p. 70) emphasises that the ability as an adult to tolerate and recover from losses largely depends on having achieved in childhood the capacity to relate to another person, originally the mother, as a whole person and to accept mixed feelings of love as well as of anger.

Winnicott (1965) has somewhat similarly drawn attention to the fact that the capacity to recover from losses like a bereavement depends on having internalised as a child a stable image of a reliable, 'good-enough' mother which serves as a lasting source of inner strength and confidence (see also p. 66).

Normal mourning

This has been described in detail by Parkes (1972, 1986). It is usual to speak of the following stages of a normal mourning reaction: shock and denial, anger and guilt, searching and pining, sadness and despair, acceptance and recovery. In practice these stages often overlap; some bereaved people may not experience each one of them, and some manifestations cannot be readily fitted into these stages. This will become clearer in the following description.

Poets and writers have described the painful nature of mourning, the despair, denial and anger, a great deal better than doctors and psychotherapists. Thus King Lear carrying the dead Cordelia in his arms exclaims:

> Howl, howl, howl, howl! – O you are men of stones:
> Had I your tongues and eyes, I'd use them so
> That Heaven's vault should crack. – She's gone forever!
> I know when one is dead, and when one lives;
> She's dead as earth. – Lend me a looking glass;
> If that her breath will mist or stain the stone,
> Why then she lives ...
> This feather stirs; she lives. If it be so,
> It is a chance which does redeem all sorrows
> That ever I have felt ...
> A plague upon you, murderers, traitors all!
> I might have saved her; now she's gone forever!

C.S. Lewis in *A Grief Observed* (1961) described his experiences following the death of his wife. The book begins as follows:

> No one ever told me that grief felt so like fear. I am not afraid, but the sensation is like being afraid. The same fluttering in the stomach, the same restlessness, the yawning. I keep on swallowing. – At other times it feels like being mildly drunk, or concussed. There is a sort of invisible blanket between the world and me. I find it hard to take in what anyone says. Or

perhaps, hard to want to take it in. It is so uninteresting. Yet I want the others to be about me. I dread the moments when the house is empty.

Susan Hill, in her novel *In the Springtime of the Year* (1974) has described vividly the numbness, searching, sorrow and despair, followed by slow recovery, of a young woman whose husband had suddenly died in an accident shortly after they had got married. The following extract describes the breakthrough of grief after a period of numbness and denial. Having stayed with relatives she returns to her empty house carrying a parcel:

She had forgotten what the room looked like. It was very cold. It might have been empty for years past. She walked around it, opened the door of a wardrobe, and then a drawer, a cupboard, looking at what was there, she picked up his hairbrush and touched the bristles to her face. None of it seemed to have anything to do with her now. Then was this all? Was there nothing more to come? Was this deadness to be what she had to live with, the absence of all grief or love or fear? Nothing more?

She took off her coat and laid it on the chair. And then because nothing was going to happen, and there seemed nothing else she had to do, she opened the brown paper parcel. She had not thought. It was so obvious and yet she had not expected it. She took them out, one by one, these clothes in which he had died, the blue shirt and the dark, woollen jersey, the corduroy trousers and thick socks, and lifted each one up, wanting to smell, beneath the wool or cotton, his own smell. She did not, and then realised that the things had been newly washed and ironed.

She put her head down and pressed her face into the pile of garments and at last the grief broke open and drowned her, for they had taken even this away from her, they had washed away his blood and now, she understood fully and finally that Ben was dead and gone from her, that she had nothing, nothing left.

Shock and denial

The initial reaction on receiving the news of the death of someone close, say a spouse, a parent, or a child, especially if it is sudden and unexpected, is one of disbelief: 'No, it can't be true; I can't believe it.' This may be accompanied by emotional numbness and a tendency to keep oneself busy with practical matters, or even to carry on one's day-to-day activities as if nothing had happened. At the same time the shock may cause a number of physical symptoms, like a dry mouth, loss of appetite, a lump in the throat, yawning and taking deep breaths, palpitations, insomnia and muscle pains, accompanied by restlessness, irritability and a vague sense of fear or dread. This may last for only a few hours or several days and will at times be interrupted by moments of realisation with sudden uncontrollable weeping, perhaps calling out for the deceased.

Anger and guilt

Sooner or later most bereaved persons will experience feelings of anger. These may be directed at the deceased: 'How could you do this to me?' Such thoughts are often experienced by a child whose mother or father has died. Alternatively the anger is directed at the doctors who are blamed for the death, or at nature or God. Not infrequently the bereaved turns the anger on himself; thus a man may blame himself for not having looked after his wife well enough or for actually having been responsible for her death by upsetting her or quarrelling with her. This is particularly common if their relationship has been ambivalent and disturbed, in which case severe guilt and self-blame may cause much further distress. An earlier fantasy of having wished someone dead is sometimes thought to be responsible for the death itself, even when this occurs months or years later, and this may lead to persistent self-accusations and guilt. It is here that the border between a normal grief reaction and depression may be difficult to define, especially if suicidal thoughts become prominent or persist.

Searching and pining

Parkes (1986) and Bowlby (1980) have drawn attention to the fact that an important aspect of mourning, which may last a long while, consists of various ways of yearning and searching for or remaining in touch with the deceased. These include constantly thinking of him, calling his name, and having imaginary conversations with him, holding on to his possessions, going into his room and looking at and touching his clothes and, in the case of a child, his toys. Or suddenly seeing him in the street or hearing his voice, e.g. when coming back to an empty home. The latter are referred to as *pseudo-hallucinations* because the bereaved quickly recognises that the person is not really there, with the result that this new realisation only causes further grief and bouts of crying and despair. Frequent visits to the person's grave, or even trying to make contact with him by attending spiritualist séances are other ways of keeping in touch or communicating with the dead. A widow may pray to God to let her die so that she can join her husband; a child may long to join his dead mother.

A related phenomenon is unconscious identification with the dead. This may take the form of behaving like or taking up the interests of the deceased, or developing physical symptoms similar to those of the deceased in his terminal illness. For example, a girl whose mother had died of cancer in a state of emaciation refused to eat because she, too, wanted to lose weight and die. Similar reactions may even occur after the death of a pet.

Dreaming of the deceased as if he were with the dreamer, alive and talking to him, is common and may continue for years. In the dream the person may feel reunited with the dead, only to feel deeply distressed when facing the reality on waking.

Sadness and despair

Sooner or later sadness and despair, often amounting to feeling hopeless and depressed, become the central feature of a grief reaction. This is usually accompanied by bouts of crying and sobbing. In fact not being able to cry, or stopping oneself from crying, may greatly prolong the grief reaction.

At first sadness and crying may only be experienced intermittently, perhaps when defences like denial or searching break down. This may occur during the funeral or at a memorial service or whenever the person is faced with the fact that the deceased will never return. It is often a great relief for the bereaved to find that close friends, or perhaps their doctor, can help them cry openly while quietly staying with them, rather than mistakenly avoid the painful subject, or even turn away because they themselves are too embarrassed.

Later on the all-pervading sense of sadness will become more persistent. This may be accompanied by feeling that life without the deceased is empty and useless, even though outwardly the bereaved person is able to carry on day-to-day tasks at home or at work, more or less normally. He may even give the impression that he has come to terms with the loss while inwardly and in private the pain and sadness remain intense for many months or longer.

This also applies to children who have lost a parent. Outwardly they may seem to have got over the painful loss quite quickly, but inwardly a desperate sense of emptiness and desolation may last for years, perhaps only to be recognised years later by a sensitive observer when as adolescents or adults they ask for help because of some emotional problems, apparently unconnected with the bereavement they experienced in childhood.

Acceptance and recovery

Slowly the acuteness and severity of grieving begins to recede. The fact that the deceased will not return becomes accepted, old interests return and new ones emerge. For example, a widow or widower may ultimately remarry. Or parents who have lost a child, one of the most painful losses of all, may feel ready to conceive again. Even then the memory of the dead child may stay with them for years, and become more vivid at each anniversary of his birth or death, the so-called *anniversary reaction*, common not only following the death of a child but also of an adult. Parents' reactions to the death of a child have been vividly described by Dominica (1987).

Of course, in other circumstances the mourning reaction may be much less turbulent and the death accepted more quickly, for example when a middle-aged person with a family of his own loses an elderly parent who has been disabled and a burden to himself and his relatives for many years.

Abnormal mourning

While the great majority of people pass through the normal processes of grieving, a small proportion develop a psychiatric illness or remain stuck in one of the stages described above. Persistent or prolonged denial of the death can be as abnormal as a prolonged severe grief reaction without any sign of recovery. In very rare cases total denial may lead to the delusional belief that, say, the husband or wife is still alive. A man whose wife had been killed in an accident three years earlier was still getting his wife's clothes ready each morning, cooked meals for both of them and refused to move because 'his wife did not want to leave their flat'.

A *depressive illness* is by far the commonest disorder, usually accompanied by persisting and sometimes delusional feelings of guilt and self-blame. Suicidal thoughts or attempts, the biological symptoms of a depressive illness, and hypochondriacal symptoms, sometimes similar to the complaints of the deceased, are common. In less severe cases it may be difficult to distinguish between a depressive illness and a prolonged, severe grief reaction.

Management

Normal mourning

Even though a proportion of people recently bereaved, women more often than men, may seek help from their general practitioner, normal mourning should not be regarded as an illness. On the contrary, it is a painful but inevitable experience which may even lead to further emotional maturation. If a general practitioner is consulted, therefore, his role will be to provide support by remaining available, willing to listen, to share what the person feels and to explain that what he is going through is not an illness but a normal though painful response to a bereavement from which he will slowly recover. Occasionally a sedative prescribed for a few days only may help him sleep.

Often there will be friends and relatives who can similarly help and support the bereaved. Loneliness and isolation make it much more difficult to work through a grief reaction and increase the risk of a depressive illness or chronic depression. Organisations like Cruse or talks with the general practitioner or a counsellor may help, and religious people often benefit from talking to a sensitive clergyman.

If there is excessive denial and the person has hardly been able to cry it may be valuable to help him express how he feels and to cry by getting him to talk in detail about the events surrounding the death and the funeral, and to recall memories of the deceased.

Counsellors used to working with the bereaved may be able to help people who are lonely and unsupported. For example, counsellors working with the bereaved at St Christopher's Hospice in London have been shown to be of help to bereaved relatives who appeared to be at risk of breakdown (Parkes 1981).

Abnormal mourning reactions

If the bereaved person has developed a depressive illness, a combination of treatment with antidepressants and counselling or psychotherapy is usually the best approach. Admission or day hospital care may have to be considered if there is a serious suicidal risk. In psychotherapy the therapist has to combine a supportive with a careful interpretive role; in the transference he may at times be experienced as filling the gap the deceased has left, while at others he may become the target of the patient's anger and frustration. To remain empathic by 'being with' the patient while he is passing through the various stages of grieving is the therapist's main task.

An abnormally prolonged grief reaction may be treated with psychoanalytic psychotherapy. Hamilton (1987) has described the psychoanalytic treatment of an adult woman who had remained chronically depressed for many years following the loss of her mother in early childhood.

DEATH AND DYING

Some of the psychological aspects of helping the dying patient and his family also require brief mention. Most of these will, of course, be handled by the patient's general practitioner, physician, surgeon or the nursing staff, but increasingly counsellors and liaison psychiatrists also become involved, and important psychological and ethical issues need to be considered (Saunders and Baines 1983; Parkes 1984).

Doctors differ as to whether or not to tell patients that they are suffering from an incurable illness, but there has been a gradual change of attitude from one of secrecy and concealment to one of greater openness. Buckman (1984) has pointed out that doctors tend to avoid breaking bad news to patients more because they are frightened of their own feelings and of not knowing how to handle those of their patients than out of concern for their patients' needs. Patients, on the other hand, differ considerably in what they feel ready to be told. The question has therefore changed from whether or not to tell the patient the truth to finding out what news a particular patient is ready to receive at a particular time during his illness.

In practice far more patients are aware of the fact that they have a fatal illness than their doctors realise. Hinton (1979) interviewed a group of 80 married patients with terminal cancer and found that two-thirds of them knew they were dying and most of them knew they would be dying soon.

Some had kept this entirely to themselves, others had shared their knowledge with their spouses.

Patients who at first deny that their illness might be fatal often change gradually as their condition gets worse and are then relieved to be able to share their anxieties with their doctors. In fact, patients who are left in ignorance until shortly before they die are likely to resent the fact that they were not told sooner. Many patients with incurable illnesses, especially if, as in the case of cancer, they may have quite long periods, say weeks, months or a year or more to live, want to use the time that is left to be close to their family, perhaps to heal misunderstandings and to make up for past estrangements. Or they may wish to finish plans or work not yet completed and to settle their personal affairs in order to do all they can to provide for those they have to leave behind. Others may value the time to resolve spiritual and religious issues, and here the help of a minister or priest may be invaluable.

When talking to a dying patient it is never enough merely to tell him the facts regarding his illness and that the outcome is going to be fatal. It is essential to give him the opportunity to talk about his hopes and fears, about past regrets and the sadness of having to leave behind those he loves and feels responsible for. It is equally important to talk about what life may still hold for him instead of just talking about the approaching end of his life.

There are however some patients who are excessively vulnerable or emotionally unstable and others who suffer from a psychiatric illness or severe anxiety so that they cannot tolerate being confronted with the fact that they are dying, and a few become severely depressed and suicidal when they discover what is wrong with them.

When faced with the task of having to tell a patient who is unaware of having a fatal illness what is the matter with him, it is important to know what kind of reaction to expect. In many ways a person's response to being told that he has a fatal illness resembles the reaction to a bereavement (Parkes 1984; Kübler-Ross 1970). The first reaction is likely to be one of *shock and denial*: 'it can't be true'. This is often followed by the second stage of *anger*, e.g. with the doctor who is telling him, or his general practitioner, physician or surgeon, and sometimes with nature or with God, for 'doing this to him'. This may be followed by the third stage of what Kübler-Ross (1970) has called *bargaining*, when the patient is convinced there must be a cure, perhaps demanding to see a series of new specialists, or looking for a cure through religious or other influences. Sooner or later the fourth stage of *sadness, dejection and despair* sets in, and finally the patient may be able to enter the last stage of *acceptance*. Those who do may accept the reality of death with a sense of calm, even enjoying what life still has to offer them, sometimes with great dignity which impresses their relatives and all those looking after them.

Individual patients differ greatly in their response to being told they are going to die. Some may at once acknowledge the truth and be grateful for being told, and after a period of grieving enter a stage of calm acceptance. In others total denial may make them forget at once what they have been told; this is best taken as an indication that they are not yet ready to face the truth. Some days or weeks later they may ask what is wrong with them and may then accept the truth as if they had never been told before. However, for some patients persistent denial may be the only way of coping. Yet others may become seriously depressed, perhaps after an initial period of anger and bargaining, and become hopeless and possibly suicidal. A few ask for euthanasia and become angry because the doctor cannot provide this.

Management

Dame Cecily Saunders, a pioneer in this field and in the development of the Hospice Movement in Britain, has been responsible for many advances in the care of the dying (Saunders and Baines 1983; Saunders 1984a, 1984b). The brief comments that follow are mainly concerned with the psychological aspects, but the relief of psychological distress cannot be separated from the relief of physical pain or other physical discomfort, so common especially in the final stages in patients dying of cancer. Analgesics should be commenced as soon as the pain becomes a troublesome symptom, mild analgesics in the early stages, building up to stronger analgesics, morphia or diamorphine, when the mild analgesics are no longer effective. It is essential to give analgesics regularly, sufficiently often and in adequate dosage to prevent recurrence of pain; to have to wait until the pain returns only causes further unnecessary distress and anxiety.

The relief of mental pain depends first of all on the provision of an environment in which the patient feels cared for, supported and understood. This may be at home with his family, provided the stress is not too great for those looking after him, in hospital or in a hospice for the dying. Wherever the patient is, it is essential for the professionals involved in his care – doctors, nurses, social workers, ministers, counsellors or others – to be ready to talk to him and members of his family and listen to their fears or hopes, bearing in mind the various issues discussed earlier. What form such talks will take depends on each individual patient. Some clearly prefer to deny what is happening to them while others, probably the majority, prefer to be told the truth and to share their anxieties. Having nobody to talk to, feeling isolated and hopeless, may in some cases even have an adverse effect on the progress of the illness itself. In some women with breast cancer an attitude of denial and a fighting spirit has been found to carry a better prognosis than an attitude of hopelessness and giving up (Greer *et al.* 1979).

Honest answers in reply to a patient's questions combined with reassurance that everything possible will be done to control the disease and to prevent pain and discomfort are essential, along with constant attention to the patient's day-to-day problems and anxieties.

Some mental symptoms require special attention. Persistent restlessness and anxiety may require treatment with one of the benzodiazepines (Diazepam, 2-10 mg) or chlorpromazine (10-25 mg) two or three times a day, or more often if required. Persistent depression, in spite of emotional and spiritual support, may respond to tricyclic antidepressants, say, amitriptyline (75-100 mg at night). An organic confusional state may respond to treatment of its underlying cause if this can be identified. Failing this, haloperidol (5-10 mg), thioridazine (25 mg) or chlorpromazine (25-50 mg) may help to relieve a confusional state.

Lastly, intensive work with dying patients and their families imposes considerable strain on the staff involved, and regular staff discussions and support from a psychiatrist experienced in this field may be invaluable.

FURTHER READING

Buckman, R. (1988). *I Don't Know What to Say: how to help and support someone who is dying*. Macmillan, London.

Kübler-Ross, E. (1970). *On Death and Dying*. Tavistock, London.

Parkes, C.M. (1986). *Bereavement: studies on grief in adult life*, 2nd ed. Penguin, Harmondsworth.

Raphael, B. (1983). *The Anatomy of Bereavement*. Hutchinson, London.

Saunders, C. and Baines, M. (1983). *Living with Dying: the management of terminal disease*. OUP, Oxford.

The following novel is also recommended:

Hill, Susan (1974). *In the Springtime of the Year*. Hamish Hamilton, London.

Part III

Examining the Patient

This part is divided into five chapters covering interviewing, history-taking, mental state examination, formulation and examination in unusual situations or of difficult patients. Each chapter sets out guidelines and general principles which should be interpreted and used with flexibility.

10

Interviewing

An interview with a patient who complains of psychological problems has many similarities to an interview with a general medical patient. In both cases good contact must be made with the patient to allow open discussion of personal or physical problems and their social and historical context. The information obtained is needed to formulate the patient's personal and physical problems and to make a diagnosis.

However, the psychiatric interview differs in important respects. First, it places more emphasis on emotional and social aspects; secondly, it becomes a major investigative and diagnostic tool in itself. The interviewing skills of the psychiatrist are therefore of primary importance. The psychiatrist can rarely rely on a physical examination and laboratory investigations to aid and verify a diagnosis. However, these may be essential, e.g. in patients complaining of physical symptoms, and can be of the utmost importance if there is any suggestion of an organic psychiatric illness.

Any psychiatric interview should be arranged so that adequate time is available for the patient to talk freely and confidentially. How this is best achieved must be left to the doctor and will depend on the circumstances under which the interview is being conducted; genuine interest, sympathetic listening and an unhurried manner are the hallmarks of good interviewing.

The following guidelines assume optimum conditions for assessment, such as the outpatient department. Assessment under different circumstances is described in Chapter 14.

AIMS AND TECHNIQUES

There are four main aims of a psychiatric interview:

(1) to collect information
(2) to assess the patient's personality and mental state
(3) to make a diagnosis
(4) to give support and establish a basis for treatment.

These are carried out simultaneously but will be considered separately here.

107

Collecting information

An accurate picture of a patient's problems must be obtained and placed in the context of his *present circumstances*, e.g. work, marriage, finances etc., and of his *past*, e.g. his family background and personal history. A detailed history has to be taken in order to achieve this. It is important to remember that the order of recording historical information in the medical notes (see p. 111), and the format of case presentation to colleagues, tend to follow a traditional pattern, but this should be distinguished from the manner in which the information is obtained from the patient. An interview which follows a fixed pattern is likely to alienate the patient. In general the patient should be allowed to lead the interview, although the doctor must retain control and clarify certain points or ask directly about experiences the patient may be avoiding or believe to be unimportant.

It is often useful at the outset of an interview to explain its purpose to the patient. For example the doctor may say: 'I would like to get a picture of your present difficulties and then try to understand how they have come about. Perhaps you could tell me what you feel your problems have been over the last few months?'

Some guiding questions will then be required, although it is a mistake to press someone too soon about sensitive matters such as sexuality, marital difficulties or paranoid beliefs. The flow of the interview should be governed by the patient, but the doctor should be alert for opportunities to ask important questions. For example a patient may mention family matters and the doctor could then say: 'Perhaps you could tell me a little more about your family' or 'I notice you have not mentioned your mother. Could you tell me more about her?' Further basic family details can thus be collected in a natural and relevant manner.

On other occasions it may be necessary to ask directly about the patient's family and background history. This is especially true in patients who are discursive, verbose and garrulous. The doctor may need to interrupt the flow of the interview under these circumstances and firmly, but tactfully, explain its purpose again.

Assessment of personality and mental state

This is the most difficult aspect of the interview. The doctor must try to assess objectively what sort of person the patient is and his present emotional state. In order to answer these questions the doctor must pay careful attention to the details of the interview. The way the patient responds to questions, his reactions to the environment, e.g. suspiciousness, the tone of his voice or facial expressions, may all provide useful clues. For example, an observation that certain questions result in a quavering voice, blushing and agitation may be gently pointed out to the patient in order to explore the area further.

Clues to a patient's general attitude may also be found in the detail of the interview. For example, some patients may attempt to answer questions with the utmost precision and become irritated when deflected from their attempts. This may suggest an obsessional personality, and further questions may clarify the picture.

An interviewer must also be able to assess his own responses to the patient. These may provide the key to the patient's problem. For example, a patient who is not overtly aggressive may make the interviewer feel frightened, and this may be the only clue to the patient's dangerousness or his inner fear of becoming violent; another patient may smile and talk easily but engender a feeling of depression in the doctor. This may be the key to the patient's underlying depression.

It is this attention to the detail of the interaction between the doctor and patient that allows a precise assessment of the patient's personality and mental state to be made.

Diagnosis

Although it may be possible to provide a label of a diagnostic syndrome, especially in organically-based illness such as senile or presenile dementia, in many cases the doctor must try to understand the patient's illness in terms of the interplay between personality and environmental factors. A diagnosis may be helpful as a label to communicate with other doctors, but it is never enough by itself to explain the patient's difficulties. For example, a diagnosis of 'depressive illness' may be appropriate, but it must then be understood in terms of the individual patient. In this context it is useful to remember the three 'P's – *predisposing factors, precipitating factors* and *perpetuating (or maintaining) factors*. In the case of a patient who is depressed, predisposing factors may include a genetic vulnerability, a previous history of depression or separation-traumata in childhood. A life event (see p. 39), such as a bereavement, may then precipitate the depression which in turn may be perpetuated, for example, by chronic marital difficulties. Careful delineation of all these factors will act as a guide to treatment. It may of course be impossible, and sometimes unwise, to search for all three factors at the first interview.

Support

The initial interview gives the doctor an opportunity to offer support and reassurance. This requires patient listening. A release of emotional tension may in itself be helpful. Appropriate reaction by the doctor, e.g. reassurance in anxiety, hope in depression, tolerance of guilt and anger, may increase the patient's confidence and provide a basis for future treatment. Furthermore, the patient may be helped to realise that his difficulties can be resolved. This is often best achieved by the interviewer showing that he has understood the situation from the patient's own viewpoint, and an explanation of the patient's difficulties may dispel tension and allow further discussion.

If this supportive work appears helpful to the patient and he is not too seriously disturbed, the doctor may not have to take any further action other than to offer the patient another appointment to see how he is then. Further steps will then be needed if he is not better. Clearly there will be some first interviews where a patient requires urgent action, e.g. if he is acutely disturbed or seriously threatening suicide. The assessment and treatment of the suicidal patient is discussed elsewhere (see p. 632).

FURTHER READING

Departments of Psychiatry and Child Psychiatry. The Institute of Psychiatry and Maudsley Hospital, London (1987). *Psychiatric Examination: notes on eliciting and recording clinical information in psychiatric patients*, 2nd ed. OUP, Oxford.

11

History Taking

The initial history should be elicited from the patient, if possible. Even if this appears adequate, other *informants* such as relatives or friends should also be interviewed. It is best to ask the patient's permission to do this and often advisable to interview the informants in the presence of the patient. This is especially true with suspicious or paranoid patients whose fears will be increased by the doctor talking about them behind closed doors. Occasionally it may be necessary to have a discussion with informants without the patient being present. This should be arranged with care and sensitivity in order not to destroy the relationship that was built up between the doctor and patient during the first interview.

Interviewing informants should be not only a fact-finding exercise but also a way of understanding how a patient interacts with others. Help in the task of history taking and the assessment of the patient may be given by the psychiatric social worker, who can see the relatives while the doctor sees the patient. Often very different views may be found and the doctor and the social worker should meet to discuss their findings before seeing the patient and relatives together. In this way a comprehensive picture of the patient, his circumstances and his relationship to others can be made. More than one interview may be necessary to obtain a full case history.

However the interview is set up, the following areas should be covered and the details recorded in the notes in the order listed in Table 11.1 (p. 112).

METHOD OF REFERRAL

A brief statement should be made as to why and by whom the patient was referred. For example, 'This patient was referred to the hospital by her general practitioner for further assessment of her depression. This followed a home visit by the GP and social worker.'

PRESENTING COMPLAINTS

These should be listed with the duration of each symptom and recorded in the patient's own words. All the patient's complaints should be recorded even if they appear minimal. For example, the patient complains of

(1) Feeling awful for the last month.
(2) Receiving messages about her husband from the post office tower for the last two weeks.
(3) Worry about her cat who fell ill two days ago.

PRESENT ILLNESS

A detailed chronological account of the illness beginning with the first change noted by the patient should be recorded here. The nature, extent, duration and effect on the patient of each symptom should be noted along with its relationship to environmental circumstances and the patient's life situation. If we take our former example – the patient complaining of receiving messages – the entry may be as follows:

> The patient felt quite well until six weeks ago when her husband was sent abroad on business. Two days later she noticed difficulty in getting off to sleep. She then began to feel awful – by which she means tired, lethargic, listless and physically weak – and nervous about going out. This did not improve and two weeks after its onset she began to suspect somebody was poisoning her and her cat. She continued work despite these symptoms. However, two weeks ago she stopped work as she received messages in her mind warning about imminent danger to herself, her husband and her cat. She believes these messages are beamed to her from the post office tower. She is unable to locate the person behind this plot, but when her cat fell ill she was convinced all her food and water were

Table 11.1. History taking: a summary

(1) Personal details: age, sex, occupation, marital status, accommodation, general practitioner.
(2) Method of referral
(3) Presenting complaints
(4) Present illness
(5) Family history
(6) Personal history: early development
                     childhood
                     schooling
                     adolescence
                     occupation
                     psychosexual history
                     marital history
                     children
                     past medical history
                     past psychiatric history
                     drug and alcohol history
                     forensic history
(7) Pre-morbid personality

poisoned. She has not eaten for the last two days. Her husband has been informed of her hospital admission and he is returning from abroad.

It is important also to record any associated changes here such as impairment of mental, occupational, social and sexual activities. Biological changes such as appetite loss, weight change or sleep disturbance should also be recorded along with any change in cigarette and alcohol consumption.

FAMILY HISTORY

In the case of adoption or fostering, details should be taken of both the real family, if possible, and the adoptive or foster family.

Mother

Her health, age, or if no longer alive, her age and the patient's age when she died and the cause of death; her occupation; her personality; past and present relationship and feelings towards her. Any mental and physical illnesses should also be noted and the patient's reaction to them, and to the mother's death, if no longer alive.

Father

As for mother.

Siblings

Listed in order of age with first names, occupation, marital status and mental and physical health. The patient's past reactions to birth of siblings and any miscarriages or stillbirths should be noted and the patient's past and current relationship with each sibling recorded.

Home atmosphere

Describe the social and economic position of the family and the emotional atmosphere in the home during the patient's childhood and adolescence. This should include details of the family relationships, e.g. who was closest to whom and how the patient and the family reacted to such problems as separations, divorce, death, unemployment etc. Note any history of violence or crime in the family.

Illness in family members

Give details of mental illnesses, alcoholism, epilepsy or known hereditary conditions in any of the relatives (including first- and second-degree relatives).

PERSONAL HISTORY

This should take the form of a biographical account.

Birth and early development

Mother's condition during pregnancy: normal or abnormal birth; feeding difficulties; milestones of development; habit training difficulties. Note that this information may only be available from an informant.

Behaviour during childhood

Play and favourite toys; any periods of separation from parents and the patient's reaction to them; temper tantrums; hyperactivity; frequent fights; violence; model child. Bed-wetting or soiling; eating problems; stammering; recurrent physical complaints, e.g. abdominal pain.

Schooling

Age of starting and finishing school; type of school; academic achievements; special abilities or disabilities; relationship to peers and teachers; school refusal; school truancy; ambitions. Obtain information for both primary and secondary schooling.

Adolescence

Attitudes to parents, authority figures and peers; reaction to growing up, puberty and bodily changes; fantasy life; attitude to sexuality including masturbation and any early homosexual and heterosexual experiences; drug taking; rebelliousness and delinquency. New interests.

Occupation

Age of starting work; jobs held in chronological order and reasons for change; satisfaction from work; work ability and ambitions; relationship to work mates, superiors and subordinates. Service in armed forces and rank achieved. Leisure activities.

Psychosexual history (see also adolescence)

Introduction to facts of life; early sexual experiences; parental attitude towards sex; sexual abuse in childhood. In girls – age at first menstrual period and reaction to it; any menstrual problems. Masturbation and sexual fantasies; homosexual and heterosexual experiences apart from marriage; emotional relationship to partners; sexual difficulties; sexual deviation; current sexual activities.

Marital history

Previous engagements and marriages; present marriage; reasons for marriage; husband's or wife's age, occupation, health and personality; marital relationship – satisfactions, dissatisfactions, any sexual difficulties; extra-marital relationships and sexual fantasy life.

Children

Chronological list of children with ages, first names and health. Miscarriages, still births or death of a child. Patient's reactions to these events and attitude to existing children.

Past medical history

Illnesses, operations and accidents in chronological order; treatment received – when and by whom. The patient's reactions to them.

Past psychiatric history

List any trea ted psychiatric conditions in chronological order with details of treatment – when and by whom. Obtain details of untreated psychiatric symptoms, e.g. behavioural problems, minor emotional reactions, anxiety or depressive symptoms and any obvious precipitants.

Alcohol and drug history

Details of smoking and drinking habits; any recent change or adverse effect on physical health or social activity, e.g. occupation, family relationships and financial situation. Use of other drugs, e.g. heroin, LSD, cocaine, amphetamines, barbiturates, cannabis, tranquillisers. How are they obtained – prescription, black market. How are they financed – crime, prostitution etc.

Forensic history

List any criminal offences in chronological order even if not convicted. Give details of borstal, probation, prison sentences. Note any violence.

PRE-MORBID PERSONALITY

The interviewer must obtain an overall picture of the patient's attitudes and patterns of behaviour in order to provide a reasonable assessment of his personality. Helpful information will already have been elicited while collecting the rest of the history, and pointers to the patient's predominant attitudes can be discerned by attending to the doctor-patient interaction. However, personality change may be part of a psychiatric illness and it is the patient's pre-morbid personality that is important here; any conclusions drawn from the interview should be checked with other informants. At the end of an interview a brief paragraph should be recorded in the notes about the patient's pre-morbid personality, giving the evidence for the conclusions. To take our example of the patient receiving messages again, the entry might read as follows:

This lady appears to have been a friendly but timid person who has been able to form long-lasting relationships – she works as a secretary in a social club and has mantained contact with friends from school. There is evidence of oversensitivity, self-consciousness and withdrawal in the past. For example she describes long-term worries over her physical appearance and has occasionally had to withdraw from company because of feelings of panic. Her religious beliefs have helped her with this and she is a regular attender at church. She has few interests of her own and her activities centre around her husband. She has no ambition and in this respect, may be considered self-effacing in view of her obvious intelligence and capabilities.

Her sensitivity and shyness was obvious during the interview and she continually apologised for being a nuisance.

It is helpful to consider the following areas when assessing personality, but they should be used as a guide to interviewing rather than as a check-list. It is important to remember that they apply to long-term functioning.

(1) Social and intellectual activities.
(2) General outlook: cheerful, despondent, anxious, irritable, tense, optimistic, pessimistic, over-confident, contemptuous, over-sensitive.
(3) Attitudes to others: timid, reserved, shy, sensitive, withdrawn, suspicious, resentful, quarrelsome, selfish, friendly, warm, demonstrative.
(4) Attitude to self: egocentric, self-indulgent, self-satisfied, vain, self-deprecating, self-effacing.
(5) Religious beliefs and moral standards.
(6) Leisure activities: hobbies, group or individual activities, creativity, sport.
(7) Habits: eating (fads), orderliness
(8) Dreams, day-dreams and fantasies. These may provide useful information about the patient's inner conflicts, fears and wishes, both past and present.

FURTHER READING

Departments of Psychiatry and Child Psychiatry. The Institute of Psychiatry and Maudsley Hospital, London (1987). *Psychiatric Examination: notes on eliciting and recording clinical information in psychiatric patients*, 2nd ed. OUP, Oxford.

Leff, J.P. and Isaacs, A.D. (1981). *Psychiatric Examination in Clinical Practice*, 2nd ed. Blackwell, Oxford.

12

The Mental State

The mental state is an objective and concise account of the patient's behaviour and psychological state, as observed and elicited during an interview. It is best described under the following headings:

(1) Appearance and general behaviour.
(2) Speech or writing.
(3) Mood and affect.
(4) Thought.
(5) Perceptual abnormalities.
(6) The cognitive state.
(7) Insight.
(8) The interviewer's reaction to the patient.

In recording the mental state the doctor must quote the patient's own words as far as possible, and include his own interpretation or opinion of the elicited data, for example whether an idea the patient holds is delusional or not. Any abnormalities should be recorded verbatim during the interview. After the interview the information should be organised under the appropriate headings.

The following is the method applied in clinical practice. A standardised structured method of examining the patient's mental state, the Present State Examination (PSE) (Wing *et al.* 1974) is available but mainly used for research purposes.

APPEARANCE AND GENERAL BEHAVIOUR

Describe how the patient is dressed and whether he appears tidy, clean, shabby, dishevelled or inappropriately dressed. Manic patients often wear bizarre combinations of dress together with clashing colours. Depressed people may pay little attention to what they wear or dress in dark, sombre colours. Note the posture, is it fixed and maintained or does the person move freely and in a relaxed fashion? Is he tense and agitated, or calm and responsive? Do movements have any apparent purpose or meaning? Is he unduly slow, hesitant or repetitive? Note whether his overall behaviour seems consistent with what he is talking about, and whether it is appropriate. Note how much eye contact he makes. Shy, nervous people may avoid eye contact, while some psychotic patients may maintain a fixed stare. Any facial grimaces or unusual body movements should be recorded here. Sometimes behaviour may suggest the patient is having psychotic experiences, e.g. someone hearing auditory hallucinations may turn his head, appear to be listening and blink rapidly.

SPEECH OR WRITING

The *form* of the patient's speech is recorded here – how he says things rather than what he says. If the patient is mute the information will have to be obtained from his writing. Abnormalities in the content of speech, e.g. delusions and obsessions, are traditionally recorded under 'thought content' (see p. 122). Neurological abnormalities of speech or writing such as dysarthria, dysphasia and agraphia are not discussed here. Full descriptions can be found in *Organic Psychiatry* (Lishman 1987).

The *form of speech* can be divided into:

(1) *Spontaneity*: does the patient instigate speech, or only give answers to questions?

(2) *Rate*: is there *pressure of speech* as in mania, where one thought follows rapidly onto the next and the patient is practically uninterruptable; or does the patient talk slowly and laboriously with long pauses in between sentences – *retardation of speech*, as in depression?

(3) *Quantity*: does the patient choose words which are to the point, or is he monosyllabic, or does he become garrulous and expansive in his description of events and people?

(4) *Volume*: does the volume of speech alter, for example does the patient's voice tail off into a whisper, or get louder when speaking about certain topics?

(5) *Tone*: is it lively and animated, or monotonous as for example in depression?

A verbatim account of what the patient says should be recorded if the speech is abnormal or inappropriate in any way.

MOOD AND AFFECT

Mood is a sustained emotional state and refers to the patient's inner, subjective experience. It can only be determined by asking the patient how he feels within himself, e.g. 'Perhaps you can tell me how you feel in your spirits'.

Affect is a more short-lived emotional state which can be observed by another person. Affect is usually in keeping with mood – someone who is smiling usually feels happy. However, in some patients this is not the case. A patient who feels depressed may cover this up by smiling. The affect is then different from the mood he is experiencing. Sometimes the affect may not be in keeping with the patient's current thoughts; for example, he may smile and look happy when talking about the death of a close friend. This is termed *incongruity of affect*.

There are many different terms to describe the quality of the patient's emotional state, and it is important to find the correct descriptive term: is he sad, happy, cheerful, anxious, irritable, suspicious, frightened, flat, perplexed? Note whether the affect is fixed or varies during the interview. If it varies, does this appear to be in response to what is being discussed? Is it appropriate or does it change rapidly for no apparent reason? Such sudden changes are termed *lability of affect* and can occur, for example, in hypomanic patients or dementia.

THOUGHT

Disorders of thought will be considered under the headings of abnormalities in the form, stream, possession and content. These abnormalities can of course only be inferred from the patient's speech or writing.

Form of thought

Disorders in the form of thought manifest themselves as changes in the structure, grammar and meaning of the patient's utterances. For example, the grammatical structure may have broken down completely so that the patient appears to be talking nonsense, e.g. 'Have a train pages, cat turn over'. This is known as *word salad*. In a less severe form the patient may coin new words, or *neologisms*, which may mean something to him but not to anybody else.

In contrast, the grammar of the patient's language may be intact, while his thoughts appear completely unconnected. This is known as *asyndetic thinking*. In a less severe form the patient's thoughts seem to link together but are directed by chance word associations, e.g. 'I had a light sleep last night because the light was on, but I made light of it – like when I light the fire at home for mother and she says I'm fit to burn.' This is called *tangential thinking* and, if accompanied by pressure of speech, *flight of ideas*. The latter is common in mania.

Sometimes the patient says something which sounds like something he or the interviewer has just said. These rhyming or punning associations are called *clang associations*; for example, when asked what time it was the interviewer said 'A quarter to two', to which the patient replied 'Buckle my shoe!' Clang associations sometimes accompany a state of excitement or heightened arousal.

Stream of thought

This refers to the rate at which thoughts come into the patient's mind. When thoughts are speeded up and come rushing into his mind, e.g. in mania, this is called *pressure of thought* and is manifest as *pressure of speech*. Conversely, when the patient has few thoughts, or thoughts come only slowly and laboriously to mind, this is called *thought retardation* and can occur in depressive illness. Many depressive patients, when asked if their thoughts have changed at all, will report that their thoughts have slowed down, or even stopped.

In *thought block* thoughts just come to a halt, often in mid-sentence, the patient feels his mind is empty, and after a pause will start talking about some unrelated topic. When this occurs the interviewer should always ask what has happened to the patient's thoughts, because it may be that the patient is responding to instructions from auditory hallucinations, rather than thought blocking. Thought blocking must be distinguished from the not uncommon experience of normal people when one train of thought is suddenly interrupted by another.

Possession of thought

Disorders of possession of thought can be divided into thought insertion, thought withdrawal, and thought broadcasting. They are characteristic of schizophrenia and usually cause the patient considerable distress.

Thought insertion

When asked whether he believes his thoughts are interfered with, the patient may report that his thoughts are no longer his own. He experiences them as being put into his mind by some external agency. This is out of his control. The thoughts are received as totally alien, quite unlike anything he himself would think, and he knows that they do not belong to him.

Thought withdrawal

The patient reports that thoughts are taken out of his mind at the moment they come into consciousness.

Thought broadcasting

The patient believes other people have access to his thoughts and therefore know what he is thinking. This is not the same as telepathy, in which thoughts are 'beamed' to another person through a wilful act of volition. In thought broadcasting it is as if thoughts are leaking out of the patient's mind so that other people, even at a distance, can somehow pick them up and know what he is thinking. The patient is totally convinced that this is what is happening and *knows* that his thoughts are no longer private to himself.

Content of thought

Abnormal thoughts include delusions, obsessions, ruminations and preoccupations.

Delusions

A delusion is a fixed, false belief which is out of keeping with the person's religious and cultural background and which is maintained even in the face of all evidence to the contrary. Religious beliefs can sometimes be mistaken for delusions; for example, a person from a different culture may hold beliefs that are perfectly acceptable within that culture, but which someone from another culture or religious background, e.g. his doctor, may mistakenly consider to be delusions (see also p. 42).

Delusions can be primary or secondary. A *primary*, or *autochthonous delusion* appears suddenly with full conviction and without any preceding events. For example, a civil servant travelling to work in the train one morning suddenly realised 'out of the blue' that a man sitting opposite him was a KGB agent assigned to follow him.

A *secondary delusion* is secondary to some other mental abnormality, such as an auditory hallucination. For example, a man was convinced that freemasons were plotting against his life because he had heard voices telling him so. Delusions can also be secondary to an abnormal mood, such as depression. For example, a man with a severe depressive illness believed his family thought him worthless and wished him dead.

There are many different types of delusions. The commonest are *paranoid delusions* in which the patient falsely believes that other people or groups of people behave in a threatening, hostile or persecuting way towards him.

Grandiose delusions may be delusions of ability or of identity. In the former the patient believes he is more powerful, influential or wealthier than is the case; in the latter that he is God, Christ, the Queen, etc. Grandiose delusions can occur in mania, schizophrenia and also in organic psychiatric disorders such as general paresis due to neuro-syphilis.

Hypochondriacal delusions can occur in schizophrenia and in depressive illness. The patient believes parts of his body are affected by illness, e.g. that his brain is rotting, his liver is riddled with worms and he has cancer from one end of his gut to the other.

Depressive delusions are delusions of guilt, worthlessness, self-blame and self-depreciation. For example, the patient believes that the world would be a better place if he were dead, having brought such misery and despair to so many people.

In *nihilistic delusions* the patient believes he is already dead, or that a part of him no longer exists, e.g. 'I have no brain – my skull is an empty vault.'

In delusions of reference events, objects or people in the patient's environment take on a very special, personal meaning for him. For example, he knows that something that is being said on the radio or television refers specifically to him.

Delusions of reference must be distinguished from *ideas of reference*, which occur in people who are abnormally sensitive and self-conscious. The person has a vague feeling that people may be looking at him or talking about him, but he realises that he is imagining it.

Another belief that must be distinguished from a delusion is an *overvalued idea*. This is a firmly held mistaken idea which is not, however, as unshakeable as a delusion, e.g. the idea of an emaciated anorexic patient that she is overweight.

Delusional perception is a special form of delusional belief. It arises for the very first time out of a normal perception, e.g. when a traffic light changed from red to green, a normal perception, a man on his way to work suddenly 'knew' this meant that his colleagues at work were all against him and were trying to make him lose his job, a delusional belief. Delusional perception strongly suggests a diagnosis of schizophrenia. The difference between delusions of reference and delusional perception is that delusions of reference arise in patients who already hold abnormal beliefs, whereas in delusional perception the delusion originates for the first time from a normal perception.

A special type of delusional belief which occurs in schizophrenia is called *delusion of passivity* or *delusion of control*. The patient believes that either the whole of his body or a part of it is not under his own control. He feels like a puppet or a robot, whose actions are controlled by an external force. Delusions of control can also affect thought processes, the patient believing that he is being made to follow certain lines of thought by some external agency.

Obsessions

Obsessional thoughts are persistently recurring thoughts, images or impulses which enter the patient's mind against his will. They are often sexual, aggressive or blasphemous in nature and are experienced as alien and unacceptable although the patient knows that they are products of his own mind. He attempts to resist having the thoughts but is unable to do so. Obsessional thoughts occur in obsessive-compulsive neurosis. They are often associated with *compulsive actions* such as compulsive handwashing, or having to check again and again whether light switches or gas taps have been turned off.

Ruminations and preoccupations

Obsessional thoughts must be distinguished from ruminations and preoccupations. *Ruminations* (literally, chewing the cud), are sequences of thoughts that occur again and again and are concerned with a particular topic or action; they often take the form of thoughts for or against a possible action like an internal debate. There is no attempt to resist them and they are not compulsive. Suicidal ruminations are an example and occur in depression. *Preoccupations* consist of being preoccupied with certain ideas or themes. For example, a housewife may become preoccupied with worries about how she will pay her bills, and at interview, although she may be distracted, her thoughts will keep returning to this topic.

PERCEPTUAL ABNORMALITIES

These are of three types:

(1) hallucinations
(2) illusions
(3) depersonalisation and derealisation

Hallucinations

Hallucinations are perceptions in any of the sensory modalities which are experienced as if they were coming from outside but occur in the absence of any corresponding external stimulus. For example, an auditory hallucination is experienced as coming from outside the patient's head, when in reality there is no one speaking to him; visual hallucinations are seen not in the imagination with eyes closed, but through open eyes in external space in the absence of any external stimulus. The patient is unable to distinguish the hallucination from reality.

Usually hallucinations occur in only one of the senses, e.g. the patient hears a voice talking to him and may even recognise to whom it belongs, but he does not see the person.

All hallucinations are sensory experiences and therefore relate to seeing, hearing, smelling, touching and tasting. They must be distinguished from delusions, which are not false perceptions but false beliefs. Thus a patient who hears a voice giving a commentary on his thoughts is not deluded. If, however, the voice keeps telling him that he is Alexander the Great, and he comes to believe this, then he has developed a secondary grandiose delusion.

It is important to distinguish hallucinations from pseudo-hallucinations. *Pseudo-hallucinations* are abnormal perceptual experiences, but they are accompanied by at least partial insight. It is as if the person knows at the time, or immediately after the experience, that it is not real. These are commonly experienced after a bereavement; a widow who has recently lost her husband may hear a door slam and her husband call 'I'm home.' However, this is a brief fleeting experience and she quickly realises that she has only imagined it.

Hypnagogic and *hypnopompic hallucinations* occur when consciousness is impaired while someone is either just falling asleep or just waking up, respectively; for example, a person may see someone sitting on his bed while he is dropping off to sleep, but he quickly wakes up and finds no one there.

Illusions

Illusions are misperceptions of a real external stimulus, e.g. the wind rustles the leaves on the trees and the patient says 'I can hear a voice talking to me', or a shadow on the wall is misperceived as a giant spider. They are distortions of a real perception.

Depersonalisation and derealisation

The term *depersonalisation* describes an experience during which the person feels himself to be unreal, not his normal self or detached from and somehow outside himself. In *derealisation* he feels that objects and people around him are unreal, e.g. buildings have a two-dimensional quality, as if part of a stage set, and people seem unreal and lifeless. These experiences are very distressing. The person has insight in as much as he recognises that these experiences are abnormal, which helps to distinguish them from delusional beliefs.

THE COGNITIVE STATE

Assessing the cognitive state includes an appraisal of the patient's orientation, memory, concentration, attention and constructional and visuospatial abilities. It also includes an assessment of intelligence, which needs to be taken into account when making an overall evaluation of the cognitive state. Cognitive abnormalities are common in organic psychiatric disorders with or without disturbance of consciousness. The patient's ability to cooperate and any impairment of consciousness, however slight, must be taken into consideration when carrying out any of the following tests.

Orientation

There may be abnormalities of orientation for time, place or person, usually in that order as the disturbance increases in severity. Does the patient know the date, the time of day, the day in the week, the season of the year? Does he know where he is? Does he know who you are, and what sort of function you have? Does he know who he is?

Memory

The history may suggest that the patient has memory difficulties, e.g. in dementia. It is clinically useful to divide memory into immediate, recent and remote.

Immediate memory can be assessed by asking the patient to repeat a name or a series of digits, such as a telephone number, immediately after being told it.

The patient's ability to retain newly learned information – his *recent* or *short-term memory* – can be assessed by giving him a name and address or a telephone number and asking him to repeat it to ensure that it has been correctly received. The interview is then continued for a further five minutes before asking the patient to recall the name and address or number. Recent memory can also be assessed by asking for news items or events in the patient's life over the past few days.

Remote or *long-term memory* can be assessed by asking the patient to describe earlier events from his personal life, say in childhood or early adult life, or recall the names of well-known public figures such as earlier prime ministers, or important public events that took place a long time ago.

More detailed psychometric testing makes use of standardised tests which provide quantitative data of memory and learning; these may help in diagnosis and allow an assessment of change over time (see p. 677).

Concentration and attention

The patient's ability or lack of ability to give a coherent, lucid and continuous account of himself will usually indicate whether there are any problems with concentration and attention. The patient should be able to respond appropriately to the interviewer's questions and keep to the topic under discussion. A simple test is to ask the patient to continue to subtract 7 starting from 100. With a patient of low intelligence it may be more appropriate to ask for the months of the year or days of the week forwards and backwards. A further test is to ask the patient to repeat a few digits both forwards and backwards, the *digit span test*. The digits should be presented at a rate of about one per second in an even tone of voice. People of average intelligence should normally be able to repeat 5 to 7 digits.

Intelligence

An evaluation can usually be based on the account given by the patient of his education, interests and achievements. However, it is important to note any discrepancies between the history and what is elicited during the interview. For example, a middle-aged publican, used to handling money and giving change, may demonstrate great difficulty with simple tests of numeracy. This indicates deterioration in his intelligence. For standardised tests of intelligence see p. 676.

Constructional and visuospatial skills

These two skills are often closely associated and may be difficult to separate. Although patients may make no complaints of difficulties in constructional and visuospatial abilities, simple tests may indicate abnormalities, especially in patients with organic psychiatric disorders.

Initially the patient may be asked to draw a straight line connecting two dots given to him by the interviewer; next he may be asked to indicate the centre of a straight line or a circle. The tests may then be made increasingly more difficult by asking him first to copy and then to draw from imagination such figures as a square, a circle, a triangle, a cube or a clock-face with figures and dials. Some patients, for example those with parietal lobe lesions, may crowd all the figures into one half of the clock-face only.

If the patient is successful in these tests, he may be asked to draw from imagination a simple picture of, for example, a house, a bicycle or a human figure.

Visuospatial ability can be tested by asking the patient to look around the room and describe the relative positions of the objects in it. He may then be asked to identify some of them and describe what they are used for. Such tests may indicate visual agnosia. Impairment of visual memory can be tested by asking the patient to close his eyes after he has looked around the room and then describe what he has seen from memory.

INSIGHT

There are three different forms of insight to assess. First, the patient may lack insight into the fact that he is ill, e.g. in hypomania and other psychotic disorders. Secondly, he may lack insight into the difference between his fantasy life and reality; by definition this is the case in delusions and hallucinations, and to varying degrees in psychotic illnesses in general. The third variety of insight is concerned with the patient's ability, or lack of it, to consider possible psychological aspects or causes of his illness. This is absent in the psychoses but may be present to some degree in the neuroses.

THE INTERVIEWER'S REACTION

The interviewer should record his own emotional responses to the patient here. Did the patient make him feel sad, sympathetic or irritated, curious or bored? Sometimes patients will evoke strong emotional responses in the interviewer, who may react to this inappropriately, e.g. by cutting short the interview or by getting angry. The interviewer must instead ask himself 'What is the patient making me feel?' and 'Why am I feeling like this about this particular person?' His feelings may turn out to be a reflection of or a reaction to the patient's feelings. For example, a doctor who was made to feel sad and hopeless by a patient commented that he wondered whether the patient felt sad or hopeless. Only then was the patient able to speak about serious problems in his marriage which had made him feel depressed for several months. It is of course important for the doctor to try to decide whether what he is feeling could be due to problems of his own or whether it is really a response to the patient.

FURTHER READING

Departments of Psychiatry and Child Psychiatry. The Institute of Psychiatry and Maudsley Hospital (1987). *Psychiatric Examination: notes on eliciting and recording clinical information in psychiatric patients*, 2nd ed. OUP, Oxford.

Hamilton, M. (ed.) (1985). *Fish's Clinical Psychopathology: signs and symptoms in psychiatry*, 2nd ed. Blackwell, Oxford.

Leff, J.P. and Isaacs, A.D. (1981). *Psychiatric Examination in Clinical Practice*, 2nd ed. Blackwell, Oxford.

13

Formulation

After recording the patient's history and mental state examination, the relevant findings and conclusions should be summarised in condensed form in what is called a formulation. This includes a brief summary of the illness and a discussion of the differential diagnosis and aetiological factors. These should be discussed in terms of the patient's personality development, social situation, reaction to life events and any significant biological factors. This should be followed by a treatment plan and an assessment of the prognosis.

The purpose of the formulation is to convey the relevant findings and the psychiatrist's opinion to all those concerned with looking after the patient, especially his general practitioner. Its length and content will vary according to the setting in which the patient was assessed. For example, it will be fuller at the end of a period of inpatient treatment than after an initial outpatient consultation, and even less complete, with much information still to be obtained, after a brief assessment in the casualty department (see p. 135). Its form and content will also vary according to whether the patient has been examined on his own, whether additional information has already been obtained from a relative or other informant, and whether the patient was assessed in a joint setting with members of his family, e.g. during crisis intervention at a domiciliary visit.

In general, the following main headings serve as a practical guide:

(1) Personal details
(2) Presenting complaints
(3) Mental state
(4) Abnormal physical findings
(5) Differential diagnosis
(6) Further information and investigations
(7) Aetiology
(8) Treatment
(9) Prognosis

In this chapter the case of 'John Smith' is used throughout as an example.

PERSONAL DETAILS

These should include the patient's name, age, marital status, present domestic circumstances, occupation, and at whose request and where he was assessed. If the patient is an inpatient, state whether he is a voluntary or compulsory patient. For example:

John Smith is a single man aged twenty who lives with his parents and works in an ice-cream parlour. He was seen in the outpatient psychiatric department, at the urgent request of his GP.

PRESENTING COMPLAINTS

Here the main complaints and the onset and course of the present illness should be described briefly, using the patient's own words where possible. The way in which the symptoms affect the patient and his family should be included:

Over the last three weeks, John Smith has felt 'strange' and 'suspicious, as if there's something going on'. This began shortly after his relationship with his girlfriend had come to an end after he had been seeing her for two years. He has been feeling tense and anxious, and is afraid to go out on his own; frequently he is unable to sleep until the early hours of the morning. For the past week he has been unable to go to work. He denied having taken any drugs. His parents have become concerned about him and took him to see their GP.

MENTAL STATE

Any *abnormal* findings should be described here, again using the patient's own words where appropriate. It is important also to mention any relevant negative findings.

The patient was noted to be tense, restless and suspicious. His speech was hesitant but coherent. He looked anxious and asked for reassurance that people at work would not know he had been to a psychiatric department. He denied feeling depressed. He believed he was being followed in the street, but he was not sure by whom. These beliefs were held with delusional intensity. He denied any perceptual abnormalities. Cognitive testing was difficult because he was easily distracted and could not concentrate. He did not think he was ill, but thought he was being victimised by some unknown agency.

ABNORMAL PHYSICAL FINDINGS

Any significant abnormalities should be described; if a physical examination has not been carried out, this should be stated:

He looks rather thin but a physical examination has not yet been done.

DIFFERENTIAL DIAGNOSIS

This should be discussed in terms of likely alternative diagnoses, with evidence in favour of or against each of them. In some cases, there will be only one possible diagnosis. In others, the condition may not fit into any clearly defined diagnostic category but may be seen as a response to stress in a vulnerable personality; e.g. in a patient with mutliple somatic and psychological complaints who has developed these symptoms when unable to cope with a stressful life situation. It must also be remembered that two diagnoses may co-exist, e.g. depression and senile dementia, or alcoholism and an anxiety state. To continue with our example:

The presence of paranoid delusions associated with marked anxiety and his lack of insight indicate that he is suffering from a psychotic illness. The absence of depressive features and of biological symptoms of depression make it unlikely that the paranoid delusions are part of a psychotic depression. The diagnosis is more likely to be that of paranoid schizophrenia of acute onset, although there is no thought disorder and no evidence of first rank symptoms. Alternatively, the condition could be due to amphetamine psychosis. Further investigations are needed to exclude or confirm this possibility.

Thus the differential diagnosis is as follows:

(1) Paranoid schizophrenia
(2) Paranoid psychosis due to drugs
(3) Psychotic depression

FURTHER INFORMATION AND INVESTIGATIONS

In order to make a choice between alternative diagnoses and get a picture of the aetiological factors involved, it is often necessary to obtain further information from relatives or other informants, or to see the patient in a joint interview, e.g. a husband together with his wife. If the patient has had psychiatric treatment before, information should be obtained about previous admissions, assessments and treatment. It may also be necessary to carry out physical and psychological investigations to assist in making a definitive diagnosis. A brief statement should, therefore, be made as to what further information and investigations are required. Returning to our example:

> In order to differentiate between these diagnoses it is important to interview his parents. This should provide information about the patient's pre-morbid personality and about any previous psychiatric illness, the family circumstances and life events at the onset of his present illness. Physical investigations should include a drug screen to exclude an amphetamine psychosis.

AETIOLOGY

The role of all relevant psychological, social and biological factors and their interaction should be discussed here. Any relevant facts concerning the patient's family history, personal development and social circumstances not yet described, should also be included. Applying these considerations to John Smith:

> A family history of his paternal grandfather and his father's brother having suffered from a schizophrenic illness has been obtained. This strongly suggests a genetic factor and supports the diagnosis of paranoid schizophrenia.
>
> Psychological factors in terms of his family background and development may have contributed to his psychological vulnerability, and recent social factors may have acted as precipitating events. Thus his parents quarrelled a lot throughout his childhood and his mother left home several times, which distressed him a great deal. When John was seven she did not return for two months, leaving him with his father; on that and other occasions he felt responsible for his two younger siblings. These separations from his mother and the emotional insecurity during his childhood may have contributed to his vulnerable, anxious and withdrawn personality, and to his difficulty in maintaining close relationships. The fact that his recent girlfriend broke off their relationship may have precipitated the onset of his present illness.

TREATMENT

This should include such decisions as whether the patient can be treated at home, as an outpatient, in a day hospital, or requires hospital admission, possibly on a section under the Mental Health Act (1983). The use of psychotropic drugs or ECT, the need for supportive therapy, psychotherapy, behaviour therapy or social rehabilitation all need to be discussed. To take our example:

The severity of his psychotic symptoms strongly suggests that, initially, he may need a period of inpatient care. However, he is very reluctant to accept this. He is not so seriously ill or suicidal that he needs compulsory admission. The next urgent step, therefore, is to discuss his management with his parents and his general practitioner, in the hope that the necessary support can be provided for him at home by his parents, possibly with the help of a community psychiatric nurse or social worker. If this is not possible, admission to a day hospital could be considered.

In either case, he needs immediate antipsychotic medication with a drug such as trifluoperazine in a dose of 5 mg three times daily. He also needs regular support from his general practitioner and others, and should be seen weekly as an outpatient to monitor his medication, if treatment is begun at home; long-term support and follow-up should be provided after recovery from his present illness.

PROGNOSIS

It is important to differentiate between the prognosis in terms of the illness itself, e.g. schizophrenia, and the prognosis in terms of the particular patient, taking into account his personal and social circumstances, strengths and weaknesses. Prognosis should be discussed from the point of view of both the *short-term prognosis*, i.e. recovery from the main symptoms or acute illness, and the *long-term prognosis*, i.e. the likelihood of relapses, persistent personality changes and abnormal social functioning. To return to John Smith:

His paranoid symptoms should respond well to antipsychotic medication. Their acute onset, clearly related to recent precipitating factors, suggests that his present illness will respond quickly to treatment.

However, his long-term prognosis is more difficult to assess. The fact that, in spite of his insecure background, he has made a reasonably good social adjustment and had been working regularly until he fell ill is in his favour. Much now depends on whether the family atmosphere remains stable and supportive; if not, he runs the risk of further psychotic breakdowns. He is clearly particularly vulnerable in intimate and close relationships, and further stressful experiences or rejections are likely to cause a relapse. Whether he could be helped with psychotherapy to resolve these difficulties can only be assessed after his recovery from the present episode. The possibility of helping the family to continue to provide a supportive atmosphere without excessive emotional involvement in order to reduce the risk of relapses should also be considered. He will in any case require long-term maintenance antipsychotic medication.

FURTHER READING

Departments of Psychiatry and Child Psychiatry. The Institute of Psychiatry and Maudsley Hospital, London (1987). *Psychiatric Examination: notes on eliciting and recording clinical informtion in psychiatric patients*, 2nd ed. OUP, Oxford.

14

Unusual Situations and Difficult Patients

The outline of history taking and mental state examination described so far has assumed that ideal conditions are available for a detailed, unhurried interview. This is not always the case. The patient may be uncooperative, the doctor may be pressed for time, or there may be no room available for a quiet, confidential consultation. In fact interviews can take place in quite bizarre situations – psychiatrists have been known to conduct an interview through the letter box while on a home visit! It is often possible to obtain enough information to make a reasonable decision even under such far from ideal circumstances. The assessment will still be based on the interview methods described earlier but will obviously need to be adapted to the particular setting and the patient's general attitude.

The examination of the mute or inaccessible patient, the restless patient and the confused patient will be considered in this chapter, along with common interview settings such as the casualty department, the patient's home and the prison hospital. We also consider the examination of medical colleagues and public figures, which may present special difficulties to the psychiatrist.

Whenever the assessment of the patient is difficult, valuable information may be obtained from informants. These may include 'passers-by', friends, the police, social workers and neighbours as well as relatives. The aim of an interview with informants under difficult circumstances is to elicit facts. This is especially true if the patient is confused, overactive or thought-disordered. It is not possible to give hard and fast rules about whether the patient or the informant should be interviewed first. This decision depends on the doctor and the particular circumstances and may be made more complicated if the patient proclaims that he does not give permission for the friend or relative to be interviewed. In general it is best to see the patient alone initially and suggest seeing the informant during the course of the interview.

THE CASUALTY DEPARTMENT

Some psychiatric departments run an emergency assessment service staffed by a doctor, nurse and social worker which is independent of the casualty department. Such a service can only be offered if staffing levels are reasonable, and in most hospitals the casualty department remains the focus of psychiatric emergency services. Although this has many disadvantages, such as extra pressure on over-stretched casualty staff, it does allow most patients presenting with a psychiatric problem to be thoroughly screened for physical illness, and enables the casualty staff to gain valuable experience in the assessment of psychiatric problems. Unfortunately this liaison between psychiatrists and casualty departments may lead to difficulties, especially when the psychiatrist is delayed in attending to a difficult or restless patient. Mutual respect for each other's skills and duties should overcome such problems.

Psychiatric patients may attend the casualty department for a variety of reasons, ranging from attempts to jump the waiting list for an outpatient appointment to sincere requests for help from a suicidal patient. The casualty officer can be very helpful in filtering these patients and may protect the psychiatrist from a great deal of unnecessary work. If the casualty officer seeks the psychiatrist's advice the request should be taken seriously.

Some patients refer themselves to casualty while others are brought by the police, e.g. on a Section 136 (see p. 706), or referred by their general practitioner, social worker, friend or relative. The casualty officer is often able to deal with self-referrals and arrange an outpatient appointment in the psychiatric department, but the more complicated problems, such as those referred by the police, often require the psychiatrist's assessment or advice.

The time available for the psychiatric assessment is likely to be short, and the activity of a busy casualty department makes a lengthy interview difficult to conduct. What then should the psychiatrist do when asked to assess a patient in casualty?

Generally speaking, it is best not to see the patient first. Initially, the opinion of the casualty staff, who will already have assessed the patient, should be sought and, if the patient has been brought by the police, the police officers should be interviewed briefly. In this way an accurate picture of the circumstances leading up to the referral, the core of the patient's problems and a little background information can be rapidly obtained. The casualty staff should also be asked about the patient's behaviour in the casualty department: Is he quiet or restless? Does he appear confused or orientated? The information obtained can then be used to focus the interview with the patient. Only when the psychiatrist feels he has as much information as possible should he go and see the patient.

The interview with the patient should be carefully focussed, goal-directed and actively controlled by the doctor, who should ask direct questions about the patient's problem, its onset, course and severity and any allied symptoms. Throughout the interview the doctor should keep certain questions in mind: Why has this patient presented now? Is the problem acute or chronic? Is hospital admission indicated? If so, will the patient accept voluntary admission? If hospitalisation is not indicated, what other possibilities are there? Would a day centre referral, day hospital assessment, social-work involvement or outpatient appointment be best? Should treatment be started now or could it wait until further assessment?

These questions can only be answered if the interview is controlled by the doctor. It is not necessary to take a detailed family and personal history, although some simple information about the patient's background and social supports may be helpful.

An example may clarify some of these points.

A patient was brought to casualty by her social worker who asked for psychiatric help for her client. The casualty officer saw the patient and was worried about her suicidal intent and so asked the psychiatrist for advice. The psychiatrist attended the casualty department and spoke first to the casualty officer and nurse and then to the social worker. Having obtained the background information, the psychiatrist opened the interview with the patient by introducing himself and saying, 'I have spoken to the casualty officer and your social worker and they have told me about your problems. Perhaps you could tell me how long you have felt so miserable.' He then led the interview by asking about somatic symptoms, feelings of hopelessness, feelings of unworthiness, guilt, and suicidal ideas. In this way the depth of the patient's depression was assessed. The suicidal ideas had not led to active plans and so the psychiatrist did not think hospital admission was necessary. He therefore asked the patient about social supports, and eventually it was agreed with the patient that she should commence antidepressant drugs and go to stay with her sister. This was supported by the social worker who undertook to make the arrangements, and the patient was given an early outpatient appointment in the psychiatric department.

Often casualty assessments are not as straightforward as this, and time may have to be spent liaising with outside agencies, relatives and other hospitals before a reasonable decision can be made. However, the interview with the patient may last only 15-20 minutes, although as much time should be allowed as is necessary to come to a decision. Following the assessment, a firm offer of help should be made. This may take the form of an outpatient appointment, referral elsewhere, inpatient admission and/or commencement of medication. Advice from senior colleagues should always be sought if the assessor is worried.

Finally the psychiatrist should write a full account in the notes, speak to the casualty officer about his decisions and contact all other agencies involved with the patient. This should invariably include the general practitioner.

THE PATIENT'S HOME

Valuable information about a patient's social circumstances and family relationships can be obtained by interviewing him at home. These *domiciliary visits* are best done together with the patient's general practitioner, who may have known the family for many years and have vital information about their circumstances. A social worker and nurse may also accompany a psychiatrist on a domiciliary visit, and it is useful for all members of a visiting team to meet before the visit and discuss its purpose; at least one member should be known to the patient. Patients are rightly suspicious of people appearing on the doorstep claiming to be doctors and nurses, so it is wise to inform the patient of the visit beforehand.

Although some visits to a patient's home will arise from a request for a psychiatric assessment by the family doctor, other visits form part of an assessment for the compulsory admission of the patient to hospital. Under these circumstances it is important that the visit is carried out with the social services and the family doctor as both will be required if compulsory admission for observation and treatment is necessary (Section 2 of the Mental Health Act 1983, see p. 704). If reports suggest that the patient is likely to be violent, the police should be informed and their help requested. It is best for the police to stay discreetly out of sight and only emerge if problems arise.

Visits to a patient's home may help the psychiatrist make a diagnosis. For example one patient, who had previously been assessed as an outpatient and considered well, was visited because of continual complaints from the neighbours about noise at night. The patient's home appeared clean and tidy and had all the trappings of a comfortable dwelling. The psychiatrist, however, noticed black polythene bags over the curtains and asked the patient about them. The patient became slightly irritated and, on further questioning, explained that the black polythene kept the laser beams out of his home. He later explained that continual noise was necessary to reduce the power of the laser beams further. Thus the polythene bags provided the key to an encapsulated delusional system and it transpired that the patient suffered from paranoid schizophrenia.

The psychiatrist needs good social skills to interview successfully in a patient's home. An ability to notice things and remark on them without appearing over-inquisitive or condescending is important, and the psychiatrist should incorporate what he sees in the patient's home into the interview. For example, many patients are quite happy to talk about photographs around the home or their reasons for keeping pets. An everyday remark about either of these may allow a natural discussion to develop about loss, social isolation and loneliness. This is especially true of the elderly and, in this group of patients, home visits may be necessary to assess the patient's ability to manage everyday activities such as cooking, shopping and cleaning. A home visit also provides a unique opportunity to observe a patient's interaction with other members of his family.

PRISON

The psychiatrist may be asked to give advice on the management of mentally abnormal offenders. These requests may take many forms, and complicated legal situations are best dealt with by forensic psychiatrists (see Chapter 61). However, the general psychiatrist may be asked to assess the mental state of an offender who has been remanded by the court to a prison hospital for medical reports. This often results in the patient being transferred from prison to the local psychiatric hospital for further treatment.

Under these circumstances the psychiatrist has to decide:

(1) Is the patient fit to plead? (see p. 693.)
(2) What is his present mental state?
(3) What was his mental state at the time of the offence?
(4) Does he require further psychiatric treatment? If so, should it be given in the local hospital or in a high or medium secure hospital?

The interview should be directed towards answering these questions. The answers may be obvious; for example, a patient suffering from paranoid schizophrenia may break a shop window as a result of abnormal mental experiences. If he is clearly psychotic at interview arrangements should be made for his transfer to hospital. Occasionally the situation may be more difficult and the psychiatrist should obtain access to all other reports, including statements from witnesses, probation officers, social workers and, if possible, relatives and other informants.

THE MUTE OR INACCESSIBLE PATIENT

The *mute patient* does not speak and seemingly makes no attempt to do so. Mutism may be total or elective, i.e. found only in particular situations or with specific people. The level of consciousness is unimpaired. Elective mutism (see p. 499) is always psychogenic.

In contrast, the *inaccessible patient* may show a change in the level of consciousness.

The early part of an interview with a mute or apparently inaccessible patient must include an assessment of the level of consciousness and a full medical and neurological examination in order to determine the presence or otherwise of an organic cause.

Reports from nurses and other informants will provide useful information about any changes in the level of consciousness; specific enquiry should be made about drowsiness, ability to understand requests, loss of concentration, and inexplicable wandering. Tests of attention, concentration and memory should be given if possible, and careful observations made of the patient's ability to attend to questions, and his awareness of the environment.

The doctor should ask himself various questions when confronted by a mute patient:

Is the patient concerned about his inability to speak?
Can he communicate through gestures or in writing?
Can he give simple answers or does he only respond to certain questions?

The answers to these questions will help to distinguish further between psychogenic mutism, organic causes of mutism and the poverty of speech or retardation of depression. The patient with psychogenic mutism may be indifferent to being speechless, the patient who is organically ill may seem distressed and attempt to speak and communicate in writing, while the depressed patient may give delayed and monosyllabic answers, and relatives may provide a history of depression.

Some patients have a delusional belief that causes their mutism; one mute patient, suffering from paranoid schizophrenia, believed that every time he spoke his life-span diminished.

Mutism may be seen in patients who are in a state of stupor. *Stupor* is a term best reserved for those patients who are in a state of total psychomotor inhibition. The concept in its historical context has been reviewed by Berrios (1981). Stuporose patients are mute and immobile but are conscious. The patient's eyes may be open and follow objects or people around the room. Unlike in coma, attempts to open closed eyelids meet resistance. It should be noted that the stuporose patient is aware of comments made about him; it should not be assumed he cannot hear.

Causes of stupor include affective disorders, depression more often than mania; catatonic schizophrenia; organic disorders such as mid-brain lesions, e.g. tumours of Rathke's pouch or cysts of the third ventricle, when the condition is referred to as *akinetic mutism*; lithium intoxication; and psychogenic reactions.

The causes of stupor must be sought urgently as prolonged stupor may result in dehydration, infection and dependent oedema. Differentiation between the various causes may be difficult clinically and information from relatives or other informants is essential. In depressive stupor there may be a history of withdrawal and increasing psychomotor retardation. The catatonic patient may assume bizarre postures and show negativism and waxy flexibility, punctuated by periods of excitement. Inappropriate affect such as grimacing, smiling and giggling may occur.

A full neurological examination, including an EEG and CT Scan, should reveal any organic cause of stupor. Psychogenic stupor is rare and can only be diagnosed if a full history is available from a reliable informant and all organic causes are excluded.

THE CONFUSED PATIENT

The confused patient is unable to think clearly and coherently. This makes interviewing difficult. The commonest causes of confusion are the acute and chronic organic reactions (see Chapter 22). Thought processes are disrupted either as a consequence of clouding of consciousness or as a result of structural brain damage or both. These changes commonly result in disorientation. In contrast, patients suffering from a functional psychosis who may present with thought disorder are rarely disorientated.

It is wise to test cognitive functions at the beginning of the interview if a patient appears muddled or bewildered. Initially the orientation of the patient should be tested. Occasionally patients may find simple questions offensive, so it is best to preface cognitive testing by a statement such as 'I would now like to ask you some rather simple but important questions – could you tell me where you are now?'

After clarifying the patient's orientation, questions about past and recent personal events should be asked to test long-term and short-term memory respectively. Finally, memory for general events, such as recent world news, should be tested. In acute organic reactions recent memories are lost early and there is a relative preservation of long-term memory. In contrast in advanced chronic organic reactions both long-term and short-term memory are defective. In all cases an informant should be interviewed in order to obtain information about the onset of the illness.

THE OVERACTIVE PATIENT

The doctor is faced with a difficult decision when confronted by an overactive patient. Restraint is likely to lead to resistance or violence, while excessive permissiveness may cause chaos in the hospital. It is best to speak firmly and politely to overactive patients and explain the purpose of any request.

Sometimes it will be necessary to follow the patient around during the interview. Careful observations of his behaviour should be made. Excessive questioning is likely to irritate the patient and only questions directed towards identifying the cause of his overactivity should be asked.

Common causes of overactivity include mania and organic states such as alcohol and drug intoxication or withdrawal. The patient's behaviour, speech and affect will usually distinguish these conditions. For example, elation and joviality are common in mania, while fear, anxiety and irritability suggest an organic cause.

The overactive patient may need to be sedated. This is discussed further in Chapter 54.

EXAMINING COLLEAGUES AND VIPs

Medical colleagues often seek the help of a psychiatrist either for themselves or for a close relative, and from time to time the psychiatrist will be asked to see a well-known public figure. Such consultations may present special problems for the psychiatrist and for the patient.

In the case of a colleague it may be difficult for either or both parties to switch from their roles as two members of staff used to working together in the same hospital, to those of patient and doctor respectively. The patient may feel embarrassed when it comes to revealing personal and often intimate problems, and he may fear a breach of confidentiality. The doctor may be in danger of colluding with this and avoid discussing embarrassing topics which may in fact be relevant to diagnosis and treatment. Sometimes the best course of action is for the psychiatrist to obtain only an outline of the patient's problem and to arrange referral to a colleague in another hospital, but this may be impossible in small communities, and the patient may insist on seeing the psychiatrist he knows and trusts.

A public figure presents somewhat different problems. He may expect to be treated as a special case and try to lay down conditions as to where and when he should be seen, what to talk about and what to conceal. The doctor on his part may be over-impressed by the status or fame of the patient he is being asked to see. This could lead the doctor to overlook or not enquire into areas that he would explore with any other patient. It is essential for the doctor not to allow such considerations or his own feelings to interfere with carrying out a full and objective psychiatric examination and assessment.

Once the psychiatrist has agreed to see either a colleague or a well-known public figure, it is helpful initially to make some allowance for the patient's position. For example, it may be appropriate to see the patient at his home so that he will not be kept waiting or be seen by a receptionist, secretary or by other patients. At the start of the interview it is often best to talk about the fact that it may not be easy for a person in his position to find himself in a situation where he has to ask for psychiatric help. This may help the patient to feel understood and express his fears and embarrassment so that he feels more at ease. The doctor can then explain to him that for the patient's sake it is essential for him, the doctor, to be as objective and thorough in his examination as he would be with anyone else who came to consult him. As a result the patient is likely to feel reassured and relieved to find that the doctor is going to treat him as a person asking for help and not as someone special who has to maintain his more customary role of a colleague or well-known figure. The interview can then proceed more or less along the usual lines of any psychiatric interview.

FURTHER READING

Leon, R.L. (1982). *Psychiatric Interviewing: a primer.* Elsevier, North Holland, New York.

Part IV

Psychiatric Syndromes

15

Classification and Epidemiology

CLASSIFICATION

Faced with any collection of individuals showing a wide variety of characteristics, a common response is to attempt to classify them into groups. One object of classification is to reduce a large number of individuals to a smaller, more manageable, number of clusters. Another object is to identify the factors or forces that have generated such a diversity of phenomena. This identification is usually reached by a two-stage process: first, the subjects are classified on the basis of superficial similarities; secondly, the underlying factors that led to the variety of surface appearances are sought. Until they are successfully identified, some clusters tend to be inappropriately lumped together on the basis of similar appearances, while others become amalgamated when the same underlying factor is recognised as responsible for their diversity.

A good example from general medicine is the nineteenth-century diagnostic category of 'dropsy'. This described swelling of the body as a result of fluid retention; it was a grouping based on similar surface appearances. When William Withering (1741-1799) discovered that foxglove extract was used by traditional healers as a treatment for dropsy and tried it on his own patients, he found that only a proportion of them responded. With hindsight, we can see that the treatment distinguished patients suffering from cardiac oedema (the responders) from those with oedema from all other causes (the non-responders).

Response to treatment *can* be used as a method of classifying patients, but it does not necessarily distinguish clear diagnostic groupings, since we know that not all sufferers from a single condition will necessarily respond to the same treatment. To develop the argument, we need to consider the nature of a clinical diagnosis. A diagnosis implies a set of hypotheses about aetiology, pathology, natural history and response to treatment. In an ideal case, all these aspects of a particular disease would be known. Thus, for tuberculosis we know the necessary cause (tubercle bacillus), the pathology, both histological and gross, the likely course, and the probable response to treatment. This pattern of factors justifies its classification as a distinct entity. By no means all diseases possess so firm a classificatory status. For example, rheumatoid arthritis has a well-known and distinctive pathology, but no known aetiology, while for the 'irritable bowel syndrome' both the aetiology and the pathology are uncertain.

Unfortunately, the aetiology and pathology are unknown for most psychiatric conditions. The few exceptions include Huntington's chorea (see p. 280), which is known to be transmitted by a single autosomal dominant gene, and Alzheimer's disease (see p. 323), where the pathological changes in the brain are characteristic, although the aetiology is obscure. For the majority of psychiatric conditions, including schizophrenia, manic-depressive illnesses and all the neuroses, no distinctive pathology has been identified, and our knowledge of aetiology is incomplete. Where some aetiological factor has been identified, it is non-specific. Thus, although patients with schizophrenia may have a family history of schizophrenia, there is also among their relatives an increased frequency of manic-depressive illness. Furthermore, a high proportion of schizophrenic patients have no family history of mental illness.

As a result of these deficiencies in our knowledge, the classification of psychiatric conditions rests heavily on patterns of signs and symptoms, and hence the categories in use are equivalent in status to the term 'dropsy'. A major advance in classification was achieved by Kraepelin (1855-1926), when he divided the global category of 'madness' into manic-depressive illnesses and dementia praecox (Kraepelin 1913a), a forerunner of the term schizophrenia. He established this distinction partly on the basis of different patterns of signs and symptoms and partly on different natural histories. The term 'dementia praecox' implied a progressive deterioration, not seen in manic-depressive illnesses. However, Kraepelin himself recognised that some patients made a good recovery from dementia praecox, so that outcome could not be used as a validation of his classification. In recent years, long-term follow-up studies and studies of schizophrenia in non-Western countries have reinforced this view. About 25 per cent of Western patients and 50 per cent of non-Western patients experiencing a first episode of schizophrenia will lose all psychotic symptoms and have no further attacks for at least five years. Furthermore, among patients remaining for many years in psychiatric hospitals are found a significant number of manic-depressives, showing that some patients with this illness have as bad an outcome as patients with schizophrenia.

If natural history cannot be used to support a classification based on signs and symptoms, can response to treatment serve to differentiate between conditions? Psychosocial treatments are clearly non-specific and may benefit patients with any psychiatric condition. Even behavioural treatments, which are specifically tailored to individual symptoms, are applicable in principle to a wide range of psychiatric illnesses. When we come to physical treatments, electroconvulsive therapy is effective for some kinds of depression and for catatonic schizophrenia. Neuroleptic drugs benefit patients with schizophrenia, mania and agitated depression in the acute stage of these illnesses. They provide effective maintenance therapy for schizophrenia and mania. Antidepressant drugs are useful in a variety of depressive conditions but may also relieve anxiety states; they can also improve the depression that afflicts some schizophrenic patients. The only specific physical treatment is lithium, which is effective for mania and depression in the acute phase and for prophylaxis, but is not beneficial in schizophrenia.

Thus, with the exception of lithium, response to treatment does not provide a useful basis for psychiatric classification. It is interesting to note that the recognition by American psychiatrists of the therapeutic value of lithium led to a major change in their classificatory system in which mania had previously played a very small part.

As a consequence of ignorance about aetiology and pathology, and the lack of characteristic natural histories and responses to treatment, classification of the majority of psychiatric disorders is based almost entirely on distinctive patterns of signs and symptoms (Kendell 1975). Such a classification is open to challenge by anyone who considers he has a better one, and there is no final court of appeal to decide between alternative systems. Hence the establishment and use of a classification in psychiatry depends entirely on professional consensus. Where this is lacking, as between America and Europe, communication between psychiatrists at the level of diagnosis is impeded. This difference has been investigated in the US-UK diagnostic project (J.E. Cooper *et al.* 1972). The way round the problem is to present data for particular groupings defined in terms of signs and symptoms, for this makes clear exactly what kind of patients are included under a rubric of, say, schizophrenia. This solution has been made possible by the development of standardised clinical assessment instruments, such as the Present State Examination (PSE) (British) (Wing *et al.* 1974) and the Schedule for Affective Disorders and Schizophrenia (American) (Spitzer *et al.* 1978; Endicott and Spitzer 1978). These have become an integral part of any research project, although they are not in general clinical use.

An ideal classification should contain categories that are *comprehensive*, i.e. encompassing the whole range of phenomena, and *mutually exclusive*, i.e. not overlapping. Standardised clinical schedules, such as those mentioned above, comprise lists of questions that cover all signs and symptoms, except excessively rare ones. They are backed up by a glossary of definitions for each sign and symptom, ensuring that the categories are distinct. However, the natural world is not easily compressed into man-made classifications, and the clinician will often encounter phenomena which straddle two categories. The task then is to match the patient's experience or behaviour as closely as possible with the ideal concept of a category as embodied in its definition.

In practice, clinicians tend to cut corners in interviewing patients. Once they have established a diagnosis to their satisfaction, they are likely not to explore the mental state further. By contrast, the use of a standardised clinical schedule forces a comprehensive enquiry into the whole range of possible signs and symptoms. As a consequence, it has become evident that patients with psychoses, such as schizophrenia and psychotic depression, suffer from a whole host of neurotic symptoms in addition to the characteristic psychotic experiences.

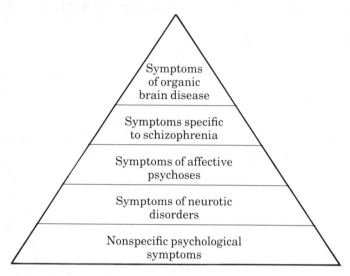

Figure 15.1. The hierarchical pyramid of symptoms

Foulds and Bedford (1975) and Foulds (1976) have proposed a hierarchical model of psychiatric symptoms, which attempts to account for this finding. An adaptation of their model is shown in Figure 15.1. The pyramid has a hierarchical structure such that symptoms at any level subsume symptoms at all lower levels. For example, patients with organic syndromes would exhibit symptoms from all other levels of the hierarchy; patients with characteristic schizophrenic symptoms would also show manic or depressive symptoms, neurotic symptoms and non-specific symptoms, such as worry and tension. When the model has been tested against clinical material, it has been found that the symptoms of the great majority of patients do conform to it. The main exception is mania, as manic patients, during the acute phase of the illness, have a strong sense of well-being and usually deny any neurotic or non-specific symptoms. The close approximation of most patients' patterns of symptoms to this model suggests that it reflects fundamental relationships between the various types of psychological dysfunction. In practice, however, diagnoses are not treated as forming a hierarchy, but as being mutually exclusive. Clinicians often deliberate between schizophrenia and manic-depressive psychosis. The occasional patient who presents an even balance of symptoms, characteristic of both kinds of illness, is often assigned to an intermediate category of schizoaffective psychosis. There is wide variation between psychiatrists in the use of this diagnosis, the status of which is consequently precarious (see p. 235).

Classificatory systems

The acceptance and use of a classificatory system depends on professional consensus. An attempt has been made to achieve widespread acceptance of a system called the International Classification of Diseases (ICD) (World Health Organisation 1978a), not just for psychiatry but for the whole of medicine. The ninth edition of the ICD is currently in use, and the tenth is in preparation (Sartorius *et al.* 1988). The section for Mental Disorders in the ICD-9 contains the following main categories:

Coding	*Psychoses*
290	Senile and presenile organic psychotic conditions
291	Alcoholic psychoses
292	Drug psychoses
293	Transient organic psychotic conditions
294	Other organic psychotic conditions (chronic)
295	Schizophrenic psychoses
296	Affective psychoses
297	Paranoid states
298	Other non-organic psychoses
299	Psychoses with origin specific to childhood

Coding	*Neurotic disorders, personality disorders and other non-psychotic mental disorders*
300	Neurotic disorders
301	Personality disorders
302	Sexual deviations and disorders
303	Alcohol dependence syndrome
304	Drug dependence

Coding	*Mental retardation*
317	Mild mental retardation
318	Other specified mental retardation
319	Unspecified mental retardation

The ICD is accompanied by a glossary which provides definitions of each diagnostic category. For example, paranoid state is defined as 'a psychosis, acute or chronic, not classifiable as schizophrenia or affective psychosis, in which delusions, especially of being influenced, persecuted or treated in some special way, are the main symptoms. The delusions are of a fairly fixed, elaborate and systematised kind.' The categories are defined mainly in terms of signs and symptoms, but these basic clinical phenomena are *not* defined, unlike the approach of research instruments such as the Present State Examination mentioned above.

Although the ICD is organised in such a way as to suggest that the categories are mutually exclusive, there is no reason why a patient should not be assigned two or more diagnoses. For instance, it would be perfectly feasible and appropriate to apply to a patient the following three categories: alcohol dependence syndrome 303, neurotic depression 300.4, and explosive personality disorder 301.3. The fourth digit in the classification is used to indicate sub-types of the main categories – for example, there are nine sub-headings of personality disorder. However, even this range fails to encompass the great variety of problematic personalities encountered in clinical practice, and the categorisation of personality disorders remains one of the least satisfactory in the Mental Disorders section of the ICD.

In America, modification of the ICD by the American Psychiatric Association (1980) led to the introduction of the Diagnostic and Statistical Manual, now in its third edition (DSM-III) and revised in 1987 (DSM-III-R). Sometimes differences between these two systems of classification cause difficulties, especially in research. The DSM-III makes use of the 'multi-axial' approach to classification in which several different elements or axes contributing to the disorder are taken into account, e.g. the clinical syndrome, personality factors, organic abnormalities, and severity. Such a multi-axial approach is now also being used in the classification of child psychiatric disorders (Rutter *et al.* 1975a; Rutter and Gould 1985) (see also p. 495).

It is worth giving some consideration to the major dichotomy into psychoses and neuroses (see also p. 156). The ICD glossary defines psychoses as 'mental disorders in which impairment of mental function has developed to a degree which interferes grossly with insight, ability to meet some ordinary demands of life or to maintain adequate contact with reality'. It acknowledges that this 'is not an exact or well-defined term'. The use of lack of insight as a touchstone for psychoses is undermined by the fact that some patients retain partial insight into their abnormal beliefs and experiences. It is true, however, that the great majority of psychotic patients suffer from delusions or hallucinations. As far as coping with the ordinary demands of life is concerned, some neurotic patients, for instance those suffering from severe agoraphobic or obsessional symptoms, can be more seriously incapacitated than many patients with psychoses. Despite these areas of overlap, the psychotic-neurotic distinction remains useful in practice. The one condition that extends across this boundary most conspicuously is depression. The issue of classification of depressive states is a particularly fraught one, and will be taken up later (see pp. 192-4).

EPIDEMIOLOGY

Epidemiology is concerned with the counting of cases and their numerical expression as a proportion of a defined population. Obviously reasonable agreement on the definition of a case must be achieved before rates can be compared across studies. The standardised assessments of symptoms and signs discussed above have enabled psychiatrists to communicate more clearly about the kind of patients they include under any diagnostic category. This enables the rates of psychiatric illness in different centres to be compared.

Rates of illness are expressed either as incidence or prevalence. *Incidence* refers to the number of new cases appearing over a given time. *Prevalence* refers to the number of all cases, new and old, detected over a specified period of time, e.g. the number of all cases of the illness detected at one point in time (point prevalence), or over one year (one-year prevalence), or throughout the lifetime of an individual (lifetime prevalence). Differences in incidence rates between centres or different countries can suggest aetiological factors, e.g. the effect of diet on heart disease, whereas differences in prevalence rates indicate factors that perpetuate the illness. Prevalence rates are also invaluable for planning services, e.g. determining the number of inpatient places required for disturbed adolescents.

Once a definition of a psychosis, such as schizophrenia, has been agreed in terms of standardised assessment, there is little difficulty in determining which patients qualify as cases. This is because the characteristic signs and symptoms are distinct phenomena which do not overlap with normal experiences. The reverse is true of the neuroses, such as anxiety states and neurotic depression, in which there is a continuum between normal fluctuations of mood and pathological mood states. The problem of where to establish a threshold is identical to that encountered with other continuously distributed variables, such as the glucose tolerance curve. In studies of glucose tolerance, if one applies the conventional threshold to a population survey, about 3 per cent of people are identified as abnormal, although they have no symptoms. In some psychiatric surveys, the threshold has been set so low that over three-quarters of the population have been identified as psychiatrically abnormal. Recent studies have employed much more conservative thresholds, but even so more than 10 per cent of all women have qualified as 'cases', mostly of depressive neurosis and anxiety states.

A major problem in psychiatric epidemiology is deciding where to look for cases. In a Western country almost all new cases of schizophrenia are referred to the psychiatric hospital services. It is very rare for a general practitioner to treat a first episode of schizophrenia without obtaining a specialist opinion. It is also unusual for sufferers to remain at home without coming to the attention of some professional, be it a health visitor or a policeman. While some schizophrenics are to be found among the population of vagrants, they have almost invariably received hospital treatment in the past. Hence it is justifiable to rely on patients known to the inpatient and outpatient services to calculate an incidence rate for schizophrenia in a Western country. Such rates vary within rather narrow limits: 10 to 15 per 100,000 population over the age of fifteen per year. The rate is related to the population over fifteen years old because schizophrenia very rarely begins below this age.

In a developing country the problem has a different dimension. Where Western-type facilities are scarce or non-existent, psychotic patients are usually treated by traditional healers, unless they present in a particularly violent or destructive way. In this case they are likely to be kept in prison, untreated, until their disturbance subsides, when they might well be allowed to return home. If their behaviour remains disturbed they could be transferred from prison to the nearest psychiatric treatment centre, which might be more than a hundred miles away. Another difference from a Western country is that psychotic patients who become vagrants are unlikely to have received treatment from the psychiatric services, although they may well have spent some time with a traditional healer. These considerations make it clear that in order to determine the incidence of schizophrenia in a developing country it is necessary to survey the hospital facilities, prisons, traditional healers and vagrants. An ambitious study of this kind has been conducted by the World Health Organisation in a variety of centres in developed and developing countries (Sartorius *et al.* 1986). A standardised clinical assessment interview, the Present State Examination, was used, which allowed a reliable system of diagnostic hierarchies to be applied to the data. It was found that if a broad definition of schizophrenia was used, the incidence varied three-fold between the highest and lowest figures. However, the application of a narrow definition resulted in very similar incidence rates across all the centres. The implication of this finding is that the cause or causes of narrowly defined schizophrenia must be common to a variety of cultures.

The epidemiology of neuroses raises very different problems. There is no question of relying on hospital statistics even in a Western country, since it has been shown that the general practitioner refers only 5 per cent of his emotionally disturbed, including his neurotic patients to a psychiatrist (see p. 644). The incidence and prevalence of neuroses can therefore only be determined by carrying out population surveys (Goldberg and Huxley 1980). A number of these, conducted in different parts of the world, have produced prevalence rates for the neuroses ranging from 0.8 per 1000 to 287 per 1000. This enormous variation is largely accounted for by technical problems of case-finding and fixing the threshold for pathology, as already discussed. Very few studies have employed the same techniques, but one that did so in two very disparate cultures, south-east London and rural Uganda, found a prevalence of neuroses that was more than twice as high among the women in Africa as among those in London (Orley and Wing 1979). This suggests that socio-cultural factors exert a considerable influence on the prevalence of neuroses, and emphasises the need for further studies of these factors.

FURTHER READING

Kendell *et al.* (1971). 'Diagnostic criteria of American and British psychiatrists'. *Arch. Gen. Psychiat.* 25, 123-130.

Kendell, R.E. (1975). *The Role of Diagnosis in Psychiatry*. Blackwell, Oxford.

Kreitman, N. (1985). 'Epidemiology in relation to psychiatry' in *Handbook of Psychiatry*, vol. 5: *The Scientific Foundations of Psychiatry* (Shepherd, M., ed.). CUP, Cambridge.

16

The Psychoneuroses

The concept of neurosis has had a stormy history, and its precise definition remains elusive. Some psychiatrists doubt the usefulness of the term because of its widespread and variable application but, despite this, every student has to grapple with the ideas that it attempts to embody.

HISTORY AND CLASSIFICATION

In 1784 William Cullen, an Edinburgh physician, used the term neurosis to describe a wide group of illnesses characterised by abnormalities of sensation and behaviour for which no physical cause could be found. Conditions such as spasm, coma, deafness, blindness and madness were included. Gradually this broad use of the term diminished, and by the nineteenth century neurosis was primarily used as a generic term associated with the illnesses 'hysteria', 'neurasthenia', 'traumatic neurosis' and 'anxiety'. The aetiology of these conditions was unknown, and the debate between supporters of somatic and psychological causes raged as strongly then as it occasionally does today. For example, neurasthenia, a condition characterised by overwhelming mental and physical fatigue, was thought by some to be a result of disordered neurochemicals, others stressed the degenerative or hereditary aspects, while others emphasised the psychological causes. However, by the end of the nineteenth century it had been gradually accepted that the neuroses were of psychological origin and, as a reflection of this understanding, they became known as the *psychoneuroses*.

Initially only hysteria and obsessional states were classified as psychoneuroses, since anxiety and neurasthenia were still thought to be caused by physical factors and were known as the *actual neuroses*. This division was soon discarded and the psychological origin of the neuroses was fully accepted. The question then arose as to which disorders should be classified under the general heading of neurosis. Anxiety, obsessional states, hysteria and neurasthenia were initially included, but during the early twentieth century psychoanalytic and psychiatric investigators began to remark on the overlap between the neuroses and abnormalities in personality. The relationship and interaction between neurotic disorders and personality have confused the issue ever since.

Originally it was thought that specific personality types were predisposed to particular neurotic illnesses. Thus hysterical personality was thought to predispose to hysterical neurosis, obsessional personality to obsessional neurosis and so on. Unfortunately the inter-relationship is not so clear and it is not known whether a person with an obsessional personality is more likely to develop an obsessional neurosis than any other neurotic disorder; conversely hysterical neurosis may arise in the context of any personality type and is not only associated with hysterical personality. It is however generally accepted that an overlap does exist between personality and neurosis, and it is useful to consider neurosis as a reaction in a vulnerable personality to stressful situations. It is important to note that the term neurosis does not cover all psychological reactions found in vulnerable personalities; it has become associated with the group of psychological illnesses which either appear out of proportion to the external circumstances or have no clear relationship to environmental events. Thus internal conflicts over aggression or sexuality may be stressful enough to precipitate a neurosis in some personalities, but not in others.

In contrast, if the stressful situations are clearly external, two categories – *acute reaction to stress* and *adjustment reaction* – may be used. An acute stress reaction is defined as a 'transient disorder which occurs in response to exceptional physical or mental stress such as natural catastrophe or battle and which usually subsides within hours or days' (ICD-9). An adjustment reaction lasts longer and is usually 'closely related in time and context to obvious circumstances such as bereavement, migration, or separation' (ICD-9). In other words, an emotional reaction which is understandable to a naïve observer and is in proportion to the individual's circumstances is probably best classified either as an acute reaction to stress or as an adjustment reaction rather than as a neurosis. For example, a student who fails his final examinations may suffer from mild symptoms of agitation, depression and anxiety lasting for a few days. This would be described as an acute stress reaction. However, if the emotional changes last longer the condition may be considered as an adjustment reaction. Unlike the neuroses, these reactions would not be considered to be of major psychopathological significance although they may of course require supportive intervention.

Clearly it is difficult to give a watertight definition of neurosis, but the following are the essential characteristics:

(1) The symptoms are experienced by the individual as arising from within and have psychological and somatic components.
(2) The symptoms are out of proportion to external circumstances.
(3) Behaviour, social relationships and personality are impaired but usually remain within socially acceptable limits.
(4) Insight is retained and the ability to distinguish reality from fantasy is unimpaired.
(5) There is no evidence of organic brain disorder.

Thus the neuroses are often seen as being similar to normal emotional reactions but differentiated from them by their severity and their lack of obvious precipitants. Anxiety, worry, tension and depression all occur in everyday life as minor symptoms and are not considered abnormal by patients or doctors until they increase in severity or interfere with social, personal or physical functioning. At this point they are often referred to as *minor emotional reactions* and may respond to simple reassurance and support. If the symptoms become more severe and debilitating, a neurosis is said to have developed, and when one particular symptom predominates, the neurosis is named after that symptom. Thus if obsessional features are most marked the illness is named an obsessional neurosis, if anxiety is to the fore it is an anxiety neurosis, and so on. In clinical practice the situation is often not so clear and symptoms may occur together. For example, a patient may complain of feeling depressed, have physical symptoms of anxiety and suffer from obsessional thought patterns. Under these circumstances it is important to determine which are the predominant symptoms and decide which syndrome – depression, anxiety or obsessional state – is primary, even though this may be a difficult decision.

Differentiation between neurosis and psychosis

A person suffering from a neurotic disorder has only part of his personality involved, is able to distinguish between inner subjective experience and outer reality, has insight into the fact that he is ill, and does not have delusions and hallucinations.

In contrast, the psychotic patient experiences delusions and hallucinations, falsifies his environment because of these experiences, suffers marked personality disturbance and loses insight into his illness. Furthermore, social adjustment is usually impaired and the capacity to make reasoned decisions is lost. Thus psychotic patients may be at great risk, become a danger to themselves or others and often require inpatient treatment.

Unfortunately these distinguishing features are not necessarily as clear cut as they may seem. For example, some psychotic patients know that they are ill, present themselves for treatment, and may even be able to carry on employment despite their illness. In contrast some neurotic patients, such as those suffering from an hysterical neurosis, may not accept that they are psychologically ill, resist all offers of treatment and withdraw from normal social interaction. The problem here is how to define insight.

Insight is not an all-or-nothing phenomenon, and it is important to gauge the degree of insight a patient has. There are three main components to insight:

(1) The degree of recognition a patient has that he is ill.
(2) The explanation he gives for his experiences.
(3) The ability he has to distinguish his inner world (internal reality) from external reality.

As a general rule neurotic patients are able to recognise that their experiences are products of their mental processes and accept that they are ill. They are also able to distinguish correctly external from internal reality. However, the explanations of their experiences may be so bizarre that they give the impression that insight has been lost. For example, patients with psychogenic pain may accept that they are ill but explain the symptom in physical rather than psychological terms and deny any psychological aetiology. In contrast psychotic patients tend to be impaired in all three components of insight. Clearly no single criterion can be used to distinguish psychotic from neurotic conditions.

The following conditions are recognised as being neurotic disorders and will be considered in more detail in this chapter:

(1) Anxiety neurosis
(2) Phobic anxiety states
(3) Obsessive-compulsive neurosis
(4) Neurotic depression
(5) Hysteria
(6) Compensation neurosis
(7) Hypochondriasis
(8) Depersonalisation syndrome
(9) Neurasthenia

The nature and causation of neurotic symptoms in general, especially those of the five major neuroses (1 – 5 above) are best understood in terms of an individual's personality development from infancy through childhood to adolescence. This requires an understanding of both conscious and unconscious conflicts, object relations and mechanisms of defence. These psychoanalytic concepts and the formation of symptoms are discussed in Chapters 5 and 6 respectively.

ANXIETY NEUROSIS

Normal anxiety, a fear of something untoward happening, is experienced by everyone; for example, mild apprehension associated with physical symptoms such as dry mouth, sweating, and urinary frequency is common before experiences such as taking examinations or giving a public lecture. These reactions, if not excessive, alert an individual and improve his performance. After appropriate action has been taken, such as having written a good examination answer, the symptoms recede and relief is experienced. Thus the anxiety does not overwhelm the individual, is short-lived, appropriate to the circumstances, and has been contained and used to advantage. Sometimes anxiety arises well in advance, alerts the individual to a forthcoming danger and provokes preparatory action. Because of its alerting quality anxiety is often referred to as *signal anxiety*.

In contrast, anxiety which overwhelms the individual and occurs in the absence of, or is out of proportion to any real threat, is known as neurotic or *morbid anxiety*. It may occur in brief episodes known as *panic attacks*, or as a persisting state, namely *chronic anxiety*. Performance, behaviour and social relationships are often impaired as a result of extreme anxiety or panic. Under these circumstances the condition is known as an anxiety neurosis; other neurotic features, such as obsessional or depressive symptoms, may be present but they do not dominate the clinical picture.

It is important to remember that neurotic anxiety, like normal anxiety, may act as a signal. It warns the individual that something is wrong. However, if the threat is unconscious, as is often the case in anxiety neurosis, appropriate action cannot be taken and this results in increasing distress. The task of psychotherapy in an anxiety neurosis is to unravel this unknown threat and make it conscious.

Psychological and somatic symptoms occur together in anxiety. When not related to any particular situation the condition is often referred to as *free-floating anxiety*. If the symptoms become attached to a particular situation, e.g. in crowds or travelling on trains, the term *situational anxiety* is used, and when that particular situation is actively avoided a phobic anxiety state has developed. *Panic attacks* may occur within the context of free-floating anxiety or situational anxiety and are defined as discrete episodes of anxiety which may be terminated by taking drastic action – for example, someone who feels trapped and unable to breathe may rush outside gasping for air.

The symptom of anxiety may, of course, also occur in almost any other psychiatric disorder or physical illness. This will be considered in more detail under the heading of differential diagnosis on p. 160.

Clinical symptoms

The symptoms forming an anxiety neurosis are conveniently divided into two major groups:

(1) Psychological symptoms
(2) Somatic symptoms

Either group of symptoms may dominate the clinical picture and each may interact with the other causing an escalation of symptoms. Thus if a patient complains that he fears he is going to die from a heart attack (a psychological symptom) he may note small changes in heart beat and this will fuel his fears and cause overbreathing leading to dizziness (a somatic symptom) which further increases the anxiety (a psychological symptom).

Psychological symptoms

The psychological symptoms give the condition its name, and fearful anticipation, or anxiety, dominates the clinical picture. Irritability, worry, feelings of nervousness and oversensitivity to normal stimuli, such as noise or light, are common, and concentration is impaired. Excessive concern over physical health may occur, but if this dominates the clinical picture the diagnosis of hypochondriasis should be considered (see p. 184). Derealisation and depersonalisation symptoms occur and they are often present together. They are described in more detail in Chapter 12 (see p. 125). It is important to remember that they are *as if* experiences: the patient knows the condition is abnormal and retains insight. In fact minor degrees of depersonalisation are experienced by many people. Sensitive ideas of reference also occur in neurotic anxiety.

The appearance of an individual may show characteristic changes if the anxiety is severe. The whole body is held alert and tense and the person may sit forward as if ready for action. The eyes are wide open, the pupils dilated, the eyebrows raised and the brow furrowed. Mouth breathing may also be observed. Agitation, the motor component of anxiety, occurs as constant fidgeting or pacing up and down and a fine tremor may be present.

Somatic symptoms

The somatic symptoms are varied and widespread and are best grouped together under the organ systems used in everyday medical practice. Generally speaking they arise from overactivity of the sympathetic nervous system and resemble a 'fight or flight' reaction. Cardiovascular symptoms include palpitations and chest pain; respiratory symptoms include breathlessness, overbreathing and difficulty in inhaling – so-called *air-hunger*; butterflies in the stomach, loose bowels and dry mouth are common; genito-urinary symptoms include frequency and urgency; impotence and loss of libido are often observed. Symptoms like dizziness and tingling sensations are commonly due to an alkalosis resulting from overbreathing which can lead to tetany. Sweating may occur and this is most common on the palms of the hand or in the axillae due to the sympathetic innervation of the sweat glands in these areas.

Musculo-skeletal symptoms are common. An inability to relax leads to muscle tension and this may result in tension headache (see p. 476). Other areas such as the neck and shoulders may be similarly affected.

Finally, the sleep pattern in anxiety neurosis shows the characteristics of initial insomnia and interrupted sleep rather than the early morning wakening found in depression. Many of these somatic symptoms may be measured by psychophysiological techniques (Lader 1969, 1975). For example, anxious patients show raised pulse rates, increased skin conductance and greater forearm blood-flow when compared to normal controls. Electromyographic recordings reflect the raised muscle tension and EEG monitoring shows decreasing alpha activity with increasing anxiety.

Differential diagnosis

In view of the varied symptoms found in anxiety states, differentiation from many physical and other psychiatric disorders may be difficult. A careful history and examination will usually suffice to distinguish the disorders but occasionally simple investigations, such as thyroid function tests to exclude thyrotoxicosis, may be needed. These should be kept to a minimum to avoid needlessly exacerbating the patient's anxiety.

Anxiety is a common feature of depression, and the agitation found in some depressive states may initially suggest a diagnosis of anxiety neurosis. Questions directed towards the patient's prevailing mood and the presence or absence of depressive features such as feelings of hopelessness and suicidal ideas will usually reveal the correct diagnosis.

Anxiety symptoms may be prominent in schizophrenia and may mask the psychotic symptoms, but careful questioning for the presence of delusions and hallucinations should clarify the clinical picture. Conversely anxiety symptoms may be so severe that schizophrenia is suspected. For example, depersonalisation and derealisation may be confused with the delusional mood that may occur in schizophrenia, but once again careful questioning should reveal the subjective 'as if' aspect of the anxious patients while patients suffering from schizophrenia will be perplexed, have no clear insight or will offer a delusional explanation for their experiences.

Physical illness may present with anxiety symptoms. Thyrotoxicosis, phaeochromocytoma, episodic hypoglycaemia and carcinoid syndrome should always be considered.

Drug and alcohol withdrawal should be kept in mind; symptoms most prominent in the mornings should arouse such suspicion.

Aetiology

As in other psychiatric illnesses, aetiological factors are best considered as arising from three main areas: biological, psychological and social. Whatever the cause, in the majority of cases of anxiety neurosis a disturbance of the patient's basic personality is an important predisposing factor.

Biological factors

There is some evidence from twin studies in support of a genetic influence in the causation of anxiety (Slater and Shields 1969). The most likely factor to be inherited may be a propensity to secrete adrenaline and noradrenaline in greater than normal amounts, but this is probably the mediator of the physical symptoms of anxiety rather than a cause of the anxiety itself.

Psychological factors

Psychodynamic theory

Freud's original view that neurotic anxiety was the result of the accumulation of repressed 'somatic sexual excitation' or libido is still often quoted and then rejected despite the fact that it was greatly modified by Freud himself and no longer forms part of modern psychodynamic theory. Freud's later formulation (Freud 1926) was that neurotic anxiety arises as a danger signal when a psychological conflict, previously repressed, is approaching consciousness. There is little doubt that many different psychological conflicts can give rise to neurotic anxiety; this is especially so when external circumstances play on an intrapsychic area of conflict. For example, a female patient who was soon to be married began to experience anxiety symptoms when she was alone with her fiancé. These developed into a chronic anxiety state. It transpired during psychotherapy that she had been subjected to a great deal of physical abuse by an alcoholic father when she was a child and this had led to an incestuous relationship. These events had been repressed and she had idealised her dead father for many years. The amorous advances of her fiancé had reawakened past repressed memories of her father's abuse and the anxiety was a signal that these painful experiences were becoming conscious.

Separation experiences or ruptured affectional ties during childhood can also predispose to the development of an anxiety state later in life (Bowlby 1979). Here, too, the anxiety arises as a danger signal, but in response to a threatened loss or separation rather than an intrapsychic conflict. An individual who has experienced traumatic losses, separations or rejections early in life later on remains over-sensitive to the threat of losses, rejection or separation. Such circumstances during adulthood, often apparently innocuous, may then reawaken the original separation anxiety and an anxiety neurosis may develop.

Learning theory

Learning theory views anxiety as a conditioned response. A painful stimulus which provokes anxiety may become paired with a neutral stimulus, and this results in the neutral stimulus engendering anxiety when it occurs again. Little support for this view-point is found in the history of patients with generalised anxiety, but it is relevant in some patients with specific phobias (see p. 165).

Social factors

It is generally accepted that external events may lead to anxiety. For example, serious illness in oneself or a relative, getting married or divorced, and moving house can all engender anxiety. These are known as life events (see p. 39). The importance of life events in the causation of the anxiety neuroses is controversial. Not everyone who experiences these events will develop an anxiety neurosis, and it is necessary to postulate an underlying vulnerable personality as a predisposing factor.

It is less certain that continuing environmental stresses such as conditions at work, living circumstances and family problems, lead to anxiety. Neurotic symptoms in general appear to be more common in people living and working under difficult conditions, and surveys of factory workers show an excess of disabling neurotic symptoms in workers performing repetitive tasks (Broadbent and Gath 1979). These are exacerbated if the work precludes direct and intimate contact with others.

Treatment

Psychological treatments

Treatment begins as soon as the interview commences. The doctor must listen carefully and offer quiet, undivided attention. This will reassure the patient that he is being taken seriously and enable trust to develop so that he can listen to the doctor's comments and accept that they might be helpful. Once the diagnosis of anxiety is established, simple reassurance about the benign nature of the physical symptoms may allow enough reduction in anxiety to facilitate further psychological exploration. For example, a twenty-eight-year-old man complaining of palpitations was gradually helped to realise by careful questioning that his symptoms only occurred when he felt anxious at parties or other social gatherings. He was then able to explore his psychological difficulties in putting himself forward and standing up for himself. The focus of attention was thus shifted from his physical symptoms to his psychological problems.

Individual or group psychotherapy or psychoanalysis all have a good deal to offer in the treatment of anxiety, depending on the patient's motivation and his ability to view his difficulties in psychological terms (see Chapter 44). Psychodynamic treatments offer an opportunity to explore the origin of the symptoms and to resolve underlying conflicts and personality problems.

Relaxation training (see p. 682) is used to decrease muscle tension, and anxiety management training (see p. 682) combines relaxation with thought-distraction techniques and self-reassurance. These techniques are simple to teach and easy to use after practice. Their main disadvantage is that patients may not persevere with them for long enough. They are usually only effective in less severe cases of anxiety.

Drugs

Benzodiazepines are often prescribed and rarely needed. They should only be used to control acute symptoms, and certainly for no longer than a few weeks at most as physical and psychological dependence rapidly develop. If they are ineffective in relieving anxiety they should be withdrawn rather than increased and an alternative treatment plan made. Diazepam orally 2 to 5 mg three times a day may be tried, although higher doses are occasionally needed.

Antidepressants have anxiolytic and sedative effects as well as antidepressant action. A sedative antidepressant such as amitryptiline orally 50-100 mg at night may be effective and quickly relieves the distress of sleepless nights. The effect occurs within a few days in contrast to the two weeks required for an antidepressant action.

Beta-blockers, e.g. propranolol, are occasionally used if somatic symptoms like palpitations are excessive, but they are of limited value and may be dangerous in high doses due to their hypotensive effect. A recent vogue for trifluoperazine and thioridazine is not recommended in view of the short-term and long-term side-effects of these drugs; their use should be reserved for psychotic illnesses.

Prognosis

Anxiety neuroses do not progress to other psychiatric illnesses, although brief, non-psychotic, depressive episodes may occur. The short-term outlook in cases of recent onset is good but depends on the severity of the symptoms; the more severe the physical symptoms the worse the prognosis, while a preponderance of psychological symptoms appears to improve prognosis. Long-term follow-up of patients suggests that about half the patients entering treatment improve substantially over a ten- to twenty-year period (Greer 1969).

PHOBIC ANXIETY STATES

Anxiety may be experienced in relation to specific situations or certain objects. When accompanied by a wish to avoid the feared situation or object, or when the situation is actually avoided, it is known as a phobic anxiety state. These are commonly divided into three groups:

(1) Simple phobias
(2) Social phobias
(3) Agoraphobia

Simple phobias

Simple phobias are experienced by everyone as children, e.g. fear of the dark, thunderstorms, animals, etc. They may either continue into adulthood or arise *de novo* in early adult life. They are more common in women. Many have, somewhat unnecessarily, been given complicated names; fear of heights is called acrophobia, fear of spiders arachnophobia, fear of enclosed spaces claustrophobia, and so on.

In view of their specificity simple phobias may not interfere with an individual's life, but occasionally the anxiety may become so severe that it begins to do so. For example, a person suffering from a fear of dogs may not dare to leave the house. In other cases daily activities may be altered to a lesser extent and situations known to provoke anxiety are avoided. For example, a fear of enclosed spaces may lead to an avoidance of lifts, small rooms, cars and so on. In another common phobia, *travel phobia*, the patient is unable to travel in cars, buses, trains or aeroplanes so that his life becomes more severely restricted.

Social phobias

These are equally common in men and women and occur most commonly in the younger age group (twenty to thirty). Anxiety occurs specifically when the individual has to meet other people and is particularly severe if strangers or distant acquaintances are involved. The condition often starts in a social situation, e.g. eating in a restaurant, going to parties or the theatre; subsequently social phobics tend to become anxious before social situations and a pattern of avoidance and withdrawal is set up. This is in contrast to socially inadequate people, who tend to become anxious after recognising their own shyness and gauche inappropriate behaviour in social situations.

Agoraphobia

Agoraphobia literally means a fear of the market place or place of assembly. It usually begins in the twenty to thirty-five-year-old age group, and two-thirds of cases occur in women. Typically its onset is sudden and appears to have no obvious precipitant, although the illness may be associated with a major life change such as marriage, bereavement, or children starting school.

The condition is commonly defined as a fear of open spaces, but usually presents clinically as an inability to leave the home or a fear of entering public places from which escape may be difficult, e.g. supermarkets, cinemas, restaurants, etc. The patient can often recall the first attack of anxiety and how leaving the situation led to relief. When the situation is re-entered, anxiety occurs again and a pattern of avoidance begins. Initially only the feared situation itself provokes anxiety, but gradually avoidance generalises and even thinking of or imagining the feared situation may engender panic. The result is an ever-increasing disability. For example, an initial panic attack in a supermarket may lead to anxiety on entering even small shops and gradually the patient becomes completely housebound; the patient is then sometimes, though unhelpfully, known as a 'housebound housewife'. Agoraphobics are often less anxious and able to go out when accompanied. Thus one housebound patient was able to go out in the company of her child or dog without experiencing anxiety and even travelled abroad accompanied by her husband. However, many agoraphobic patients also develop a travel phobia, as described above. Agoraphobics are often considered to have passive, anxious and dependent pre-morbid personalities. There is often a childhood history of separation experiences or emotional deprivation which may play a significant role in the later development of the condition. Marital conflicts play an important part in some cases.

Aetiology

There is no single satisfactory explanation for the occurrence of phobic anxiety states. There is some evidence of a genetic influence on their severity (Torgerson 1979). Although simple phobias may be left over from childhood, this neither explains their original onset, even though they may be considered normal in childhood, nor offers a reason for their persistence. It is likely that a vulnerable, anxious personality is a predisposing factor in many cases.

Learning theory suggests that classical conditioning occurs in the formation of phobic anxiety states. If this were the case a traumatic event should commonly be found associated with the onset of the phobia, e.g. a fear of entering shops might have developed after being present in a shop during a bomb explosion. However this simple pairing of situation and traumatic event does not seem to be the case.

Psychoanalytic theory suggests that the phobic situation is a symbolic representation of an inner conflict; in an attempt to escape that conflict the anxiety attached to it becomes displaced onto a more easily avoidable external object or situation.

The best explanation probably takes all these features into account. For example, a person with psychological difficulties over his sexuality may be vulnerable to mild anxiety when physically close to other people. This may occur for example in lifts and, instead of facing the anxiety associated with the original sexual difficulty, it becomes attached to this more neutral or manageable situation and the patient therefore begins to avoid lifts. The choice of feared object or situation is thus linked, albeit symbolically, to the original conflict and the fear then becomes reinforced or generalised by a process of conditioning. Whatever the cause of phobic states, it seems unlikely that severe phobic anxiety can ever arise without some underlying psychological conflict or personality disorder being present as a predisposing if not causative factor.

Treatment

A variety of treatment approaches is commonly used, and each is directed towards a different aspect of the condition – psychotherapy to help resolve the psychological conflicts underlying the disorder, behavioural techniques to modify the avoidance responses, and drug therapy to relieve the acute distressing symptoms of anxiety.

Behavioural techniques commonly used include desensitisation, modelling and flooding. These are described elsewhere (see Chapter 46), but in essence they involve exposure of the patient to the phobic stimulus until his anxiety decreases and the avoidance response ceases. In simple phobias this may be done in imagination alone, but this is unlikely to be effective in more diffuse states such as agoraphobia. Here a structured, hierarchical programme of increasing exposure in reality to the feared situation is developed with the patient; nowadays, the nearest relative or a close friend, often also bound up in the disorder, is asked to participate in the treatment programme (Mathews *et al.* 1981). This *systematic desensitisation* may be combined with relaxation training and drugs, and is well suited for use by general practitioners (Marks and Horder 1987).

Drug therapy is probably only of help as an adjunct to behaviour therapy, e.g. benzodiazepines may relieve anxiety during a programme of desensitisation and antidepressants may be required to alleviate any depressive features. Phenelzine, a monoamine oxidase inhibitor, has been suggested to be of use in agoraphobia, but the evidence for this is inconclusive (Tyrer *et al.* 1973).

Even if phobic symptoms are relieved by these techniques, *psychotherapy* – individual, group or family therapy – may then be required to resolve underlying conflicts, marital and other problems which may have given rise to or perpetuated the phobic disorder. This applies particularly to agoraphobia.

It is of interest to note that Freud pointed out as early as 1919 that in the case of agoraphobic patients the analyst has to 'induce them by the influence of the analysis to go out alone' and that 'only when that has been achieved at the physician's demand will the associations and memories come into the patient's mind which enable the phobia to be resolved' (Freud 1919, p. 166). Freud was thus the first to advise a combination of a behavioural with a psychoanalytic approach.

Prognosis

Phobias tend to persist in spite of active treatment. Simple phobias have the best prognosis, while the more widespread conditions, such as agoraphobia and the social phobias, are more difficult to treat. However, behavioural treatment for agoraphobia may be successful and the initial benefits maintained for up to nine years (Munby and Johnston 1980).

OBSESSIVE-COMPULSIVE NEUROSIS

The term obsessive-compulsive neurosis, or obsessional neurosis for short, encompasses a number of conditions characterised by the presence of obsessions or compulsions. The balance of these symptoms may vary from patient to patient but the phenomena are often isolated from the rest of the patient's mental activity, although depression is a common associated feature. The illness usually starts in the late teens or twenties and appears to be equally common in both sexes. Some definitions may help the understanding of the obsessional neuroses.

Obsessions are defined as recurrent persistent thoughts, ideas, images, or impulses which are perceived by the patient as inappropriate or absurd and recognised as a product of his own mind. They can be very distressing and may be resisted.

Compulsions are motor acts which are resisted but carried out despite being regarded as senseless. They are accompanied by a subjective sense of compulsion and any resistance leads to increasing tension which can only be relieved by carrying out the motor act. They are often associated with obsessions but may occur alone.

Rituals are often considered to be the same as compulsions, but they should be differentiated. Rituals have a magical quality attached to them, are not necessarily accompanied by a sense of compulsion and, furthermore, may have group or cultural acceptance. For instance the theatrical world has a number of examples, e.g. the ritual of going outside, turning around three times and spitting if the title of the play *Macbeth* is mentioned in the theatre during its production. This differentiation between rituals and compulsions is somewhat blurred and the two terms are often used synonymously.

Bearing these definitions in mind, we can list the important features which characterise obsessive-compulsive disorders. They are as follows:

(1) The symptoms show a sense of compulsion, persistence and insistence.
(2) The symptoms are resisted but usually without success.
(3) The patient acknowledges the alien quality of the symptoms but recognises that they originate within the self.

Clinical features

Obsessional thoughts, ideas, images and impulses are often aggressive, sexual or obscene in nature and are unpleasant and disturbing to the patient. For example, a religious person may suffer recurrent blasphemous thoughts and fear shouting them out in church; obsessional images may take the form of vividly imagined car crashes involving the whole family, or obscene sexual acts; obsessional impulses may be horrific, e.g. a recurring impulse to pick up a knife and stab a member of the family. These disturbing characteristics lead to anxiety and depression, and attempts may be made to reduce the anxiety by replacing the thoughts by more pleasant ones or by resorting to compulsive motor acts in the belief that, in this way, the harmful effects can be prevented – so-called 'magical undoing' (see p. 56).

Compulsive acts may occur singly or repeatedly in a particular order and often happen without the patient being aware that they have any relation to obsessional thoughts. For example, a patient may take several hours to undress and get into bed due to a compulsion to do up and undo his buttons over and over again without knowing why. Alternatively, compulsions may be clearly associated with obsessional thoughts such as fear of contamination from touching everyday objects leading to a hand-washing compulsion in which the hands are washed over and over again.

Compulsive checking is another symptom: for example, the patient may find he cannot leave the house as he feels compelled over and over again to check the gas taps or the light switches even though he knows this is irrational. Prevention of or resistance to these compulsive acts always causes great anxiety, but performing them offers only temporary relief.

Differential diagnosis

The diagnosis is seldom in doubt when the condition is severe, although in milder cases anxiety neurosis and phobic disorders should be ruled out by taking a careful history and mental state.

Obsessional symptoms may complicate a depressive illness or depression may occur in an obsessional neurosis. The relationship of the two disorders is unclear, but obsessional symptoms probably occur in about a third of patients with a depressive illness.

Interestingly, obsessional states may be confused with schizophrenia; this is especially so when the obsessional ideas or imagery become complex, intricate and well-developed. The presence of other psychotic symptoms will usually reveal the correct diagnosis, and it should be remembered that obsessional features occur in about 3 per cent of schizophrenic patients (Rosen 1957).

Occasionally obsessional symptoms form part of an organic disorder such as presenile dementia or following encephalitis lethargica, but the other features of the organic condition usually reveal the correct diagnosis.

Aetiology

Although constitutional and organic factors may play a part in the causation of obsessional states, the basis for the development of an obsessional neurosis probably lies in a disturbance of personality development.

Psychodynamic theory

This lays emphasis on the role of disturbance in personality development. Most patients with an obsessive-compulsive neurosis have an over-developed conscience, often because they have been brought up in an excessively strict and puritanical manner. This leaves them with exaggerated guilt feelings, especially about aggressive and sexual impulses. According to classical analytical theory, fixation at and regression to the anal stage of development (see p. 71) may play a part in the development of their symptoms, especially the need to control their unacceptable sexual and aggressive feelings and fantasies. For example, compulsive checking of gas taps or light switches may represent the need to control their unconscious destructive impulses. These patients may have had to battle for their autonomy in childhood, and persistent aggressive and rebellious impulses may be responsible for their obsessional symptoms. However, similar observations apply to other psychoneurotic disorders and our understanding of the origins of this condition remains incomplete.

Learning theory

Learning theorists have tried to account for obsessional disorders in terms of avoidance responses (Rachman 1971; Rachman and Hodgson 1980). However, these do not account fully for obsessional ideas, images, thoughts and impulses which are not accompanied by a compulsion.

Other theories

Various neuropsychological theories propose defects in the patients' arousal systems as being the primary abnormality (Beech 1978). Thus minor stimuli cause a sensitive arousal system to over-react and the individual must then take massive action to contain the anxiety. Other theories suggest a mood change as the primary disturbance. This is important since it follows that treatment would have to be directed towards the mood of the patient rather than the thoughts or compulsive acts. These theories probably underestimate developmental factors and the complexity of the disorder.

Treatment

Obsessional neuroses are difficult to treat. The main available therapeutic approaches are listed below. A combination of treatment methods, say drugs and behaviour therapy, may be required if treatment is to be successful (Marks *et al.* 1988).

Psychotherapy

This may initially be on a supportive basis and, although unlikely to lead to the disappearance of the obsessional symptoms, may help the patient to feel understood. Doctors must at all costs avoid antagonising the patient by telling him to 'pull himself together'. The patient knows better than the doctor what useless advice this is as he has already tried unsuccessfully to resist his obsessional thoughts or compulsive acts. Further tension will only increase already exaggerated guilt feelings.

More formal psychoanalytic psychotherapy aims to help the patient understand the unconscious meaning of his symptoms while taking other aspects of his illness and underlying personality problems into account.

This may allow the symptoms to become less of a preoccupation, but unfortunately the rigidity, rationalisation and intellectualisation of obsessional patients frequently act as resistance to psychotherapy. Furthermore any intellectual insight may be incorporated into the obsessional thinking rather than becoming a vehicle of change.

Behaviour therapy

Behavioural treatments (see Chapter 46) are primarily directed towards the removal of compulsive acts. Flooding, modelling, exposure in vivo and response prevention techniques are all used and may be helpful in about two-thirds of cases (Marks *et al.* 1975). Often close family members are asked to take part in the treatment programme; they have to be trained to stop the patient from carrying out his compulsive acts.

Patients with obsessional thoughts are notoriously difficult to treat, but behavioural treatments such as thought stopping have been tried (see p. 587).

Drugs

These have little to offer, but occasionally, if the symptoms are part of a depressive illness, they may respond to treatment with an antidepressant drug. Clomipramine has been suggested as the drug of choice for obsessional symptoms even if depression is absent.

ECT and psychosurgery

ECT should only be considered if depression is the primary diagnosis and obsessional symptoms are a secondary phenomenon. Psychosurgery has been tried but its long-term effects remain uncertain. Such treatment can only be justified after all other treatments have failed and the disorder is seriously interfering with the patient's life. At the present time the operation is restricted by the Mental Health Act (1983) which requires the patient's consent and a second psychiatric opinion (see p. 707).

Prognosis

Most psychiatrists are pessimistic about the outcome of the obsessional neuroses as at least half have an unremitting course despite active treatment (A. Black 1974). The rest follow a fluctuating course, although personality and environmental factors probably influence the final outcome. The prognosis is worse in patients with a pre-morbid obsessional personality, and stressful events, such as increasing responsibility at work, may exacerbate the symptoms.

NEUROTIC DEPRESSION

The problem of how to classify the depressive disorders is at present a controversial and confusing issue within psychiatry and is discussed more fully in Chapter 18, where psychotic depression will also be described in detail.

There are many patients who complain of feeling moderately or even seriously depressed but who have no psychotic features, i.e. they have no delusions or hallucinations and have insight into their disorder. This is why their condition is called a neurotic as opposed to a psychotic depression.

Further, it is usually easy to identify a stressful life event which has preceded the onset of the illness so that the latter can readily be seen to have developed as a reaction to that event. Such events include losses like a bereavement, an illness affecting the patient or a close relative, divorce, separations, the end of important relationships, moving house, serious disappointments and so on. Neurotic depression is therefore also called reactive or exogenous depression.

An important feature of neurotic or reactive depression is that, like other neurotic symptoms, the degree of depression and its persistence are out of proportion to the loss sustained. This corresponds to an anxiety neurosis where the degree of anxiety is out of proportion to the threat the patient faces. Unlike anxiety, depression occurs as a reaction to a loss that has already taken place, whereas anxiety develops in anticipation of a threatening event. One of the difficulties in diagnosis is how to decide where normal human sadness ends and abnormal or excessive sadness, i.e. neurotic depression, begins. Of course this difficulty also applies to other neurotic disorders, especially anxiety neurosis.

It should also be noted that while psychotic depression used to be thought of as entirely endogenous, i.e. not associated with external life events, it is increasingly being recognised that even in psychotic or endogenous depression a stressful event may have precipitated the onset of the illness (Brown and Harris 1978) (see p. 200). Moreover, some endogenous predisposition, either genetic or more often a vulnerable personality due to emotional deprivation in childhood, or both, may be present in reactive depression. In clinical practice, therefore, it is often more useful to ask oneself in each individual case of depression to what extent exogenous and to what extent endogenous factors may have contributed to the patient's depressive illness.

Clinical features

In neurotic or reactive depression the patient complains of a sense of sadness, misery, depression or despair which continues unabated, despite occasional temporary relief brought about by everyday distractions or pleasant events. Diurnal variation of mood tends to be absent, but if it occurs the depression is usually worse towards the end of the day. This is in contrast to endogenous or psychotic depression, in which the depression is worse in the morning and improves towards the evening. Ideas of guilt, self-reproach and unworthiness, common in psychotic depression, may be absent or, if present, less severe. Self-pity and a sense of hopelessness are common, and patients are unable to feel pleasure (anhedonia) or look forward to the future. They often blame others for their predicament and feel that life has treated them unfairly.

Patients often wish they were dead but tend to be less actively suicidal than those with psychotic depression. Thoughts of suicide and suicidal attempts are, however, quite common and should be specifically asked for. By definition delusions and hallucinations are absent. Biological symptoms may be absent but if they occur they tend to be less severe than in psychotic depression. Thus there may be some loss of appetite and weight loss, although in neurotic depression increased appetite, even compulsive over-eating and weight gain may be seen instead. Tiredness, poor concentration and loss of libido are common. Sleep disturbance, if present, may take the form of initial insomnia or early morning wakening or both, or there may be a tendency to sleep for hours in the morning, perhaps in an attempt not to have to face another day.

Anxiety is often an associated feature, making the differential diagnosis between an anxiety state and neurotic depression more difficult. Usually, however, the preponderance of depressive symptoms helps in making the correct diagnosis provided it is realised that symptoms of anxiety are common in neurotic depression.

Aetiology

The aetiological role of losses and disappointments in neurotic depression has already been described. Psychodynamic considerations provide an understanding of the reasons why some people react to such life events by becoming neurotically depressed, as opposed to others who respond to similar events with normal degrees of sadness and then make a gradual recovery.

There is ample evidence that parental death before the age of eleven (see p. 40) or severe emotional deprivation in childhood result in a personality which remains excessively vulnerable to later bereavements, separations, rejections or other disappointments. Any such loss tends to reawaken the earlier feelings of desolation and misery the person was exposed to at a much earlier age. Moreover in childhood we normally internalise those aspects of mother and father which helped us as infants and children to cope with and contain such painful affects as sadness, guilt and anxiety. The lack or loss of such parental figures prevents such internalisation so that the adult later on does not have the internal capacity to contain and recover from such painful affects. In psychotherapy of patients with neurotic depression it is the stable, containing relationship with the therapist that may lead to the growth of an inner source of strength and survival when faced with serious losses and disappointments.

Another important consideration is that life events involving losses like a bereavement often play on inner emotional conflicts which are then responsible for feelings of guilt and depression. For example, many patients with neurotic depression suffer from an over-developed conscience so that when a close relative dies the patient blames himself for not having looked after him well enough, or even of having been responsible for his illness and death. The resultant feelings of guilt and self-blame then aggravate his grief and impede the normal process of gradual recovery.

In 1917 Freud drew attention in *Mourning and Melancholia* to the close similarity between mourning on the one hand and melancholia, now called depression, on the other. The more ambivalent the person's feelings towards the deceased have been before he died the more likely he is to enter a state of depression rather than work through a normal grief reaction (see also pp. 94-5).

Sometimes, when a person's conscience and moral standards are over-developed, even a relatively minor event like a sexual misdemeanour or having hurt someone close to him or failed to achieve some ambition may lead to excessive self-blame and the development of neurotic depression.

Careful exploration of psychodynamic factors in terms of personality development, unresolved conflicts and their relation to recent life events is essential in every patient suffering from neurotic depression and in deciding on his treatment.

Treatment

Psychotherapeutic support is particularly important in the management of patients with neurotic depression. Antidepressant medication is only needed if biological and depressive symptoms are severe, and should be avoided in milder cases. If there is a serious risk of suicide hospitalisation may be necessary, but adequate support by relatives and by the general practitioner, psychiatrist, social worker, community nurses and, perhaps, day hospital care may make this unnecessary. If there are recognisable psychological factors such as long-standing emotional conflicts, a disturbed personality make-up or marital disharmony, formal psychotherapy – individual, group or marital – may be helpful, provided the patient is sufficiently motivated.

HYSTERIA

Hysteria is not a clear-cut clinical entity, and the word is used in several different ways. Its most widespread application is as a term of abuse, and this has led some psychiatrists to suggest abandoning it as a diagnostic category altogether. Unfortunately this does nothing to clarify the concept; it merely deals with a difficult problem by avoiding it or pretending that the disorder does not exist. It is more sensible to attempt to understand what aspects of the human mind and behaviour the word hysteria attempts to encapsulate.

It is most important that hysteria is not confused with hysterical personality. Hysterical personality is a personality disorder (see p. 330) and hysteria does not necessarily arise within the context of an underlying hysterical personality although it may occasionally do so. Conversely, a person with an hysterical personality is no more likely to develop an hysterical neurosis than any other of the neuroses.

Historical background

Hysteria was first described by Hippocrates, and the ancient Greek view is well described by Plato in the *Timaeus*:

> The womb [*hystera* in Greek] is an animal which longs to generate children. When it remains barren too long after puberty it is distressed and sorely disturbed and strays about in the body cutting off the passages of breath, it impedes the respiration and brings the sufferer into the extremest anguish and provokes all manner of disease besides. The disturbance continues until the womb is appeased by passion and love. Such is the nature of woman and all that is female.

Thus hysteria was thought only to occur in women with unsatisfactory sex lives or virgins and widows; for a cure they should seek sexual satisfaction. The relationship between hysteria and sexuality has continued ever since. During the Middle Ages, as described in the *Malleus Maleficarum* (Summers 1971), the defect that predisposed women to hysteria was supposed to be 'wanton sexuality rather than virginity'; sexuality became an 'evil which predisposed lascivious women to seduction by the devil'. This opinion gradually fell into disrepute. Charcot (1825-1893), the French neurologist, emphasised the importance of suggestibility in hysteria and the possibility of an organic brain defect, while Pierre Janet (1859-1947), a French psychologist and psychiatrist, drew attention to dissociative phenomena in hysteria (Janet 1907). However it was Freud's work (Breuer and Freud 1895) with patients suffering from hysteria which re-emphasised abnormal psychosexual development as an important factor in the genesis of the condition (see also pp. 541-3). This was eventually to lead to his exploration of unconscious mental processes and hence to psychoanalysis. Knowledge of the unconscious and associated mental mechanisms is fundamental to contemporary understanding of hysteria (see Chapters 5 and 6).

Varieties of hysteria

There are several conditions subsumed under the term hysteria. They may be distinguished by their clinical manifestations:

(1) Hysterical neurosis
(2) Epidemic hysteria
(3) The Ganser syndrome
(4) Multiple personality
(5) Briquet's syndrome

By far the commonest of these is hysterical neurosis.

Certain symptoms and signs are common to these five conditions and therefore provide the core for any definition of hysteria:

(1) The unconscious formation of the symptoms.
(2) The presence of dissociation (see below).
(3) Evidence of primary and secondary gain, with the proviso that the latter is not used as a diagnostic criterion on its own.
(4) The absence of any physical pathology to account for the symptoms.

Hysterical symptoms are often divided into two groups:

(1) Dissociative phenomena (mental symptoms)
(2) Conversion phenomena (physical symptoms)

Dissociation is a mental mechanism which occurs in the face of unacceptable conflict. Certain mental activities are split off from others, although a person may be aware of one or the other at different times. The result is an apparent restriction of conscious awareness so that only certain themes are available to the patient while other themes of emotional importance, such as recent emotionally disturbing events, are inaccessible to him. Intellectual ability and motor skills may be retained. A severe example of this process occurs in multiple personalities, as R.L. Stevenson described in fictional form in *Dr Jekyll and Mr Hyde*. The two personalities differ in almost every respect and each is unaware of the other.

Conversion refers to another process that occurs in an attempt to solve a mental conflict; severe mental conflict leads to anxiety, and in order not to have to experience this the conflict is repressed (see p. 54) and becomes *converted* into a physical symptom which relieves the anxiety. This is known as *primary gain* and is a compromise as one symptom is replaced by another, a mental by a physical one. *Secondary gain* then becomes possible as the patient may use the physical symptom to avoid difficulties or gain attention. Of course secondary gain is a phenomenon that may occur in any illness; for example, a patient with a peptic ulcer may use the condition to remain off work. Although it is common in hysteria it is not specific to this illness and cannot therefore be used as a diagnostic criterion. It is the primary gain that is characteristic of hysteria, and this should always be looked for as a positive diagnostic sign. Despite this, the term secondary gain has become associated with hysteria rather than other illnesses, and this has led doctors and others wrongly to dismiss patients as 'being hysterical' when they appear to 'use' their physical symptoms to their advantage.

Hysterical neurosis

Clinical features

Dissociative symptoms

These include amnesia and fugue states.

Hysterical amnesia shows all the features of a psychogenic amnesia (see p. 34) and is usually sudden in onset, often following a stressful event. The memory loss is either global or restricted to certain emotionally charged events. In global amnesia even knowledge of personal identity and past life are lost. These gross symptoms are inconsistent with the good preservation of intellect and other cognitive functions, and an organic cause of such severe symptomatology would be accompanied by a change in the level of consciousness. Often patients with hysterical amnesia may be able to retain new information despite the global amnesia, and this should arouse suspicion; for example, they may be able to look around a room and recognise that they are in a hospital; they may deny that an event has happened while simultaneously insisting they have amnesia for the period in question. Sometimes a relative may help to confirm the diagnosis.

In *fugue states* the patient not only loses his memory but undertakes complicated actions such as leaving home and travelling from one place to another. Although the actions take place in clear consciousness and the person is able to obtain money, buy tickets, enjoy conversation, etc., during the episode, he may be surprised to find himself in a strange place, not knowing where he is, and present at a police station or hospital suffering from amnesia. Once again the distinguishing features of hysterical amnesia should be looked for and must be differentiated from lying or malingering (see p. 182).

Fugue states may also occur in depression, epilepsy, alcoholism and after head injury, and these should be considered in the differential diagnosis. Sometimes only inpatient observation will reveal the true diagnosis, perhaps only after contact has been made with relatives who can provide the necessary information.

Conversion symptoms

Conversion symptoms are motor, sensory or visceral. Motor symptoms include fits, tremors, faints, paralysis of one or more limbs, difficulty in walking and aphonia. Sensory symptoms include anaesthesia, paraesthesia, pain, blindness and deafness. Visceral symptoms include hysterical vomiting and urinary retention. Gross conversion symptoms such as paralysis appear to be less frequent now than at the turn of the century.

Conversion symptoms show some typical characteristics, and if hysteria is suspected the following clinical features may help to make a positive diagnosis:

(1) The physical symptoms do not correspond in nature and extent with any known somatic illness but with a false idea of illness in the patient's mind.

(2) The physical signs which one would expect to accompany an organically determined symptom are not found. For example, an hysterical aphonia will not be accompanied by paralysis of the vocal chords, and the patient may be able to cough or hum; an area of anaesthesia follows no known nerve distribution; or a paralysis shows no muscle wasting (except in chronic disuse), reflex changes or abnormal plantar responses.

(3) The patient may exaggerate or dramatise the symptoms. This is especially clear in disorders of gait, in which the walk may take bizarre forms and bear no resemblance to the patterns found in neurological disorders.

(4) The severity of the symptoms is not always matched by appropriate concern and the patient's affect may be calm and bland. This is known as *belle indifférence*. It is due to the fact that the underlying unconscious conflict which is threatening to become conscious has been converted into the physical symptom so that the anxiety originally associated with the conflict has declined or disappeared.

(5) The symptom may represent the underlying conflict in a *symbolic* manner. For example, a paralysis of the right arm may represent an unconscious conflict between wanting to but being afraid of hitting someone; or aphonia may represent a conflict between wanting to shout at someone but feeling frightened and guilty of wanting to do so.

(6) A history of a precipitating threatening situation may be elicited from the patient or a relative, e.g. a sexual assault or encounter, or a breakdown of a close relationship. Sometimes these events will have been completely repressed but may be brought back into consciousness by analytical psychotherapy, hypnosis or abreaction (see p. 182).

Despite these positive features, hysterical conversion symptoms put the doctor in a dilemma. He is rightly afraid of missing some organic complaint, yet knows that excessive or repeated physical investigations may focus the patient's attention more firmly on his symptoms. A middle course is probably best: as full a physical examination as the symptoms warrant should be combined with a full psychiatric assessment.

Slater (1965) followed up a group of patients diagnosed as suffering from hysteria and found that 60 per cent later developed organic disease.

This study was based on a group of patients who had been referred to a specialist hospital for patients with neurological disorders. Such a group is bound to be highly selective and differs markedly from other patients with hysterical symptoms seen in general practice and elsewhere, where hysteria in the absence of organic disease is much more common. Slater, however, also found that among the remaining 40 per cent, some, mainly younger patients, had conversion symptoms and did not develop organic disease. The diagnosis of hysteria should therefore rarely be made for the first time in any patient over the age of thirty-five. After this age the possibility of an associated organic condition such as dementia or a cerebral tumour should be seriously considered even if positive features of hysteria are also present.

The picture is further complicated by the fact that patients with well-established hysterical conversion symptoms may, of course, also develop an organic illness, and thus an incipient carcinoma or other serious disease may be missed. Conversely hysterical symptoms may also arise as a functional complication of an organic disease; for example, a patient who has epilepsy may also have hysterical fits. The chances of the development of organic disease going unrecognised will be less if any marked change in the nature of the patient's symptoms is taken as an indication for further psychological and physical investigation.

Once a diagnosis of hysteria has been made, further questions must be asked: why did these symptoms occur when they did? Will the patient be happier without them, or better with them? Will he be able to cope with the underlying repressed emotional conflicts if they are brought back into consciousness, or is he likely to become depressed or suicidal? In that case might it be safer not to explore the underlying psychopathology or treat his hysterical symptoms? What effect are the symptoms having on other people?

The doctor must also take notice of his own reactions to the patient. Hysterical behaviour may make him feel helpless and angry, and hence less objective and inclined to criticise. No doubt some misconceptions also arise in this way. One misconception is that hysteria is the same as malingering. In fact *malingering* is the conscious simulation of an illness which the individual knows is not present; hysteria is unconscious and the patient believes he is ill. In some patients hysteria and malingering may of course co-exist; they are hard to separate, especially if either or both are superimposed on an organic ailment or follow an injury, e.g. in a compensation neurosis (see p. 183). The distinguishing features between malingering and hysteria are discussed later in this chapter (see p. 182).

Epidemic hysteria

This remarkable phenomenon is observed in all cultures. It occurs most often in close-knit communities such as schools, colleges, nurses' homes and religious communities. Outbreaks appear to have become more common and certain features suggest the diagnosis. Girls or young women are most commonly affected, and the 'illness' tends to start in the younger age group (twelve to fifteen). It may follow community apprehension about an illness such as poliomyelitis or worry about forthcoming examinations. College staff and associated adults such as parents or teachers are rarely affected.

Symptoms often include abdominal pain, faintness, dizziness, nausea, headache and weakness, and their severity outweighs any abnormal physical signs. Usually a single vulnerable girl is affected first and other girls then succumb to similar symptoms, often as a result of seeing other affected children. Inevitably the spread of symptoms causes alarm and the outbreak may be explosive. For example, a sixteen-year-old girl, a member of a group of drum majorettes, fainted during a march in Newcastle. A few minutes later six other girls complained of dizziness and abdominal pain. Shortly afterwards a large number of girls clutched their abdomens and started crying. The march was abandoned and all the children were taken to three different hospitals. As soon as the children were separated the symptoms subsided. No physical cause, such as food poisoning, was found for the symptoms despite zealous investigation (Smith and Eastham 1973).

Treatment involves firm reassurance regarding the nature of the problem; if this fails more drastic action has to be taken, such as closing a school.

The Ganser syndrome

This is a rare condition first described by Ganser (1898), characterised by the presence of hysterical symptoms, an apparent disturbance of consciousness, hallucinatory, usually visual, experiences, and the giving of absurd or approximate answers. For example, a patient was asked, 'How many legs has a horse?' His answer was 'Three.' When asked, 'How many legs has an elephant?', his answer was 'Five.' These approximate answers indicate that the patient has understood the question, but the answers are striking in their absurdity. The condition is usually followed by an amnesia for the whole episode. While a few cases may be due to organic brain dysfunction or psychotic thought disorder, it is probable that Ganser's syndrome has a complex psychogenic basis, similar to that found in hysteria. Some cases occur in prisoners who may be suspected of simulating madness. Lack of understanding should not lead to an assumption that the syndrome is a result of malingering if the nature and consistency of the clinical picture is more suggestive of an hysterical condition. The condition and its management have been discussed by Carney *et al.* (1987).

Multiple personality

Multiple personality is probably related to fugue states (see p. 176). A sudden unconscious switch occurs between two or more alternative personalities as a result of dissociation. Neither personality 'knows' the other, and they tend to differ markedly in their behaviour, attitudes, abilities and social functioning. A remarkable example is described by Schreiber (1975) in her book *Sybil*, in which a patient has no fewer than sixteen personalities. This book describes the psychoanalytic treatment of the case and is recommended to anyone interested in the condition.

Briquet's syndrome (St Louis hysteria)

This syndrome was originally described by Briquet in 1859 and resurrected by psychiatrists in St Louis (Purtell *et al.* 1951). Patients are usually female and the condition starts below thirty years of age. They complain of long-standing multiple somatic symptoms, which are described in dramatic terms and affect almost any part of the body. Sexual and gynaecological complaints are common, and surgical procedures are often performed despite the absence of organic pathology. The women are often highly manipulative and refuse to consider psychological explanations. They continue to consult doctors for many years without getting relief. The diagnosis is more often made in the USA than the UK.

Treatment of hysterical disorders

The aim of treatment of hysterical disorders is to remove the symptoms and bring about changes in the patient's personality so that he learns to experience and express his problems directly instead of developing symptoms as an indirect means of communication. Sometimes, however, this may be impossible or even unwise as the underlying repressed emotional conflicts may be so severe that treatment leads to depression or suicide. Furthermore the secondary gain may be so great that the patient is unwilling to lose his symptoms. The following treatment methods should all be considered and adapted to the personality and motivation of the patient. A combination of methods may be required.

Psychotherapy

The first step in treatment is to help the patient understand his symptoms in terms of his relations with others; only later will he begin to understand the meaning of his symptoms in terms of his own personality and inner conflict. This early stage of treatment is often unsuccessful as the patient may lack motivation and insist his illness is of physical rather than psychological origin. In that case he may refuse psychotherapy or, if an outpatient, stop coming after a few sessions. Whatever the attitude of the patient, it is wise for the therapist not to focus on the physical symptoms but direct attention towards interpersonal and intrapsychic problems. If the patient begins to respond to a psychotherapeutic approach, more long-term analytic psychotherapy, individual or group, may help to resolve his underlying conflicts and personality problems.

Marital and family therapy

After a full family and personal history has been taken it may become clear that other members of the family are perpetuating the patient's hysterical symptoms. In this case a marital or family approach may be helpful. For example, a female patient with an hysterical aphonia felt unable to go out without her husband as she could not speak to shopkeepers and other people. As a consequence her husband had stopped work and accompanied her everywhere. He seemed quite happy about this despite having little conversation at home and having to interrupt his successful career. Marital therapy, combined with speech therapy for the wife, gradually helped disentangle the husband's involvement, and eventually the patient ventured out on her own and began to recover her voice. In this case the husband's own compliant character was perpetuating the patient's symtoms. Of course marital treatment may put the marriage in jeopardy, and occasionally this risk outweighs any potential benefit.

Reassurance and support

A patient may be reassured that he is not seriously ill. If possible a simple explanation of the symptoms should be given accompanied by a pronouncement about an optimistic prognosis. Part of the explanation should be couched in terms of the patient's emotional difficulties or life stresses. For example, a patient who has a paralysed arm and also has marital difficulties may be reassured there is nothing seriously wrong with her arm and that the muscle weakness she experiences is occurring because of emotional upset about her marital difficulties. This may encourage further ventilation of her emotional problems. If the patient questions this simple explanation the doctor may acknowledge that, although the process linking the emotional upset and the physical symptoms is not fully understood, the association is well known. He may then reassure the patient that a few sessions of physiotherapy are all that is required for treatment. This will introduce an element of suggestion. Suggestion is only likely to be effective if perpetuating factors, in this case the marital difficulties, are also dealt with simultaneously. Regular encouragement and support are essential even if simple physical treatments such as physiotherapy are used as an adjunct.

Abreaction

This may be used if the patient is suffering from total or partial amnesia. Hypnosis or a short-acting barbiturate such as methohexitone sodium or amylobarbitone, or a tranquilliser like diazepam is used to lower the patient's state of consciousness in an attempt to facilitate the return and expression of repressed memories and their associated emotions. This may release great anxiety and depression which require further care and treatment.

Drugs and behavioural treatments

There is little place for either of these methods in hysteria and its associated syndromes.

Prognosis

It is difficult to give an overall prognosis for the hysterical disorders in view of their heterogeneity. Epidemic hysteria tends to resolve as rapidly as it develops, but the other disorders are difficult to treat and their outcome probably depends more on the underlying personality, the amount of secondary gain and the environmental circumstances of the patient than on treatment. Briquet's syndrome tends to have an unfavourable outcome, and this perhaps reflects the severity of the underlying personality disorder found in these patients. Conversion symptoms seem to have a better prognosis; some studies (Ljungberg 1957) have reported an 80 per cent recovery rate within a year of the onset of symptoms in patients without severe underlying personality disorder and only transient precipitating life events. In other cases the symptoms may persist for years or indefinitely.

Distinguishing between malingering and hysteria

The distinction between malingering and hysteria can be very difficult; it may only be possible when adequate information is obtained from relatives or other informants. It is worth noting that malingering is a rare condition; if it is suspected, think again!

The following clinical features may help to distinguish malingering from hysteria:

(1) A malingerer is more commonly anxious, attempts to avoid inconsistencies and becomes angry or irritable when these are pointed out to him. In hysteria any inconsistencies are often gross, and when they are pointed out to the patient the reaction may be one of indifference.

(2) Hysterical patients accept suggestions and may consider them, while the malingerer tends to reject suggestions and fails to cooperate in any enquiry.

(3) A malingerer may have a markedly abnormal personality as evidenced by a history of self-mutilation or drug abuse.

(4) Malingering is more likely to arise when the patient feels trapped in an obviously threatening situation, e.g. in the armed forces during wartime or in prison.

Despite these differences misdiagnosis is common. The best known example of malingering, to be distinguished from hysteria, is Munchhausen's syndrome. This will be briefly described here as it is well known to all medical students and doctors despite its rarity.

Munchhausen's syndrome

Patients with Munchhausen's syndrome, described by Asher (1951), usually present themselves in the casualty department simulating an acute illness like renal colic or an acute abdomen supported by a dramatic history, just plausible and perhaps partly based on truth; this leads to extensive investigation and sometimes to surgery. They tend to move from hospital to hospital, creating first interest, then suspicion and annoyance, and finally exposure and triumph on the part of the doctor. This may lead to the patient being discharged with ignominy but with the reasons for his complaints still undiscovered and his emotional needs unsatisfied. The patient usually has no wish to talk about his psychological difficulties; instead he appears to enjoy the sheer pleasure of a war with doctors, and the syndrome then becomes a way of life. In other cases there is considerable misery and isolation on the part of the patient and frustration on that of the doctor; this might in a few cases have been prevented by an earlier effort to understand its psychological basis. The patient, however, usually resists any attempt to discuss possible psychological reasons for his behaviour and refuses to accept help. These patients are most commonly men; they go to extreme lengths to imitate illness, and it is likely that the syndrome is part of a severe personality disorder.

COMPENSATION NEUROSIS

This condition is rare. The term is only used when a patient complains of intractable mental and physical symptoms following an accident which resulted in a claim for compensation. A similar syndrome may occur in the absence of a claim for compensation and is known as post-traumatic neurosis. The syndrome is most commonly seen following an accident in which the patient considers another party, e.g. his employers, a public company such as the railway, or the council, to be responsible. It is also seen in patients whose pension depends on regular review of the consequences of their injury. It may follow a head injury (see p. 274), although any part of the body can be involved.

The most common physical symptoms are dizziness, headache and loss of energy. Mental changes such as irritability, intolerance of noise, anxiety and depression are equally common. It may be difficult to distinguish between the development of neurotic symptoms and the continuation of organically based symptoms; in some cases both may be present. Trimble (1981) has reviewed the disorder.

Miller (1961) a neurologist, reviewed 200 cases which followed a head injury and were specifically referred for medico-legal examination. He found that the development of 'indubitably neurotic complaints' was inversely related to the severity of the injury. Unskilled workers formed the largest proportion of this group and industrial accidents were twice as common as road accidents. He considered that compensation neurosis was often a result of conscious simulation of symptoms or malingering, especially as the symptoms often only improved when the compensation claim had been settled or dropped. In many cases, however, the patient's symptoms are more likely to be a result of unconscious processes as in the other neuroses. In cases following a head injury organic changes in the brain may also play a part, especially in the early stages after the injury (Lishman 1988) (see also p. 274).

Treatment of the condition is difficult. Severe psychiatric problems such as depression should be treated in their own right. However, in the vast majority of cases the patient will require long-term support. Every effort should be made to have any claim for compensation settled as soon as possible, as this may help recovery. Patients who are young or middle-aged are said to do well, while elderly unskilled men with a previously good employment record do badly.

HYPOCHONDRIASIS

Hypochondriasis shows all the features of worrying; a worry is a series of unpleasant thoughts which are beyond voluntary control and out of proportion to the subject matter. Hypochondriasis is a worry specifically concerned with the possibility of disease or malfunction of parts of the body. Of course physical illness may co-exist with hypochondriasis, but in that case the worry or preoccupation with illness is out of proportion and unresponsive to reassurance. The patient has insight into the fact that his constant anxiety about physical illness is abnormal or excessive, but he is unable to control it. Hypochondriasis must not be confused with psychosomatic illness in which an organic illness is caused or influenced by the psychological state of the individual (see Chapter 37).

Clinical features

Hypochondriacal symptoms may take many forms, but the commonest symptom is preoccupation with pain. The pain tends to be poorly localised, diffuse, not clearly described and linked with many other physical complaints. Preoccupation with heart disease, chest disease, respiratory symptoms and gastrointestinal disturbance are common.

Differential diagnosis

Hypochondriasis can be secondary to depression and anxiety, and these conditions should be excluded before a treatment plan is made. More often it presents as a primary disorder associated with an anxious personality and stresses within the family.

Hypochondriasis must also be distinguished from hypochondriacal delusions which occur in psychotic depression, schizophrenia and dysmorphophobia (see p. 258).

Aetiology and prognosis

The cause of hypochondriasis is uncertain. There is evidence that it is common in men of low socio-economic class, and it is possible that it occurs in people who are unable to communicate their difficulties in any other way. Clinically there appears to be a psychological withdrawal from the outside world and greater investment in 'the self', and psychoanalysts have tended to view this neurosis as related to the narcissistic disorders. The prognosis is poor even with long-term psychotherapy.

Treatment

If the condition is secondary to anxiety or depression, treatment is directed towards the primary illness. Patients suffering from primary hypochondriasis are best treated with supportive or analytic psychotherapy after a full explanation that no organic disease is present. Attention should be directed away from the physical complaints and towards the rest of the patient's life. It is important not to repeat examinations or investigations once the diagnosis has been established. Drugs and other treatments are contra-indicated.

DEPERSONALISATION SYNDROME

Depersonalisation and derealisation (see p. 125) occur in anxiety neurosis, depression and other disorders, e.g. temporal lobe epilepsy, and may, for brief periods, appear in normal people under stress. However depersonalisation occasionally presents as a primary disorder, and then it is called depersonalisation neurosis or depersonalisation syndrome. A depersonalisation neurosis is defined as 'an unpleasant state of disturbed perception in which external objects or parts of the body are experienced as changed in their quality, unreal, remote, or automatised' (ICD-9). Insight is retained and the subjectivity of the experience is recognised by the patient. Anxiety and other symptoms may be absent.

The disorder is said to be commonest among young females who complain of an inability to feel normal emotions such as pleasure, dislike, love and hate. There is often an associated sense of being cut off from other people, and the whole experience is distressing and painful.

Most cases are secondary to an anxiety neurosis or depression, and the treatment and prognosis is then that of the primary condition. The prognosis of depersonalisation neurosis itself is poor and most cases persist for many years with only short periods of relief. Treatment is difficult and patients are best helped by supportive psychotherapy and encouragement to lead a normal life.

NEURASTHENIA

This condition, originally described by Beard (1880), still retains a place in the International Classification of Diseases but its use has diminished as doubts about its validity have increased. It is characterised by overwhelming fatigue and muscle weakness associated with sleeplessness, appetite loss, irritability and poor concentration. These symptoms are so common in other disorders such as depression and anxiety that it is difficult to distinguish neurasthenia as a distinct disorder. Furthermore such symptoms are more likely to present to the physician than the psychiatrist, and this has led to attempts to find muscle abnormalities such as defective mitochondria or to ascribe the origin of the symptoms to some organic cerebral disorder such as encephalitis. Overall, the diagnosis is best avoided, but attempts should be made to look for possible underlying psychological problems that could account for the symptoms.

FURTHER READING

Krohn, A. (1978). *Hysteria: the elusive neurosis. Psychological Issues*, Monograph 45/46. International Universities Press, Inc., New York.

Marks, I.M. (1987). *Fears, Phobias and Rituals*. OUP, Oxford.

Mathews, A.M., Gelder, M.G. and Johnston, D.W. (1981). *Agoraphobia: nature and treatment*. Tavistock, London.

Merskey, H. (1983). *Does Hysteria Still Exist?* SK&F Publications, vol. 2, no. 4. Smith Kline & French Laboratories, Welwyn Garden City.

Nemiah, J.C. (1985). 'Anxiety states (anxiety neuroses)' in Kaplan, H.I. and Sadock, B.J., *Comprehensive Textbook of Psychiatry*, 4th ed., vol. 1, 883-894. Williams & Wilkins, Baltimore/London.

Nemiah, J.C. (1985). 'Obsessive-compulsive disorder (Obsessive-compulsive neurosis)' in Kaplan, H.I. and Sadock, B.J., *Comprehensive Textbook of Psychiatry*, 4th ed., vol. 1, 904-917. Williams & Wilkins, Baltimore/London.

Rycroft, C. (1983). *Anxiety and Neurosis*. Allen Lane, London.

17

Disasters and the Post-Traumatic Stress Disorder

DISASTERS

Major disasters and their catastrophic effects have been known throughout the history of mankind. They usually take place suddenly and unexpectedly and often involve large numbers of people or whole communities, leading to loss of life, serious injuries and sometimes also loss of home and property. They can, however, develop more slowly, e.g. during famines, or affect only one or a small number of individuals. What such disasters have in common is that they are so catastrophic and overwhelming that they go beyond anything the individuals involved would normally have to cope with, so that their psychological capacity to function is stretched beyond their limits of endurance. Kinston and Rosser (1974) have reviewed some of the earlier literature on the mental and physical effects of disasters.

Some disasters are due to natural events, e.g. fires, earthquakes, floods, volcanic eruptions, drought or famine, others are due to diseases, and yet others are man-made, e.g. wars, major accidents, fires and industrial disasters such as leakage of nuclear materials.

The bombing of Hiroshima and Nagasaki by the atomic bomb and the effects on the survivors, the Hibakusha, have been vividly described by Lifton (1967). The deaths and suffering during trench warfare in the First World War have been imaginatively recounted in a novel, *Strange Meeting*, by Susan Hill (1971). The effects of the bombing of civilian populations during the Second World War serve as another example. Many Vietnam veterans have been found to suffer from the after-effects of their overwhelming experiences during the war.

In 1966 the waste from a giant tip above the Welsh mining village of Aberfan suddenly collapsed and hit the village school, killing 116 schoolchildren. Almost every family in the village was bereaved and the effect on all the inhabitants persisted for months and even years (Lacey 1972). The sudden collapse in 1972 of the Buffalo Creek dam in West Virginia led to torrential floods which carried with them whole communities, houses and all their inhabitants. Both this disaster and that at Aberfan were made all the worse in the eyes of the survivors because in each case the disaster could have been prevented if only proper precautions had been taken in time.

The fire in the Cocoanut Grove night club in Boston in 1942 caused many deaths and severe burns among young people. The victims were taken to the Massachusetts General Hospital. Cobb and Lindemann (1943) and Lindemann (1944) have described the grief reactions and other psychiatric effects among the survivors and relatives whom they saw there and later followed up. The recent deaths by drowning of 193 people when the channel ferry Herald of Free Enterprise suddenly capsized outside Zeebrugge in March 1987, the deaths of 31 people during the fire at the Kings Cross Underground Station in London in November 1987, the devastating earthquake in Armenia and the destruction of the Pan Am jet above Lockerbie in 1988 remain very much in people's minds today.

The literature on the effects of disasters and how to provide the help that is needed has been reviewed by Raphael (1986). She describes the effects of Bush fires in Australia, including the Ash Wednesday fire which threatened and destroyed some of the suburbs of Adelaide, and also discusses some of the factors that have helped people survive such long-drawn-out disasters as the Holocaust.

Behaviour during the disaster

If the disaster starts suddenly and unexpectedly, as is often the case, those involved experience intense fear, but panic is rare. Fear of death and an intense wish to escape usually predominate. Individuals become alert and hypervigilant, searching for a way out, protecting themselves with their hands, crouching and holding on to others. Panic is more likely to ensue when people are unsure what is happening and become confused or isolated. Often they hold on to family members, e.g. parents to their children, in a desperate attempt to protect them. Some heroically try to save others although this applies more often to rescuers when they reach the scene than to the victims.

The flight itself can be most distressing. Some of the survivors of the recent Kings Cross fire in London who were familiar with the underground station and tried to find the exits through dense smoke and fire knew that they were scrambling over the bodies of injured or dying people in order to escape.

Some victims become helpless, stunned and apathetic as a result of the severe shock and confusion, so that they wander around dazed and unable to help themselves, the so-called 'disaster syndrome', and this may persist for hours or even days if they are brought to safety.

Immediate after-effects

Those who have escaped death, including some who may be seriously injured, are likely to remain preoccupied for some time with how near to dying they have been. They keep going over the events wondering how they managed to survive, but perhaps feeling guilty and deeply distressed that others close to them, say their parents, children, husband or wife, have died. In the days following the disaster survivors may re-experience the trauma by having *flashbacks* which are intrusive, uncontrollable and disturbing. This may happen when awake, or during sleep as dreams or nightmares. These flashbacks, sometimes accompanied by panic, may be triggered by stimuli that are reminiscent of the disaster, e.g. a sudden noise or an explosion, the screeching of brakes, the smell of burning or the sound of running water. As a result some survivors attempt to avoid exposure to anything that might remind them of the disaster, and become withdrawn and isolated.

Others may experience a sense of vulnerability and remain frightened of a similar event happening again, or they may anticipate new dangers. General irritability and anger at the senselessness of the disaster are common, and may be directed at people's lack of understanding or at the inefficiency and failure of a system that went so tragically wrong.

It is important to note that not only the victims but also the rescuers may be affected, and of course the relatives of some of the victims who died. For example, having to identify the mutilated body of a relative can be extremely stressful. So may the waiting period when relatives do not yet know whether someone close to them has died in the disaster, or perhaps the fact that his body has never been found.

POST-TRAUMATIC STRESS DISORDER

While professionals like social workers, psychologists and counsellors, as well as other volunteers, are often involved in helping victims in the early stages after a disaster, psychiatrists are more often called in later to help those who have symptoms for longer periods. In an attempt to classify these after-effects psychiatrists have coined the term post-traumatic stress disorder (PTSD), which is now included in the DSM-III. The literature on PTSD has been reviewed by Andreasen (1985). In summary, the criteria for a diagnosis of PTSD laid down by the DSM-III, and recently revised in DSM-III-R, include the following:

(1) The person has experienced a stressful event that is outside the range of usual human experience and would be markedly distressing to almost anyone.

(2) The event is being re-experienced in vivid dreams, intrusive recollections and flashbacks, usually in response to some triggering stimulus. Illusions and short-lived hallucinatory experiences may also occur.

(3) The person avoids stimuli which could be reminiscent of the disaster, leading to numbness, unresponsiveness and withdrawal.

(4) The person experiences increased arousal which was not present before the event. This includes difficulty in going to sleep or staying asleep; irritability or outbursts of anger; difficulty in concentrating;

hypervigilance and an exaggerated startle response. Guilt about survival and memory impairment may also be present.

The DSM-III-R (American Psychiatric Association 1987) also distinguishes between an acute PTSD of early onset that clears up within six months of the traumatic event and the chronic syndrome whose onset may be delayed and from which the person may never fully recover.

While such definitions are useful for purposes of psychiatric classification they contribute little to our understanding of the suffering and experience of the individual victims. Moreover the PTSD is often associated with other symptoms, e.g. those of depression and of grief reactions if the survivor has lost relatives or friends in the disaster, or lost his family, his home, his property and perhaps his physical health as the result of injuries.

Management

Immediately after the disaster the survivors need a great deal of physical, psychological and social care. Increasingly health-care professionals are organising bodies of helpers who can be called upon to go and help at the site of the disaster at the earliest possible moment. Their help will be needed not only by the survivors but also by some of those who were involved in the rescue operations and by relatives of the victims.

Those who are still shocked and apathetic need comfort and physical care, followed by psychological support to help them recover and get in touch with their feelings. Others may be acutely distressed, anxious and confused and need to be given every opportunity to talk freely to a helper about what happened to them, what they now feel about themselves, and perhaps about those who they fear have died in the disaster. If victims, relatives and rescuers can thus be encouraged on several occasions to share their feelings early on with a helper whom they are getting to know and whom they can trust, this may not only bring much relief at the time but also prevent the development of persistent suffering later on.

Helpers may also need to accompany relatives when asked to identify the body of someone they have lost, or when they first see someone close to them who is severely injured and likely to die. Such work can be extremely stressful for the helpers, and they in turn may need support and help from other professionals, individually or in groups.

During the first few days some survivors may need sedatives to help them sleep, and those who are injured and in pain, e.g. from severe burns, need strong and regular analgesics. Thereafter the victims and relatives should gradually be encouraged to cope with their problems of readjustment and grief while being given all the practical and psychological support they still need.

Treatment of the various manifestations of the PTSD usually involves counselling, support and psychotherapy. Tranquillisers and sedatives may be needed for short periods. Depressive symptoms may require treatment with antidepressants. Some of the victims may be helped by psychotherapy during which they can reveal the intensity of their suffering and sometimes also much earlier memories which are being re-experienced following the disaster.

FURTHER READING

Lifton, R.J. (1967). *Death in Life: survivors of Hiroshima*. Random House, New York.

Raphael, B. (1986). *When Disaster Strikes*. Hutchinson, London.

Wolfenstein, M. (1957). *Disaster: a psychological essay*. Glencoe Free Press, New York.

18

Affective Disorders

Affective disorders are disorders of mood. They are extremely common and include all forms of depression and mania. Anxiety states used to be included but are now usually grouped with the other psychoneurotic disorders (see p. 157).

CLASSIFICATION

The affective disorders are best considered under two main headings: depression and mania. Depressive illnesses are dominated by a depressed mood, mania by an elated mood or elation. There is general agreement about this basic subdivision, but considerable controversy exists about further subdivisions, especially of the depressive disorders (Kendell 1976). Aubrey Lewis (1934) discussed the manifestations and classification of severe depression, then still called melancholia, and pointed out that both constitutional and environmental factors play a part in most cases of depression.

Depressive illnesses are often subdivided either according to their supposed aetiology, or according to their symptomatology. From an *aetiological* point of view it is common practice, especially in the UK, to talk of either *reactive* or *endogenous depression*. In the former, the depressive illness follows readily identifiable, stressful life events, usually a loss like a bereavement, separation or disappointment to which the patient reacts by getting depressed. In endogenous depression the illness is said to appear in the absence of external precipitating events, as the result of biological changes. The difficulty with this subdivision is that, in patients with a reactive depression, constitutional factors usually also play some part, while in endogenous depression preceding life events are now known often to be present as well (Paykel 1974; Brown and Harris 1978). The distinction in terms of aetiology is therefore often far from clear-cut. In spite of this, the categories of reactive and endogenous depression remain widely used in the UK. In clinical practice it is preferable to ask oneself, in each patient with a depressive illness, to what extent external and to what extent endogenous factors – genetic, biochemical or constitutional – have contributed to the illness.

Looked at from the *symptomatic* point of view, depressive illnesses are subdivided into *psychotic* and *neurotic depression*. This is further complicated by the fact that the term psychotic depression tends to be used in at least two different ways. Strictly speaking it should refer to an impaired sense of reality and the presence of delusions or hallucinations, as opposed to neurotic depression where these are absent by definition. However the term psychotic depression is often used to describe a depressive illness in which the depressed mood is persistent and severe, and in which there are marked biological symptoms, such as early morning waking, loss of appetite and loss of weight, loss of libido and diurnal variations of mood, even when the sense of reality is maintained. In neurotic depression both the depressive and biological symptoms are usually less severe, and the latter may be absent or take a different form, e.g. the patient may overeat or sleep longer than usual (see p. 171).

A further difficulty arises from the fact that the subdivision in terms of supposed aetiology – endogenous versus reactive – does not always coincide with the subdivision in terms of symptomatology – psychotic versus neurotic. In general, an endogenous depression is more often psychotic in nature so that the terms endogenous and psychotic are often used interchangeably; and a reactive depression is usually less severe and neurotic in nature so that the terms reactive and neurotic depression also tend to be used interchangeably. The clinical descriptions of endogenous depression in this chapter and reactive (neurotic) depression in Chapter 16 illustrate this further.

Because of these problems of classification, attempts have been made to use statistical analyses to decide whether or not the endogenous and reactive types of depression do in fact constitute separate categories. The findings of Kiloh and Garside (1963) and Carney *et al.* (1965) in Newcastle supported the existence of two separate disease entities, while Kendell (1968) and Kendell and Gourlay (1970) found that the categories formed a continuum in their groups of patients. The controversy has therefore not been resolved.

A different classification, proposed by the St Louis group in the USA (Spitzer *et al.* 1978), divides depressive illnesses into *primary* and *secondary*, depending on whether or not the depressive illness is the result of some other psychiatric or physical disorder. This subdivision is useful in research but of little clinical value and has not thrown any light on the problems surrounding the endogenous versus reactive classification.

Some patients with depressive illnesses of the endogenous type also have episodes of mania. This led Kraepelin (1913a) to introduce the term *manic-depressive psychosis*, a diagnosis which has remained important within the group of affective disorders and will be considered later in this chapter (see pp. 206-11). Nowadays, following the work of Leonhard (1979, first published in 1961) and Perris (1966), patients who suffer from both depressive and manic episodes at different times in their lives are said to be suffering from the circular or *bipolar* type of manic-depressive psychosis. Those patients who have recurrent depressive episodes only are said to have *unipolar depression*. Patients who have recurrent episodes of mania used to be classified as suffering from unipolar mania, but it is now recognised that patients with recurrent mania will almost always eventually develop a depressive illness; they are therefore now usually classified in the bipolar group of manic-depressive psychosis (Winokur *et al*. 1969). This division of the affective disorders into unipolar and bipolar is now widely accepted in clinical practice.

AETIOLOGY

No one aetiological theory can account for all affective illnesses and their multifaceted manifestations. All or any of the hypotheses discussed below may be relevant. The clinician should keep this considerable range of causative possibilities in mind in the assessment of each individual patient and avoid too narrow a preconception which, in the present state of knowledge, will limit has ability to help the patient. Whybrow *et al*. (1984) in a detailed, historical review have put forward the view that mood disorders can best be understood by integrating psychodynamic, biological, social and behavioural approaches.

The following account is mainly concerned with the aetiology of endogenous depression and manic-depressive psychosis.

Genetic factors

Family studies have shown that close relatives, i.e. children, siblings, or parents, of a patient with endogenous depression have an increased incidence of affective disorders.

The relatives of patients with bipolar affective illness are likely to suffer from a bipolar illness, should they develop an affective disorder. Bipolar patients thus appear to pass on a specific vulnerability to the development of a bipolar disorder. Patients with a unipolar depressive illness pass on a vulnerability to affective illness, but this may be either unipolar or bipolar (Bertelsen *et al*. 1977).

Recent molecular genetic studies have thrown new light on the genetic predisposition to bipolar affective disorders (manic-depressive psychosis). Egeland *et al*. (1987) studied families with bipolar affective disorders in the Old Order Amish population, a closed, genetically isolated community in Pennsylvania. Genetic linkage studies using recombinant DNA techniques have led to the localisation of a dominant gene on chromosome 11, which was linked with a strong predisposition to bipolar affective illness in the families they studied. It should be noted, however, that similar genetic studies in Iceland have not shown this linkage between bipolar affective illness and abnormalities on chromosome 11; studies in Israel have suggested that in some families with bipolar affective illness the responsible gene may be situated on the X-chromosome. It seems that the gene may be localised on different chromosomes in different families (Baron *et al*. 1987; Robertson 1987).

Biochemical factors

The monoamine hypothesis

The monoamine hypothesis postulates that depression is associated with decreased activity of monoamine neurotransmitter substances at the synapses in certain, as yet not clearly identified, sites in the brain, while mania may be associated with increased monoamine activity. This hypothesis arose from the chance observation that when reserpine was given as a hypotensive agent to patients with hypertension some of them became depressed. In animal experiments reserpine was found to lower the concentration of monoamines in the brain. It was also found that certain antidepressant drugs, the monoamine oxidase inhibitors (MAOIs) raised the level of monoamines at the synapses by their inhibitory effect on the enzyme monoamine oxidase. Similarly, the tricyclic antidepressants were found to increase the monoamine level in the synaptic cleft by preventing their re-uptake by presynaptic neurones (see also p. 604).

A great deal of further research has been done since the monoamine hypothesis was first put forward by Schildkraut (1965). Some of the findings are inconclusive, and it is likely that in its original form the monoamine hypothesis of depression is oversimplified. This applies especially to its role in the aetiology of mania.

First, it is not yet clear which of the monoamine neurotransmitters – noradrenaline, 5-hydroxytryptamine (5-HT, serotonin) or dopamine – are involved, or whether depression results from a relative imbalance between the levels of two or more of these neurotransmitters. Present findings suggest that noradrenaline and 5-HT are more likely to be involved than dopamine. It has also been suggested that different clinical types of depression, e.g. endogenous or reactive, psychotic or neurotic, bipolar or unipolar, agitated or retarded, might be specifically correlated with decreased activity of one or other of these neurotransmitters. However, so far there is no convincing evidence that this is the case.

Another difficulty has arisen from the finding that some of the more recent antidepressants, e.g. the tetracyclic drug mianserin (see p. 606), have little effect on the re-uptake of noradrenaline or 5-HT by the presynaptic neurones. They appear instead to act on the receptors of the presynaptic neurones.

The monoamine hypothesis has also been extensively investigated by looking for direct evidence of abnormalities of the monoamines and their metabolites in the brain, or in the cerebrospinal fluid, blood or urine. The metabolite of 5-HT that has been studied is 5-hydroxyindole acetic acid (5-HIAA), that of noradrenaline is 3-methoxy-4-hydroxyphenylethylene glycol (MHPG) and that of dopamine is homovanillic acid (HVA). Some observers have reported reduced levels of some of these metabolites either in parts of the brain of depressed patients who had committed suicide, or in the cerebrospinal fluid, blood or urine of patients with depressive illnesses. Others have failed to do so and at present findings are inconclusive; this applies particularly to changes observed in the cerebrospinal fluid, blood or urine, as it is often unclear to what extent the changes observed reflect changes in brain metabolism or elsewhere.

Attempts have been made to treat depressed patients by administering precursors of monoamines. Levodopa, the precursor of dopamine, does not relieve depression but has precipitated the onset of a manic illness in some patients with a bipolar affective disorder. The administration of the aminoacid L-tryptophan, the precursor of 5-HT, has in some patients with depression enhanced the effectiveness of MAOIs or of the tricyclic antidepressant clomipramine. Coppen *et al.* (1967) have claimed that L-tryptophan on its own can also act as an antidepressant.

The present state of the monoamine hypothesis has been reviewed by Ashcroft (1982). One possibility is that reduced monoamine activity is one of several mechanisms associated with a depressed mood but not necessarily of primary aetiological significance, except in some patients with a bipolar affective illness.

Endocrine factors

Further evidence for a biochemical basis of affective disorders stems from the fact that some endocrine disorders, e.g. hypothyroidism, hyperparathyroidism and Cushing's disease can produce a prolonged affective illness, which may only respond when the underlying endocrine disorder is treated.

About half of the patients with endogenous depression are found to have increased secretion of cortisol and raised plasma cortisol levels. In normal subjects the plasma cortisol level falls during the afternoon and evening, whereas in depressed patients it remains high. Cortisol secretion can be suppressed in normal subjects by giving dexamethasone, a synthetic corticosteroid, 12 hours previously. About a third of depressed patients do not show this suppression of cortisol secretion when given dexamethasone. The significance of this finding is not yet clear, but failure to respond to the dexamethasone suppression test may be more common in patients with severe unipolar than other forms of depression.

Psychodynamic factors

In 1917 Freud turned his attention to depression and summarised his findings in *Mourning and Melancholia*. He pointed out that in both mourning and melancholia, now called depression, there was a 'profoundly painful dejection, cessation of interest in the outside world, loss of capacity to love and inhibition of all activity' as a result of loss. However, Freud believed that the two conditions could be distinguished. Patients with melancholia showed lower self-regard and greater ambivalence towards the lost person than patients in mourning. The low self-regard 'finds utterance in self-reproaches and self-revilings, and culminates in a delusional expectation of punishment'. These severe inner self-criticisms were thought to arise from an overdeveloped conscience or super-ego and were fuelled by ambivalence, i.e. the more the individual had hated the lost person, the more severe the self-accusations. In their most severe form, the inner self-reproaches may be projected and experienced as auditory hallucinations, coming from outside. In essence, melancholia was thought to be similar to psychotic depression, normal mourning more akin to neurotic depression.

These early views were later modified by Freud when he realised that the differences between mourning and melancholia (depression) were not so clear-cut. He suggested that normal mourning, as an adult, could only take place if an individual had developed a stable inner world, as a result of satisfactory development during childhood. Failing this, severe depression could take the place of normal mourning after the loss of a loved one. Freud also suggested that, in melancholia, the loss was not necessarily external, but could be an imagined or internal loss, say a loss of faith or identity.

Melanie Klein's concept of the depressive position (Klein 1952) and Winnicott's concept of the stage of concern (Winnicott 1963b) have contributed further to our understanding of the nature of depressive illnesses. These concepts have been described in Chapter 7 (see p. 70). In essence, if a child has learnt to relate to his mother – and later to others – as a whole person, to have concern for her and to tolerate his mixed feelings of love and hate without excessive guilt, he is more likely to cope with losses later in life without becoming depressed. Winnicott has pointed out that 'good-enough' mothering (see p. 66) helps a child to develop a stable, inner image of a mother who can survive his anger and destructiveness, who forgives and continues to love him. It is this stability which protects against depression following a loss or disappointment later in life. Failure to achieve this inner stability, either as the result of loss of or separation from his mother, or as the result of emotional deprivation in his relationship to her, leaves the child and future adult vulnerable to excessive guilt and depression following a loss. These theories have received some confirmation from recent epidemiological studies. For example, Brown and Harris (1978), studying a group of women in Camberwell, have shown that the loss of mother before the age of eleven is a vulnerability factor predisposing to depression.

Although these early childhood experiences are important in the development of both endogenous and reactive depression later in life, it remains unclear what particular psychological or biological, including genetic, factors will determine what kind of depression the individual patient is likely to develop.

Learned helplessness

From his experimental work on animals, Seligman (1975) has described a behavioural syndrome which he calls *learned helplessness*. This occurs when animals are placed in situations associated with some noxious stimuli, e.g. electric shocks, from which they cannot escape. They become withdrawn, retarded, reduce their food consumption and have disturbed sleep. He has suggested that learned helplessness in animals is the counterpart of depressive disorders in man, and that such helplessness may have aetiological significance in humans.

Cognitive theory

Beck (1967) has proposed a cognitive theory of depression. The suggestion is that gloomy, negative thoughts about oneself and the world are not secondary to the depressed mood but of primary aetiological significance. Beck suggests that people who habitually think in this way are more likely to become depressed following minor rejections and emotional trauma. However, there is as yet no evidence that these cognitive changes precede rather than follow the onset of the depressive illness.

Social factors

The onset of depression can be precipitated by life events, especially those associated with loss. Although this applies to all patients with reactive depression it is also true of many cases of endogenous depression (see p. 192).

As well as having a precipitating effect, life events also have a predisposing effect. As mentioned earlier, Brown and Harris (1978), in a study of depressed women, have demonstrated that loss of mother, by death or separation, before the age of eleven, makes an individual more susceptible to developing depression in later years. Brown also cites other vulnerability factors from his work among working-class women living in London. These include being unemployed outside the home, having young children to look after and the absence of a confiding relationship.

Physical illness

Not surprisingly, having an illness or developing a physical disability can lead to depression, but some illnesses, such as glandular fever and influenza, appear to have a particularly strong association with depression. Affective disorders can also be associated with neoplasms (see p. 278).

Seasonal Affective Disorder

The fact that the mood of an individual may change according to the season was noted by Kraepelin (1921) in relation to some manic-depressive patients. Recently groups of patients have been described who become depressed only during the winter months and recover spontaneously in the spring (Rosenthal *et al.* 1984; Thompson and Isaacs

1988). Their depression occurs regularly at this time and never in the summer months. These patients are said to suffer from Seasonal Affective Disorder (SAD). They become depressed, irritable, lethargic and withdrawn, and lose their normal sexual desire. In contrast to endogenous depression they sleep more, crave carbohydrate food and put on weight.

Some similarities between SAD in humans and hibernation in animals have led to the theory that the condition may result from a decrease in the length of daylight, the so-called *photoperiod*. In animals the effect of light on behaviour is diverse. For example, in deer a decrease in length of the day stimulates rutting behaviour, while in hamsters it induces weight gain, infertility and hibernation. These effects in animals are probably mediated via a pathway linking the retina, the hypothalamus and the pineal gland, which secretes melatonin. By altering the length of the photoperiod experimentally the behaviour of animals can be changed and the amount of melatonin secreted can be varied. In both humans and animals prolonging the photoperiod reduces the secretion. However, no abnormality of melatonin secretion has been found in patients with SAD (Murphy *et al.* 1988).

Despite this, it has been shown that patients with SAD improve if they are exposed to bright light for several hours, usually between 2 and 6 hours daily. Full-spectrum light is given from a fluorescent box. The patient sits about three feet away and looks at the light about every half minute. For light treatment to be effective looking at the light is essential. Treatment is equally effective if given in the middle of the day instead of the early morning or at night, so that it is not related to the duration of exposure to daylight (Thompson and Silverstone 1988). The possibility that light exposure acts as a placebo cannot be excluded. There is no evidence that it works by reducing secretion of melatonin in patients with SAD.

It should also be noted that some patients suffer from depression regularly but at times other than the winter months, e.g. each spring or summer. In these patients factors other than light exposure must therefore be responsible.

ENDOGENOUS DEPRESSION

Clinical features

The psychotic or endogenous type of depression often presents for the first time in mid-life, although it can start earlier. It is more common in women. There is often, but not invariably, a family history of depression.

When taking a careful history, particularly from a near relative, it is sometimes discovered that the patient has had undulating moods since early adulthood, with times of greater enthusiasm or productivity alternating with fallow periods of relative inertia. The term cyclothymia has been used to describe this, but there is no convincing evidence that cyclothymic personality disorders (see p. 332) necessarily predispose to affective illnesses.

The onset of a bout of endogenous depression may be precipitated by a significant life event and may develop over a matter of days or, more commonly, over a week or so.

The patient lacks his usual enthusiasm and retreats from normal activities. His demeanour becomes gloomy and morose and he sees little point in work or pleasurable activities. His sleep may be impaired even before the mood change is noted. Characteristically, the patient will wake up in the small hours full of worries and depressive thoughts. This is often the worst time of the day for him. He wakes with gloomy, restless despair about the disasters he feels will take place during the coming day. He feels lonely and ill-understood. As the depressive illness gathers momentum, so these feelings continue throughout the day. His appetite fails and he often eats because others insist, but with no relish at all. His weight falls rapidly and, as a result, his appearance changes markedly. He looks haunted and sad; even a contrived smile does little to modify this. His enjoyment of all aspects of living is decreased and his interest in sex subsides. His concentration is markedly impaired and he cannot work. Each attempt to focus his thoughts is foiled by intrusion of depressive thinking or by *hallucinations*. The patient will often complain of memory loss but, on close examination, this is seen to be the result of failure to concentrate rather than a loss of storage or recall. The patient often expresses self-blame, guilt and unworthiness. He may exaggerate minor misdemeanours or develop *delusions*. For example, he may believe that he is evil or has cancer or venereal disease and that he is an intolerable burden on others and on society. When these delusions are coupled with total despair about the future, suicidal thoughts and actions are common and should be specifically asked for (see p. 214).

There may be marked motor abnormalities. The patient may become increasingly slow in his movements; this is known as *motor retardation*. He may even become totally immobile, so-called *depressive stupor* (see p. 140). After recovery, the patient may recollect that, at the time, he felt as though he were dead to the world. Alternatively, the disorder of movement takes the form of agitation due to severe accompanying anxiety, so called *agitated depression*. This is particularly common in the elderly depressed patient. In this state the patient is unable to keep still. He will constantly pace about the room, wringing his hands or twisting his arms. If he tries to keep still, he almost immediately becomes restless and, once more, paces the room. This restlessness, coupled with anorexia, may lead to extreme emaciation. The speed of thinking and talking are similarly affected. In the retarded patient there is little or no spontaneity of speech, and responses to questions are very delayed, almost as though the questions had not been heard. The patient appears totally wrapped up in his own depressive world. The agitated patient may constantly repeat anxious self-derogatory statements, sometimes pleading for help and yet unable to bring himself to accept it. Interestingly enough, tearfulness and sadness are not inevitable correlates of severe depressive illness. Very often the patient wishes to cry but feels he cannot. He may experience an absence of feeling and say that he has no feeling of affection or love; this can be very hurtful to concerned relatives.

Many patients complain of physical symptoms and consider that it is the pain or discomfort which is causing their depression. Gastrointestinal disturbance, headache, migraine, tinnitus, back pain and weakness may all be part of the picture. It is important to carry out a physical examination and, if necessary, investigations to exclude organic disease. There then comes the difficult task of establishing a meaningful connection between the symptoms and the patient's mood. Sometimes the physical symptoms may have a symbolic meaning, but more often it seems as if the depressive illness lowers the threshold of pain or other bodily sensations so that hitherto minor discomforts are perceived as extreme. Sometimes physical symptoms, e.g. severe and uninterrupted *facial pain*, disappear completely after treatment with antidepressants; such symptoms are referred to as *depressive equivalents*. Patients often assume that a psychiatric diagnosis implies that they are imagining the symptoms. In fact psychogenic pain is just as real as pain due to organic disease, and it is important to explain this to the patient. The interaction can be complex. For example, prolonged tinnitus can produce profound depressive feelings, and the depression in turn can exacerbate the awareness of the tinnitus.

This description of the clinical features of episodes of endogenous depression, with the ever-present risk of suicide and the effects of the illness on other family members can be highlighted by considering the life of Virginia Woolf (1882-1941). Throughout her life she suffered from severe bouts of psychotic depression, the first of which occurred at the age of thirteen. The last, at the age of fifty-nine, ended in suicide by drowning. Throughout these years she continued to write her novels, finishing *Between the Acts* only a few weeks before the onset of her last bout of depression. Her husband Leonard Woolf took continuous care of her during all these recurrent illnesses, persuading her to eat, taking her to doctors, and constantly watching her to prevent yet another suicidal attempt, often feeling desperate at not knowing how to help her more. To quote Quentin Bell's biography (1972, vol. 2, p. 226):

On the morning of Friday 28th March, a bright, clear, cold day, Virginia went as usual to her studio room in the garden. There she wrote two letters, one for Leonard, one for Vanessa [her sister] – the two people she loved best. In both letters she explained that she was hearing voices, believed that she could never recover; she could not go on and spoil Leonard's life for him. Then she went back into the house and wrote again to Leonard:

Dearest
I feel certain I am going mad again. I feel we can't go through another of those terrible times. And I shan't recover this time. I begin to hear voices and I can't concentrate. So I am doing what seems the best thing to do. You have given me the greatest possible happiness ... If anyone could have saved me it would have been you. Everything has gone from me but the

certainty of your goodness. I can't go on spoiling your life any longer. I don't think two people could have been happier than we have been.

V.

She put this on the sitting-room mantelpiece and at about 11.30 slipped out, taking her walking stick with her and making her way across the water-meadows to the river ... Leaving her stick on the bank she forced a large stone into the pocket of her coat. Then she went to her death, 'the one experience', as she had said to Vita, 'I shall never describe'.

Treatment

Before the introduction of effective treatments for endogenous depression, patients often remained in a state of suicidal hopelessness for many months or even years. Fortunately, the full extent of their illness can now be modified or cut short; there are few things in psychiatry so gratifying as to see a patient emerging from a disastrous depression.

Some patients can be well cared for at home during a depressive illness, although their withdrawal, lethargy and lack of spontaneity often make life difficult for friends and relatives. However, most patients suffering from severe depression require hospital admission either because of the risk of suicide or because of their reluctance to eat and drink. The assessment of suicidal risk is discussed elsewhere (see p. 632).

There are many different drugs and other physical treatments used in the treatment of endogenous depression. However, it is of immense importance to the patient to sense that his doctor understands how he feels and is helping him through his depression in a personal and caring way. Even though some patients prefer to think of their illness as a chemical one, over which they have no control, others will wish to explore the nature of their vulnerability and the way in which they can avoid or deal with the precipitating factors. It is the doctor's task to develop a supportive relationship with the patient in order to determine which of these approaches is most likely to help. Of course, some patients, who initially appear to prefer a 'chemical approach', may later feel that other difficulties have contributed to their illness and wish to discuss and get help with these.

Physical treatments

Drugs

Tricyclic antidepressants. There are many different tricyclic antidepressants and they are discussed in more detail in Chapter 49. In general, it is best to be familiar with one or two that are sedative in their action and one or two that are more activating. Amitriptyline is a sedative antidepressant and therefore useful in those patients whose depressive illness is accompanied by anxiety and agitation. A dose of amitriptyline orally 150 mg at night is usually adequate.

Imipramine has less sedative and more activating properties and is a better choice of drug for those patients who show withdrawal and retardation. In view of its activating effect, it is best given only during the day, e.g. imipramine orally 25 mg three times daily. For a maximal antidepressant action the dose may be increased or another antidepressant with sedative properties given at night. Trimipramine orally 75 mg at night is often used for this purpose. All patients given antidepressants should be informed about their side-effects. The most common of these are constipation, dry mouth, mild blurring of vision and drowsiness.

Patients with a psychotic depression respond better to tricyclic antidepressants than to placebos (Morris and Beck 1974), but the response varies in different patients. Failure to respond may be due to a number of factors. An inadequate dose of medication is one possible reason but often other factors such as personality, social circumstances, or family and marital difficulties may perpetuate the illness. In those patients who improve it is advisable to continue the drug for some months after symptomatic recovery as this reduces the risk of relapse. However, the length of time may have to be curtailed as a result of unpleasant side-effects. Once the decision to stop antidepressants has been taken, they should be reduced gradually over a period of several weeks.

Tetracyclic antidepressants. This group of antidepressants have fewer anticholinergic effects than the tricyclic antidepressants. Patients therefore tend to suffer from fewer side-effects and find them more acceptable. A further advantage is the fact that they are less cardiotoxic than tricyclic antidepressants and so safer if taken in an overdose. Although the antidepressant action of tetracyclic drugs is said to be as great as that of the tricyclic antidepressants, many psychiatrists doubt this and prefer the older tricyclic compounds. The most widely used tetracyclic is probably mianserin. This has sedative properties and is therefore usually given at night, e.g. mianserin orally 30-60 mg.

Monoamine oxidase inhibitors (MAOIs). These are rarely used nowadays because of the danger of a hypertensive crisis occurring when they are mixed with certain other drugs, e.g. cough medicines and certain foods containing tyramine, e.g. cheese, marmite, game and some alcoholic drinks. They may however, occasionally be useful if the patient has failed to respond to tricyclic antidepressants or in the treatment of depression associated with multiple neurotic symptoms, such as hypochondriacal worries, irritability, tension, lethargy and phobic symptoms. The MAOIs most often used are phenelzine, a hydrazine derivative, 45-75 mg daily in divided doses, and tranylcypromine, which is related to the amphetamines. The mode of action of MAOIs is discussed further in Chapter 49.

Miscellaneous antidepressants. Various other drugs are used in the treatment of depression. These include L-tryptophan, tranquillisers, lithium and psychostimulants. They are discussed further in Chapter 49.

ECT

Before antidepressant drugs were introduced ECT was the most commonly used effective treatment for patients with a severe depressive illness. Nowadays it is used for patients who are seriously depressed, e.g. those with a high suicide risk and those who are grossly retarded or in depressive stupor, so that rapid improvement is essential. ECT is likely to start being effective after only one or two treatments, as compared with antidepressants which take from ten days to two weeks to act (see also Chapter 50). ECT is also used in patients who have failed to respond to antidepressants. However, many patients are afraid of ECT, especially those who rely on their imaginative abilities like artists and writers, because they fear that ECT might impair their memory and creativity. Their fear, which may be unjustified, has to be carefully balanced against the disabling and dangerous effects of severe persistent depression. In practice the undoubted efficacy of ECT is sometimes not utilised because of the often unfounded worries that surround its use. Many patients may as a consequence endure considerable suffering when antidepressant medication is not effective.

Psychosurgery

This is still occasionally used as a treatment for a depressive illness that has failed to respond to all other treatments. It is discussed further in Chapter 51.

Sleep deprivation and continuous narcosis

Some psychiatrists used to advocate the induction of a state of narcosis as a treatment for depression. Sedatives were used to induce sleep for a continuous period of a few days but light enough to allow feeding. There is little evidence that this is an effective treatment for depression and it has fallen into disuse. Surprisingly enough, the opposite suggestion has also been made, i.e. that sleep deprivation might relieve depression. This is still being investigated.

Psychological treatments

Psychotherapy

Since the introduction of the antidepressant drugs the use of psychoanalytic psychotherapy as the sole treatment for endogenous depression is no longer justified. It may, however, be helpful in milder cases in conjunction with drug therapy or, in more severe cases, when the patient has begun to improve as a result of drugs or ECT. Long-term individual psychotherapy, marital therapy or group therapy may be indicated following recovery from a depressive episode to help with conflicts, personality problems or disturbance in the family. Even when formal psychotherapy is not indicated, a supportive psychotherapeutic approach is essential in combination with physical treatment. The place of psychotherapy in neurotic depression is discussed in Chapter 16 (see p. 173).

Cognitive therapy

Patients who are depressed have particular ways of thinking about themselves and the outside world. The aim of cognitive behaviour therapy is to change the patient's erroneous assumptions about himself in the belief that the depressed mood will then improve (Beck *et al.* 1979). For example, a depressed patient may forget a business appointment and conclude that he is, and always has been, a useless businessman and company director. This way of thinking is known as over-generalisation. Other abnormal cognitions include 'magnifying' negative events and 'minimising' the importance of pleasant events. These habitual ways of negative thinking are identified with the patient, who is then offered alternative ways of thinking about himself and the outside world.

The effectiveness of cognitive therapy in endogenous depression remains uncertain, but similar approaches have always played some part in supportive and to a lesser extent in insight-directed psychotherapy.

Prognosis

Even before effective antidepressant treatment was introduced most patients with endogenous depression improved over time if they did not kill themselves, but the duration of each episode varied from a few months to several years. With treatment the duration has been shortened, but depressive illnesses of this kind often recur. Approximately 90 per cent of patients with unipolar depression will suffer further depressive illnesses at some point during their life. Each patient seems to have his own pattern which can sometimes be predicted. For example, the illness may start every autumn or spring, and sometimes it is useful to reinstate antidepressant therapy before the expected recurrence. Overall, approximately 15 per cent of patients who have suffered a psychotic depression eventually kill themselves.

In spite of this relatively poor long-term prognosis, the outcome of a single episode of endogenous depression is favourable with modern treatments. Furthermore, the combination of physical treatments, such as medication, with psychotherapy may improve the prognosis by decreasing vulnerability to life events, such as disappointments, moving house, bereavement or other losses. Family therapy has also been used in the hope of lowering the risk of relapses, as in schizophrenia (see p. 252).

Resistant depression

Some patients do not respond to treatment with drugs or ECT. In these cases a further reappraisal should be made to identify factors which may originally have been overlooked, e.g. factors intrinsic to the patient's personality, related to social circumstances or the result of interpersonal difficulties within a marriage or family. If such exacerbating or perpetuating factors are present, treatment will need to be directed towards alleviating them through psychotherapy or social measures. Sometimes such compounding factors cannot easily be discerned or removed and then the doctor and patient may either hope for a spontaneous remission or try a combination of drug treatments. A tricyclic antidepressant, e.g. clomipramine, combined with lithium and L-tryptophan, has been recommended. Some psychiatrists combine a tricyclic antidepressant with an MAOI, but such a combination may cause serious side-effects. When all treatments have failed over a period of time psychosurgery may have to be considered (see Chapter 51).

MANIC-DEPRESSIVE PYSCHOSIS

As we have seen, patients who develop endogenous depression may at other times in their lives also develop attacks of mania, and vice versa. They are therefore said to be suffering from manic-depressive psychosis, circular type (ICD-9). Some patients only have recurrent attacks of endogenous depression; these are said to be suffering from manic-depressive psychosis, depressed type (ICD-9). Others suffer from recurrent attacks of mania only and are said to be suffering from manic-depressive psychosis, manic type (ICD-9).

As mentioned earlier, an alternative way of subdividing manic-depressive psychoses is into bipolar and unipolar (see p. 193). The *bipolar* type corresponds to the circular type. The *unipolar* type was, until recently, applied to those patients who had only depressive or only manic attacks. However, as almost all patients who appear only to have manic episodes ultimately also develop depressive episodes, patients who only have manic episodes are now included in the bipolar group (Winokur *et al.* 1969).

Clinical features of mania

The onset of mania is characterised by a change in mood, and the manic swing may start insidiously, sometimes following a stressful life event. This may be an exciting event such as promotion or a new relationship, but it may also be a loss or disappointment. Initially the patient is joyous, almost exalted, and his enthusiasm is often quite contagious. Colleagues are swept along, amazed at the patient's activity, although, perhaps with hindsight, they later become aware that he was 'over the top'. The patient is aware that his thinking seems accelerated, as does his speech. His movements are rapid and restless. His productivity is great and his social life gathers momentum. His appetite for life seems to increase, so that initially he over-indulges in food and perhaps alcohol, and might start to become over-demanding sexually or promiscuous. His sleep becomes impaired but he may enjoy this since it allows him more time for his activities. For example, a businessman organised a secretary to take dictation from 6 a.m. to 9 a.m. before his regular secretary came into work.

The patient's thoughts begin to fly from one subject to another, leaving seemingly superb schemes in mid-air. Gradually he becomes intolerant of friends and family, who cannot keep up with him and do not help him complete his projects. As the illness progresses over days or weeks, he becomes bombastic, grandiose and intolerant of the apparent slowness of others. Increasingly, therefore, he feels frustrated at petty restrictions and his mood shifts from joy to anger. He accuses others of interfering with his plans by thwarting them, and he becomes paranoid. By this time his sleep has deteriorated further; he believes he only needs a few hours of sleep, goes to bed late and gets up in the early hours to resume his important activities. He is constantly on the move and has little time for food and drink. His weight may decrease to the point of emaciation and dehydration.

His grandiosity may become so extreme that he considers himself an heroic figure of historical importance, such as the Messiah. These ideas may eventually be held with delusional intensity and insight may be lost.

As the illness progresses further, the patient tends to over-spend, as befits his exalted position, and he often enters into unwise business deals, or grandiosely distributes largesse which he does not possess. His job is clearly in jeopardy because of his poor judgment. His marriage is threatened because of his behaviour, his unreasonable demands and, perhaps, because of his infidelity. The destructive nature of the illness is, therefore, apparent to everybody except the patient himself. Sometimes he has enough insight to realise that he is becoming exhausted or overtaxing himself, but he rarely considers himself in need of medical treatment. Unless helped, however, financial circumstances and marriage may be irreparably destroyed, leading to a prolonged period of realistic despair as the illness subsides. The manic swing may last many months if untreated.

At its earlier, less severe stage, the condition is often called hypomania, the term mania being used only when the condition is severe, but little is gained from this distinction.

From the above account, it follows that the patient may show the following features on *mental state examination*. He may have been brought along to see the doctor by a relative and, when asked if he has any difficulties, deny there is anything wrong. Further close questioning only leads to irritability or contempt and, although the patient may initially be elated, jovial and bombastic, misery and unhappiness may not be far beneath the surface. The patient's clothing is often over-colourful or eccentric and markedly different from his normal attire. There may be evidence of flight of ideas and pressure of speech. Thoughts may be tangential, rapid and experienced as being of exceptional clarity. Occasionally, colours appear brighter and contours of objects are more clearly defined. Finally, insight may be lost and *grandiose* and *persecutory delusions* develop. *Auditory hallucinations* may also occur. Underlying misery, even tearfulness, may be fleetingly expressed during an interview before being hidden once again behind a happy façade. Overactivity, grandiosity and *elation* may be used as a massive defensive organisation against a threat of depression. This is sometimes referred to as *manic defence*. Many patients become depressed following treatment for their elation and overactivity, and it may be difficult to determine if their depression is predominantly an endogenous swing, a collapse of the manic defence, or a realisation of the destruction brought about in their lives during their manic illness.

Treatment

At an early stage of a manic mood swing, it may be possible to persuade the patient to accept treatment. He may retain some insight and, with tact and guile, the doctor may be able to help him understand that he is ill. Unfortunately, the patient has 'never felt better in his life' and his feeling of well-being and self-importance may be difficult to overcome. However, some patients may accept medication, and haloperidol orally, 5 mg four times daily, may subdue the elated mood without causing intolerable drowsiness. Relatives or other caring individuals involved with the patient should be encouraged to monitor his activities discreetly and prevent his personal excesses. Normal working should be discouraged until the patient's mood is stable.

At a later stage of illness, the patient will require hospital admission. This should occur before irreparable damage has been done to his personal and professional life, and sometimes requires compulsory admission under the Mental Health Act (1983) (see Chapter 62).

Physical treatment of acute mania

Drugs

Phenothiazines and butyrophenones are both used in the treatment of acute mania. For example, chlorpromazine orally 100 mg four times daily, or haloperidol orally 10 mg four times daily, may be necessary to calm the patient. Pimozide orally 10-15 mg daily is sometimes used instead. Lithium carbonate can undoubtedly be effective in the treatment of acute mania, but its action may take a week or more to develop. It is therefore usually best to get the acute symptoms under control first with haloperidol or chlorpromazine.

ECT

ECT has been recommended for the treatment of mania which has been unresponsive to drugs. There is no general agreement as to its usefulness in this condition and it is rarely used nowadays.

Psychological treatment

Psychological treatment methods are ineffective during the acute phase of a manic illness. The overactivity, the grandiosity and irritability of the patient all work against a constructive therapeutic relationship. These symptoms, as well as other features of the illness such as thought disorder, also make the management of the patient on a hospital ward extremely difficult. Challenging the patient, for example by trying to restrict his activities, leads to arguments and possible violence. His grandiosity enables him hurtfully to insult staff, and manic patients are often able quickly to pick up on staff differences. In general, the staff of the ward have to work as a closely co-ordinated team who are quite clear on their management policy and firm about its implementation. After recovery from the acute episode long-term support is essential in the hope of preventing relapses or treating them at the earliest opportunity.

Prophylaxis of manic-depressive psychosis

Lithium

There is now ample evidence that lithium carbonate is effective in preventing recurrent affective changes, depression or mania, in patients with manic-depressive illness (Johnson 1980: Strinivasan and Hullin 1980). As a general rule, lithium prophylaxis is only started if the patient has suffered at least two major affective swings within two years. Approximately two-thirds of patients suffering from a bipolar illness respond well and show either a reduction in severity or shortening in length of each episode. Some of these patients may cease to have major affective swings altogether. The remainder, especially those with rapidly cycling mood swings, do not respond. There is less evidence that lithium carbonate is effective in preventing episodes of depression in patients with a unipolar depressive illness.

The plasma level of lithium required for effective prophylaxis is uncertain and probably varies from patient to patient. A blood level between 0.4-1.0 mmols/litre is usually recommended, as high levels may cause dangerous toxicity. A typical initial dosage, giving an appropriate plasma level, is lithium carbonate orally 800 mg at night, but this may have to be increased. More detailed information on the uses, side-effects and pharmacology of lithium is found on p. 610.

Major tranquillisers

Some psychiatrists recommend the use of major tranquillisers, at low doses, for those patients with a bipolar affective illness who have failed to respond to lithium carbonate. Flupenthixol decanoate intramuscularly 10-20 mg fortnightly or monthly may be effective in some patients, but further studies are needed to confirm this.

Carbamazepine and other anticonvulsants

Carbamazepine and sodium valproate have recently been recommended as useful in the prevention of recurrent affective swings. Carbamazepine may also increase the efficacy of lithium therapy (see p. 612).

Psychotherapy

Formal psychotherapy may be useful for patients after recovery from an acute episode of mania or depression, especially to help them with underlying conflicts and depressive feelings related to losses or other life events. Some may benefit from individual psychotherapy during a period of remission, directed at personality difficulties or associated problems which may exacerbate their manic-depressive illness. If a patient with manic-depressive psychosis is accepted for psychotherapy, it may need to be combined with drug therapy, and facilities for readmission to hospital must be readily available in case of relapse. Others may benefit from marital or family therapy if there are significant interpersonal problems.

Prognosis

Before the introduction of effective prophylaxis for manic-depressive illness, the prognosis was poor. Most patients suffered from recurrent depressive episodes, often with suicide attempts, and showed social decline resulting from their behaviour during the attacks of mania. However, in contrast to schizophrenia, the personality of the individual did not appear to deteriorate between these episodes. Fortunately the prognosis now appears much better, and at least two-thirds of patients improve with appropriate treatment and show fewer disabling symptoms or relapses. However, there is some evidence that affective swings may get worse as the patient becomes older.

FURTHER READING

Burton, R. (1621). *The Anatomy of Melancholy*. Reprinted 1955. Tudor, New York.
Murphy, E. (ed.) (1986). *Affective Disorders in the Elderly*. Churchill Livingstone, Edinburgh and London.
Paykel, E.S. (ed.) (1982). *Handbook of Affective Disorders*. Churchill Livingstone, Edinburgh and London.

Whybrow, P.C., Akiskal, H.S. and McKinney (1984). *Mood Disorders: towards a new psychobiology*. Plenum Press, New York and London.

19

Suicide and Acts of Self-Harm

Psychiatrists are frequently asked to assess patients who are either threatening to kill themselves or have already attempted to do so. Any threat of suicide or act of self-harm must be taken seriously. In the case of those who threaten suicide the initial task is to decide how great the risk is of their carrying out the threat. In the case of patients seen after an attempt at suicide – an act of self-harm – the task is to decide whether they had intended to die, in which case they are likely to make further attempts, or whether they had, at least in part, expected to survive.

As a general rule patients who show the features described below under the heading 'Suicide' are at high risk, while those showing the features described under 'Acts of Self-harm' (pp. 216-23) are at lesser risk. Inevitably there is overlap between patients who commit suicide and those who harm themselves but do not die. One per cent of patients who initially harm themselves without intending to die successfully commit suicide within a year of the act. Acts with death as an intended outcome may accidentally fail; conversely acts not meant to result in death may do so, e.g. a patient who takes an overdose of paracetamol may succumb to liver failure. Despite this overlap, the characteristics of patients who kill themselves and those who harm themselves differ and for clarity they will be considered as separate groups in this chapter.

SUICIDE

Suicide may be defined as 'a wilful self-inflicted life-threatening act which has resulted in death' (Beck *et al.* 1976). It is more common in men than in women. As a generalisation, patients who kill themselves tend to be middle-aged or elderly men, to have a history of mental illness or alcoholism, to be living alone and to have reacted badly to setbacks in life. Twenty per cent leave a suicide note. The methods used to commit suicide differ between the sexes; men are more likely to use a violent method such as hanging, jumping from a high building or using firearms and knives; women tend to use drug overdose. Analgesics, hypnotics, antidepressants and tranquillisers are the commonest drugs used; they will often have been prescibed by a doctor. The use of vehicle exhaust gas is increasing (Bulusu and Alderson 1984).

Epidemiology

The official figures for suicide in England and Wales give an incidence of approximately 10 per 100,000 population, but the true rate is probably higher; some car accidents and other apparently accidental deaths are almost certainly due to suicide. When in doubt, coroners do not record a verdict of suicide. Other countries have different methods of collecting data on suicide, which makes comparison of figures difficult (Sainsbury *et al.* 1980). However, it is generally accepted that rates are high in Hungary (40 per 100,000 population) and East Germany (36 per 100,000 population) but low in Spain (3.9 per 100,000 population) and Greece (2.8 per 100,000 population).

The suicide rate shows not only differences between nations but also fluctuations within a population over time. For example, in Britain a peak occurred during the economic depression of the early 1930s, while a trough was noted during both world wars. More recently there was a decline in the suicide rate during the 1960s. This may have resulted from improvements in the treatment of psychiatric illness. However, the fall in the number of deaths from carbon monoxide poisoning following the introduction of natural gas between 1958 and 1971 may partly account for it (Kreitman 1976).

Other associations

Suicide is commonest during the spring in both hemispheres; it is commonest in men; in socio-economic classes I and V; among the divorced, widowed and single, in decreasing order; in urban areas and among the unemployed (see Table 19.1). These demographic features suggest that social deprivation and personal isolation are important predisposing factors. They are clinically important as they point to identifiable 'at risk' groups. Suicide is common among doctors, especially anaesthetists and psychiatrists (Rich and Pitts 1980).

Table 19.1. Comparison of patients who kill themselves
with those that harm themselves

	Suicide	*Acts of self-harm*
Age	over 50	under 35
Sex	males	females
Social class	I and V	IV and V
Marital status	divorced>widowed>single	single>divorced teenage wives
Employment	unemployed/retired	unemployed
Psychiatric illness	common	rare
Physical illness	occasional	poor association but greater than expected for age group
Alcohol dependence	15%-20%	15%

Causes

There is little doubt that in most cases an individual who commits suicide must have succumbed to a massive intrapsychic struggle. This struggle may either have arisen within the context of a psychiatric illness such as depression or be due to a long-standing personality disorder. These two aspects, along with the psychodynamic and social causes of suicide, will be considered separately – although it must be borne in mind that personality characteristics, psychiatric illness and social circumstances all interact.

Psychiatric factors

The most frequent psychiatric disorders associated with suicide are depression and alcoholism. Approximately 50 per cent of suicides are associated with a *depressive illness* (Roy 1982). Excessive guilt, biological symptoms, previous suicide attempts and being single, separated, widowed or divorced increase the risk of suicide in depressed patients (Sainsbury 1978). This marked association between suicide and depression is of considerable clinical importance, as the early recognition and treatment of depression offers ample opportunity for the prevention of suicide. Furthermore, 90 per cent of suicides contact either their general practitioner or a psychiatrist in the year before their death and 48 per cent do so within one week before the act (Barraclough *et al.* 1974).

The incidence of suicide in *alcoholics* is 80 times greater than that found in the general population (Kessel and Grossman 1961) and drinkers are especially at risk if they have other difficulties such as physical illness, unemployment, marital problems and associated drug abuse. Overall, 10-15 per cent of male alcoholics kill themselves (Nicholls *et al.* 1974). Drug abusers also show an increased suicide rate, though the true incidence in this group remains uncertain as drug overdose, a common cause of death, may be accidental (Bewley *et al.* 1968).

Personality factors

At least 50 per cent of people who kill themselves suffer from a personality disorder (Ovenstone and Kreitman 1974). The commonest personality disorder associated with suicide is the antisocial or psychopathic type. This is considered in detail elsewhere (see p. 336). Other personality characteristics are considered in the next section.

Psychodynamic factors

Several psychodynamic factors contribute to our understanding of why patients kill themselves. Among these, the way people handle their aggressive fantasies, wishes and feelings is particularly important. Aggression may find expression in many different ways. It may be directed outwards, leading to overt hostility, physical violence or even murder; it may be incorporated into sexual behaviour, leading to rape and sado-masochistic relationships; or it may be directed against oneself leading to self-hatred and self-destructive acts. It is this last expression of aggression that is relevant to suicide. For example, if in a close relationship between, say, boyfriend and girlfriend or husband and wife, one partner resents the other one and feels angry but is too frightened or guilty to express his aggression, he may eventually turn the hatred and aggression against himself and commit suicide. If the attempt is unsuccessful and he survives, it is helpful to try to discover towards whom he had felt so resentful or harboured conscious or unconscious death wishes.

Sometimes a patient, say a girl who feels rejected by her boyfriend, may take an overdose not only because she has turned her anger against herself but also in order to manipulate her boyfriend and make him come back to her, or to punish him and make him feel guilty. The decision to kill oneself is therefore often over-determined, i.e. it results from several conflicting conscious and unconscious wishes. In fact there may be a split in the personality, one part wanting to die while another part maintains the fantasy of still being alive after the act and of having successfully manipulated or punished the partner.

There are other fantasies that commonly contribute to and precede acts of suicide. For example, after a bereavement the surviving partner may identify with the deceased and wish to be dead too. This is often linked with the hope and fantasy that by dying they will be reunited.

Suicide is often experienced as the only way of getting rid of intolerable psychic pain. This is seen particularly in those personality disorders that result from early emotional deprivation. At early stages of development it is the mother who provides the necessary support for the child by helping him to contain feelings of frustration, anger, sadness or despair. Gradually the child internalises his mother's capacity to contain psychic pain so that later in life he himself can contain and tolerate sad and painful feelings (see p. 70). If such early internalisation has failed, perhaps due to the mother's failure, separation or death, the adolescent or adult is unable to tolerate psychic pain and death by suicide is then seen as the only solution. In patients with such long-standing personality problems suicide as a way of escaping from psychic pain may be considered for many years before the act is carried out. For example, one patient who took a massive overdose of aspirin at the age of twenty-one had first considered suicide at puberty. She had harboured this secret thought throughout her adolescence and found it of great comfort as it offered a final solution to any distressing insoluble problem she might encounter.

The internal struggle between a desire to live and a wish to escape from intolerable pain indicates that the suicidal patient may not actually want to die but can find no other solution. Death provides the only relief. Once a decision is made the conflict is relieved and calm may follow. This calmness may be misinterpreted by others if it follows a long period of agitation and depression; it only suggests that a decision has been made but does not indicate in what direction. It may therefore reflect an increase rather than a decrease in suicidal intent. Thus the patient who appears to have recovered after a suicide attempt may continue to require psychiatric treatment and support to prevent another, possibly successful attempt.

Another form of disordered personality structure that may predispose to suicide is found in patients suffering from a severe split in their personality, one part of the self being experienced as bad and the other as good (see p. 70). Such patients may become preoccupied with the bad parts of the self and experience themselves as unlovable, hateful and bound to be rejected. When faced with an actual rejection they take this to be another confirmation of how bad and unlovable they are. Their self-hatred, directed towards the bad parts of themselves, then leads them to suicide which is seen as a way of getting rid of the bad parts. The fact that the split-off good parts will inevitably be destroyed as well is denied. In order to prevent suicide in patients with such character disorders psychotherapy has to be concerned with healing the split between the good and bad parts so that the patient learns to see himself as a whole person who can accept and integrate his good and bad aspects.

These psychodynamic factors of suicide are important in that they emphasise the inner reality of the patient rather than just the external factors. It is the fantasies behind the suicidal act which are important in predicting further suicide attempts and, as such, should be looked for in every suicidal patient and addressed in psychotherapy.

Social factors

The demographic and epidemiological features mentioned earlier have led sociologists to offer explanations of the causes of suicide. Durkheim (1897) spoke of 'anomic' and 'egoistic' suicide. When a society or social group to which a person belongs disintegrates the individual feels deprived of the social structure and norms he used to rely upon. Durkheim called this state of social disintegration *anomie*; if the individual then killed himself he called this *anomic suicide*. On the other hand, if a person left the social group or community he belonged to and as a result felt isolated and killed himself, he called this *egoistic suicide*.

There is some evidence that excessive publicity about suicide may result in subsequent suicides. For example, in England in 1978 a spate of self-burnings followed widespread media reports about two women who burned themselves to death (Ashton and Donnan 1981). However, suicide by example is rare.

ACTS OF SELF-HARM

There has been a dramatic increase in the number of patients who harm themselves without necessarily intending to die. For example, during the decade 1963-73 there was a four-fold increase in the number of patients admitted to hospital following an act of self-harm (Kreitman 1977). A number of terms have been used to describe this behaviour:

(1) Attempted suicide
(2) Parasuicide
(3) Deliberate self-harm: (a) deliberate self-poisoning;
                           (b) deliberate self-injury.

None of these terms is wholly satisfactory. 'Attempted suicide' (Stengel and Cook 1958) suggests that a desire to die accompanies the act; this is not necessarily the case. 'Parasuicide' avoids this problem and was defined by Kreitman (1977) as 'a non-fatal act in which an individual deliberately causes self-injury or ingests a substance in excess of any prescribed or generally recognised therapeutic dose'. Unfortunately the name itself continues to suggest suicidal intent even though the intended outcome of the act is not part of the definition. 'Deliberate self-harm' (Morgan *et al.* 1975) avoids these problems and refers to all patients who try to harm themselves irrespective of the purpose of their act, even if the act turns out not to have been harmful. The term is further subdivided according to the method used in the act. Thus the term 'deliberate self-poisoning' is used for those patients who ingest tablets or chemicals, and 'deliberate self-injury' for those who cut themselves. Unfortunately these terms also have their drawbacks. First, they minimise the possibility of suicidal intent and this may encourage the belief that patients who harm themselves are never suicidal. In fact, as mentioned earlier, 1 per cent of patients who commit an act of self-harm will kill themselves within a year following the act, and in approximately 20 per cent of patients the intent to die is serious. Secondly, the word 'deliberate' implies a purely conscious motivation on the part of the patient. This is unfortunate as these patients feel *compelled* to harm themselves, often for unconscious reasons. This is often not understood and may lead doctors and nurses to adopt an unsympathetic attitude.

In order to avoid some of these difficulties the term 'act of self-harm' will be used here as it implies neither motivation nor intent.

The nature of the act

Ninety per cent of patients who attend hospital after harming themselves have taken an overdose of drugs (Morgan *et al.* 1975). Minor tranquillisers, aspirin, paracetamol and antidepressants are the commonest drugs used. In many cases the patient has little knowledge of the likely effects of the drug he has taken.

The remaining 10 per cent of patients have injured themselves, most commonly by self-laceration, but occasionally by a violent method such as shooting or jumping in front of a train. Patients in the latter group are usually male and seriously suicidal. On rare occasions violent attacks on the body result from delusions or hallucinations. For example, a patient suffering from schizophrenia believed that his penis was an instrument of the devil and he decided that he should cut if off to protect the world from evil. The delusional belief thus caused a serious act of self-injury.

The rest of this section focuses on those patients who take overdoses. The few remaining patients who harm themselves by self-mutilation will be considered later in this chapter (pp. 223-5).

Epidemiology

Acts of self-harm are twice as common in women than men, representing the most common single reason for admission to a medical ward for women and second only to myocardial infarction in men. Overdoses are particularly common among fifteen to thirty-five-year-olds: approximately 1 per cent of women of this age group take an overdose in any one year. The act is rare after middle age.

Other associated features include low socio-economic status, social deprivation, single or divorced status, unemployment, family discord and physical illness or disability such as epilepsy (see Table 19.1). Early parental loss and child abuse are predisposing factors. Alcohol consumption precedes 50-60 per cent of acts of self-harm, but alcohol dependence is only present in approximately 10-15 per cent of cases. This figure may be higher for men.

Acts of self-harm have shown a marked increase since 1960 and are ten times more common than suicides. Although the overall rates have fallen over the period 1980-1985, the rates in adolescents continue to increase (Hawton 1982).

Clinical features

The patient is typically a young, socially deprived woman who is experiencing difficulties in relationships, often in relation to her mother or sexual partner. The act of self-harm is usually impulsive and may be precipitated by the breakdown of a close relationship. Commonly the patient has been rejected and, after an altercation with her partner, starts drinking to excess. The overdose is then taken, sometimes even in the presence of her rejecting partner. Young adolescents may use their mother's medication.

Relief may not be felt following the overdose; this is in contrast to the decreased tension often experienced after self-mutilation (see p. 224). Some patients experience fear and remorse soon after the overdose and obtain medical help.

The individual's motivation may be conscious, unconscious, or both. Only the conscious motives behind acts of self-harm will be considered here. The unconscious motives, which give the acts their compulsive quality, are similar to those discussed in relation to suicide (see p. 214). Patients who have taken an overdose of tablets give many reasons for their act. Twenty-five per cent insist that they wished to die at the time of the act, but only half of these patients are considered suicidal when assessed by a psychiatrist. The remainder deny any intent to die and give one or more of the following reasons for the act:

(1) A wish to escape from emotional turmoil or an unbearable situation.
(2) A wish to make another person feel guilty.
(3) A desire for help and attention. The patient hardly ever admits this although the doctor or psychiatrist may suspect it.

The reasons given by a patient for taking an overdose are of interest but should be treated with caution. Suicidal patients may deny suicidal intent in order to obtain release from hospital; conversely some patients may report suicidal ideas merely to give a satisfactory and acceptable explanation for their behaviour. The fact that most patients do not admit a desire for help or attention may make treatment difficult.

Causes

Acts of self-harm usually take place within the context of an abnormal personality. Although a definite diagnosis of personality disorder is made in only about 50 per cent of patients who have taken an overdose (Kreitman 1977), it is likely that most if not all of them have a character or personality disorder which leaves them abnormally vulnerable to stressful circumstances and makes them harm themselves.

Patients who harm themselves by taking an overdose almost always have a childhood history of emotional deprivation (see Chapter 7), often due to parental discord, separation or divorce. Loss of a parent through death is less common. These early developmental problems lead to persistent difficulties in relationships during adolescence and adulthood. Consequently, acts of self-harm often take place in the context of *family discord*, including marital difficulties, sexual problems and *social isolation*. *Unemployment* may also be a predisposing factor. A tendency to commit self-damaging acts increases with the length of time out of work.

During the six months before an act of self-harm, stressful *life events* (see p. 39) are four times more common than in the general population (Paykel *et al.* 1975). Personal rejection, such as failure of a relationship, loss of employment or separation from a loved one are particularly common, and overdoses tend to occur within one month of the event.

Psychiatric illness

Most patients who harm themselves do not suffer from a psychiatric illness. Depressive symptoms may be present but form part of a transient emotional reaction rather than a depressive illness. Feelings of nervous tension, frustration, helplessness, irritability and despair are particularly common (Newson-Smith and Hirsch 1979). Overall only 5 per cent of patients who harm themselves suffer from a severe psychiatric illness such as psychotic depression or schizophrenia. A further group, representing about 15 per cent of cases, have severe problems with alcohol. It is the patients in these last two sub-groups who are at particular risk of subsequent suicide.

Treatment

The majority of patients who have taken an overdose require admission to hospital for immediate medical care. Subsequently 10 per cent of patients require admission to a psychiatric ward. The remaining 90 per cent require some form of outpatient treatment or follow-up.

Admission to a psychiatric ward may be necessary to make a full assessment of a patient's problems or to allow a crisis to resolve. However, inpatient management is usually reserved for patients with severe psychiatric illness and those at high risk of suicide. Nurses and doctors should cooperate closely to ensure that the observation and supervision of these patients matches their suicidal risk. Occasionally a patient requires compulsory admission under the Mental Health Act (1983).

Treatment is initially directed towards alleviating any psychiatric illness. For example, antidepressants or ECT may be required in depression. As the patient improves careful nursing and support should continue as suicidal ideas may not resolve as rapidly as other depressive symptoms. All too often a patient thought to be better leaves hospital only to kill himself soon afterwards. Suicides in patients recently discharged from hospital have increased over the last decade, and careful follow-up and support are essential. This should be planned in conjunction with the general practitioner, relatives, social workers or community psychiatric nurses.

Outpatient treatment should be planned with the patient soon after the act of self-harm. Three broad approaches to treatment are available:

(1) Psychological treatment
(2) Social support
(3) Physical treatment

These should be arranged so that a patient recognises them as relevant to his particular problem.

Psychological treatment

This usually involves one of the following: individual psychotherapy, group psychotherapy, marital therapy, family therapy, supportive therapy and counselling. These treatments are discussed in more detail elsewhere (see Chapters 44 and 45).

Many patients who harm themselves have difficulties in expressing themselves verbally and emotionally. This is not necessarily a contra-indication to psychotherapy. On the contrary, individual or group psychotherapy may be the best treatment to help patients overcome these problems. Psychotherapy allows an understanding of conscious and unconscious motives which led to the act of self-harm; it also promotes more appropriate ways of relating to people and of expressing feelings instead of distress being communicated only through further acts of self-harm.

Psychotherapy with patients who harm themselves is difficult, and in view of the likelihood of recurrent acts of self-harm, hospital admission may be necessary for short periods. Appropriate arrangements with a hospital should be made at the beginning of therapy and not left until a crisis arises. Counselling may be helpful for those patients who need only short-term help. In counselling the major problems of the patient are clarified and constructive ways of tackling them explored. The approach is a practical problem-orientated one rather than an attempt to explore underlying emotional difficulties. It is important that the counsellor gives regular encouragement as each problem is tackled.

Social support

Financial and housing problems are common in patients who harm themselves and social intervention is often essential. Social problems need to be alleviated before any psychological treatment is possible. Occasionally a hostel or day centre is necessary to provide social stability. Only then can psychological problems be dealt with.

Physical treatments

Physical treatments such as the use of drugs or ECT are only used if an underlying psychiatric illness is present. For example, antidepressants may relieve the distressing symptoms of an endogenous depression. As the majority of patients who harm themselves without wanting to die do not suffer from a psychiatric illness, physical treatments have little place in their treatment. Anxiolytics to reduce tension are likely to lead to drug dependence and are rarely of help. Moreover, prescribing drugs provides the means for subsequent overdoses.

The role of the general practitioner

The general practitioner should be informed in all cases of self-harm and he should be involved in planning treatment. He will be the first to respond if another crisis arises and he often has detailed family and social information which would otherwise not be available. Close cooperation between the general practice team and the hospital is particularly important when dealing with manipulative patients if a cohesive treatment plan is to be prevented from breaking down.

General practitioners have an important preventive role, as 60 per cent of patients who harm themselves consult the doctor during the month before the act and 40 per cent do so during the preceding week (Hawton and Blackstock 1976). Unfortunately limited consultation time often prevents adequate assessment of suicidal intent and general practitioners may be better placed to prevent recurrent acts of self-harm rather than pre-empt the first attempt. Careful prescribing is an obvious precautionary measure to prevent patients using the medication for an overdose. A history of a previous act of self-harm is an important warning signal.

Difficulties of treatment

The problem of denial

Many patients who harm themselves deny their difficulties. For example, a patient who takes an overdose may calmly inform the doctor a day later that the act was foolish and will certainly never be repeated. The doctor may be tempted to collude with this denial and feel reassured that the patient can be safely discharged without further action being taken. This is a mistake. All patients who harm themselves should be taken seriously even if they themselves describe their difficulties as trivial. A major task of an initial assessment is to help the patient understand the seriousness of what he has done. The doctor may need to confront the patient with this. All too often doctors and other professionals encourage the patient quickly to return to normal life, which minimises the seriousness of the overdose. This is dangerous and only leaves the patient with his difficulties unresolved. More than one interview may be necessary to overcome denial, and the doctor must establish enough rapport with the patient to ensure that further appointments are kept. Treatment will only be possible if denial on the part of both patient and doctor is overcome.

Children and young teenagers

This group of patients should be seen in conjunction with child pyschiatrists or other specialists working with children or adolescents. The child's family needs to be fully involved and the school may need to be contacted. Case conferences between all those who are involved may need to be convened.

Recurrent acts of self-harm

Patients who repeatedly harm themselves engender anger and frustration in everyone involved in their welfare. This should not lead to despair and hopelessness on the part of the therapist and others looking after them. Long-term support of this group of patients over a period of years may bring about remarkable changes. In this group the high risk of suicide must always be borne in mind. A list of factors associated with a high risk of suicide is found in Table 54.1 (p. 632).

Prognosis

Twenty per cent of patients who commit an act of self-harm do so again within one year and 10 per cent will eventually take their own lives. The risk of suicide in the year following the act is approximately 1 per cent (Morgan *et al.* 1976). Factors associated with risk of repeated self-injury are listed in Table 19.2.

Table 19.2. Factors associated with recurrent acts of self-harm

Psychopathic personality
Criminal record
Unemployment
Low socio-economic class
Alcohol and drug problems
Previous psychiatric treatment
Previous acts of self-harm
Problems of sexual identity

SELF-MUTILATION

The vast majority of patients who harm themselves and attend hospital have taken an overdose of drugs. However, a small proportion, probably 5-10 per cent of all patients who commit acts of self-harm, do so by self-mutilation. The actual figure may be higher as many such acts, e.g. cutting onself, may not be brought to medical attention.

Self-mutilation usually takes the form of superficial cuts or scratches on the wrists, arms or abdomen. Self-inflicted cigarette burns on the back of the hands and arms are also common. Occasionally it consists of serious self-inflicted wounds such as deep cutting of tendons, nerves and arteries. The more violent the attack on the body, the more serious is the suicidal intent. Such serious acts of self-mutilation are more common in men. Occasionally severe self-mutilation may accompany a psychotic illness such as schizophrenia and be a result of delusions or hallucinations. These more serious attacks on the body are rare and will not be considered further here. The remainder of this section deals with those acts of self-cutting which are superficial and appear to involve little or no suicidal intent.

Characteristics

Patients who cut themselves show similar characteristics to those who take overdoses, but they tend to be younger. All have severe personality disturbances, especially borderline personality disorders (see Chapter 27).

The following are important associations. Eating disorders such as anorexia nervosa and bulimia are common, as are drug and alcohol abuse (Simpson 1976). Psychological distress over menstruation can be a factor; for example, dislike of menstruation and adverse reactions to the onset of menstruation in adolescents and of the bodily changes of puberty are frequent (Laufer and Laufer 1984). Patients who cut themselves often show confusion over sexual identity, and sexual problems are common (Rosenthal *et al.* 1972). Interestingly, there is a greater than expected incidence of hospitalisation before the age of five for the surgical correction of congenital malformations in these patients. Persistent disturbance of the patient's body image may be a significant factor in such cases (Simpson 1976).

Clinical features

The 'typical' patient tends to be female, young, lacking in self-esteem and showing persistently disordered or aggressive behaviour. Family disturbance and difficulties with relationships are particularly common.

The act of self-mutilation tends to follow circumstances which have made the patient angry, frustrated or disappointed. A sense of inexorable mounting tension develops and the patient is unable to relax. Depersonalisation or other dissociative experiences may occur. At this point the patient cuts herself in an attempt to dispel the excessive tension. Cutting may be done with razor blades or knives, but often glass or crockery is smashed first to provide a sharp cutting edge. The cuts are usually superficial and may be multiple; ten to twenty parallel cuts on the forearms, wrists, or abdomen are common. At this point dissociation may be severe; patients often feel no pain and may be surprised at the sight of blood a few seconds later. Dissociation at the time of cutting is short-lived and the same mental process does not occur when suturing the wound. The surprising practice of some doctors of suturing self-inflicted wounds without a local anaesthetic is therefore punitive and unjustifiable.

At the sight of blood the patient often feels relief and may then take appropriate action such as clearing away broken glass, stopping the bleeding or attending casualty.

Treatment

The treatment of patients who cut themselves is difficult. There are two major approaches – a symptom-oriented approach, using supportive techniques and relaxation, and a psychotherapeutic approach, aimed at bringing about changes in personality. A combination of both methods may be required. Treatment is impossible unless the patient has stable social circumstances. Those patients whose social circumstances are severely disordered may require admission to a day centre, a day hospital or hostel while treatment is carried out. This requires careful liaison with other agencies. For example, a social worker may provide practical, everyday support, while the psychotherapist helps the patient with her emotional problems. Close interdisciplinary work is needed throughout treatment as patients may manipulate staff and foster disagreement among them.

Support and relaxation

Patients who cut themselves provoke anger and frustration in people around them and, as a result, feel isolated, rejected and deprived of affection. An offer of emotional support from a doctor, nurse, social worker or other professional may alleviate some of this distress and be the first step in helping the patient find new ways of dealing with her problems. The next step is to help the patient to control frustration. Tension mounts in patients who cut themselves whenever unfavourable events occur. The patient has no way of reducing the tension other than by cutting herself. Relaxation techniques (see p. 682) may help decrease tension before it becomes unbearable. The patient must practise relaxation exercises regularly and needs support and encouragement to do this. All too often the patient gives up the practice too early.

Psychotherapy

Patients who cut themselves have severe personality problems and psychotherapy or psychoanalysis may be the treatment most likely to offer a possibility of change. The aim of therapy is to help the patient understand the unconscious conflicts and motivation underlying her acts, to outgrow the effects of early emotional deprivation, and to learn better ways of expressing her emotional difficulties. Long-term commitment on the part of the patient and therapist is required, but some of these patients are not sufficiently motivated to accept such a commitment when they are first seen. In such cases a period of initial support is needed.

A major problem of therapy is the patient's inability to express emotions in any way other than by cutting herself. Any rejection or frustrating experience leads to anger and helplessness which can only be communicated by cutting herself again. The capacity to contain and tolerate emotional distress is absent. Thinking and symbolisation are needed by everyone in order to contain painful feelings such as those of helplessness, loss, separation, anger and frustration. The relative failure of these processes in patients who cut themselves is usually the result of difficulties in the early relationship between mother and child. These severe personality deficits can only be overcome in long-term psychotherapy or psychoanalysis.

Prognosis

There is little accurate information about the prognosis for patients who mutilate themselves. Almost all continue to mutilate themselves at intervals over long periods and some also take overdoses from time to time. Some gradually recover over a period of years, especially those who are in long-term psychotherapy. Even with treatment some end their lives by suicide (Nelson and Grunebaum 1971). The outcome probably depends on the severity of the underlying personality disturbance.

FURTHER READING

Alvarez, A. (1974). *The Savage God: a study of suicide*. Penguin, Harmondsworth.

Hawton, K. (1986). *Suicide and Attempted Suicide among Children and Adolescents*. Sage, London.

Hawton, K. and Catalan, J. (1982). *Attempted Suicide: a practical guide to its nature and management*. OUP, Oxford.

Roy, A (ed.) (1986). *Suicide*. Williams & Wilkins, London.

20

Schizophrenia

The word 'schizophrenia' conjures up a wide variety of images of madness in the layman's mind, for example people talking to themselves, behaving abnormally, being out of touch with reality and raving. A common misconception is that people with schizophrenia have a split personality, like Jekyll and Hyde. This is not the case. The belief probably arose from the term itself, which was coined from the Greek *schizein* (to split) and *phrên* (mind), and is often misinterpreted as meaning 'split mind'. In fact it refers to a person whose mental functions – thoughts, feelings and perceptions – have become disintegrated and fragmented, whose behaviour has become abnormal, and who has lost touch with reality.

Clinical descriptions of what would now be called schizophrenia were not formulated until the nineteenth century. Before then few, if any, attempts were made to distinguish between different forms of madness. It was a French physician, Morel (1809-1873), who reported a case study of an adolescent, aged fourteen, who he thought was dementing; subsequently he named this condition, which we would now call schizophrenia, 'démence précoce', a precocious dementia which occurred in earlier rather than later years (Morel 1852, 1860). Morel's concept of a premature dementia was taken up by the German psychiatrist Emil Kraepelin (1855-1926), who used the term *dementia praecox* and distinguished it from manic-depressive psychosis (Kraepelin 1913a) He did, however, realise that this was not a true dementia in that not all aspects of personality function were necessarily affected and the condition did not always progress to mental deterioration. The word 'schizophrenia' was coined in 1910 by a Swiss psychiatrist, Eugen Bleuler (1857-1939), largely to get away from the idea of a dementing process and stress instead the disintegration or splitting of mental processes (Bleuler 1911).

Schizophrenia is one of the two major functional psychoses, the other being manic-depressive psychosis (see p. 206). It is an umbrella term, covering a number of conditions which differ in their clinical presentation but which are thought to have a related aetiology. Many psychiatrists nowadays talk about 'the schizophrenias'.

EPIDEMIOLOGY

The epidemiology of schizophrenia has been reviewed by Hare (1982).

Age and sex

Schizophrenia is hardly ever seen before the age of fifteen. The commonest time of onset is between twenty and thirty-nine, but it can start after forty-five, and also in the elderly. Paranoid symptoms are more common when it starts later in life. The overall sex incidence is about equal, but there is a slight preponderance of men before and of women after thirty-five.

Prevalence

By definition the prevalence of schizophrenia involves a head count of all cases, either at a single point in time or over a stated period, say one year. There are problems in arriving at an accurate figure, partly because not all people who have schizophrenia are in contact with a counting agency, e.g. general practitioner, psychiatrist, hospital or day centre. There are also problems in deciding whom to include, e.g. whether to include an individual who has just recovered from an acute episode but still has some minor disability, and in defining the diagnostic criteria to be used (see p. 43). Figures therefore differ, but the one-year prevalence rate for the UK, derived from pooled data, is 3.3 per 1000. The range in different countries, including Japan, China, India, the USA, and Western countries varies from 2 to 4 per 1000; the rate quoted for the USSR is 5.1 per 1000 (B. Cooper 1978), probably because wider criteria are used there for the diagnosis of schizophrenia.

Incidence

This refers to the number of new cases seen over a given period of time. Figures for the annual incidence rate differ widely as they also depend on the diagnostic criteria used and on the method employed to find new cases, e.g. all those admitted to hospital or all those seen by general practitioners with a first attack. Figures for first contact rates in two districts in England, Camberwell and Salford, using strict diagnostic criteria (see p. 147) were 0.14 and 0.11 per 1000 population (Wing and Fryers 1976). In the USA, where much wider diagnostic criteria were used in the past, figures as high as 0.25 per 1000 have been quoted. The incidence was remarkably similar in nine different developing and developed countries when strict diagnostic criteria were used (Sartorius *et al.* 1986) (see p. 152).

Lifetime expectancy (morbidity risk)

This is defined as the risk which any individual has of developing schizophrenia during his lifetime. The figure for the UK is 0.85 per cent. This figure is remarkably constant throughout the Western world. However, a higher figure has been found in northern Sweden (Böok 1953). It has been suggested that people predisposed to schizophrenia prefer to live a withdrawn, isolated existence. This might lead to people with such a predisposition migrating into or remaining in such an extremely isolated environment as the northern parts of Sweden and might account for the higher lifetime expectancy in such areas. Conversely, the lower than average lifetime expectancy of schizophrenia found in the close-knit Hutterite communities in North America could be due to the fact that people who prefer an isolated existence have left these communities.

CLINICAL FEATURES OF ACUTE SCHIZOPHRENIA

It is important to distinguish between the features of the acute syndrome and those of the chronic syndrome. The latter is discussed on p. 235.

Four major aspects of mental function can be affected to a greater or lesser extent in acute schizophrenia: behaviour, mood, thought and perception. The majority of patients lack insight into the fact that they are ill. The onset of the psychosis may be preceded by a feeling that something strange or sinister is about to happen. This is called a *delusional mood*.

Behaviour

The degree to which behaviour is affected varies from patient to patient and in different types of schizophrenia. The type of schizophrenia in which behaviour is most affected is catatonic schizophrenia (see p. 234). During this illness, the patient may spend long periods of time in a *catatonic stupor*, absolutely motionless, neither speaking nor responding to an observer. However, psychophysiological measurements show that people in a catatonic stupor are influenced by what is going on around them; for example, skin conductance level, pulse rate and blood pressure change in response to external stimuli, such as someone talking to the patient. Indeed, patients will sometimes give a clear description of what was happening during their stupor after they have recovered. Sometimes people in this state will adopt the most bizarre and uncomfortable-looking postures, such as standing on one leg with both hands stretched above their head for hours on end, or lying on their bed with their head three inches above the pillow all night long. If muscle tone is examined, a smoothly-increased resistance to movement may be noticed. Limbs can be placed by the examiner in awkward positions which are then maintained without apparent distress, and only slowly is the resting posture reassumed. This is called *waxy flexibility* (flexibilitas cerea).

Sometimes the stuporose condition is interspersed suddenly and unpredictably by periods of excitement. This is a state of uncontrolled purposeless motor activity, in which patients can harm themselves by running into walls or doors. Stupor may return equally quickly and unpredictably.

Catatonic schizophrenia is observed much less commonly nowadays than 70 or 80 years ago. However, it should always be considered as a diagnosis when examining a patient who is mute and unresponsive.

Other disorders of movement occur in schizophrenia, e.g. mannerisms and stereotypies. A *mannerism* is defined as a movement which is understandable to others but appears odd and out of context, e.g. the patient who makes the sign of the cross in blessing, or who gives a military salute to anyone who speaks to him. A *stereotypy* is a repeated, apparently purposeless movement which usually has some meaning for the patient, but may be incomprehensible to anybody else. A rare disorder of movement is *Mitgehen*. This is the continued movement of a limb in response to light pressure by the examiner, despite the patient being told to resist the pressure. The movement resembles that of a finely-balanced anglepoise lamp which continues to move after a light touch.

Mood and affect

The patient's mood and affect may be abnormal in schizophrenia. A major disturbance of affect is *flattening* or blunting. Here there is no affectual tone or emotional investment in what the patient is saying. The speech is monotonous. Everything is said in the same flat way so that, for example, there is no change in affect whether the patient is talking about going shopping or about the recent death of a close friend. Sometimes the affect is inappropriate to the mood the patient is expressing, for example a patient who was restless and tense and appeared close to tears, when asked how he was feeling, replied 'Great! Never felt better – this is the happiest day of my life!'

Occasionally the affect is *incongruous*. This means that it cannot be understood by the observer as arising from what the patient is talking about, or from what is happening to him. The person may grimace or laugh for no apparent reason. Sometimes a range of affect is displayed; for example, the patient may begin by being cheerful and good-humoured, then become guarded and perplexed, then anxious, then terrified, shouting and screaming and crawling under the table, then burst into tears and rock backwards and forwards – all for no apparent reason. Often the patient is unable to explain these feelings afterwards but seems to have been overwhelmed by them.

Thought

In schizophrenia, abnormalities occur in the form, stream, possession and content of thought (see p. 120).

Disorders in the *form of thinking* (thought disorder) are common. In the severest form of thought disorder all coherence of thinking is lost. This is called word salad, in which words and utterances are jumbled. In a less severe form, there appears to be no logical connection between successive thoughts or sentences. In the least severe form of thought disorder, the patient may coin a few new words, or neologisms, which have some meaning for him but not for anybody else, e.g. the word PROCALATION in the letter quoted below.

The following extract from a letter of a young schizophrenic woman written during an acute episode illustrates some of these forms of thought disorder:

> Apologise; and I might find some new fun, I.
> NO PROMISES MIND YOU
> WITH LOVE AND MORNINGTON CRESCENT.
> I find the going hard, will heart and mind and
> body please be sufficient for the intellectual
> on the found on the street one. I met your
> secretary at the MORE House and did SOWE
> promised he help with a PROCALATION and then
> never saw her again to hear if she was in the
> left mind. Hope your RIVERS for a long time.
> Come and drink tea, sea and have a bite to eat
> on Thursday 6.30. And if you NEED to get rid of
> that painting now's the chance. I'll introduce
> you as the painter so as to enable you to put
> sickness out of your mind for at least ½ an hour.
> Natalia (also Natalie).

The *stream of thinking* refers to the rate at which thoughts flow. In schizophrenia, *thought block* may occur (see p. 121). Thoughts just come to a halt, and the patient's mind feels empty until he starts talking again about some unrelated topic. Healthy people can experience something similar, e.g. when very tired or under great pressure. When thought block occurs as part of the schizophrenic syndrome, it occurs repeatedly and is associated with other schizophrenic signs and symptoms.

Disorders of *thought possession* occur, when thoughts are perceived as no longer private and under the patient's control. For example, he may think his thoughts are not his own, but have either been put into his mind or taken away or broadcast to others. Further descriptions of thought insertion, thought withdrawal and thought broadcasting are given on p. 121.

The most common disorders of *thought content* found in schizophrenia are delusions (see p. 122). Both primary and secondary delusions can occur in schizophrenia. The most common types of delusion are paranoid, grandiose, religious and sexual. Delusional perception may occur (see p. 123) and delusions of reference are common. Sometimes a patient with schizophrenia will believe that either his body or his actions are not under his own control. This experience is a type of delusion, called *delusion of control* or *passivity* (see p. 123). The following comment from a patient illustrates this phenomenon: 'I know you thought I wrote that note to you yesterday, but it wasn't me – they were using my hand to hold the pen to write with.'

Perception

In schizophrenia the commonest perceptual abnormalities are *auditory hallucinations* (see p. 124). These also occur in many other psychiatric conditions, but in schizophrenia they have certain characteristics. Patients commonly hear a voice, or voices, which refers to them in the third person, i.e. as either he, she or it, and this voice may give a running commentary on the patient's thoughts or actions. Sometimes the voice will say aloud a thought the patient has just had (*Gedankenlautwerden*) and sometimes it becomes authoritative, giving commands or orders. *Somatic hallucinations* refer to changes within the body, e.g. feeling one's liver suddenly turn into gold, or feeling electricity running up and down the spine. Visual hallucinations can occur but are rare in acute schizophrenia; as they also occur in other conditions, e.g. organic psychiatric disorders, they have no diagnostic value by themselves.

Criteria for diagnosis

These, then, are the major abnormalities which can occur, to a greater or lesser extent, during the course of an acute schizophrenic illness. How do clinicians go about making a diagnosis?

During the early twentieth century, the clinical observations of Eugen Bleuler were used by many clinicians to make a diagnosis of schizophrenia. Bleuler described four fundamental features, often referred to as the four 'A's of schizophrenia: autism, affective incongruity (see p. 120), loosening of associations and ambivalence. He used the term autism to refer to a process by which a patient withdraws from the external world into an inner world of his own; loosening of associations implied disordered thought processes; and ambivalence referred to the presence of both negative and positive attitudes towards a person, an action, or an idea. Bleuler considered that the delusions and hallucinations found in schizophrenia were not of diagnostic significance and were merely 'accessory symptoms'.

In contrast, the German psychiatrist Kurt Schneider (1887-1967), working in Heidelberg in the 1940s and 1950s, proposed that the delusions and hallucinations found in schizophrenia were of diagnostic significance and that the features described by Bleuler were of secondary importance. Schneider originally put forward eleven symptoms which he considered to be characteristic of acute schizophrenia. These are known as *Schneiderian first-rank symptoms* and are still used today to make a diagnosis of schizophrenia (Schneider 1959). They may be grouped together into five main categories.

(1) Passivity feelings – the delusional belief that either a part or the whole of one's body or mind is controlled by some external agency.

(2) Auditory hallucinations – voices talking about the patient in the third person; voices which give a running commentary on the patient's thoughts or actions; voices which repeat the patient's thoughts out loud (*Gedankenlautwerden*).

(3) Delusional perception – a delusion which arises for the first time out of a normal perception.

(4) Disorders of thought possession – thought insertion; thought withdrawal; thought broadcasting.

(5) Somatic hallucinations – unusual feelings inside the body, usually attributed to some force acting over a distance.

According to Schneider, only one first-rank symptom needs to be present to make a diagnosis of acute schizophrenia. It is important to note that first-rank symptoms do not refer to chronic schizophrenia, in which negative symptoms (see p. 235) predominate. However, even in acute schizophrenia, first-rank symptoms are only present in 80 per cent of cases. In the remaining 20 per cent the diagnosis of acute schizophrenia has to be made in their absence. A history of previous schizophrenic episodes and a family history of schizophrenia may assist in making the diagnosis in such cases.

Whatever the criteria on which the diagnosis is based, it can only be made in the presence of clear consciousness. The diagnostic criteria, including Schneiderian first-rank symptoms, can occur in conditions other than acute schizophrenia, especially in the acute organic psychiatric reactions, but in these there is evidence of clouding or more severe disturbance of consciousness, which does not occur in schizophrenia. It is particularly important to exclude toxic causes, especially amphetamine and alcohol, both of which can cause a schizophrenia-like syndrome, sometimes called symptomatic schizophrenia. Occasionally other organic cerebral disorders, such as space-occupying lesions or systemic diseases affecting the brain, e.g. systemic lupus erythematosus, can cause a schizophrenia-like syndrome; these must be looked for and the underlying condition treated, if present. Patients who have had temporal lobe epilepsy for several years may also develop a schizophrenia-like syndrome (see p. 317).

For research purposes standardised assessment criteria such as the Present State Examination are now being used (see p. 147).

Cultural and diagnostic differences

The International Pilot Study of Schizophrenia (WHO 1973) investigated how the diagnosis of schizophrenia was made in nine countries and found similar diagnostic criteria in seven of them, the exceptions being Washington and Moscow where the criteria were much broader (see also p. 43). At two-year follow-up the course and outcome were more favourable in developing than in developed countries (WHO 1978b; Sartorius *et al.* 1986). The reasons for these differences were unclear.

Another cross-national study, the UK-US Diagnostic Project (J.E. Cooper *et al.* 1972), also showed that the concept of schizophrenia was much wider in New York than in Britain. Many of the patients receiving a diagnosis of schizophrenia in the US would have been considered to be suffering from depressive illness, mania or personality disorder in Britain. The difference may partly be due to the influence of Bleuler and psychoanalytic thinking on the diagnosis of schizophrenia in the United States, whereas British psychiatrists have restricted themselves to the narrower diagnostic criteria of Kraepelin and Schneider. This divergence in diagnosis is now being rectified by using stricter criteria in both countries.

Types of acute schizophrenia

Traditionally, acute schizophrenia has been subdivided into catatonic, hebephrenic, paranoid and simple.

Catatonic schizophrenia is characterised by marked changes in behaviour, as described earlier. Other schizophrenic features can occur, but are usually less obvious.

Hebephrenic schizophrenia usually occurs in younger people. Hebe was the Greek goddess of youth, who spent much of her time playing practical jokes. Hebephrenic patients often appear silly or childish, as a result of inappropriate affect and gross thought disorder. Delusions and hallucinations are common.

Paranoid schizophrenia is a type of schizophrenia in which paranoid delusions predominate. The personality is usually better preserved than in the other types. The diagnosis cannot be made on the presence of paranoid delusions alone, since these occur in many other psychiatric conditions (see p. 255). Some other features of schizophrenia must also be present, such as the characteristic auditory hallucinations. Paranoid schizophrenia tends to run true to form, in that relapses are usually of a paranoid type.

Simple schizophrenia tends to have an insidious onset. It usually arises in adolescents or young adults. It is characterised by social withdrawal, failure at work or study, loss of motivation and unusual behaviour. It appears to have more in common with chronic forms of schizophrenia, but positive symptoms can emerge. When it occurs during adolescence, it can be difficult to differentiate from identity crises or other forms of adolescent disturbance.

This type of sub-grouping has more historical than practical value, and clinicians rarely use it. Furthermore, some patients exhibit symptoms of the different types of schizophrenia at various stages of their illness.

Schizoaffective disorder

In 1933 Kasanin described nine patients who, in the context of either persistent or recent emotional difficulties, developed a sudden psychosis characterised by fantastical delusions, hallucinations and affective symptoms. The combination of schizophrenic and affective symptoms in the acute illness led him to coin the term schizoaffective disorder. All these patients recovered within a few months. Since then the term has been used in various ways. It has been used in the past to describe patients who have schizophrenia and later become depressed, a condition now known as post-psychotic depression (McGlashan and Carpenter 1976); or as a category into which patients are placed if their diagnosis is unclear.

Nowadays, only those patients who simultaneously have the characteristic symptoms of schizophrenia and of either mania or depression merit the diagnosis (Spitzer *et al.* 1978). Thus there are two sub-categories of schizoaffective disorder, namely schizoaffective mania and schizoaffective depression.

It remains unclear whether patients who fall into these categories constitute a separate group or represent a sub-group of either schizophrenia or the affective psychoses. At present the evidence suggests that schizoaffective mania is a variant of affective psychosis, while schizoaffective depression is more closely related to schizophrenia (Brockington and Meltzer 1983).

CLINICAL FEATURES OF CHRONIC SCHIZOPHRENIA

Some patients who have had episodes of acute schizophrenia from which they never fully recovered may go on to develop chronic schizophrenia. The main features of chronic schizophrenia consist of withdrawal, social isolation, flattening of affect, poverty of speech and ideation, and lack of drive or motivation. This is called the *clinical poverty syndrome*. In contrast to the so-called positive symptoms seen in acute schizophrenia, the symptoms of the clinical poverty syndrome are described as negative. The more positive, florid symptoms seen in acute schizophrenia, e.g. delusions and auditory hallucinations, may sometimes be present as well. For example, some chronic schizophrenic patients continue to hear voices and these may become treasured companions, so that the patient misses them when they disappear. Others continue to feel persecuted by their voices.

Negative symptoms are often seen in patients who have become institutionalised in mental hospitals. Studies of people with chronic schizophrenia who have become institutionalised over many years have demonstrated that the severity of negative features is related to the lack of social stimulation they receive and the number of personal possessions they have (Wing and Brown 1970). However, the clinical poverty syndrome can develop and persist even under favourable social conditions. It should also be noted that chronic schizophrenia can develop insidiously in people who have not been psychiatric patients before.

The diagnosis of chronic schizophrenia cannot be made on the clinical poverty syndrome alone, since there are many other causes of communication problems and social withdrawal. The syndrome is frequently coupled with some form of schizophrenic thought disorder, e.g. a loosening of thought associations; sometimes speech is entirely incomprehensible. The combination of thought disorder with the clinical poverty syndrome strongly supports a diagnosis of chronic schizophrenia. There may, of course, have been previous episodes of acute schizophrenia, but the chronic syndrome can develop without there having been an earlier acute episode.

AETIOLOGY OF SCHIZOPHRENIA

It is important to separate factors thought to play a major role in causing schizophrenia from factors which have a crucial bearing on the course of the condition, affecting relapse and remission. The two will interact, but causation and course may have different determinants. The following are the main aetiological theories of schizophrenia.

Genetic factors

There is strong evidence that genetic factors play an important role in the aetiology of schizophrenia. One of the major issues in research is to try to separate inherited from environmental factors and to study their interactions. These issues have been reviewed by Shields (1978) and Rainer (1982).

The early studies were concerned with determining the life-time risk of developing schizophrenia for members of families in whom one or more members were known to have schizophrenia, compared with the life-time risk in the general population. The latter is now known to lie between 0.8 and 1 per cent. Slater and Cowie (1971) and Shields (1978) have reviewed the data from a variety of studies. The risk of developing schizophrenia among close relatives of someone who is schizophrenic is as follows:

Siblings of one schizophrenic person, neither parent affected:	9%
Children of one schizophrenic parent, mother or father:	12%
Children of two schizophrenic parents:	40%

While these figures strongly suggest a genetic basis, the possibility that they could be due to environmental influences could not be excluded as in these studies family members were all brought up in the same family. The figures are however useful in genetic counselling, whatever their origin.

In order to separate genetic from environmental factors researchers have turned to twin studies, comparing rates of schizophrenia in monozygotic and dizygotic twins. Monozygotic twins are genetically identical. As they are brought up in the same environment, they also share the same environmental factors. Dizygotic twins do not share the same genetic make-up, but do share the same environment. The *concordance rates* for schizophrenia between the two groups have therefore been compared. If we considered ten pairs of twins and found that one of each of these pairs had schizophrenia and every one of the co-twins also developed schizophrenia, the concordance rate would be 100 per cent. If, out of the ten pairs of twins, only five pairs were concordant, i.e. both twins were affected in only five out of the ten pairs, the concordance rate would be 50 per cent.

There is general agreement that the concordance rate for monozygotic twins is considerably greater than for dizygotic twins. However, the figures differ widely in different studies. This is partly due to the fact that in earlier studies monozygosity was not always clearly determined, but also because different criteria and degrees of severity were used for the diagnosis of schizophrenia. To give two examples, in a study by Gottesman and Shields (1972) the concordance rate was 50 per cent for monozygotic and 12 per cent for dizygotic twins; in a Norwegian study (Kringlen 1967) the concordance rate was 25-38 per cent for monozygotic and 4-10 per cent for dizygotic twins.

While these findings strongly support the importance of genetic factors, environmentalists have argued that the very nature of twinship, especially identical twinship, causes problems in the development of twins. 'Sameness' is often encouraged in identical twins, e.g. in dress and education, and the influence of the one on the other is very great. As a result, mutual dependence, jealousy and difficulty in achieving a sense of separate identity can cause serious emotional problems, which might contribute to the development of schizophrenia.

In order further to distinguish between genetic and environmental factors, studies have been carried out in which children born to a schizophrenic mother but separated from her a few days after birth and subsequently brought up in foster homes or institutions or adopted, were compared with a control group of children of non-schizophrenic mothers similarly separated from their mothers and reared in similar placements (Heston 1966; Heston and Denney 1968). In Heston's studies, conducted in Oregon, USA, there was further clear evidence of a genetic basis. Of 47 children of schizophrenic mothers who had been separated from their biological mother within a few days of birth, 5 later developed schizophrenia; none of the control children of non-schizophrenic mothers developed schizophrenia. These findings have been confirmed by studies by Rosenthal *et al.* (1968, 1971) who studied children reared in adoptive homes in Denmark. These authors used rather wide diagnostic criteria, including in their group of patients not only those diagnosed as schizophrenic but also some borderline (see p. 342) and schizoid personality disorders, a group they called 'schizophrenia spectrum' disorders, which makes comparison with other studies difficult. However, this does not detract from their finding that adopted children of schizophrenic parents have a significantly greater risk of developing schizophrenia or related disorders than adopted children of non-schizophrenic parents, when brought up by non-schizophrenic adoptive parents.

The same group of Danish and American workers (Kety *et al.* 1968, 1971) have also carried out different kinds of adoption studies, using the Danish adoption register. They compared the biological and the adoptive families of adoptees who had become schizophrenic with the biological and the adoptive families of non-schizophrenic adoptees. Their most significant finding was that the biological families of schizophrenic adoptees showed a significantly higher prevalence of schizophrenia and related disorders than their adoptive families.

Recently Sherrington *et al.* (1988) have actually been able to localise a susceptibility focus for schizophrenia on the long arm of chromosome 5 in two British and five Icelandic families with multiple members suffering from schizophrenia and so-called schizophrenia-spectrum disorders. However, no such abnormality on chromosome 5 was found by Kennedy *et al.* (1988) in a large Swedish pedigree. It seems likely that a variety of abnormal genes may be involved in the susceptibility to schizophrenia (Gill 1988).

In summary, there can no longer be any doubt that genetic factors play a very important role in the aetiology of schizophrenia. At the same time the fact that over half of monozygotic twins born to two schizophrenic parents *do not* develop schizophrenia suggests that environmental factors also play a part in determining whether or not a genetically predisposed individual will develop the disorder. Further research on the nature of the interaction between environmental and genetic factors is required.

Biochemical factors

Genetic abnormalities often express themselves through biochemical abnormalities, and in schizophrenia at present the most prominent biochemical theory of aetiology is the dopamine hypothesis.

The *dopamine hypothesis* arose out of studies which investigated the actions of neuroleptic drugs used in the successful treatment of schizophrenia. The phenothiazine group of drugs act on the dopaminergic system by blocking post-synaptic dopamine receptors, and in some cases this gives rise to Parkinsonian and other extrapyramidal symptoms. Indeed the therapeutic potency of the drugs appears closely related to the degree of dopamine blockade they produce.

It was therefore originally postulated that people with schizophrenia have an excessive turnover of dopamine in the brain, but there is little experimental evidence to support this. There is no excess of homovanillic acid, the main dopamine metabolite, in the cerebrospinal fluid of schizophrenic patients and no increased excretion of dopamine or its metabolites in the urine. The hypothesis that schizophrenia might be due to excessive dopaminergic activity in the brain is also difficult to reconcile with the fact that dopaminergic neurones are widely distributed in the brain, including especially the basal ganglia, the substantia nigra, the mid-brain and the hypothalamic-pituitary pathways. Any excess of dopaminergic activity would have to account for the specific symptoms of schizophrenia, possibly by affecting some particular parts of the dopaminergic system, but as yet there is no evidence for this. Furthermore antipsychotic drugs do not have effects specific to schizophrenia, but are equally effective in mania. It would appear that, although dopamine receptors are blocked by drugs which control schizophrenic symptoms, there is no proof that increased dopaminergic activity is the central aetiological mechanism in schizophrenia.

Another theory, the *transmethylation hypothesis*, arose from the finding that certain hallucinogenic drugs, e.g. mescaline and lysergic acid diethylamide (LSD), are methylated derivatives of dopamine and of indoleamine respectively. It was postulated therefore that abnormalities in neurotransmitter metabolism might result in the production of endogenous hallucinogenic substances, which might then give rise to the symptoms and signs of schizophrenia. However, the drug-induced psychoses produced by mescaline and LSD differ in many ways from a schizophrenic psychosis, and the search for toxic metabolites of neurotransmitters has proved unsuccessful.

Psychodynamic factors

The descriptive or phenomenological approach has provided the criteria needed to make a diagnosis of schizophrenia and to distinguish it from other psychiatric disorders; in the last few decades research has also provided essential information on the genetic and biochemical factors which are involved in the aetiology of the disease, as outlined above.

However, there is a widespread tendency to use the symptoms of schizophrenia – the thought disorder and the delusions and hallucinations – merely to make the diagnosis, while ignoring the meaning of these symptoms. Psychological understanding of the form and content of schizophrenic symptoms can add considerably to our knowledge of the relationship of the symptoms to the patient's personality, and his present or past experiences, and thus to better understanding of the illness as it affects the individual.

It is the psychodynamic and, more specificially, the psychoanalytic approach which has provided such psychological understanding. Whether this also contributes to our knowledge of the aetiology of the disorder remains uncertain.

At the beginning of this century, Jung (1907) began to study schizophrenic patients in depth while working with Bleuler at the Burghölzli Hospital in Zurich (see p. 562). In essence Jung considered that in schizophrenia, then still called dementia praecox, unconscious material entered consciousness and that, as in dreams, analysis of the content and nature of the symptoms could lead to psychological understanding of the meaning of the patient's symptomatology and abnormal behaviour. Later on he acknowledged that organic factors may also be involved in the causation of the disorder, and that this might determine whether a patient develops a psychotic rather than a neurotic disorder when unconscious conflicts enter consciousness.

Freud did not treat any psychotic patients by psychoanalysis. He did, however, make a contribution to the understanding of the psychoses by applying the psychoanalytic concepts he was using at the time to an autobiographical account by a man suffering from a severe paranoid psychosis. The name of the author was Schreber and the detailed study by Freud (1911) of Schreber's description of his illness is referred to as the Schreber case (see p. 260). Nowadays, Schreber's illness would probably be diagnosed as paranoid schizophrenia.

Briefly, Freud considered that, in response to unacceptable and hence anxiety- and guilt-provoking impulses, the schizophrenic withdraws from real people and objects in the outer world, and compensates for this by living in a fantasy world of internal images or objects. The psychotic person's delusions and hallucinations and the fantasised people or objects then fill the gap left by the loss of real relationships in the outer world. Such withdrawal into a fantasy world could, Freud thought, be understood in a way similar to that in which neurotic symptoms could be understood. For example, he explained the development of paranoid delusions in terms of the defence mechanism of projections; the patient projects his own aggressive impulses into others and feels himself to be the victim of their aggressive attacks against him. Freud also considered that the schizophrenic patient regresses to earlier narcissistic stages of development so that he himself instead of others becomes the centre of his attention or 'libido'.

Since then several psychoanalysts have made important advances towards the psychological understanding of schizophrenia. Freeman in this country has studied acute and chronic schizophrenic patients by observing their behaviour and communications during interviews and analytical psychotherapy (Freeman et al. 1965; Freeman 1969, 1988). He considered that the symptoms could best be understood in terms of disturbed object-relationships, including transference phenomena, the meaning to the patient of his delusions and hallucinations, the kind of defence mechanisms, primitive or more mature, which are being used, disturbed cognitive and perceptual functions, and the nature of the super-ego. Searles (1965) in the USA has carried out similar studies in chronic schizophrenic patients in psychoanalytic treatment as inpatients at Chestnut Lodge, Rockville, Maryland, USA.

Further advances have been made by those psychoanalysts who use the concepts of Melanie Klein (see p. 70), especially Rosenfeld (1965, 1987) and Bion (1967) in this country and Kernberg (1977b) in the USA. These concepts include the role of primitive defence mechanisms like splitting and projective identification (see pp. 49, 56), and regression to the paranoid-schizoid position (see p. 70). This has thrown new light on the nature of the patient's symptomatology and his disturbed relationship to others. The following examples will illustrate this further.

When a schizophrenic patient uses modes of functioning characteristic of the earliest, symbiotic stage of development (see p. 65), i.e. a sense of fusion with mother, he is unable to experience himself as separate from other people. Thus he may feel identified with, say, his doctor or nurse, or with Christ or the Devil, or with his therapist in the transference. When he relates to others in a manner corresponding to the beginning of the separation-individuation phase (see p. 66), his ability to distinguish between himself and others, his so-called ego-boundary, will be ill-defined. He may then feel that his thoughts are known to others (thought broadcasting), or put into his mind by others (thought insertion). He may feel unsure whether he is a man or a woman, still easily identifying with a person of the opposite sex, and suffer from confusion as a result. When he regresses to the paranoid-schizoid position he will experience the world as entirely hostile and persecutory. And when he uses the mechanism of projective identification he may, for example, project all the destructive parts of his own personality into his therapist who will then be experienced as dangerous and destructive.

Bion (1967) has suggested that a schizophrenic person may feel that his own thoughts and words are destructive so that he dares not make normal use of words or sentences and thus develops thought disorder.

What light does such psychodynamic understanding of schizophrenic symptoms and behaviour throw on the aetiology of the disorder? The genetic basis of schizophrenia and the effectiveness of antipsychotic drugs in the control of the acute symptoms and prevention of relapses make it clear that psychological factors alone cannot account for its origin. Interaction between organic and psychological factors provides a more likely explanation. One possibility is that disturbed cerebral function, of genetic and biochemical origin, could lead to the abnormal psychological functions described above. In some patients, emotional disurbances in early childhood combined with serious present-day stresses could lead to regression, resulting in the use of primitive mental mechanisms. This, in genetically predisposed individuals, could then precipitate the onset of the psychotic illness. An integrated approach, which combines psychodynamic understanding with knowledge of biological factors, is more likely to lead to better understanding and management of the illness in each individual patient than either a biological or a psychodynamic approach on its own.

Family influences

It has been claimed that abnormal family influences and disturbed parent-child interactions are significant factors in the causation of schizophrenia. For example, it has been suggested that a cold, rejecting mother and an indifferent, passive father predispose a child to the development of schizophrenia. An American psychoanalyst, Fromm-Reichman (1948) even coined the unfortunate term 'schizophrenogenic mother'. There is no evidence to support these views.

It was Gregory Bateson, an anthropologist, who first put forward another theory, that of the *double-bind* (Bateson *et al.* 1956). Essentially, a double-bind consists of the child repeatedly being given one set of instructions, usually verbal, by a parent, while all the non-verbal clues imply the opposite. The child is literally 'bound' and does not know how to respond or what is expected of him. An example may help to illustrate this point: a teenage girl asks her mother if she can go out with her friends to the cinema. Her mother replies, 'Of course dear – do go', but in a tone of voice which clearly indicates how unhappy it makes her to be left alone all evening. However, double-binding takes place in ordinary families, and there is no convincing evidence that it causes schizophrenia.

Other family theories of schizophrenia are those of Lidz, Wynne, and Laing. Lidz has described two typical kinds of family structure (Lidz *et al.* 1957; Lidz 1975). One type is called 'marital skew'. Here one dominant parent has a pathological hold on the child which the other parent is too passive to prevent. The other type is called 'marital schism' in which constant conflict between the parents leads each to belittle the other, so that the child is caught in the middle. Again, these kind of abnormalities have been found in many families and are not specific to schizophrenia.

Wynne has suggested that disordered communication occurs among the parents of people who later develop schizophrenia, notably 'vague, indefinite and loose' communications (Wynne *et al.* 1958, 1977). These studies suggest that such disordered communications were more common in parents of schizophrenic than in parents of neurotic offspring. It is, however, possible that these abnormalities could be a reaction to, rather than a cause of the illness. Other studies have failed to confirm these findings (Hirsch and Leff 1975).

Laing (1960) and Laing and Esterson (1964) believed that schizophrenia should not be viewed as an illness at all. Instead of considering the individual schizophrenic person as being the sick member of the family, they considered that it was the whole family, and society, who were sick. The pressures of a sick society are exerted through the family, and result in one family member becoming schizophrenic. The person labelled schizophrenic is then seen as struggling to maintain his autonomy within a sick family. Laing's theories are interesting and provocative hypotheses but they are of little value in clinical practice when faced with a schizophrenic patient. His clinical observations (Laing 1960) are more helpful when trying to understand patients with schizoid personality disorders (see p. 330).

Life events

As with other psychiatric illnesses, in schizophrenia there is convincing evidence that life events may be precipitating factors. A life event may involve some type of loss, e.g. moving house, losing a job, illness or death in the family. Alternatively, it may be an emotionally charged event, e.g. marriage or the birth of a child. It is important to distinguish dependent from independent life events in the onset of schizophrenia. If somebody loses his job as a result of early symptoms preceding the onset of schizophrenia this would represent a life event dependent on the illness. If, however, everyone at work was made redundant, this would represent an independent life event.

Brown and Birley (1968) compared the incidence of independent life events in a group of fifty patients admitted for an acute episode of schizophrenia with a group of control subjects. Three times as many of the schizophrenic patients (60 per cent) had experienced such life events over a three-week period before the onset of their first attack or relapse of acute schizophrenia, compared with the control group (20 per cent).

Social factors

First attacks of schizophrenia are known to occur more commonly in people of lower socio-economic status. At first this was thought to be due to the stresses people are exposed to in such low-status groups. However, it was then found that social distribution of the fathers of these schizophrenic patients was evenly distributed throughout the socio-economic classes. The greater incidence of first attacks of schizophrenia in these lower status groups, therefore, appears to represent a drift down the social scale before the onset of the illness (see also p. 38).

It is also known that schizophrenic patients are over-represented in under-priviledged inner-city areas with a high proportion of single-person households; moreover, a higher proportion of schizophrenic patients are unmarried and live alone, when first admitted, compared with non-schizophrenic controls. There is evidence (see p. 38) that the higher incidence of first attacks of schizophrenia in inner-city areas is confined to migrants, who have come from more privileged areas during the last few years before the onset of the illness.

These findings indicate that the drift down the socio-economic scale, social isolation and migration into inner-city areas all precede the onset of schizophrenia, perhaps due to pre-morbid problems in interpersonal relations and poor social functioning. However, the resultant social isolation, life in unfamiliar surroundings and poor socio-economic conditions may, in turn, act as precipitant factors, initiating the first attack in people already predisposed to schizophrenia.

Predisposing factors

As described in the section on genetics, hereditary factors undoubtedly predispose a person to schizophrenia. Whether early family influences affecting personality development can also act as predisposing factors, increasing a person's vulnerability to schizophrenia, remains uncertain.

There is some evidence that schizophrenia is more common among later-born siblings in large families; this is necessarily associated with greater maternal age. There is also a trend towards a greater incidence of winter births, but the reason for this association remains unknown.

Research has also been done on the possible influence of pre-natal, obstetric and post-natal complications. Retrospective studies of schizophrenic patients are limited by the difficulty in obtaining accurate data of perinatal complications. Attempts have therefore been made to carry out prospective studies of people at high risk of developing schizophrenia, e.g. children born to a schizophrenic parent. Such studies are so far inconclusive.

Neurological factors

Minor neurological abnormalities, without localising significance, have been reported in some patients with schizophrenia. The most common are those of balance, proprioception and stereognosis. None is of diagnostic value.

Non-specific EEG abnormalities have also been reported. CT scans of the brain have revealed more abnormalities in schizophrenic than normal subjects. For example, there is evidence of ventricular enlargement in some patients with chronic schizophrenia (Farmer et al. 1987). Larger ventricular size among the siblings of schizophrenic people has also been reported; the significance of these findings is unclear (Weinberger et al. 1980). The important association between schizophrenia and epilepsy is discussed on p. 317.

TREATMENT OF ACUTE SCHIZOPHRENIA

Patients with acute schizophrenia usually need to be treated as inpatients, although there are exceptions to this. The main reasons for admission are the following:

(1) Appearance or reappearance of acute schizophrenic symptoms.
(2) Unpredictable or threatening behaviour by the patient, which has led to anxiety in others.
(3) Lack of family or social support.

In practice, admission is more often needed when two of these situations occur together (Sturgeon and Bowman 1977). Admission to hospital may in itself be therapeutic. Taking someone out of an environment which may have helped to precipitate the illness can diminish the intensity of the symptoms and lead to their eventual resolution. In the days before effective antipsychotic medication, there was little else that could be done, although insulin coma and ECT were tried.

Drugs

Before the introduction of phenothiazine medication in the 1950s, episodes of schizophrenia lasted for months or years. The new drugs have revolutionised treatment, as psychotic symptoms were found to respond rapidly. A wide range of phenothiazine drugs with different properties is now available (see p. 612).

Patients often need high doses of antipsychotic medication during an acute florid episode of illness, e.g. 200 mg of chlorpromazine four times a day. This dosage may need to be maintained for several days or even weeks until the florid symptoms begin to fade. The dosage can then be gradually reduced as improvement occurs, but in order to reduce the risk of relapses it is advisable for the patient to continue taking a small maintenance dose of antipsychotic medication for a considerable time after the acute episode (see also p. 252).

Some patients tolerate the phenothiazine group of drugs poorly, and may do better on haloperidol, a butyrophenone (see p. 614). Recently there has been some suggestion that the anti-epileptic drug carbamazepine, in high doses, has an antipsychotic effect. However, it may prove more effective in the control of manic than schizophrenic symptoms.

Schizophrenic patients who need long-term antipsychotic medication are often advised to take depot preparations, such as fluphenazine or flupenthixol decanoate (see p. 615). These are given by intramuscular injection once every two to three weeks. This avoids the need to take daily oral antipsychotic medication. Oral medication has however been shown to be as successful in preventing relapse as depot preparations, provided the patient is willing to take it and remembers to do so.

Side-effects

The phenothiazines have many untoward side-effects. The most common of these are the extrapyramidal effects which result from the fact that the phenothiazines act by blocking the effect of dopamine on dopamine receptors. They include drug-induced Parkinsonism, acute dystonia, akathisia and tardive dyskinesia (Marsden and Jenner 1980; Marsden *et al.* 1975).

Drug-induced Parkinsonism

Parkinsonian features usually develop a few weeks after starting treatment. They consist of facial immobility, lack of movement, muscular rigidity and increased salivation. In schizophrenia the antipsychotic effects of phenothiazines are so important that treatment should be continued though at reduced dosage if possible. If Parkinsonian symptoms persist these should be treated with an anti-parkinsonian agent such as procyclidine 5-10 mg or benzhexol 2-5 mg three times daily. Anti-parkinsonian drugs should not be given routinely as not all patients develop Parkinsonian symptoms while on phenothiazines, and they have their own side-effects; they may also increase the risk of developing tardive dyskinesia.

Acute dystonia

This consists of the sudden onset of involuntary muscular spasms, e.g. of the muscles of the face, tongue, jaw or neck, leading to torticollis, or of the spine. An oculogyric crisis is another manifestation. The dystonic symptoms usually start within a few days of starting treatment with phenothiazines and occasionally after only one or two doses. The symptoms are relieved by the intramuscular injection of procyclidine or benzhexol.

Akathisia

This usually starts within a few days of starting treatment and consists of acute restlessness. Patients are unable to sit down or to keep still. It may be accompanied by increased salivation and an unpleasant sensation of the tongue being drawn back into the mouth. Treatment is the same as for acute dystonia.

Tardive dyskinesia

This occurs later in treatment (hence the term 'tardive') when high doses of antipsychotic drugs are given over long periods, especially in the elderly, in those who have previously had akathisia, and in patients with associated organic cerebral disorder. It is characterised by lip-smacking, chewing and sucking movements, grimacing, and sometimes choreo-athetoid movements of the trunk and extremities. This is a serious complication because it frequently persists even when the drugs are stopped (Barnes et al. 1983; Stahl 1986). Recent reports suggest that it improves or disappears in only about half the cases. Tetrabenazine 25-100 mg has helped some patients.

It has been suggested that tardive dyskinesia may be due to hypersensitivity of or an increase in the number of post-synaptic dopamine receptors in the striatum following long-term dopamine blockade. A rare complication, the *neuroleptic malignant syndrome*, is discussed on p. 616.

Other side-effects

Galactorrhoea with engorged breasts, due to increased secretion of prolactin, and *amenorrhoea* occur in some women. Men may develop enlarged breasts and decreased libido or impotence.

Postural hypotension occurs particularly after intramuscular injection of chlorpromazine, or when high doses are used, and in the elderly.

Cardiac arrhythmias may occur, probably as the result of the anti-adrenergic action of some phenothiazines, especially those with a piperidine side chain.

Cholestatic jaundice is most likely to occur when chlorpromazine is used; it usually clears up when the drug is stopped. If necessary, another antipsychotic drug should be substituted, e.g. trifluoperazine. 5 mg of trifluoperazine is equivalent to 100 mg of chlorpromazine.

Anticholinergic effects. These include a dry mouth, urinary retention, constipation and blurred vision. Ejaculation may be retarded.

Inhibition of melanin reactivity. This can lead to photosensitivity and skin rashes, especially in patients on chlorpromazine. They should be told to avoid exposure to direct sunlight.

Deposition of pigment, causing purple patches in the skin, has been described. Pigment deposits in the cornea and lens can cause visual disturbance. Thioridazine can cause pigmentary retinopathy, leading to blindness.

The *seizure threshold* can be lowered and this can lead to epileptic fits, especially in patients with epilepsy.

Social and occupational therapy

During their inpatient stay, it is most important to encourage patients to develop relationships with staff and other patients. This can be very difficult initially because much of the patient's thinking may be preoccupied with hallucinations and delusional beliefs and his behaviour may be very disturbing to the other patients and staff. However, every effort should be made to ensure that the patient does not remain withdrawn and isolated as this may delay recovery. It is also important that the medical and nursing staff try to understand, as far as possible, the nature of the patient's psychotic beliefs and the reasons for his disturbed behaviour, so that they can establish a helpful relationship, however difficult this may be.

Many activities in occupational therapy (see Chapter 60) are designed to create a focus for the patient's thoughts and provide an outlet for them; to give the patient an opportunity to interact with other people; and to help him to attain a sense of achievement. Work-like activities may reduce the frequency and intensity of hallucinations. Some patients find relief through painting, which may give them an opportunity to express their thoughts and fantasies. Several impressive collections of schizophrenic art exist in centres throughout the world. However, some creative artists lose their creativity when they become schizophrenic, for example the dancer Nijinsky (1890-1950) and the poet Hölderlin (1770-1843). Van Gogh (1853-1890) continued to paint during his psychotic episodes, but his illness was probably not schizophrenia but due to manic-depressive psychosis or the toxic effects of absinthe (Hemphill 1961).

As the psychosis fades and insight begins to return, patients are often confused and upset by what has happened to them. It is important to give them the opportunity to talk about the realities and frightening aspects of their illness with a sensitive and exerienced person who can go on supporting them after discharge from hospital. A combination of antipsychotic medication, social measures and supportive psychotherapy is more effective than medication alone.

Psychotherapy

Before the discovery of antipsychotic drugs in the 1950s, no effective treatment for schizophrenia was available. Various forms of psychotherapy, especially psychoanalytic psychotherapy and psychoanalysis were therefore used to try to help patients with acute or chronic schizophrenia, both in the USA (Fromm-Reichman 1954; Searles 1965; Arieti 1974) and the UK (Rosenfeld 1965; Freeman 1988). As described earlier (see p. 239), while this has led to greatly increased understanding of the meaning of the symptoms and behaviour, the effectiveness of psychoanalytic psychotherapy in schizophrenia has remained controversial.

Freud himself held the view that psychoanalysis could not be used to treat schizophrenic or other psychotic patients because he considered that they, unlike psychoneurotic patients, were unable to develop a transference, which had by then been recognised as an essential condition for successful psychoanalytic treatment (Freud 1916, pp. 438-439, 447). Since then the work of Rosenfeld (1965, 1987), Searles (1965) and others has shown that schizophrenic patients do in fact develop a strong transference towards their therapist, but this differs in important respects from the transference of patients with psychoneuroses and other non-psychotic disorders The psychotic patient is unable to distinguish transference from reality; he may, for example, consider his therapist *in reality* to be his hostile, frightening father instead of seeing that he is reacting to him *as if* he were his father. This absence of the capacity for insight and self-observation in the psychotic therefore makes it difficult, or impossible, for the therapist or analyst to sort out with the patient what is happening in their relationship. Such a *psychotic transference* makes work in the transference extremely difficult, and this in turn leads to corresponding problems in the counter-transference; the therapist may feel confused, useless, persecuted, frightened, angry and at times even identified with his patient's madness. Psychoanalysts who treat psychotic patients differ in their view of how to handle patients with a psychotic transference. Rosenfeld (1965, 1987), considered that in spite of the serious difficulties involved the analyst should rely on the use of interpretations, while others modify their technique and use a more flexible and supportive approach. In either case the aim is the same, i.e. to help the patient regain insight and a sense of reality.

The present position can be summarised as follows. There is now strong clinical evidence that for acute episodes of schizophrenia, analytical psychotherapy or psychoanalysis by themselves do not constitute adequate treatment. If attempted, they need to be combined with antipsychotic medication. During the acute stage the patient will probably have to be treated in hospital and, once discharged, the psychotherapist must have access to further management as an inpatient if the patient's symptoms recur. Some patients benefit from a combination of psychoanalytic treatment with drug therapy and find the growing understanding of the meaning of their symptoms and the relationship to the therapist helpful. The advances in our understanding of the symptomatology of schizophrenia which have arisen from such psychoanalytic treatment have already been described (see p. 240). Other patients find the close emotional involvement with their therapist too disturbing and either break off treatment or suffer a relapse. It has been claimed that analytical psychotherapy may prevent relapses, but this needs further study.

Even though in clinical practice psychoanalytic psychotherapy is rarely indicated in the treatment of schizophrenic patients, the majority of patients benefit if those who look after them, be it in hospital or in the community, can understand the meaning of their patients' disturbed behaviour and apply this in day-to-day management alongside any other treatment methods.

TREATMENT OF CHRONIC SCHIZOPHRENIA

Drug treatment in chronic schizophrenia is much less successful than in acute schizophrenia. Although the positive, florid symptoms respond to medication, the negative features often show no improvement. The treatment of chronic schizophrenia relies mainly on social interventions, encouraging the patient to be more active and less withdrawn, and aims to redevelop his skills, e.g. by using industrial and social and rehabilitation programmes. Day-care programmes can often provide the support many patients need, and community care schemes can bring considerable improvements to their daily lives. However, it should be remembered that too much pressure can precipitate relapse.

In the longer term, many chronic patients need sheltered accommodation to provide support and some degree of supervision. This is often necessary to maintain the patient at his optimal level of functioning, and withdrawal of social support often leads to clinical deterioration. Relatives of patients also need counselling, help and practical guidance.

COURSE AND PROGNOSIS

It is important to note that 25 per cent of patients who present for the first time with acute schizophrenia make a complete and permanent recovery. In about another 50 per cent of cases there will be relapses, without progression to chronic schizophrenia. In the remaining 25 per cent of cases, recurrent relapses lead to personality deterioration with impairment of social function and behaviour, culminating in the development of the chronic syndrome. As described earlier, it is possible to develop chronic schizophrenia without ever having experienced an acute episode. Acute episodes can also be superimposed on the chronic syndrome. This may lead to an exacerbation of chronic schizophrenia with intensification of the negative symptoms. Given adequate social and rehabilitative interventions, marked improvements can occur. Manfred Bleuler (1974; 1978) has followed up over 200 patients for twenty years and has described the course of their illness in detail.

How, then, can we predict which patients are likely to become more severely or less severely handicapped by schizophrenia? Certain factors seem to be of some help as indicators of prognosis:

(1) *Age*: the younger the person is when he first becomes ill, the worse the prognosis.

(2) *Onset*: a rapid onset, over a few days or a week or so, carries a better prognosis than a gradual onset over months or years.

(3) *Affect*: preservation of affect during the acute episodes has a better prognosis than flattening of affect. Depressive symptoms carry a better prognosis, excitement a poorer prognosis.

(4) *Family history*: a family history of schizophrenia carries a worse prognosis.

(5) *Intelligence*: higher intelligence appears to be associated with a better prognosis.

(6) *Pre-morbid personality*: a person with a 'good' pre-morbid personality, i.e. an ability to socialise, form relationships and a good work record, has a better prognosis.

On average, the florid symptoms of an acute episode treated with antipsychotic drugs (see p. 245) will have disappeared in eight to twelve weeks. The patient will then be put on a maintenance dose of antipsychotic medication, which should be the smallest dose necessary to prevent symptom re-emergence. Patients with good prognostic indicators may only need to take medication for six months. There is, however, strong evidence that patients who continue to take antipsychotic medication for at least two years after the acute episode have lower relapse rates than those who do not take medication over this period.

Many patients, on leaving hospital, can benefit from spending time in after-care homes or hostels, such as the Richmond Fellowship provides. Here, patients are given a structure to their day and are also helped to talk through any emotional or practical problems which arise. Many people find this transition between the hospital and the community helpful and reassuring.

Family life and relapse rate

It has been mentioned that 75 per cent of patients who present with a first episode of schizophrenia are at risk of relapse. Much work has been done to establish the reasons for this and how it can be prevented.

Brown *et al.* (1958) discovered that the relapse rate for schizophrenic patients who, after discharge from hospital, returned to live with a relative, was significantly higher than the relapse rate for those who lived either in lodgings or with a non-relative. Research workers then investigated the reason for these differences. The emotional atmosphere in the family appeared to be of prime importance. An index of *expressed emotion* (EE) was developed as a measure of the emotional atmosphere in the family (Brown and Rutter 1966). This is done by giving a semi-structured interview called the Camberwell Family Interview to the patient's relatives in their own home. The interview is recorded and subsequently analysed for four features: critical comments, hostility, warmth and over-involvement. Relatives can thus be assigned to either a 'high EE' or a 'low EE' category (Vaughn and Leff 1976a, 1976b; Leff and Vaughn 1981). It was found that relapse was far more likely if the patient lived in a family with high EE. The effect of expressed emotion and the amount of contact

Fig. 20.1. Percentage of patients who relapsed during a nine-month follow-up

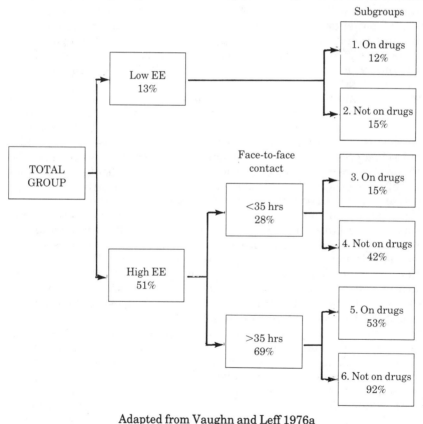

Adapted from Vaughn and Leff 1976a

between patient and relative on the rate of relapse is shown in Figure 20.1. Those patients who are in high contact, defined as more than 35 hours per week of face-to-face contact, with high EE reatives are at the greatest risk of relapse. If patients take antipsychotic medication, their relapse rate falls from 92 per cent to 53 per cent; if they also reduce the amount of social contact with their high EE relatives to below 35 hours a week, the relapse rate falls even further to 15 per cent. This is directly comparable to that of the low risk group (Leff and Vaughn 1981; Leff *et al.* 1983). There are also psychophysiological differences between the two groups (Sturgeon *et al.* 1984).

Leff *et al.* (1982) have been able to change the expressed emotion of relatives from high to low and to reduce the amount of social contact between patient and relatives by educating the relatives about the nature of schizophrenia, by providing a relatives' group where they could discuss difficult issues, and by working with the families in family therapy sessions.

Over the course of nine months, 75 per cent of the high EE relatives either changed to low EE or reduced the amount of social contact with the patient to below 35 hours a week. The relapse rate in this experimental group of patients, all of whom, like those in the control group, were maintained on antipsychotic medication, was 8 per cent compared to a relapse rate of 50 per cent in the control group. The effects of this intervention programme were still significant at a two-year follow-up (Leff *et al.* 1985).

It is important to stress that the intentions of high EE relatives are not 'bad'. They are concerned and worried about the well-being of their schizophrenic family member, doing the best they can with the means at their disposal. Relatives often receive little or no advice or counselling about schizophrenia from professionals, and are sometimes made to feel guilty or responsible for having in some way brought about the condition. They often feel socially isolated, unsupported and poorly understood. Relatives often need as much help and support as the patient.

However, even under the most favourable circumstances, some patients still relapse. It seems likely that this is, at least in part, due to the impact of life events. Patients living with low EE relatives show a clear association between relapse and life events. However, those patients at high risk of relapse, i.e. living in high contact with high EE relatives and not on medication, show no such association. They are presumably so close to the threshold of relapse for most of the time that no life event is needed in addition to cause a relapse.

Leff *et al.* (1983) propose a hypothetical interaction between life events, medication and expressed emotion in the relative to account for a schizophrenic patient's vulnerability to relapse (see Figure 20.2, in which the curves represent a patient's likelihood of relapse). The likelihood is increased by either a life event, or by living with a high EE relative. The curve rises steeply in response to a life event, more gradually in response to contact with a high EE relative, until it reaches the level at which schizophrenic symptoms appear – at the line marked (a). Maintenance treatment with antipsychotic drugs raises the threshold of relapse to the line marked (b). However, the new elevated threshold may still be exceeded when a patient, living with a high EE relative, experiences a life event.

Fig. 20.2. Life events, relatives' expressed emotion and drugs in schizophrenia.

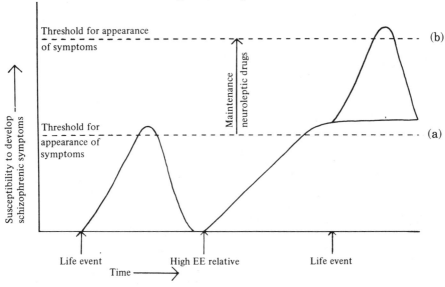

Adapted from Leff *et al.* 1983

These findings are of considerable help in clinical practice as they indicate ways of reducing the relapse rate in schizophrenia.

FURTHER READING

Arieti, S. (1974). *Interpretation of Schizophrenia*. Basic Books, New York.

Creer, C and Wing, J. (1975). 'Living with a schizophrenic patient'. *Brit. J. Hosp. Med.* 14, 73-82.

Freeman, T. (1988). *The Psychoanalyst in Psychiatry*. Karnac Books, London.

Hamilton, M. (ed.) (1984a) *Fish's Schizophrenia* 3rd ed. Wright, Bristol. (An up-dated edition of Fish's original account of schizophrenia, published in 1962.)

Rosenfeld, H. (1987) *Impasse and Interpretations*, Tavistock, London.

Wing, J.K. (ed.) (1978) *Schizophrenia: towards a new synthesis*. Academic Press, London.

The following novels are also recommended:

Head, Bessie (1973). *A Question of Power*. Heinemann, London.
White, Antonia (1954). *Beyond the Glass*. Virago, London.

21

Paranoid States

Historically the word paranoid, which derives from the Greek words *para* (beside) and *nous* (mind), was used to describe thinking and experiencing the world in a manner which was 'out of mind', or mad. The corresponding noun, paranoia, was similarly used in the last two centuries as almost synonymous with madness. Nowadays paranoid has acquired a much more specific meaning, describing people who experience the world as hostile and persecutory, while the term paranoia is used as a label for only one specific, rare psychiatric disorder, described later in this chapter.

In clinical practice the term paranoid is now used to describe first, certain mental symptoms – paranoid ideas and paranoid delusions – and secondly, certain psychiatric disorders in which these symptoms are prominent.

Paranoid ideas are experienced by many people who are over-sensitive and self-conscious. They consist of feeling that other people are taking undue notice of one, e.g. when in public places or under stress. Such people feel that they are being watched and criticised or that others suspect something they want to keep secret, e.g. that they might be homosexual. Such ideas tend to fade when the person is no longer in the stressful situation. Paranoid ideas differ from delusions in that the person is aware of the fact that he may be imagining these experiences but he cannot control them. Such ideas are common in people with paranoid personality disorders (see p. 330).

Paranoid delusions are firmly held delusions of hostility and persecution (see also p. 122). Grandiose delusions sometimes co-exist so that the patient may feel that he is someone special who is being persecuted; or the delusion of being admired and loved may change into the opposite belief of being hated and persecuted.

By themselves paranoid delusions cannot be used to make a diagnosis because they occur in a variety of psychiatric conditions. These include paranoid schizophrenia, affective disorders and organic psychiatric disorders, e.g. the effects of chronic alcoholism, drug intoxication and acute confusional states, as well as a group of conditions called *paranoid states*, to be considered next. These are rare conditions in which paranoid delusions occur but which do not fit into any of the above categories of organic or affective disorders, nor can they be diagnosed as paranoid schizophrenia, at least not when they first present. They include:

Paranoia
Paraphrenia
Morbid jealousy
Erotomania
Induced psychosis (folie à deux)
Capgras syndrome
Fregoli's syndrome
Dysmorphophobia.

Nowadays it is thought that some of these may be more closely related to schizophrenia than was believed originally; this will be referred to under the individual headings when appropriate.

PARANOIA

This condition was first described by Kraepelin (1921). The central core of paranoia is a well-organised and often elaborate system of paranoid delusions. These are of insidious onset and are not secondary to other conditions, such as alcohol dependence or affective disorder; the delusions run a chronic course, usually without remission. One differentiating feature from schizophrenia is that the delusions are not accompanied by other schizophrenic features and there is no deterioration in the patient's personality.

There is now considerable doubt about the existence of this disorder as a separate entity since, if followed up for long enough, many patients eventually develop schizophrenic features.

PARAPHRENIA

In this condition the paranoid delusions are accompanied by hallucinations, often in several senses. The personality and intellectual functions are well preserved and patients may be able to carry out their day-to-day life reasonably well. Paraphrenia usually starts later in life and may be associated with loneliness and impaired sight or hearing. It is more common in women. The condition responds to treatment with antipsychotic medication, and attempts should be made to improve the sensory deficits and social isolation. It is now thought that this condition may represent the late onset of paranoid schizophrenia, and may not constitute a separate diagnostic entity.

MORBID JEALOUSY

Morbid or pathological jealousy is sometimes called the *Othello syndrome* because the central feature is a delusional belief that one's sexual partner is being unfaithful. The condition has been reviewed by Shepherd (1961).

It is more common in men than in women. The patient often gives a history of having felt inadequate for many years before the onset of the condition, especially in his sexual role.

As a result of his delusional belief, the morbidly jealous person will make life a misery for his partner, and may not allow her out of his sight for more than a few minutes at a time. He will subject her to nothing less than an interrogation whenever he believes she cannot adequately account for her movements. He may frequently search the bed linen or undergarments for signs of sexual infidelity. As a result the partner becomes so desperate that she may agree with his accusations even though she knows they are untrue. This only increases her partner's jealousy, leading to outbursts of rage and violence. In some cases the morbidly jealous man may murder his partner.

Although pathological jealousy may be a distinct syndrome, it can also occur as part of a number of other psychiatric conditions, such as paranoid schizophrenia, depressive illness, alcohol dependence and organic psychiatric disorders. Treatment should then be directed at the underlying cause.

In the absence of any of these associated psychiatric disorders the patient's personality, especially his long-standing sense of inadequacy, plays a major role. Consequently the treatment of the distinct syndrome is more difficult. Antipsychotic medication may be used initially in an attempt to control the delusions. Unfortunately this often fails. The partner also needs help, either individually or by seeing her and the patient together. If the problem continues and the risk of violence remains high, the partner may have to be advised to separate for the sake of her own safety.

EROTOMANIA

(de Clérambault's syndrome)

This is a rare condition described in 1921 by de Clérambault. It is more common in women than men and is characterised by a delusional belief that someone who is either famous or socially superior is passionately in love with her. Sometimes the patient pesters the person she believes loves her. If her demands remain unanswered, her love may turn to hatred and she may believe that, instead of loving her, he hates or deliberately persecutes her. For example, a receptionist suddenly became convinced that the Mayor was deeply in love with her, following his formal visit to the department where she worked. She wrote to him almost every day for a year, urging him to declare his love, to divorce his wife and to marry her. The Mayor's refusal to respond to her letters led her to believe that he was deliberately prolonging her state of unhappiness. The dynamic psychopathology of erotomania has been discussed by Christodoulou (1986) and Freeman (1988).

Erotomania may be a symptom of paranoid schizophrenia, but

characteristic symptoms of schizophrenia may only appear after many
months, if at all.

INDUCED PSYCHOSIS
(folie à deux)

This condition is characterised by the development of a paranoid
delusional system shared by two people who live together, say husband
and wife, two siblings, or parent and child. Very rarely more than two
people may be involved in the shared delusion. Usually one person
develops the delusional system first and the other suggesible partner
develops the same delusion later. For example, a couple in their sixties
were convinced that the neighbours kept them awake at night by placing
a machine against the adjoining wall which sent high-pitched frequencies
into their house. The man, who had developed the delusion first, would
try to detect where the machine was located; he would then make his wife
place a piece of metal sheeting over the spot to reflect the frequencies
back. When her husband was subsequently admitted to hospital, the
wife's belief in the delusion began to fade until she eventually thought it
was silly. The husband's delusions persisted and he was found to be
suffering from schizophrenia. In other cases the partner who first
develops the delusion may not have an identifiable psychiatric disorder
responsible for his delusional system.

Treatment usually requires separation of the two partners in addition
to antipsychotic medication for the more severely affected partner if his
delusions persist.

CAPGRAS SYNDROME

In this condition, described by Capgras and Reboul-Lachaux (1923), the
patient believes that someone she knows well is not in fact that person
but has been replaced by a double. For example, a patient in hospital told
her husband that she knew he was not her husband although he looked
like him and behaved like him; but she 'knew' he was his double. This is a
very rare condition and is more common in women than in men. It may be
associated with schizophrenia or affective disorders. If this is the case,
treatment is that of the underlying condition.

In a related condition, known as *Fregoli's syndrome*, the patient thinks
that people he meets are identical with a person he knows well and
considers to be his persecutor. The conditions are characterised by
misidentification, and their psychodynamic and organic causes have
been discussed by Christodoulou (1986).

DYSMORPHOPHOBIA

This condition is included here as it is often, though not always,
associated with paranoid ideas or paranoid delusions. It is characterised

by the patient's conviction that a part of his own body is misshapen or is too large or too small. Usually only one part of the body is involved, e.g. the nose, ears, mouth, breasts, buttocks, or external genitalia. In fact the observer will not be able to detect any or at most only minimal deformity. The conviction may be delusional or it may be an overvalued idea (see p. 123). It often dates from adolescence, when the patient may report having been teased or having overheard derogatory remarks about his appearance. The patient firmly believes that others are put off by his appearance, and he may be convinced that they are making adverse comments about him. He puts any problems in his personal and social relationships down to his deformity and insists that only plastic surgery can solve his difficulties. The condition is sometimes associated with schizophrenia or depression. More often it is a part of a severe personality disorder (Hay 1970) in which case the mistaken belief takes the form of an overvalued idea rather than a delusion. Birtchnell (1988) has reviewed the disorder.

Treatment of dysmorphophobia is difficult. If there is an underlying psychiatric illness like schizophrenia or depression this should be treated in its own right, but even then patients often remain very resistant to giving up their belief. Surgery is contra-indicated in such cases. Antipsychotic medication, e.g. pimozide, should also be tried in those severe cases of dysmorphophobia in which the delusion is firmly entrenched and persistent, even in the absence of evidence of schizophrenia.

In those patients in whom dysmorphophobia is the result of an underlying personality disorder, and when the belief takes the form of an overvalued idea rather than a delusion, psychotherapy is sometimes worth attempting. The aim of psychotherapy in these cases is to help the patient to recognise that he is displacing unacceptable aspects of his personality into what he considers to be misshapen body parts and to help him resolve the underlying dislike of aspects of himself as a person. If psychotherapy is successful the patient may agree that surgery is no longer necessary. Such a satisfactory outcome of psychotherapy is rare and cosmetic surgery may have to be given a trial. Surgery is more likely to be successful if there is at least some objective evidence of deformity, e.g. a slightly deformed nose. If, as is often the case, the patient is dissatisfied with the result of the operation, severe neurotic symptoms, depression, paranoid or schizophrenic symptoms may develop (Connolly and Gipson 1978). Such patients may then demand further surgery or threaten the surgeon with litigation. If psychotherapy, pimozide and surgery fail the dysmorphophobia may persist and long-term support may be needed.

PSYCHODYNAMIC ASPECTS

Many of the psychodynamic concepts described in Chapter 20 on schizophrenia (see p. 239) also apply to the paranoid states. Only some additional comments need be made here. The psychopathology of paranoid personality disorders is discussed separately in Chapter 26 (see p. 334).

Projection is the mechanism of defence which is prominent in all paranoid disorders; unacceptable sexual or aggressive impulses are projected into others. If aggressive feelings are projected others will be experienced as being aggressive and persecutory.

In the Schreber case (Freud 1911) (see p. 240), Freud postulated a link between the patient's unconscious passive homosexual fantasies and his delusions of being persecuted by men. He considered that Schreber was unable to accept his repressed homosexual wishes. Instead of consciously acknowledging that he loved men and wanted to be loved by them, he unconsciously turned these wishes into the opposite feeling of hating men; he then projected this hatred and felt himself to be hated and persecuted by them. While this mechanism may have played an important role in the case of Schreber, it does not necessarily follow that repressed homosexual desires are present in all cases of paranoia or other paranoid states. They do, however, play a significant role in some cases. As they are unconscious they may only emerge during psychodynamically orientated psychotherapy.

It is important to note that since Freud published the Schreber case there has been increasing recognition by both Freud and others of the importance of destructive and aggressive impulses in human mental functioning. Projection of destructive rather than sexual fantasies may be the main factor in some cases of paranoid psychosis, while in others, e.g. erotomania, sexual fantasies may be more important; in some cases both may play a part, e.g. in morbid jealousy. It is, in fact, unlikely that all paranoid patients have identical psychological conflicts.

MANAGEMENT

Some comments on treatment have already been made in relation to the individual paranoid disorders. The management of paranoid disorders in general is exceedingly difficult. The patient is usually guarded, suspicious, mistrustful and quarrelsome. He may not see the need for treatment and adamantly refuse it. The initial aim of management must be to gain and maintain the patient's trust without colluding in his paranoid delusions. This can be very difficult. It is imperative not to challenge the patient's paranoid belief. It is best to convey to the patient that you believe what he is telling you is true for him, and understand how very distressing it must be. Decisions about whether to admit the patient to hospital depend upon how the symptoms affect him or others. Occasionally compulsory admission is necessary, e.g. if he is a danger to others, as in morbid jealousy. During treatment, which usually includes the use of antipsychotic drugs, patients need support and encouragement, especially when the paranoid delusions lessen and insight begins to return. Formal psychotherapy is rarely indicated, except in paranoid personality disorders (see p. 330) and occasionally in dysmorphophobia (see p. 259).

FURTHER READING

Christodoulou, G.N. (ed.) (1986). *The Delusional Misidentification Syndromes.* Karger, Basel.

Enoch, M.D. and Trethowan, W.H. (1979). *Uncommon Psychiatric Syndromes*, 2nd ed. Wright, Bristol.

Freeman, T. (1988). *The Psychoanalyst in Psychiatry*, Karnac Books, London.

Hamilton, M. (1984b) 'Paranoid states', ch. 5 in *Fish's Schizophrenia* (Hamilton, M., ed.), 3rd ed. Wright, Bristol.

22

Acute and Chronic Organic Mental Reactions

The terms *organic psychiatric disorders* and *organic psychiatric reactions* are widely used to refer to all those acute and chronic psychiatric conditions that are due to known organic disturbances of the brain, either arising in the brain itself or secondary to systemic disease elsewhere. The alternative term *organic mental reaction* is useful in so far as it implies an organic cause which manifests itself in mental functioning and is a reaction to a physical cause which needs to be determined in each case.

In general, most gross and identifiable physical disturbances of the brain produce syndromes which have a good deal in common. The rapidity with which the brain itself becomes affected rather than the type of noxious agent alone tends to determine the clinical picture, although the pre-morbid personality may also play a part. It is useful therefore to distinguish the clinical pictures of acute organic and chronic organic mental reactions; some patients may show intermediate or subacute forms. Organic reactions due to abnormalities of the brain itself can be either diffuse or localised. Localised cerebral lesions such as a cerebral tumour may give rise to focal signs and symptoms which point to the site of the pathology. These are referred to as organic disorders or reactions with *regional affiliations* and are described in Chapter 3.

ACUTE ORGANIC MENTAL REACTIONS

These are often referred to briefly as acute organic reactions. An alternative term in common use is *acute confusional state*, but as confusion, though common, is not always present, the term acute organic reaction is preferable.

The term *delirium* is also sometimes used to describe all types of acute organic reactions, but is better confined to describing a particular sub-group of severe acute organic reactions in which impaired consciousness is associated with hallucinations and delusions, mood changes, usually fear and excitement, and restlessness, e.g. in delirium tremens. However, in the USA the term delirium is applied to all acute organic reactions. Another term used occasionally is acute organic psychosis, but as the patient is not necessarily psychotic this label is best avoided.

Aetiology

As mentioned above, acute organic mental reactions can be due to disorders of the brain itself, or secondary to disease elsewhere in the body. Acute organic reactions may also be superimposed on and aggravate a chronic organic reaction; for example, a patient with chronic mental symptoms due to Alzheimer's disease may suddenly develop a superimposed acute organic reaction due to a chest or urinary infection.

Table 22.1. Causes of acute organic reactions

1. Degenerative	Presenile or senile dementia when complicated by infection, anoxia, etc.
2. Space-occupying lesions	Cerebral tumour, subdural haematoma, cerebral abscess.
3. Trauma	Acute post-traumatic psychosis.
4. Infection	Encephalitis, meningitis, subacute meningovascular syphilis, exanthemata, streptococcal infection, septicaemia, pneumonia, influenza, typhoid, typhus, cerebral malaria, trypanosomiasis, rheumatic chorea.
5. Vascular	Acute cerebral thrombosis or embolism, episode in arteriosclerotic dementia, transient cerebral ischaemic attack, subarachnoid haemorrhage, hypertensive encephalopathy, systemic lupus erythematosus.
6. Epileptic	Psychomotor seizures, petit mal status, post-ictal states.
7. Metabolic	Uraemia, liver disorder, electrolyte disturbances, alkalosis, acidosis, hypercapnia, remote effects of carcinoma, porphyria.
8. Endocrine	Hyperthyroid crises, myxoedema, Addisonian crises, hypopituitarism, hypo- and hyperparathyroidism, diabetic pre-coma, hypoglycaemia.
9. Toxic	Alcohol – Wernicke's encephalopathy, delirium tremens Drugs – Barbiturates and other sedatives (including withdrawal), salicylate intoxication, cannabis, LSD, prescribed medications (anti-parkinsonian drugs, scopolamine, tricyclic and MAOI antidepressants, etc.) Others – lead, arsenic, organic mercury compounds, carbon disulphide.
10. Anoxia	Bronchopneumonia, congestive cardiac failure, cardiac dysrhythmias, silent coronary infarction, silent bleeding, carbon monoxide poisoning, post-anaesthetic.
11. Vitamin lack	Thiamine (Wernicke's encephalopathy), nicotinic acid (pellagra, acute nicotinic acid deficiency encephalopathy), B12 and folic acid deficiency.

From Lishman (1987)

Table 22.1 gives a list of causes, both intracerebral and extracerebral, of acute organic reactions. It will be obvious from this list that correct diagnosis of the underlying cause of an acute organic mental reaction requires wide knowledge of general medicine and neurology, and close collaboration between physician and psychiatrist is often essential.

Clinical features and assessment

The onset is fairly rapid or sudden, depending on its cause. Impairment of consciousness is present to varying degrees. In severe cases of sudden onset, say after a head injury, the patient may at once lose consciousness completely and be in a state of coma. Much more often the condition develops over a period of a few hours or days. The patient may at first be aware of feeling generally ill, weak and listless and may find it difficult to give a clear history. He may admit to feeling muddled and unable to concentrate even if this is not at once obvious to the observer. This is common when the organic reaction is due to a high temperature. At this stage the physical symptoms, e.g. cough and pain in the chest, may overshadow the mental symptoms and lead to the correct diagnosis and treatment of the underlying cause.

As the level of consciousness becomes progressively more impaired the patient enters a state of *clouding of consciousness* or 'drowsy numbness', sometimes known as 'twilight state'. At this stage it may be difficult to rouse him; he may sleep for long periods unless he is woken; and when awake he may be dazed, bewildered and unable to concentrate. Characteristically his state of consciousness will vary, with *lucid intervals*; his confusion and any accompanying fear or restlessness are often worse at night. Memory is impaired at this stage with failure of registration due to lack of attention, and *impairment of recent memory* so that the patient becomes *disorientated* in time and space. He may not remember the names of his doctor or nurses or ultimately even of his friends and relatives. In a medical ward, he may get out of bed and wander about, unable to find his own bed again, and if not watched he may leave the ward.

Perceptual abnormalities such as illusions are common. The patient may misinterpret what he sees in the ward or what the nurses, doctors or other patients are doing so that he gets frightened, irritable or aggressive. Even parts of his own body may appear to undergo frightening alterations. *Hallucinations*, more often visual than auditory, sometimes tactile as in delirium tremens (see p. 380), are common, adding to his state of confusion and terror.

The thinking processes become slowed down, illogical and disconnected. Reality testing becomes impaired and *delusions* may be present, often paranoid in nature. As a result the patient may become terrified and scream, or, if too weak, mutter incessantly without being understandable. This may be accompanied by tachycardia and sweating. It is to this advanced stage that the term delirium is often applied.

Such clouding of consciousness, when severe, may make it very difficult to elucidate the underlying cause as the psychiatric symptoms outweigh any physical symptoms and it may be impossible to obtain a history. Information from relatives or other informants, a full physical, including neurological examination, and investigations are essential. The latter may include a chest X-ray, urine tests, blood culture, haematological investigations, estimation of electrolytes, serology for syphilis, thyroid function tests, drug scan, EEG, lumbar puncture, skull X-ray and CT scan. Unless a correct diagnosis is made and appropriate treatment instituted the condition may progress to total loss of consciousness or coma.

If the patient recovers he usually has an amnesia for the period of impaired consciousness, although sometimes an isolated experience like a delusion or hallucination may be remembered. For example, a patient who had a period of severely impaired consciousness for 48 hours due to acute septicaemia subsequently had no memory for these two days, other than a conviction that the hospital in which he was being treated had been pulled down except for a narrow vertical part of the building on top of which his bed was precariously perched, so that he had felt in danger of falling to the ground many floors below.

Laurie Lee in *Cider with Rosie*, his autobiographical account of his childhood, gives a vivid account of his own experience of 'delirium' while suffering from a high fever due to pneumonia:

> By nightfall I was usually raving. My limbs went first, splintering like logs, so that I seemed to grow dozens of arms. The bed no longer had limits to it and became a desert of hot wet sand. I began to talk to a second head laid on the pillow, my own head once removed; it never talked back, but just lay there grinning very coldly into my eyes. The walls of the bedroom were the next to go; they began to bulge and ripple and roar, to flap like pastry, melt like sugar, and run bleeding with hideous hues. Then out of the walls, and down from the ceiling, advanced a row of intangible smiles; easy, relaxed, in no way threatening at first, but going on far too long.

Differential diagnosis

It is important to distinguish an acute organic mental reaction from other psychiatric disorders. If delusions and hallucinations are prominent the condition may be mistaken for acute schizophrenia, but clouding of consciousness and impairment of memory do not occur in schizophrenia. Furthermore, visual hallucinations more often occur in acute organic reactions, often in association with auditory and tactile hallucinations, while in schizophrenia visual hallucinations are rare. Slowing down of thought processes and motor activity, with lack of interest in the environment, combined with apathy and depression, may simulate a depressive illness; here again it is the impairment of consciousness and memory loss that should lead to the correct diagnosis. Occasionally an acute hysterical reaction with pseudo-hallucinations (see p. 124) and fluctuating bizarre behaviour may simulate an acute organic reaction. In general, the history and absence of any signs of organic disease in these other disorders should help to avoid such mistakes, but sometimes observation and investigations over a period of days are needed to establish the diagnosis.

Management

This depends primarily on the treatment of the cause (see Table 22.1). Nevertheless much needs to be done to help not only the patient but also the relatives. The general atmosphere surrounding the patient should be calm and orderly. Investigations should be performed rapidly, efficiently and with minimal fuss. Anxiety on the part of the doctors or nurses is easily transmitted to the patient and his relatives; they should be told why investigations are carried out and what is being done to help the patient.

The patient is best nursed in a side room, as the ceaseless activity on the ward acts as a stimulus to further confusion, perceptual disturbances and delusions. The amount of unfamiliar apparatus should be reduced to a minimum, and the level and kind of illumination should be adequate and so arranged as to dispel shadows. Noise should also be kept to a minimum. Frequent changes of staff should be avoided and, however difficult it may be, nurses familiar to the patient should stay with him. Calm reassurance by a firm yet sympathetic nurse known to the patient is most important. The presence of a relative who is familiar to the patient can help considerably, but if relatives are too anxious or intrusive they may make things worse. Sources of additional pain and discomfort must be avoided or dealt with; these may include cracked lips secondary to dehydration, pain surrounding injection or infusion sites, constipation, retention of urine or difficulties with micturition. The loss of spectacles may make the world look even more distorted. Any of these circumstances can hamper recovery and make the acute organic mental syndrome worse.

Fever, if present, can be reduced by non-specific means such as tepid sponging until its cause is identified and appropriate treatment given. Dehydration and thirst make the condition worse and an adequate fluid intake must be maintained. In the elderly patient particular attention should be paid to the presence of urinary tract or respiratory tract infections. These can be additional causes of severe deterioration of the mental state. If the acute organic reaction is unresponsive to these measures the patient may require sedation for symptomatic relief. It should always be remembered, however, that excessive psychotropic medication may exacerbate the syndrome and cause respiratory depression and hypotension. Drugs that can be helpful include thioridazine and haloperidol, starting with a low dose and increasing if necessary.

If, as is often the case, the acute organic mental symptoms occur in the context of a terminal illness, e.g. advanced cancer with secondaries, so that there is no treatment available for the underlying condition, it is essential to relieve all physical and psychological discomfort by means of full and effective doses of tranquillisers and analgesics, like chlorpromazine and morphia or heroin (see p. 102).

CHRONIC ORGANIC MENTAL REACTIONS

These are also referred to as *chronic organic psychiatric reactions* or chronic organic reactions for short. Other less helpful labels are chronic confusional state, chronic organic psychosis, or dementia; the former two are best avoided because the patient is not necessarily confused or psychotic, while dementia is best avoided as a general label for all the chronic organic reactions as it is also used as a diagnostic label for a particular sub-group, i.e. the irreversible senile and presenile dementias (see Chapters 23 and 25). Moreover, unlike the latter, a few rare chronic organic reactions, e.g. general paresis and normal pressure hydrocephalus, are treatable (if diagnosed in time), so that permanent damage to the brain can be avoided and normal function restored. The term chronic organic mental reaction is used here as it stresses the need in each case to search for the underlying cause and because it emphasises that these reactions give rise to mental symptoms but without any particular implications concerning symptomatology or prognosis.

Table 22.2. Causes of chronic organic reactions

1. Degenerative	Senile and presenile Alzheimer's disease, arteriosclerotic dementia, Pick's, Huntington's, Creutzfeldt-Jacob, normal pressure hydrocephalus, multiple sclerosis, Parkinson's disease, Schilder's, Wilson's, progressive supranuclear palsy, progressive multifocal leucoencephalopathy, progressive myoclonic epilepsy.
2. Space-occupying lesions	Cerebral tumour, subdural haematoma.
3. Trauma	Post-traumatic dementia.
4. Infection	General paresis, chronic meningo-vascular syphilis, subacute and chronic encephalitis.
5. Vascular	Cerebral vascular disease, état lacunaire.
6. Epileptic	Epileptic dementia.
7. Metabolic	Uraemia, liver disorder, remote effects of carcinoma,
8. Endocrine	Myxoedema, Addison's disease, hypopituitarism, hypo- and hyperparathyroidism, hypoglycaemia.
9. Toxic	Alcoholic dementia and Korsakoff's psychosis, chronic barbiturate intoxication, manganese, carbon disulphide.
10. Anoxia	Anaemia, congestive cardiac failure, chronic pulmonary disease, post-anaesthetic, post-carbon-monoxide poisoning, post-cardiac arrest.
11. Vitamin lack	Lack of thiamine, nicotinic acid, B12, folic acid.

From Lishman (1987)

Aetiology

Chronic organic mental reactions are a result of gradual damage to the brain, usually by diffuse pathological processes but sometimes accompanied by or commencing with focal lesions or *regional affiliations* (see Chapter 3). Table 22.2 provides a list of underlying causes.

Clinical features

By far the commonest causes of a chronic organic reaction are Alzheimer's presenile and senile dementia, and multi-infarct dementia. These are considered further in Chapters 23 and 25, but the following gives a detailed clinical account of the symptoms of *senile dementia*. It also serves as a useful model for the other chronic organic reactions, since the symptoms are similar whatever the cause. In each individual case the history, examination and investigations may however reveal important and sometimes diagnostic features pointing to one or other treatable underlying disorder, as opposed to the irreversible conditions of senile and presenile dementia.

It should be emphasised first of all that in spite of the serious and progressive symptoms about to be described there is no impairment of consciousness in dementia or in other chronic organic reactions, in contrast to the acute organic reactions. The onset is insidious so that no exact time of onset can be given by relatives or the patient. Not infrequently subtle changes in personality and behaviour or slight forgetfulness remain unnoticed until a sudden deterioration occurs as a result of some environmental change, such as moving house or changing job, or a bereavement. Any of these events may disturb the patient's routine and thus bring the problem to the surface. An illness, say an infection or an accident, perhaps leading to admission to hospital, may have the same effect. A careful history, best taken from a close relative, may then reveal that minor abnormalities had in fact been developing over a period of months or more and antedated the apparent recent onset. Occasionally, however, the condition has followed directly on some acute episode like a cerebrovascular accident, a head injury or anoxia due to a severe chest infection or cardiac arrest.

The commonest abnormality first noted by the relatives, rather than by the patient himself, is *impairment of memory* and some falling-off of intellectual function. The patient may become absent-minded, forget names and what he has to do outside his usual routine. He may start to prepare lists which he feels will help him to remember, only to forget where he has put the scrap of paper. When going shopping he may not be able to cope with money and obtain the correct change. He may begin to make mistakes at work which are noticed by his work-mates or superiors rather than by himself. At home he may repeat the same action several times, having forgotten that he has already done it; or he may repeat the same question or tell stories repeatedly to the same audience in a perseverative manner.

As the condition progresses, loss of memory for past events may become as affected as that for more recent events. As a result the patient may lose his way even in quite familiar surroundings, and he may be unaware of the day of the week, the date or even the month, the season or the year. He may even forget his own address and fail to recognise close friends and relatives. Quite commonly the patient will invent accounts of events in order to fill in gaps in his memory. Such confabulation can sometimes be quite elaborate, with fanciful stories or translocations in time. On other occasions a simple excuse is made. Quite often the patient will respond to a question about current events or the date by saying that he has mislaid his spectacles and cannot be expected to know the contents of the newspaper or the date, or he may simply state that he is not interested in the answer. He may on the other hand become very upset and angry at his inability to function properly and flare up in an outburst of rage, the so-called *catastrophic reaction*. Fortunately the majority of patients are either unaware of the extent of their difficulties or unconcerned about them. A minority, however, are all too painfully aware of their deficiencies and become tearful and despairing. This seems to occur particularly in patients whose older siblings or parents have shown similar symptoms and have gradually deteriorated to helplessness, thus indicating the path the patient realistically fears he may be following.

Another common early sign first noted by the relatives may be a subtle *change in personality*. The patient may become a caricature of his pre-morbid self. Character traits of irritability, inflexibility, intolerance and querulousness may be accentuated. Perhaps they were not particularly noticeable before, or well controlled. Perhaps they were only evident on rare occasions, but with the onset of the chronic organic mental syndrome they become more prominent. Sometimes close relatives, particularly the husband or wife, maintain that there is a lack of empathy where it certainly existed before. There may be an inability or a lack of willingness to appreciate the feelings of others. The patient's world contracts so that he is preoccupied with his own apparently minor problems to the exclusion of concern over external major events. This may lead to preoccupation with and total absorption in physical discomforts. Problems with dentures, spectacles, bowels or feet, all become a subject for continuous concern and debate. Diminishing interest in the external world often results in the patient sitting inert for long periods, perhaps occasionally nodding off into sleep.

Sometimes the patient's personality changes lead to *disinhibition*. Unusually for the patient, he may recount bawdy stories inappropriately in front of the grandchildren at tea, or worse, he may act in a disinhibited fashion sexually. This sexual disinhibition may take the form of exposure or indecent assault; or he may be seen to pass urine in public. Occasionally he may be caught shoplifting.

On the other hand, personality changes may be characterised more by rigidity and an increase in obsessional traits. Orderliness and routine become paramount and any disturbance of this can produce extreme distress and a catastrophic reaction, as described above. Many daily activities are ritualised so that meals have to be taken at certain times and in special ways. A routine of watching television and going to bed at a special time must be adhered to and weekday outings become totally predictable. If these enforced routines are interrupted by, say, admission to hospital or a vacation, this causes acute anxiety, sometimes panic, and usually a worsening of the disorder. In some cases even the failure of a regular visitor, delay in mealtimes or the lateness of transport to attend outpatients will produce a catastrophic reaction. The family often feel forced to fall into the routine themselves, and sometimes they need help in extricating themselves from this situation.

Abnormalities of *mood* are common in the chronic organic mental reactions. The patient, perhaps aware of his difficulties, may present with a chronic depressive picture, characterised by apathy, lack of volition, hypochondriacal concern, insomnia and an altered sleep pattern. The clinical picture can be similar to that of a depressive illness, and the differential diagnosis is often very difficult, depending more on the assessment of the clinical picture than on special psychological or physical tests. It is particularly important to look for evidence of memory and intellectual impairment; a positive family history of depression, or a lack of such a history, may be helpful. Of course, a patient may have both a depressive illness and a chronic organic mental disorder, and if in doubt it may be worthwhile instituting a trial of antidepressant treatment.

Other abnormal affective states are seen in the chronic organic mental reactions. Reference has been made to the outbursts of rage, the catastrophic reaction, which occur when the patient finds himself unable to perform a previously familiar task, or to reply to a question which he could easily have answered in the past, or when his routine is upset. Even if there are no episodes of catastrophic reaction the mood of the patient can be very labile. Characteristically these mood changes are abrupt and short-lived, lasting a few minutes or hours at the most. The mood may quickly fluctuate from incongruous exuberance to tearful despair. Uncontrollable tears flow at emotional scenes, e.g. visits from the family or some sad tale on television. The patient often realises the inappropriateness of his response and covers up his tearfulness with enforced coughs or covers his face with a newspaper. If this occurs frequently close relatives may become concerned at the possibility of severe depression and need reassurance.

The general impairment of cerebral function is also manifest in the patient's *thinking* and *speech*. There is a diminution in spontaneity; new ideas hardly occur and decisions about what is right or wrong become impossible. There is a perseverative return to earlier ideas which become fossilised, and all this leads to serious problems in a working situation, perhaps on a committee on which the patient may still be sitting. Speech becomes *stereotyped*, *perseverative* and filled with platitudinous comments. Sometimes the ability to discuss abstract thoughts is so impaired that the speech becomes totally *literal* and *concrete*. Perhaps because the patient can no longer deal with the subtleties of communication and thought, he becomes suspicious and frankly paranoid. Unable to reason correctly, delusions may gain a hold. Defective hearing or sight may exacerbate these paranoid tendencies. More severely affected patients will not be able to maintain consistent delusional ideas, which then become transient and ill-formed and may slowly fade as the disorganisation of thinking becomes more severe.

Course, diagnosis and prognosis

In the early stages neurotic symptoms like anxiety, depression and obsessionality may predominate and conceal the underlying disorder. In particular, hysterical conversion symptoms may occur, perhaps because his failing inellectual capabilities may make it more difficult for the patient to cope with stressful situations. This is why the onset of hysterical symptoms for the first time in middle or old age should always lead one to search for a possible underlying organic cerebral disorder (see p. 178). Sometimes the course of a chronic organic reaction like dementia may suddenly be exacerbated by a superimposed acute organic reaction, perhaps due to a chest or urinary infection. Such sudden deterioration of mental function is usually accompanied by impairment or clouding of consciousness, not otherwise present in chronic organic reactions. If the correct diagnosis is made and the cause of the acute reaction treated, the patient's mental state will usually revert to its previous state.

The majority of chronic reactions are due to senile or presenile Alzheimer's disease and hence irreversible and progressive. Provided the patient lives long enough all his mental functions will deteriorate. His memory loss becomes global, affecting remote as well as recent memory, so that he recognises no one; his mood becomes empty and shallow, and his speech meaningless and incoherent. This leads to total social decline ultimately accompanied by physical weakness and deterioration so that he has to be permanently nursed and looked after.

Occasionally, however, the cause of a chronic mental reaction is treatable (see Table 22.2) Hence the importance, in the early stages, of searching for any underlying condition other than Alzheimer's disease. Treatable causes include a benign cerebral tumour, e.g. a frontal meningioma, subdural haematoma, normal pressure hydrocephalus, general paresis and meningovascular syphilis, metabolic and endocrine disorders, especialy myxoedema, lack of vitamins, etc. Detailed physical, including neurological examination and investigations, as outlined for the acute organic reactions (p. 265) are essential if these admittedly rare but treatable causes are not to be missed.

FURTHER READING

Lishman, W.A. (1987). *Organic Psychiatry: the psychological consequences of cerebral disorder*, 2nd ed. Blackwell, Oxford.

23

Organic Psychiatric Disorders

The changes that occur in acute or chronic organic mental reactions were described in general terms in the previous chapter. The individual organic psychiatric disorders and their particular presentation will be considered here. Emphasis will be placed on their psychiatric rather than their medical and neurological manifestations. Senile dementia due to Alzheimer's disease has already been described (see p. 268) and is considered further in Chapter 25. The organic complications of alcoholism are dealt with in Chapter 30.

In several of the conditions to be discussed physical symptoms predominate so that the patient may first be seen by a physician, while in others the psychiatric symptoms are more prominent so that the psychiatrist is likely to be involved first. The general practitioner is usually consulted first of all and may be confronted with a confusing mixture of physical and mental symptoms. The organic psychiatric disorders often present difficult diagnostic problems, and collaboration between the general practitioner, physician or surgeon, neurologist and psychiatrist may be essential.

Even if a definite diagnosis of a medical or neurological disorder has been established, the question often arises as to whether any accompanying mental symptoms are the direct consequence of the organic disorder, e.g. depression due to myxoedema. The mental symptoms may be coincidental, e.g. a patient with a carcinoma who has psychotic symptoms due to co-existent chronic schizophrenia. Or they may be due to the patient's psychological reaction to a disabling physical disease, e.g. depression following a myocardial infarction. Some of these difficulties will be discussed further in Chapter 39.

HEAD INJURY

Psychiatrists are rarely consulted in the management of the acute effects of head injuries. It is the chronic after-effects which frequently come to their notice, but as these are often influenced by the preceding acute effects the latter will be referred to briefly.

Acute effects

The immediate effect of a head injury is usually some degree of impairment of consciousness, so-called *concussion*. This may vary from feeling momentarily dazed, to a brief period of loss of consciousness, to prolonged coma. As consciousness returns the patient may develop the various symptoms described earlier (p. 264) under the heading of acute organic mental reaction; in the case of a head injury this is sometimes referred to as an acute post-traumatic confusional state. Its duration depends on the nature and severity of the injury and may last from a few minutes to days or weeks.

Some impairment of memory or amnesia is almost invariable in all but the mildest cases. The period of amnesia that extends from the time when the injury took place to the complete return of normal memory function is referred to as the duration of *post-traumatic amnesia*; there is often also a period of *retrograde amnesia* covering the interval between the head injury and the last event clearly remembered before it occurred; this is usually of relatively short duration and may be absent. The length of post-traumatic amnesia and the duration of post-traumatic loss of consciousness or disorientation are important prognostic indicators; the longer their duration the greater the likelihood of prolonged or lasting psychiatric after-effects. If there is severe brain damage the patient may be left with permanent dementia or varying and less severe degrees of cognitive impairment. It is obvious that the immediate psychiatric and neurological effects and the prognosis are affected by any localised damage to the brain; this applies to both closed and open head injuries and will not be considered further here.

Chronic effects

Not surprisingly severe head injuries are often followed by persistent psychiatric and neurological sequelae (Lishman 1968, 1973). The psychological and social sequelae have been reviewed by McClelland (1988). After minor head injuries many patients make a complete recovery, but in others chronic symptoms may develop. It is particularly in these cases that it is difficult to assess whether the symptoms are of physical or psychological origin or a mixture of both. Many patients experience a head injury as a stressful life event, especially if it is followed by concussion; all the more so if it was accompanied by emotional shock or associated with circumstances that led to guilt or resentment. In that case anxiety, preoccupation with symptoms like headache and dizziness, irritability, poor concentration, insomnia, frightening dreams, and some degree of depression may persist for months or even years. This is more likely to occur in people who were overanxious and had other personality problems or neurotic symptoms before the accident.

In others the head injury may be followed by more clearly defined psychiatric disorders. These include anxiety states, depressive reactions, symptoms of conversion hysteria, obsessional symptoms and personality changes. Psychotic illnesses, such as an affective psychosis, schizophrenia or a paranoid psychosis can also be precipitated by a head injury. In all these cases it may be difficult to decide whether some persistent organic cerebral abnormality is contributing to the psychiatric disturbance and to what extent pre-morbid personality disorders and the emotional impact of the injury, or a combination of these are responsible. Obviously, a history of severe head injury followed by prolonged post-traumatic amnesia and evidence of neurological sequelae or persistent intellectual impairment indicate that organic factors play a major role.

It is important to note that *epilepsy* is a common consequence of head injury, occurring in 5 per cent of closed, and 30-40 per cent of open head injuries. The development of epilepsy often leads to further psychological and social problems, which in turn aggravate the psychiatric after-effects (see Chapter 24).

Post-traumatic syndrome

Headache and dizziness are common symptoms in the first few days or weeks during recovery from any head injury. However, in some patients headache and dizziness, accompanied by irritability, insomnia, poor concentration and fatigue, can cause marked disability and persist for months or years. This condition is called the *post-traumatic* or *post-concussional syndrome*. In some patients it develops after an interval, the patient having apparently made a good recovery from the head injury.

It now seems likely that this syndrome is partly of organic and partly of psychological origin. Lishman (1988) considers that organic factors may play a more important part in the early stages following the injury while secondary neurotic factors become more prominent in long-continued cases. In some cases the syndrome develops in patients who consider, often with good cause, that the injury was the result of negligence on the part of their employer or due to an accident for which the other party is held responsible. As a result they seek compensation and get involved in litigation. When, after prolonged delay, the case for compensation is finally settled the symptoms may clear up. The term *compensation neurosis* or *accident neurosis* is often used under these circumstances (Trimble 1981) (see also p. 183). Miller (1961) considered that these symptoms were of psychological origin. It is likely that conscious or unconscious factors play a part in causing these symptoms, but organic factors may also be involved. Kelly (1975) has pointed out that the symptoms may clear up before the claim for compensation has been settled. However, the syndrome is rarely seen in patients with gross brain damage and cognitive impairment; it is more common after minor head injuries and in patients with a past history of psychoneurotic symptoms.

When the patient is first seen it is important to exclude a subdural haematoma, which could be responsible for the headache. Vestibular damage needs to be excluded as a possible cause of dizziness. This may, for example, occur following a whiplash injury. In practice the vague and unremitting nature of the headache, the absence of true vertigo and normal vestibular tests, and the persistent complaints of fatigue, inability to go to work or to concentrate usually make the diagnosis clear, especially if the symptoms have remained unchanged for a long time. In some cases emotional distress, e.g. guilt concerning the circumstances of the accident, plays a significant role.

Management of chronic after-effects

Only the psychiatric aspects will be considered here. The first task is a full assessment of all physical and psychological aspects followed by support, reassurance and practical help with any remaining disabilities. This will involve collaboration with the patient's family, and often also with his employers. If there is persistent intellectual or physical impairment, prolonged re-education and rehabilitation are essential.

If the symptoms are mainly or entirely of psychological origin, a psychotherapeutic approach, sometimes involving other family members, combined with encouragement and practical support is required, often over a long period. If the patient is involved in litigation, every effort must be made to encourage lawyers and others involved in the case to settle the claim at the earliest opportunity.

Boxing and head injury

There is now ample evidence that professional boxers are in danger of developing both neurological and psychiatric abnormalities, sometimes referred to as 'punch-drunkenness', as a result of repeated damage to the brain over a period of several years. Neurologically there may be evidence of mild or severe pyramidal, extrapyramidal and cerebellar involvement. Psychiatric manifestations include impairment of memory and intellectual function, and such personality changes as irritability, morbid jealousy, outbursts of temper or apathy. The condition may progress to severe dementia unless boxing is discontinued, in which case the condition may be arrested. Investigations may show evidence of cerebral atrophy, and at post-mortem there are degenerative changes in the cerebral cortex, the brain stem and in the hippocampal system, sometimes in association with perforation of the septum pellucidum.

Chronic subdural haematoma

Head injuries sometimes give rise to the development of a subdural haematoma. If this follows shortly after the injury the condition is usually suggested by persistent impairment of consciousness, perhaps leading to coma, sometimes accompanied by localising signs, and this should lead to surgical exploration and treatment. It will not be considered further here.

A chronic subdural haematoma is much more difficult to diagnose and may present with psychiatric symptoms. It may follow a minor head injury that has been forgotten, e.g. in the elderly or in an alcoholic who had a fall when drunk; or after a major head injury from which the patient has apparently made a good recovery.

Symptoms may not develop for some weeks or even months after the injury. Characteristically there may be fluctuating changes in consciousness, varying from mild drowsiness to clouding or more severe impairment. Impairment of memory and intellectual function may occur and lead to a mistaken diagnosis of primary dementia, especially in the elderly. These symptoms may be accompanied by disturbed behaviour simulating hysterical fugue states. The condition is more often suspected if headache is a prominent symptom, but this may be absent or mild and varying in degree. Neurological signs and evidence of raised intracranial pressure may also be absent, or may only develop when the condition has reached an advanced stage. In some patients the diagnosis may therefore be missed altogether unless neurological investigations, including a CT scan, are carried out.

CEREBROVASCULAR ACCIDENTS

Cerebrovascular accidents due to cerebral thrombosis, embolism or haemorrhage are usually seen and treated by physicians but, if recovery occurs, persistent or progressive psychiatric symptoms often become of major importance and may require psychiatric treatment and rehabilitation, alongside treatment of the physical sequelae.

The main disorders include impairment of cognitive function, affective disorders, mainly depression, personality changes and more specific localising symptoms such as disturbances of language or apraxia, depending on the regions of the brain involved.

Impairment of memory and intellectual function is common and usually becomes apparent after recovery from the initial period of loss or impairment of consciousness. The degree of recovery is very variable, depending on the region of the brain affected and its extent. The condition may progress to severe dementia; this is particularly common after repeated minor cerebral infarctions as in *multi-infarct dementia* (see p. 324). This may be associated with changes in personality and behaviour, as well as emotional lability leading to catastrophic reactions (see p. 269). Reactive depression following a stroke is common and is naturally influenced by the degree of physical and mental disability. Poor or slow recovery, inability to resume work, lack of the necessary support from family members and social isolation all contribute to the depression. In treatment attention has to be paid to all these factors.

Less often the patient may develop an endogenous depression which may respond to treatment with antidepressants.

CEREBRAL TUMOURS

The majority of patients with cerebral tumours, primary or secondary, present with physical rather than mental symptoms, or a combination of both. It is rare therefore for them to be referred first to a psychiatrist. Only those psychiatric aspects will be considered here which may be important for early diagnosis and in the differentiation from other psychiatric disorders.

Clouding or more severe impairment of consciousness may be an early symptom, especially in rapidly growing tumours, as a result of raised intracranial pressure. It may occur before there are any other neurological abnormalities.

Cognitive impairment, especially of memory and orientation, associated with personality changes, is common if the tumour is slow growing and especially if it is situated in the frontal or temporal lobe. The resulting picture of progressive dementia without abnormal or neurological signs can then lead to a mistaken diagnosis of presenile or senile dementia unless investigations, including a CT scan, are carried out.

> For example, a man of fifty-two who had become demented over a period of nine months was diagnosed as suffering from presenile dementia. During the next six months his dementia rapidly progressed and his level of consciousness began to fluctuate, but there were no abnormal neurological findings. A CT scan showed a large anterior frontal lobe tumour, which turned out to be a meningioma and was successfully removed. His mental function returned almost completely to normal in the next few weeks except for a period of amnesia covering several months before the operation.

The mental symptoms and signs, like the neurological, are to some extent dependent on the site of the tumour. The psychiatric characteristics of lesions and hence of tumours in the frontal, temporal and parietal lobes were described in Chapter 3, where attention was also drawn to the severe amnesic syndrome that can result from lesions, and hence also from tumours in the hypothalamic-diencephalic region surrounding the third ventricle or in the hippocampal formation in the temporal lobes (see p. 34). Tumours affecting the hypothalamus may also be associated with hypersomnia, i.e. greatly prolonged but otherwise normal sleep, voracious appetite, diabetes insipidus, and other disturbances of hypothalamic function. Tumours or cysts in the region of the third ventricle can present with *akinetic mutism* (see p. 140); this is characterised by immobility, the patient lying almost completely still and gazing into space, mutism and failure to respond to external stimuli. This rare condition is mentioned here because it may be difficult to differentiate from depressive or catatonic stupor. Occasionally a cerebral tumour, especially of the temporal lobe, may present with symptoms that resemble a schizophrenic syndrome or a depressive illness.

In general, it is rare for patients with a psychiatric illness to be discovered to have a cerebral tumour but, if the psychiatric picture is atypical, the possibility has to be borne in mind. Careful and repeated neurological examination and investigations are essential in such cases if the correct diagnosis is not to be missed.

NEUROPSYCHIATRIC COMPLICATIONS OF CANCER

Cerebral metastases arising from a primary carcinoma elsewhere, e.g. the bronchus, breast, prostate gland, pancreas or gastro-intestinal tract, can give rise to the symptoms described above.

Occasionally neuropsychiatric symptoms can be the result of a carcinoma elsewhere but in the absence of cerebral secondaries; this applies particularly to carcinoma of the bronchus. The symptoms are usually those of widespread neurological abnormalities, but occasionally mental symptoms may predominate or precede any neurological changes, or even any evidence of the primary carcinoma. The mental symptoms may take the form of impairment of memory and dementia, or of mood changes, especially depression and anxiety. At post-mortem there are widespread degenerative and inflammatory changes in the brain, sometimes involving the limbic system, including the hippocampus and other parts of the inferior medial portion of the temporal lobes, areas known to give rise to severe memory loss (see p. 33). Whether these changes are due to encephalitis, possibly of viral origin, immunological abnormalities, or some abnormal metabolite produced by the primary carcinoma is unknown. These rare complications of a carcinoma elsewhere must be considered in the differential diagnosis of cerebral tumours and of dementia or affective disorders.

Lastly, *depressive symptoms* may occasionally develop for the first time some months or even longer before the appearance of a carcinoma; this applies particularly to carcinoma of the pancreas. In these cases there are none of the pathological findings in the brain described above.

SENILE AND PRESENILE DEMENTIAS

Dementia in patients over the age of sixty-five, so-called senile dementia, falls into two categories: Alzheimer's disease, also called senile dementia of Alzheimer-type, and multi-infarct dementia. These are discussed in Chapter 25. A detailed clinical description of Alzheimer's disease is also given on p. 268.

The term 'presenile dementia' is used to describe the dementias that occur before the age of sixty-five.

Presenile dementia

Dementia which develops before the age of sixty-five, usually between forty and sixty, is called presenile dementia. In addition to multi-infarct dementia starting before the age of sixty-five, three different types of presenile dementia used to be described as disorders distinct from senile dementia: Alzheimer's disease, Pick's disease, and Creutzfeldt-Jakob disease. However the pathology and clinical features of Alzheimer's disease in patients over sixty-five and of the Alzheimer variety of presenile dementia are now recognised to be indistinguishable.

The *Alzheimer type of presenile dementia* will therefore not be described in detail here. Suffice it to say that its course is similar to that of the Alzheimer type of senile dementia but starting at an earlier age. The patient may lose insight into the failure of his intellectual function early on; as the disease progresses dysphasia, extrapyramidal and pyramidal abnormalities and epileptic fits may develop, and within a few years the patient will die in a state of gross dementia. There is a somewhat increased familial incidence in presenile Alzheimer's disease, but much less so than in Pick's disease.

Pick's disease

This much rarer form of presenile dementia usually starts in the fifties but may commence as early as the twenties. It is more common in women than men and there is a strong genetic tendency.

Clinically it tends to differ from Alzheimer's disease by the early development of *personality changes*, antisocial behaviour and disinhibition, often preceding the appearance of memory loss and progressive dementia. Mild euphoria is common in the early stages. It leads to gross dementia and death, usually after several years.

Pathological changes differ from those seen in Alzheimer's disease. The cerebral atrophy affects especially the frontal and temporal lobes, which may account for the severe early personality changes. Histologically the plaques and neurofibrillary tangles characteristic of Alzheimer's disease (see p. 323) are absent. Instead there may be large balloon-shaped neurones alongside widespread loss of neuronal cells and gliosis, as seen in other forms of dementia.

Creutzfeldt-Jakob disease

This rare form of presenile dementia is of particular interest because it has been shown to be due to a *transmissible agent* with the properties of a slow virus. The disorder has been transmitted by direct inoculation of infected brain tissue into chimpanzees, other monkeys and guinea pigs, and also by intravenous and other parenteral routes. The disorder has also been transmitted from one infected animal to another by injecting material from other organs such as lymph nodes, the liver or spleen. A few cases have been reported where the disease was surgically transmitted accidentally from a patient with the disease to another individual during neurosurgical or ophthalmic procedures (Gajdusek *et al.* 1977).

Creutzfeldt-Jakob disease usually starts with general symptoms of weakness, fatigue and mood changes. This is soon followed by widespread neurological abnormalities, hallucinations, delusions and severe dementia, ending in death within a few months up to a year or two, often after a period of impaired consciousness and delirium. The cerebrospinal fluid is often normal except for a rise in protein, but the EEG is almost always grossly abnormal; in the later stages of the illness characteristic triphasic sharp wave complexes appear; these stand out against generalised suppression of cortical activity.

Changes in the brain include severe degeneration of neurones that gives rise to characteristic gross spongy appearances in the cortex.

Kuru

The discovery that Creutzfeldt-Jakob disease is due to a transmissible virus followed a similar discovery in the case of kuru, a rapidly progressive and fatal neurological disease leading to dementia that affects members of a tribe in New Guinea. When brain tissue from these patients was inoculated into chimpanzees either intracerebrally, intramuscularly or intravenously, and subsequently from an affected chimpanzee to others, the animals also developed a rapidly fatal neurological disorder. At post-mortem the brain showed extensive degenerative changes similar to those seen in humans. It is thought that cannibalism may have played a part in the origin and spread of this disorder in humans as female members of the affected tribe who ate portions of human brain showed the highest incidence of kuru. The incidence has declined as cannibalism has been given up (Gajdusek 1977). Genetic factors may also play a part.

HUNTINGTON'S CHOREA

This disorder, described by George Huntington in 1872, although relatively rare, is responsible for a great deal of suffering in affected individuals and their families. Huntington, his father and grandfather, all doctors practising in Long Island, USA, observed several affected families over a period of 78 years (Huntington 1872). The origin of some of the families in the USA has since been traced back to immigrants from England.

The condition is caused by a dominant autosomal gene with 100 per cent penetrance so that each child, boy or girl, of a parent who carries the gene stands a 50 per cent risk of developing the disease. Recent studies have shown that the abnormal gene is located on chromosome 4 (Gusella *et al.* 1983).

The prevalence varies from place to place, depending on the presence of affected families in different regions. In the UK as a whole the prevalence is 4 to 7 per 100,000 population, with a very high prevalence of 560 per 100,000 in a small community on the east coast of Scotland.

There is now some post-mortem evidence that the level of the inhibitory transmitter substance gamma aminobutyric acid (GABA) in the basal ganglia is reduced, a finding which may account for the appearance of involuntary movements in Huntington's chorea. Degenerative changes are especially marked in the caudate nuclei although the cortex, especially in the anterior frontal region, is also affected. Cerebral atrophy with dilatation of the ventricles can usually be demonstrated on a CT scan.

Clinical features

In the majority of patients the condition starts in middle age, although it can commence in childhood or old age. Owing to its relatively late onset many people who carry the gene may produce children before they know that they are affected and that their children stand a 50 per cent chance of developing the disease. This is more likely to happen when the fact that other family members have been affected has been kept secret, or when the parent does not know his biological parents because of adoption or illegitimacy.

The earliest sign may be the appearance of slight jerky movements which over the years develop into severe, uncontrollable *choreiform movements* with disturbance of gait and inability to carry out even the simplest tasks. Rigidity may be associated with the choreiform manifestations. Classically this is followed after some years by progressive *dementia*. Insight is often maintained, leading to anxiety, depression and suicide. Occasionally *personality changes* with loss of emotional control and early signs of dementia precede the onset of the choreiform movements.

The nature of the progressive dementia in Huntington's chorea differs from that seen in Alzheimer's disease in several respects. Apathy and slowing down of all cognitive functions with loss of efficiency and disihibition are often more prominent than memory loss, and such neurological abnormalities as dysphasia and apraxia, so often seen in Alzheimer's disease, do not occur. In the terminal phase apathy and mutism may develop even in the absence of total memory loss. This type of dementia is now often referred to as *subcortical dementia* (Cummings 1986), as compared with the cortical dementia seen in Alzheimer's disease; the implication is that the dementia is largely due to degenerative changes in such subcortical structures as the basal ganglia, including the caudate nuclei which are severely affected in Huntington's chorea.

Some patients develop paranoid ideas or frank psychotic illnesses of a depressive or schizophrenic type, either before the appearance of any other symptoms or during the slowly progressive course of the illness, which may vary from a few years to several decades.

Effects on the family and prevention

It is not surprising that both affected and unaffected members of the family may show severe anxiety, depression, attempted suicide and other disturbed behaviour, partly as the result of the presence of affected members within the family. This may lead to the fear of developing or passing on the disease. Martindale (1987) and Martindale and Yale (1983) have pointed out that professionals involved in caring for these families, doctors included, often use defences like denial and rationalisation in an attempt to protect family members from the realisation that they might be at risk of developing or passing on the disorder. This may lead to failure to obtain genetic counselling early on, especially before the age of childbearing. Such counselling is essential if the incidence of the disease and the suffering of affected individuals and their families is to be reduced, at least until some form of biochemical control or prevention of the disorder may be found. If pregnant, a woman and her husband may decide to ask for a termination rather than bring a child into the world who may stand a 50 per cent chance of developing this serious and devastating disease.

In fact, the recent discovery of genetic markers for Huntington's chorea may soon make it possible to determine whether or not an individual actually carries the gene, and whether the foetus is affected. At present the accuracy of such a test is still under investigation. Moreover, there are considerable ethical implications in the use of such predictive tests. A negative test result would clearly relieve the anxiety of members of a family in which others are already affected. However, a positive result given to a person who is not yet suffering from the disease could lead to great distress, anxiety and depression with which the individual might find it very difficult to cope. These issues are discussed by Craufurd and Harris (1986).

NORMAL PRESSURE HYDROCEPHALUS
(adult communicating hydrocephalus; normal pressure or intermittently raised pressure hydrocephalus)

This rare disorder is described here because it is one of a few causes of a dementing process which, if diagnosed correctly, sometimes responds to treatment. Essentially it consists of gross symmetrical dilatation of the ventricular system which gives rise to secondary cerebral atrophy, as compared with the enlargement of the ventricles in Alzheimer's disease where the dilatation is secondary to the primary cerebral atrophy. Normal pressure hydrocephalus differs from obstructive hydrocephalus where the ventricles are enlarged as the result of obstruction to the outflow of cerebrospinal fluid from the ventricular system into the subarachnoid space. In normal pressure hydrocephalus there is no obstruction to the flow of CSF from the ventricles so that there is free communication between the ventricles and the subarachnoid space; hence the term communicating hydrocephalus. There is, however, a block in the subarachnoid space at the base of the brain, usually in the basal cisterns, preventing the upward flow of cerebrospinal fluid and hence its re-absorption into the superior saggital sinus.

The cause of obstruction at the base of the brain is often unknown but it is sometimes due to adhesions following previous head injury, sub-arachnoid haemorrhage or meningitis.

Clinical features

The condition presents with gradual onset of *memory loss*, slowing of mental processes, apathy and progressive dementia. Characteristically this is accompanied by a slow, *shuffling gait* with unsteadiness and a tendency to fall, and sometimes by *urinary incontinence*. It is this combination of symptoms and a somewhat fluctuating course that should alert one to the correct diagnosis and differentiation from Alzheimer's disease. Rarely a schizophrenia-like picture may develop, with delusions and hallucinations. The condition usually starts in elderly patients of sixty and upwards, but it can start earlier.

Investigations used to include air encephalography which showed the grossly enlarged ventricles but no or very little air in the subarachnoid space above the basal cisterns. This has been replaced by the CT scan which similarly shows gross symmetrical enlargement of the ventricles with atrophy of the brain but, unlike in Alzheimer's disease, the sulci are usually not widened. Recently continuous recording of the intracranial pressure over a period of two days or more has shown that the pressure is in fact not permanently normal or even low, as used to be thought, but that there are intermittent periods during which it is raised, and a characteristic pattern of raised pressure waves has been demonstrated. This is why the previous term 'normal pressure hydrocephalus' no longer seems appropriate; alternative terms have been suggested, e.g. 'intermittently raised pressure hydrocephalus' or 'adult communicating hydrocephalus' (Pickard 1982). The periods of raised intra-ventricular pressure are probably responsible for the dilatation of the ventricles. Increased pressure and high pressure waves are not found in Alzheimer's disease.

Treatment

This consists of creating a shunt between one of the lateral ventricles and the superior vena cava through the jugular venous system by means of a catheter with a one-way low pressure valve. These shunt operations are not always successful but are more likely to succeed if periods of raised pressure with high pressure waves have been demonstrated when monitoring the intracranial pressure. Blockage of the catheter, infection or formation of a subdural haematoma may complicate the procedure later on. If successful, the psychiatric symptoms may improve markedly within a few days or weeks after introduction of the ventriculo-caval shunt, but the unsteady gait may only improve slightly or remain unchanged.

NEUROSYPHILIS

The incidence of neurosyphilis has decreased greatly, mainly as the result of early treatment of primary or secondary syphilis. Of the three syphilitic disorders of the central nervous system – meningovascular syphilis, tabes dorsalis and general paresis – it is the latter which causes mental symptoms that can mimic many other psychiatric disorders. *General paresis*, sometimes called general paralysis of the insane or GPI, will therefore be considered briefly here.

In 1913 Noguchi and Moore demonstrated the presence of treponema pallidum in the brains of patients who had died of GPI. This constituted an important historical event in psychiatry (see also p. 12) as it was the first psychiatric disorder whose aetiology was definitely shown to be due to an identifiable organic cause, even though the association of GPI with syphilis had been suspected long before. The infection also accounted for the macroscopic and microscopic changes in the brain. In essence these consist of thickening of the meninges which become adherent to the brain, and extensive inflammatory and degenerative changes within the brain which lead to cerebral atrophy, dilatation of the ventricles and widening of the sulci.

Psychiatric manifestations

Classical descriptions of general paresis emphasised the appearance of psychotic manifestation, characterised by *grandiose delusions, euphoria* and expansive behaviour, followed by the gradual development of cognitive impairment, loss of memory and progressive *dementia*.

This picture is much less common nowadays. Instead, the patient may develop all the characteristics of *psychotic depression* with depressive delusions, either associated with or followed by progressive dementia. In others symptoms of dementia develop first, simulating alcoholic, presenile or senile dementia. Sometimes the condition may first present with a schizophrenic or paranoid psychosis, or as a sudden acute organic reaction with clouding of consciousness. Rarely it may commence with the gradual onset of fatigue and personality changes like irritability and vague somatic complaints.

General paresis, rare though it is nowadays, can therefore simulate many psychiatric disorders and should be considered in the differential diagnosis. In many but not all cases some abnormal neurological findings like minor pupillary irregularities will be present early on, but the fully developed Argyll-Robertson pupil may not develop until later. Optic atrophy, dysarthria and tremor may be present, as may be early signs of pyramidal involvement. *Epileptic fits* may also occur. However, none of these signs may be present in the early stages and serological tests for syphilis in the blood and cerebrospinal fluid will be needed. In the days before effective treatment the disorder gradually led to gross dementia, ataxia, progressive spastic paralysis, generalised weakness and death.

Treatment

Large doses of penicillin, at least 600,000 units given intramuscularly daily for a period of up to twenty-one days, usually arrest the progress of the disease. Occasionally symptoms may get worse temporarily within the first few days of treatment, the so-called *Herxheimer reaction*. This may be accompanied by fever or epileptic fits, and should be controlled with oral prednisone and by discontinuing the penicillin. Penicillin should be recommenced within a few days while treatment with prednisone continues. The more long-term effect of treatment should be monitored by examination of the cerebrospinal fluid at intervals, usually two months, six months and a year after the first course of treatment, and then yearly for five or more years. If the cell count in the CSF rises to more than five cells per ml a further course of penicillin is needed.

Rehabilitation, support and assistance with personal and social problems is essential to bring about maximum improvement of psychiatric symptoms and social functioning. The prognosis is largely determined by the severity and duration of symptoms when the disease is first diagnosed. The earlier in the course of the disorder treatment is instituted the better the long-term outlook.

MYALGIC ENCEPHALOMYELITIS

This disorder, sometimes also called benign myalgic encephalomyelitis, has been of interest to psychiatrists since the outbreak of an epidemic affecting the staff, mainly women, at the Royal Free Hospital in London in 1955. That epidemic, sometimes referred to as the Royal Free disease, was characterised by a variety of symptoms which consisted mainly of painful muscles, a sense of exhaustion after even minor physical exertion or mental stress, headache and sometimes also pain in the chest, vertigo and tinnitus, anxiety and depression. Low-grade fever was present in some patients. Symptoms often lasted or fluctuated for a year or longer, but the patients ultimately recovered and there were no fatalities.

The absence of abnormal neurological signs, failure to identify an organic cause and preponderence in females later led to the suggestion that the disorder might have been of psychological origin, in the nature of an epidemic of hysteria (McEvedy and Beard 1970a, 1970b).

Since then further similar epidemics have been described by Fagan *et al.* (1983), as well as some sporadic cases (Keighley and Bell 1983;

Winbow 1984). In these recent outbreaks there was evidence of viral infection. In particular, elevated neutralising antibody titres to Coxsackie B viruses have been demonstrated. It therefore now seems likely that myalgic encephalomyelitis (ME) can in some cases be of viral origin.

The differential diagnosis does, however, continue to present considerable problems, especially in isolated cases. Patients who present mainly with depression, anxiety and vague muscular pains may be wrongly diagnosed as suffering from ME, and the correct diagnosis of a depressive or other psychiatric illness may be missed, sometimes with serious consequences, e.g. if the depression remains untreated. A clear relationship between muscular effort, fatigue and myalgia should suggest ME. The possibility also remains that some outbreaks of epidemic hysteria (see p. 178) could be wrongly diagnosed as being due to ME or vice versa.

There is no effective treatment for myalgic encephalomyelitis, but if the depressive symptoms predominate they sometimes respond to antidepressants such as flupenthixol or lofepramine.

AIDS

The acquired immune deficiency syndrome (AIDS) can give rise to psychiatric problems at all stages of its development. Even individuals who are not infected but are afraid of catching it may develop psychological symptoms. Accounts of the medical aspects of AIDS will be found in medical textbooks, but a brief description of the different stages of the disorder will be helpful here.

The first of these stages is infection with the human immuno-deficiency virus (HIV) so that the person becomes seropositive but is symptom-free, though he is now infectious to others. In the individual case it cannot be predicted when symptoms of clinical AIDS will develop, but the proportion of patients who, after having become seropositive, progress to the full syndrome of clinical AIDS increases over the years. In a study of homosexual and bisexual seropositive men in the USA 36 per cent had developed AIDS 88 months after having become infected. It has also been estimated that 30 per cent of haemophiliacs over the age of twenty-one developed AIDS within six years after infection from infected blood products (Curran, Jaffe et al. 1988).

The next stage is the AIDS related complex (ARC) characterised by general lymphadenopathy, fever, weight loss and fatigue but as yet no secondary infection. A proportion of these patients will after varying lengths of time develop the syndrome of clinical AIDS with a variety of opportunistic infections, e.g. pneumonia due to pneumocystis carinii or neoplasms like Kaposi's sarcoma. Once this stage has been reached the outcome is fatal, although every effort is being made to develop effective treatment methods. It is important to note that the brain may be infected directly by HIV, causing dementia or other organic psychiatric disorders, as described below.

Psychological and psychiatric aspects

The 'worried well'

Psychological problems may be encountered in people who are not infected with HIV but who are worried that they might be, or are afraid of contracting the disorder. This applies particularly to those who belong to a high-risk group like homosexuals, bisexuals, intravenous drug abusers and haemophiliacs. These fears have been increased by the knowledge that the incidence of AIDS is increasing, even in heterosexuals, especially in Africans, and that there is, as yet, no effective treatment for it. Guilt about promiscuous sexual behaviour or drug abuse and the frequent moralising attitude of society, stigmatising or even blaming homosexuals, has further contributed to their anxieties.

Anxiety, panic attacks, depression, somatic preoccupations, e.g. misinterpreting minor physical complaints as signs of AIDS, are among the symptoms with which they present. They often request tests for AIDS but even when these are negative their anxiety soon returns. Others are afraid of being tested in case the result is positive and refuse to have it done.

These patients require a great deal of support from their doctor or from counsellors skilled and trained in dealing with AIDS-related problems.

The seropositive but symptom-free

Those who have been found on immunological testing to be sero-positive have many serious psychological problems to face. Perhaps the most worrying aspect for such people is the uncertainty as to what is going to happen to them. As a third of seropositive but symptom-free people will develop the disease over the course of the next few years, and an increasing proportion as time progresses, each individual is faced with the fact that no one can tell him whether, and if so when, he may develop the clinical AIDS syndrome and die. Anxiety, depression, suicidal ideas and sometimes suicidal attempts are common. So may be constant preoccupation with and obsessional ruminations about physical health, watching for any signs of the illness.

At least as serious is the knowledge that he has now become infectious to others so that he lives in fear of passing the virus on to his sexual partner or partners. Homosexual, bisexual or heterosexual people, if promiscuous, may try to control their promiscuous behaviour. Failure to do so further increases their anxiety and guilt. Even those who have only one permanent partner are understandably afraid of passing the infection on to him or her; many avoid intercourse or become preoccupied with the thought that the condom they were using may not have provided adequate protection to their partner. However, a few individuals may take revenge on society by becoming irresponsible in their sexual behaviour.

Self-blame about their earlier promiscuous sex life is very common. Some may blame themselves for being homosexual or drug abusers. Such feelings of low self-esteem are often reinforced by the prejudices of society, which have been increased by the rapid spread of AIDS. The sense of being outcast or isolated is made worse by the fact that others, even close friends and relatives, may shun their company because they are under the misconception that AIDS can be passed on by ordinary social contact. Even doctors and nurses have at times avoided contact with patients who are seropositive and even more so with sufferers from clinical AIDS. The increasing tendency of some life insurance companies to reject those who belong to one of the high-risk groups further adds to their sense of rejection and isolation, and makes them feel understandably angry and resentful.

The clinical AIDS syndrome

From the psychiatric point of view the most important manifestations of AIDS are those which arise from *direct infection of the brain by HIV* (Ho *et al.* 1985), resulting in both neurological and psychiatric symptoms. The latter involve particularly cognitive functions, giving rise to slowing of mental processes, apathy, lack of interest and inaccuracy in performance. Gradually memory will become more obviously impaired and ultimately the picture will be one of dementia, similar to the subcortical type of dementia as seen in Huntington's chorea and Parkinson's disease.

This condition is now known as the *AIDS dementia complex* (ADC) (R.W. Price *et al.* 1988; Fenton 1987). Psychotic symptoms resembling schizophrenia or an affective disorder may also be present. In addition motor functions may become impaired with unsteadiness of gait, ataxia, paralysis and the appearance of extrapyramidal signs. The CT scan shows evidence of cortical atrophy and the cerebrospinal fluid may show an increase of cells and protein though this may not be present in the early stages. At post-mortem there is evidence of encephalopathy and direct infection of the brain with HIV. ADC usually develops in the advanced stages of clinical AIDS when there is evidence of secondary infections, but it may precede such infection. The brain itself may, in addition to the direct infection with HIV, also be affected by secondary infection e.g. by toxoplasmosis, cerebral abscesses or meningitis, as well as by neoplasms, e.g. primary or secondary lymphoma.

Quite apart from these organic psychiatric manifestations, patients with the fully developed syndrome suffer from similar but much more serious psychological problems and symptoms than those seen in the earlier stages. Being severely ill physically and having to be admitted to hospital, combined with the knowledge that they are going to die, inevitably causes a great deal of emotional distress. As in other terminal illnesses the patient will pass through the stages of shock and denial, anger, despair and depression, but in patients with AIDS this is made much worse by feelings of guilt and self-blame and often by feeling isolated, rejected and an outcast, as described above. These devastating psychosocial aspects are well described by Deuchar (1984), and the painful personal experiences of a patient with AIDS are described by Madeley (1987).

In the clinical management of these patients, be it at home or in hospital, the professional staff need to be sympathetic and well informed about AIDS. As far as possible the patient should be treated as any other patient, although gloves must be worn when handling blood samples or other body fluids or specimens; masks and protective clothing need only be worn when surgical or invasive procedures are being carried out. It should be made clear to friends and visitors that AIDS is not contracted through ordinary social or physical contact. It is all the more important at this stage of the disease to make the patient feel supported and cared for instead of being shunned or rejected (Adler 1987).

The staff may be helped in this difficult task, which is bound to arouse their own fears and influence their feelings towards the patients, by attending staff groups run by counsellors or liaison psychiatrists familiar with AIDS. Self-help groups such as 'Body Positive' are often of help to AIDS sufferers, and the Terrence Higgins Trust, in addition to providing information and running self-help groups, gives courses for counsellors and staff involved in the treatment of patients with AIDS.

SOME NEUROLOGICAL DISORDERS

The importance of the inter-relationship between disturbance of cerebral structure and function on the one hand, and of mental function on the other is apparent from the various organic psychiatric disorders discussed so far. The same applies to a number of neurological disorders, e.g. Parkinsonism, multiple sclerosis and Friedreich's ataxia. These and other neurological conditions are commonly thought of as disorders which cause a variety of physical symptoms, but it is not always appreciated that they too often give rise to mental symptoms. Many of these are directly due to organic changes in the brain, but others such as anxiety, depression and hysterical manifestations may be caused by the patient's reaction to his disability. Moreover, some of the drugs used to treat neurological disorders, e.g. levodopa in Parkinson's disease, may give rise to mental changes as a result of their effect on cerebral function.

Parkinson's disease

This disorder is called after James Parkinson who first described it in 1817 under the name of 'shaking palsy' or paralysis agitans. The exact aetiology is often not known, in which case the diagnosis is one of idiopathic Parkinsonism. However, following the epidemics of encephalitis lethargica, or sleeping sickness, between 1917 and 1920 and the sporadic appearance of this form of encephalitis in the 1930s, it was observed that a number of patients developed symptoms of Parkinson's disease either while they were ill with sleeping sickness or afterwards, sometimes after an interval of many years. These patients are said to be suffering from post-encephalitic Parkinsonism.

In both cases the cerebral lesions affect the extrapyramidal system. The substantia nigra is particularly involved, as are the putamen, the globus pallidus and caudate nuclei. Further, it is now known that in Parkinson's disease there is gross *diminution of the neurotransmitter dopamine* in the affected areas, especially the basal ganglia, probably as a result of the degeneration of the melanin-containing cells in the substantia nigra. The dopamine deficiency appears to be responsible for a variety of psychiatric and neurological symptoms. It is, of course, well known that the use of phenothiazines in the treatment of schizophrenia and other psychiatric disorders can cause Parkinsonian symptoms, probably by blocking dopamine receptors at the synapses (see p. 245).

Clinical features

The physical symptoms and signs of Parkinsonism essentially consist of a rapid tremor at rest, most often seen in the hands, cog-wheel rigidity, and slowness and difficulty in initiating movements, referred to as hypokinesia; they are described fully in textbooks of neurology.

The psychiatric aspects of Parkinson's disease include disturbance of mood, cognition and occasionally hallucinatory phenomena. The latter may also occur as the result of treatment with levodopa or anticholinergic drugs.

First, it is important to note that in spite of severe physical disability many patients with idiopathic Parkinsonism show a remarkable capacity to remain effective and successful in their work, some of them continuing to be creative and original, and to lead a satisfying life, including their personal relationships. The same applies to some patients with post-encephalitic Parkinsonism, but many of the latter group ultimately entered a state of almost total immobility, withdrawal and apathy, quite unable to respond or to relate to anyone. Oliver Sacks (1982) has described the experience of several of these patients who remained in this state, sometimes accompanied by visual hallucinatory experiences, over many years. He also described their dramatic response to levodopa (see below, p. 291).

Mood changes

Some degree of depression and irritability is common in patients with Parkinsonism and may be a reaction to their symptoms and the knowledge that they have developed the disease. Exacerbation of their symptoms and failure to respond to treatment are often responsible.

More severe depressive illnesses may occur, sometimes with psychotic features. These may be directly related to the organic cerebral changes and often respond to antidepressant drugs or ECT.

Cognitive changes

It is now know that some patients with Parkinsonism who have had the disease for many years and who have severe motor disability may develop *impairment of memory and thought processes*, progressing to dementia. Slowness of thinking is common, and the condition resembles that of *subcortial dementia* as seen in Huntington's chorea (see p. 281) rather than the Alzheimer type of dementia. In patients who are virtually immobile and unresponsive to their surroundings it may be very difficult to decide to what extent a dementing process may be partly responsible for their condition. Sacks (1982) has described how some patients with severe, chronic post-encephalitic Parkinsonism regained normal mental functioning when treated with levodopa, though often only temporarily.

Hallucinations

Some patients with advanced post-encephalitic Parkinsonism may develop visual hallucinations without impairment of consciousness. Some of these may be pleasant, perhaps consisting of experiences that the patient has been deprived of by the profound physical disability. Sacks (1982) described a woman with post-encephalitic Parkinsonism who had been confined to an institution for many years and who got pleasure from hallucinations of men coming to visit and caress her. However, the hallucinations may have a frightening character.

In other patients the hallucinations may be part of an acute organic psychiatric reaction, the result of treatment with levodopa or anticholinergic drugs.

Psychological effects of levodopa

Although anticholinergic drugs like benzhexol or procyclidine are effective in the treatment of the physical symptoms in less severe cases, levodopa, the immediate precursor of dopamine, is now recognised as the more effective drug, giving rise to considerable improvement in about two-thirds of cases (Parkes and Marsden 1973). It is sometimes used in conjunction with anticholinergic drugs or amantidine. However, some patients cannot tolerate levodopa, which can cause many untoward side-effects, both physical and psychological. The former include nausea, vomiting, severe dyskinesia and hypotension.

The psychological effects of levodopa can be highly beneficial in some patients, while others develop severe side-effects. Apathy and depression may improve markedly, and Sacks (1982) has described how some patients with post-encephalitic Parkinsonism who had been totally withdrawn and irresponsive became alert, interested and alive for the first time after many years when treated with levodopa. However, they often relapsed or developed severe side-effects if kept on levodopa, although some could tolerate the drug in reduced dosage. Levodopa can also cause improvement in intellectual function. This, combined with the relief from depression, may make it possible for some patients to return to almost normal mental functioning.

Unfortunately levodopa can also cause severe psychological disturbances. These include acute confusional states with *delusions* and *hallucinations*, as mentioned earlier, with or without clouding of consciousness, sometimes associated with agitation and aggressive outbursts. Levodopa can also cause severe *depression*. In some patients levodopa will therefore have to be discontinued. Some may be able to tolerate it in smaller doses, or for short periods at a time. It should also be noted that the beneficial psychological and physical effects of levodopa may cease abruptly so that the patient suddenly feels completely immobile, totally unable to communicate with anyone, depressed and hopeless. This may last for a few hours or several days, and the patient may then equally suddenly return to his previous state of relative well-being. These so-called 'on-off effects' may be very frightening and distressing.

Treatment with levodopa therefore requires close attention to each individual patient's psychological and physical tolerance and response to the drug, and modifications of the treatment regime are often required.

Multiple sclerosis

As the widespread demyelinating lesions of multiple sclerosis (MS) can affect the brain as well as the spinal cord, mental changes of organic origin are commonly seen in this disorder. Equally important is the fact that psychological reactions may occur as the result of the patient's reaction to the disorder.

The commonest are *mood changes*. It used to be said that mild euphoria often occurred in patients with MS, but a depressed affect is equally common. The depression may be partly due to the patient's reaction to his illness and the knowledge that temporary improvement may be followed by the appearance of new symptoms. In others the mood changes may be organic in origin.

Some degree of *impairment of memory* and of intellectual function occurs in a high proportion of cases, but it is often mild and may only be discovered on psychological testing. More advanced and progressive changes leading to dementia can occur but they are rare and may show fluctuations like the neurological symptoms.

Psychotic illnesses, more often schizophrenic than depressive in type, have been described but these are rare. They may occur before the development of neurological abnormalities, or the neurological signs may be so slight that the diagnosis of MS is overlooked.

The relationship between MS and *hysterical conversion* symptoms may lead to difficulties in diagnosis. Such symptoms as ataxia, muscular weakness, paraesthesiae or sensory loss may appear early in MS, and if neurological signs are absent at that stage a diagnosis of conversion hysteria may be made and shown to be mistaken later when signs of MS become apparent. Associated euphoria may be mistaken for belle indifférence and appear to confirm the diagnosis of hysteria.

In other patients in whom the diagnosis of MS is clearly established hysterical conversion symptoms may become superimposed, perhaps as the result of denial or repression of associated anxiety. In some patients with MS the impaired cognitive function and mood changes of organic origin may interefere with the patient's ability to cope with stressful situations and thus lead to hysterical conversion symptoms.

While the frequency of hysterical manifestations in patients with MS remains uncertain, they undoubtedly occur and it is sometimes difficult to decide which symptoms are of organic and which are of psychological origin. The psychosomatic aspects, including the possible role of psychological factors in the origin and course of MS, have been discussed by Paulley (1985).

Friedreich's ataxia

This neurological disorder is mentioned briefly because it is occasionally accompanied or even preceded by a psychotic syndrome resembling schizophrenia, associated with paranoid features and sometimes with violent behaviour. If this precedes the onset of the typical symptoms and signs of involvement of the cerebellar and pyramidal tracts, the diagnosis is almost certain to be missed, but a family history of the disorder or pes cavus and kyphoscoliosis may lead one to suspect the diagnosis.

Myasthenia gravis

This condition must be considered for several reasons. First, in the early stages there may be considerable difficulty in distinguishing between myasthenia and psychoneurotic symptoms. The common early complaints of being easily fatigued and of brief periods of muscular weakness can easily be mistaken for functional symptoms, especially if they are preceded by emotional stress which sometimes precipitates the onset of myasthenia. Once such symptoms as ptosis, diplopia, or difficulty in chewing, aggravated as the patient continues to eat, make their appearance, and when it becomes more obvious that the muscular weakness follows use of the muscles involved, the diagnosis becomes clearer. Rapid improvement after injection of choline esterase antagonists like neostigmine methyl sulphate (prostigmin) or edrophonium chloride (tensilon) may confirm the diagnosis.

Secondly, emotional stress, anxiety and life events may not only precipitate the onset of the disorder but also influence the course of the disease by aggravating the symptoms.

Lastly, it is not surprising that in turn myasthenia gravis often causes considerable anxiety, panic and depression as a reaction to the disabling and often frightening symptoms such as severe muscular weakness, inability to swallow or to speak, or even difficulty in breathing (Sneddon 1980). Supportive psychotherapy therefore plays an important role in management alongside medical treatment with neostigmine or pyrido-stigmine, or by thymectomy.

ENDOCRINE DISORDERS

The relationship between endocrine disorders and psychiatric distur-bance is complex. On the one hand endocrine disorders can cause abnormal mental function, e.g. thyrotoxicosis, myxoedema, Cushing's disease, Addison's disease, hypo- or hyperglycaemia due to diabetes, phaeochromocytoma, and hyper- or hypoparathyroidism. In the majority of these conditions the mental changes are due to the organic effects of disturbed hormonal function on the brain. Occasionally, it is the psychological effect of the illness, e.g. the person's reaction to the discovery that he is diabetic, or a woman's reaction to the development of hirsuties due to Cushing's disease, which may act as a stress factor and precipitate the development of, say, an anxiety state or depression.

On the other hand, emotional disturbance due to stressful life events may sometimes precipitate the onset of an endocrine disorder like thyrotoxicosis or diabetes or aggravate the disorder.

Thyrotoxicosis

The fact that thyrotoxicosis is sometimes precipitated by an acute emotional disturbance or stressful life event has already been mentioned. In spite of earlier claims, there is no evidence that there is a characteristic personality type that predisposes to thyrotoxicosis, although there may be a history of long-standing emotional instability. It is more common in women.

Once established, anxiety and emotional lability are prominent features, as are overactivity and difficulty in concentration, sometimes associated with mild cognitive impairment. Rarely the labile mood manifests itself as depression.

At this stage thyrotoxicosis must be differentiated from an anxiety state (see p. 160). This may be made more difficult if the condition has followed a precipitating life event in a person with long-standing emotional insta-bility. Weight loss in spite of increased appetite, preference for cold weather, warm and sweaty rather than cold hands, persistent tachycardia even when asleep, in conjunction with positive eye signs and other physical signs of thyrotoxicosis, usually help in diagnosis. If in doubt, thyroid func-tion tests should be carried out early to determine the correct diagnosis.

In severe untreated cases the thyrotoxic patient may develop an acute organic psychiatric reaction with confusion, extreme restlessness or mania, a so-called *thyroid crisis*. Rarely the patient may become apathetic and stuporose, resembling depressive stupor. Psychotic reactions, affective or schizophrenic, have been described but are more likely to occur in patients already predisposed to these disorders.

The psychiatric symptoms usually respond to medical treatment of the thyrotoxicosis.

Hypothyroidism

Like thyrotoxicosis, hypothyroidism or myxoedema is much more common in women than men. It can occur at any age but is commoner in middle age and in the elderly.

The onset is gradual and it is always accompanied by some mental abnormalities. If, as often happens, the characteristic physical features are overlooked, the correct diagnosis may be missed or delayed, with serious consequences due to failure of early treatment with thyroxine. The physical features to look out for are the typical puffy facial appearance with baggy eyelids, loss of hair and eyebrows, rough, dry skin, a hoarse voice and general slowness of speech and movements. There may be cardiac enlargement, and angina is a common complaint.

In the early stages the mental changes consist of gradual slowing of all mental processes, impairment of memory, lethargy, sometimes accompanied by increased sleep, poor appetite and mood changes, usually mild depression or apathy, but sometimes irritability and aggressiveness. It is particularly at this stage that a wrong diagnosis of depression or of early dementia is often made. Such mistakes can be avoided by carrying out thyroid function tests.

As the condition worsens psychotic symptoms may develop, producing a picture of *myxoedema madness* (Asher 1949). This may take the form of an acute organic psychiatric reaction with *clouding of consciousness* and *paranoid delusions*, or of a *psychotic depression*, again with paranoid features, or a *schizophrenia-like psychosis*. Sometimes the features of *dementia* predominate, and if a mistaken diagnosis of presenile or senile dementia is made the condition deteriorates over months or years.

Neurological abnormalities may be present. These include slowing of ankle jerks at an early stage, epileptic seizures, cerebellar ataxia, and sometimes the development of coma with hypothermia.

All these mental and physical changes clear up within a few weeks of starting treatment with thyroxine, except when the diagnosis has been delayed for more than a year or two, in which case symptoms of dementia may only partially recover. This once more underlines the importance of carrying out thyroid function tests at the earliest possible stage.

Diabetes

Psychological considerations are important in diabetes in two respects. First, in the influence that emotional factors can have on the onset and course of the disorder; secondly, in the effect of diabetes on mental function.

Genetic factors are of major importance in predisposing a person to the development of diabetes, but there is some clinical evidence that emotional stress may occasionally precipitate its onset. In middle age obesity, which may itself be due to overeating of emotional origin, is another predisposing factor.

Once the disease is established emotional stress can increase the blood sugar level and hence insulin requirements. If not recognised in time this may lead to increased levels of blood ketones and result in the development of diabetic coma.

Equally important is the fact that the experience of being diabetic and of needing insulin, or of having to adhere to a diet, can cause emotional problems which may interfere with adequate control and thus affect the course of the disorder. For example, in children, having diabetes and the treatment regime may lead to problems between the child and its parents. Parents are likely to be overanxious if their child becomes diabetic and their insistence on the necessary dietary control and regular injections of insulin may make the child rebellious and resentful. His refusal to comply, combined with increasing tension and unhappiness, may lead to poor control and thus to further parental anxiety and frustration.

Similarly, adolescents and sometimes adults may deny the need to adhere to their diet or to give themselves regular injections, perhaps because these interfere with their social life. Occasionally a child or adolescent may on purpose give himself too much insulin or omit a meal to induce a hypoglycaemic attack in order to get out of a situation he dislikes. In adults anxiety about possible impairment of sexual function due to diabetes or a sense of inadequacy associated with being diabetic may cause problems in intimate relationships or in marriage.

In diabetic patients attention needs to be paid to the interaction between these physical and psychological aspects (Tattersall 1981); both must be considered if proper control is to be established and maintained. A good relationship between the patient and his doctor is essential to help the diabetic to come to terms with his disorder and lead a normal life. This is equally important if in long-standing diabetes such complications as symptoms due to arteriosclerotic changes or ocular involvement develop and require appropriate treatment.

The mental changes which occur as the result of either hypoglycaemia or hyperglycaemia and ketosis, leading to diabetic coma, are well known. Both present with the symptoms of an acute organic mental reaction. In hypoglycaemia anxiety, irritability, a sense of unreality and mild confusion with impairment of thinking and speech, are among the early symptoms. These quickly progress to more severe impairment of consciousness and ultimately to coma, sometimes associated with an epileptic fit. They respond rapidly to the administration of glucose.

Other causes of hypoglycaemia

Hypoglycaemia in diabetics rarely comes to the notice of a psychiatrist, but there are several other causes of hypoglycaemia presenting with mental symptoms which lead to the patient first being referred to a psychiatrist. The psychiatric manifestations of hypoglycaemia are sometimes referred to as *neuroglycopenia* and have been reviewed by Marks and Rose (1981). The conditions causing hypoglycaemia, apart from diabetes, include the following:

Insulinoma of the pancreas

This islet cell tumour of the pancreas is composed of beta cells: it is benign in 90 per cent of cases, but malignant, sometimes giving rise to secondaries, in 10 per cent. Varying amounts of insulin are secreted by the tumour cells so that the blood sugar fluctuates markedly from normal to very low levels.

The psychiatric symptoms are extremely variable and may be present for several years before the correct diagnosis is made. Although typical acute hypoglycaemic attacks may occur from time to time these are often absent. In long-standing cases there may simply be a gradual change in personality, leading to emotional lability and occasionally to paranoid ideas. Alternatively, impairment of memory and intellectual function may develop. In other patients the periods of hypoglycaemia may lead to recurrent episodes of anxiety or panic, or of bizarre, sometimes violent or disinhibited behaviour accompanied by confusion and loss of contact with the surroundings. These may last for an hour or longer and are usually followed by amnesia for the attack after recovery. As the condition progresses these attacks of grossly disturbed behaviour may become more frequent. Sometimes typical hypoglycaemic attacks of the kind seen in uncontrolled diabetics, with impairment or loss of consciousness, with or without fits, occur in addition or by themselves, and point to the correct diagnosis. The symptoms of an insulinoma can therefore resemble personality disorders, anxiety or depressive states, hysterical conversion symptoms, fugue states or epilepsy. It is a rare disorder but should be considered in the differential diagnosis of unusual psychiatric presentations, especially if these take the form of episodic behaviour disturbance. The blood sugar is usually but not always low during acute attacks. Other tests, including the effect of prolonged fasting and the tolbutamide test, are described in medical textbooks.

Postprandial (reactive) hypoglycaemia

Here the drop in blood sugar is not due to excessive production of insulin but follows the intake and rapid absorption of carbohydrates. The blood sugar, after its initial rise, falls to below normal levels usually 1½-4 hours after a meal. The symptoms are not relieved by glucose nor are they produced by fasting. The condition occurs in otherwise healthy individuals, but it can be due to rapid absorption of carbohydrates, e.g. following a gastrectomy.

The psychiatric symptoms usually consist of sudden weakness and faintness, accompanied by anxiety 1-4 hours after eating. Fully developed attacks of hypoglycaemia hardly ever occur. These patients often show evidence of mild anxiety and irritability between attacks, and it may be difficult to decide whether the symptoms are due to hypoglycaemia or psychoneurotic in origin, or a combination of both. Treatment with a low carbohydrate diet usually helps to prevent attacks.

Alcohol

Hypoglycaemic attacks can occur some hours after excessive alcohol consumption, especially if the person is under-nourished, as may be the case in chronic alcoholics.

Self-induced hypoglycaemia

Occasionally hypoglycaemia is self-induced in diabetic or non-diabetic people who have access to insulin, such as doctors or nurses, either as an overdose or to draw attention to themselves when under stress.

Cushing's disease

Whether this disorder develops as the result of a pituitary adenoma or an adrenal tumour or over-production of ACTH by the pituitary, the persistently high level of cortisol and often also of other steroids and androgens cause not only physical but also psychiatric symptoms. The latter may be the earliest signs of Cushing's disease. The commonest mental symptoms are changes in mood, especially *depression*. Anxiety, restlessness and irritability are also common. If the mental symptoms develop before the characteristic physical features the diagnosis is easily missed. In other cases the moon-shaped face, hirsuties and obesity, associated with hypertension, develop first and the only mental changes may be those of mild depression and anxiety, perhaps in part due to worry about the unsightly changes in appearance. Impotence in men, sometimes accompanied by testicular atrophy, and amenorrhoea in women may be other or additional causes of emotional distress.

It should be noted here that the mental changes due to the persistently high levels of cortisol in Cushing's disease are usually more severe than the changes observed in patients who are taking corticosteroids for therapeutic purposes. In the latter the mood changes are usually less severe and consist of depression or elation; psychotic symptoms are rare.

Once the diagnosis of Cushing's disease is made and the condition satisfactorily treated, the psychiatric complications usually clear up rapidly. However, if the disease was caused by a pituitary tumour and the pituitary had to be removed, the necessary replacement therapy with steroids, and sometimes also thyroxine, may cause psychological problems. Some patients try to deny the need for regular replacement therapy and for increased doses of steroids at times of stress or other illness; as a result they may develop symptoms of adrenal insufficiency. Others become anxious and depressed on account of the need to remain on steroids, and some keep watching themselves for possible signs of recurrence of Cushing's disease.

Addison's disease

Here the atrophy or destruction of both adrenal cortices leads to a fall in production of all adrenal steroids, including cortisol, corticosterone, aldosterone and androgens, giving rise to a physical syndrome which is the opposite of that seen in Cushing's disease. Loss of appetite and weight, nausea, general weakness, loss of libido, impotence and inability to cope with any forms of stress, physical or psychological, are common early symptoms; they are accompanied by low blood pressure, hypothermia and the characteristic hyperpigmentation of the skin and oral mucosa. At this stage mild depression, a sense of exhaustion, lack of energy and of initiative are present in most patients with Addison's disease. Poor concentration, impaired memory and slowing or poverty of thought processes are common. If untreated an Addisonian crisis will develop, often preceded by nausea and vomiting, and leading on to an acute organic psychiatric reaction with impairment and ultimately loss of consciousness, hypotension and sometimes epileptic fits.

All the psychiatric manifestations respond to replacement therapy; glucocorticoids seem to be more important for the correction of the mental symptoms than the correction of the electrolyte disturbance with mineralocorticoids.

Phaecochromocytoma

This rare condition, caused by a tumour of the adrenal medulla, is important from the psychiatric point of view because it enters into the differential diagnosis of anxiety states and panic attacks. It almost always presents with episodic attacks of suddenly feeling very distressed and anxious, often amounting to severe panic, and accompanied by pallor, palpitations, severe headache and sweating. These attacks are often provoked by exercise, postures which raise the intra-abdominal pressure, or by emotional stress or excitement. They last from a few minutes to several hours, and are followed by weakness and exhaustion. They are caused by increased secretion of adrenaline and noradrenaline, and are therefore accompanied by marked hypertension. In about half the cases the blood pressure is also raised between attacks.

Although the condition is rare it should be considered in the differential diagnosis of anxiety attacks. The raised blood pressure during attacks should alert one to the possibility of a phaeochromocytoma. Estimation of the 24-hour excretion of vanilmandelic acid in the urine and other investigations should be instigated to confirm or disprove the diagnosis, as described in medical textbooks.

Hyperparathyroidism

Here the raised serum calcium due to a parathyroid adenoma can give rise to psychiatric symptoms in addition to the characteristic physical symptoms, such as those due to osteoporosis, renal colic due to renal calculi, muscular weakness, thirst and anorexia.

The psychiatric symptoms are often those of lethargy and depression, which may be present for years before the correct diagnosis is made; later on there may be evidence of poor concentration and impaired memory and intellectual function. The severity of the mental symptoms appears to be determined by the height of the serum calcium level. At levels above 16 mg per 100 ml acute organic confusional states are common, leading ultimately to impairment of consciousness and coma. Once the correct diagnosis is made, usually by finding a high level of serum calcium and a low level of serum phosphorous, and once the serum calcium has returned to normal after surgery, the mental symptoms usually subside rapidly.

Hypoparathyroidism

This is either idiopathic in origin or may follow accidental removal of the parathyroid glands or interference with their blood supply during thyroidectomy or other surgical procedures. It can occur at any age, including childhood. Attacks of tetany, cataracts developing early in life, and sometimes epilepsy may suggest the diagnosis. In addition to the low serum calcium and raised serum phosphorus levels there may be calcification in the basal ganglia visible in the skull X-ray.

If the condition develops rapidly after an operation on the neck the mental symptoms may be those of an acute organic mental reaction with impairment of consciousness, confusion and hallucinations. If the condition is of gradual onset and has been present for several years, neurotic symptoms like irritability, anxiety and depression are common and may vary in intensity over time. Children may be acutely anxious or prone to unexplained outbursts of temper. Alternatively the symptoms may be those of poor concentration, memory loss and impaired intellectual function, resembling mental handicap in children or dementia in adults. Epilepsy may be associated with these symptoms, as may attacks of tetany.

Treatment with vitamin D or dihydrotachysterol and a high calcium intake leads to marked improvement of the psychiatric manifestations, usually even after the diagnosis has been delayed for several years.

VITAMIN DEFICIENCIES

Deficiencies of the following vitamins of the B group are known to give rise to psychiatric as well as physical symptoms: thiamine (vitamin B1), nicotinic acid amide (nicotinamide), pyridoxine (vitamin B6), cyanocobalamin (vitamin B12) and folic acid. These disorders are more often seen in under-developed countries, especially at times of famine, than in Western countries. In the West they can occur as the result of self-neglect, e.g. in elderly, demented patients living alone, or in the mentally handicapped living in the community without adequate personal or financial support. Chronic alcoholism associated with under-nourishment is another relatively common cause. Vitamin deficiency can also be due to prolonged vomiting or malabsorption caused by gastrointestinal disorders, and occasionally by severe, prolonged dieting. In clinical practice a patient often shows evidence of several vitamin deficiencies at once, as well as other signs of malnutrition, e.g. hypoproteinaemia.

Thiamine (vitamin B1) deficiency

Vitamin B1 deficiency was first described as *beriberi*, caused by a prolonged inadequate diet consisting mainly of highly polished rice. Beriberi is characterised by cardiac failure, oedema and peripheral neuritis. This may be preceded or accompanied by lethargy, depression, poor concentration and forgetfulness, resembling a neurasthenic syndrome.

In the West thiamine deficiency is usually due to chronic alcoholism associated with an inadequate diet. It presents with the fairly sudden onset of Wernicke's encephalopathy followed by Korsakoff's psychosis (see Chapter 30, p. 381). Occasionally it is the result of anorexia and vomiting, caused, for example, by cancer of the stomach. Patients with beriberi sometimes also show some of the symptoms of the Wernicke-Korsakoff syndrome.

Whatever the cause, thiamine needs to be given initially by intravenous or intramuscular injection of 100 mg daily for several days, as the amount that can be absorbed from the gut is limited. Wernicke's encephalopathy can be fatal unless treated early, and thiamine is essential in the treatment of the Wernicke-Korsakoff syndrome. Parentrovite is often used to correct any other vitamin B deficiencies in addition to that of vitamin B1.

Nicotinic acid deficiency

Pellagra is the classical syndrome caused by prolonged lack of nicotinic acid. In addition to the physical symptoms of dermatitis on exposed skin surfaces, diarrhoea and a sore red tongue, psychiatric symptoms constitute an important aspect of pellagra. In the early stages these consist of a neurasthenic syndrome of mental fatigue, anxiety, depression and impaired concentration, similar to that seen in thiamine deficiency. *Depression* may be severe and may lead to a diagnosis of a depressive illness. Progressive memory loss may suggest early *dementia* if the mental symptoms appear before the dermatitis and diarrhoea. In the more advanced stages an acute organic mental reaction with psychotic features, severe memory impairment and clouding of consciousness may develop.

Nicotinic acid deficiency is particularly common in a population whose staple diet consists mainly of maize. A high proportion of the daily requirement of nicotinic acid is derived from tryptophan, which is lacking in maize. In the UK and USA chronic alcoholism, poor dietary intake in the elderly, and malabsorption are among the more common causes.

Although lack of other vitamins of the B complex is often associated with nicotinic acid deficiency, both the mental and physical symptoms of pellagra usually respond rapidly to parenteral administration of 100 mg of nicotinic acid alone, given every hour for ten hours on the first two days, followed by six-hourly administration orally or parenterally once improvement has commenced. In practice parentrovite is commonly used and ensures that all the B-vitamins are included.

Pyridoxine (vitamin B6) deficiency

This has been suspected of playing a part in the causation of depressive states (Carney *et al*. 1982). It can also cause convulsions in infancy.

Cyanocobalamin (vitamin B12) deficiency

There used to be some uncertainty whether deficiency of vitamin B12 could cause mental symptoms directly by affecting cerebral function or only indirectly by causing pernicious anaemia, when the anaemia may be responsible for such symptoms as general weakness, fatigue and depression. There is, however, now sufficient evidence that long-standing deficiency of vitamin B12, even in the absence of anaemia, can cause early signs of dementia, such as memory loss, especially in the elderly; and occasionally it can be responsible for an acute organic psychiatric reaction or for a depressive illness or paranoid psychosis. It should therefore be considered in the differential diagnosis of these psychiatric conditions; estimation of the serum B12 level should assist in making a diagnosis, especially if there are no signs of pernicious anaemia or subacute combined degeneration of the spinal cord. The possibility of vitamin B12 deficiency should be considered particularly if there is a history of gastric surgery or of chronic gastrointestinal disorder leading to malabsorption.

The difficulty in diagnosis is made worse by the fact that low serum B12 levels are commonly found in psychiatric patients, especially the elderly, so that it may be difficult to decide in the individual case whether the B12 deficiency is the result of the disorder, e.g. in elderly demented patients living on an inadequate diet, or the cause of it. When in doubt treatment with parenteral neocytamen (hydroxocobalamin) is worth a trial, using the same dosage as in the treatment of pernicious anaemia or subacute combined degeneration of the cord.

Folic acid deficiency

This is briefly referred to here although there is still some doubt whether folic acid deficiency by itself can cause psychiatric disorders. As with vitamin B12, a low serum folate level in psychiatric patients can be the result of anorexia or self-neglect caused by, say, dementia or depression, rather than its cause. However, occasionally a patient with all the symptoms of dementia may respond to treatment with folic acid. It has also been claimed that folic acid deficiency may on rare occasions play a part in the aetiology of depressive illnesses. Treatment of epileptics with phenytoin, phenobarbitone or primidone can also cause folic acid deficiency and megaloblastic anaemia. Some of the mental symptoms seen in epileptics might therefore be due to folic acid deficiency caused by these anticonvulsant drugs.

A trial of treatment of folic acid, 5 mg three times daily, is worth considering if a patient with dementia or depression is found to have a low level of serum folate. The same applies to epileptic patients who develop mental symptoms while taking anticonvulsant drugs. Folic acid should however not be given if vitamin B12 is also deficient as only B12 but not folic acid is effective in the treatment of pernicious anaemia or subacute combined degeneration; both these conditions can in fact be made worse by the administration of folic acid unless the B12 deficiency is treated first.

SYSTEMIC LUPUS ERYTHEMATOSUS

There is a high incidence of neurological and psychiatric symptoms in systemic lupus erythematosus (SLE). They usually occur during the acute stages of the illness and during relapses, although on rare occasions they may precede the development of symptoms outside the central nervous system. Usually the polyarthritis, skin lesions, renal involvement and prolonged or intermittent fever will point to the diagnosis, which can then be confirmed by the demonstration of antinuclear antibodies in the serum and of LE cells in the blood. The former test gives a positive result in a greater number of patients with SLE than the LE cell test, and is therefore preferred.

The psychiatric manifestations can take many different forms. About a third of patients with SLE develop acute organic psychiatric reactions at some stage of the disease, often with paranoid or depressive delusions or hallucinations. A chronic organic reaction with impairment of memory and cognition is less common but can lead to a picture of dementia. Alternatively the picture may be one of psychotic depression, or it may present with schizophrenic symptoms. Sometimes neurotic symptoms of depression, anxiety or hysterical features predominate; these may in part be due to the patient's psychological reaction to this prolonged, disabling and relapsing disease which interferes with his, or much more commonly, her personal and social life.

The organic psychiatric reactions are almost certainly due to widespread lesions of small blood vessels in the brain, with haemorrhages and necrosis of surrounding tissues. These are also responsible for the occurrence of neurological symptoms and signs, such as cranial nerve lesions, extrapyramidal signs and occasionally dysphasia or hemiparesis. Peripheral neuropathy may also occur.

The psychiatric and neurological symptoms, like the systemic manifestations, usually respond well to treatment with steroids, but the prolonged use of steroids in large doses, essential though it is to control the disease, may itself give rise to depression and psychotic manifestations.

Other collagen diseases, e.g. polyarteritis nodosa, can give rise to similar psychiatric symptoms but will not be discussed further here.

ACUTE INTERMITTENT PORPHYRIA

As acute porphyria often presents with psychiatric symptoms and may lead to considerable difficulties in diagnosis, it is briefly discussed here. Description of the medical aspects and of other varieties of porphyria will be found in medical textbooks. The condition is due to an inherited dominant gene of incomplete penetrance causing enzyme deficiency which leads to failure of synthesis of porphyrins and hence to excess production of porphobilinogen. The mental symptoms may occur on their own or accompany the physical symptoms. The latter often take the form of acute attacks of abdominal pain with nausea, vomiting and constipation. Pain in the limbs, muscular weakness, headache, or an acute peripheral neuropathy are alternative symptoms, sometimes leading to respiratory paralysis.

The mental symptoms may vary from emotional lability with depression, outbursts of violence and bizarre behaviour, to an acute organic mental reaction with delusions, often of paranoid type, and impairment or loss of consciousness. Epileptic seizures may also occur.

Attacks are commonly provoked by an infection or by drugs, especially the barbiturates, but also by amitriptyline welldorm, sulphonamides, steroids, anticonvulsants and oestrogen, e.g. in the contraceptive pill. Alcohol can also precipitate attacks.

Excess of porphobilinogen and d-aminolaevulinic acid in the urine during attacks should lead to the correct diagnosis. Characteristically the urine, which may appear normal on passing, turns red on standing. However, there does not appear to be a direct relationship between the amount of porphobilinogen in the urine and the development or severity of the attacks. In fact there may be high levels of porphobilinogen in between attacks.

A mistaken diagnosis of hysterical conversion symptoms or of a personality disorder is easily made, especially if there is a history of obscure attacks of abdominal pain in the past for which no cause was found, or of a laparotomy which revealed no abnormality. When acute psychotic symptoms predominate the picture may simulate acute schizophrenia or psychotic depression.

While there is no specific treatment, the acute psychiatric symptoms may require medication. Promazine and chlorpromazine are safe drugs to use, as is paraldehyde; morphia or pethidine can be used to control severe pain.

SLEEP DISORDERS

Sleep disturbances are common and may be associated with psychiatric disorders. The commonest symptom is insomnia. Narcolepsy, sleep walking and night terrors are rare but will also be referred to briefly.

Neurophysiology of sleep

Normal sleep in man and other mammals comprises two types of alternating sleep: REM (rapid eye movement) sleep and non-REM sleep. REM sleep, in which there are rapid conjugate eye movements, is associated with dreaming; when woken while in the stage of REM sleep the subject will on 80 per cent of occasions report that he has just been dreaming. It used to be thought that dreaming was confined to REM sleep, but rarely, on less than 10 per cent of occasions, the subject when woken during non-REM sleep may also have just been dreaming. The psychological significance of dreams is discussed in Chapter 5 (see p. 50) and will not be described further here.

EEG studies recorded in sleep laboratories show that on falling asleep the subject rapidly passes from the fast (about 10 cycles per second), low-voltage alpha-rhythm, characteristic of the relaxed waking state with eyes closed, into stage 1 of non-REM sleep with desynchronised low-voltage activity. This is rapidly followed by stage 2, in which 'sleep spindles' (brief episodes of fast activity) make their appearance. After a few more minutes the subject enters the deeper stages of non-REM sleep, stages 3 and 4. In these, especially stage 4, the EEG shows 1-4 cycles per second, high voltage delta waves.

Approximately every 90 minutes the EEG pattern reverts to that of stage 1, but now sleep is associated with rapid conjugate eye movements which are superimposed on the EEG. This is the *REM phase*, during which dreaming occurs. Each REM phase usually lasts about 20 minutes, after which the EEG once more reverts to that of deeper stages of non-REM sleep.

During a night of 8 hours' sleep the subject will on average pass through four or five such phases of REM sleep, making a total of about 90 minutes. Adults therefore spend about 20-25 per cent of the night in REM or dream sleep. Neonates spend considerably longer, 45-65 per cent, infants and young children 25-40 per cent, and people over sixty rather less, 12-20 per cent, of the night in REM sleep.

REM sleep is a necessary part of total sleep. This has been

demonstrated by the fact that subjects who are deprived of REM sleep by being woken up each time they enter a REM phase for several nights in succession become irritable and tense during the intervening days although they have had about 6-7 hours of non-REM sleep each night. Moreover, once they are allowed to sleep normally they make up quantitatively during the first few nights of uninterrupted sleep for the amount of REM sleep lost.

The REM or dream state of sleep also differs from non-REM sleep in other biological respects. There is marked autonomic arousal with frequent changes in pulse and respiratory rates as well as blood pressure. The measurements vary from abnormally high to normal levels. These peripheral changes are often related to the dream content. In males, infants and children included, REM sleep is often accompanied by penile erection, and ejaculation may occur in response to dreams with a sexual content.

There are also changes in muscular tone and activity. During REM sleep muscle tone is markedly diminished, sometimes almost amounting to paralysis, especially in the neck muscles and the muscles necessary to maintain an upright posture. There may be increased activity of smaller muscles as evidenced by twitching of the hands, feet and face, and, of course, by the rapid movements of the ocular muscles themselves.

Insomnia

The complaint of not getting enough or interrupted sleep is very common, both among patients with psychiatric disorders and among people who are not otherwise ill.

Age has an important influence on the duration of sleep. Infants and children sleep much longer than adults, and with increasing age the amount of sleep is reduced. Many people over the age of sixty-five have difficulty in going to sleep and may wake frequently. Some elderly people accept this as part of normal ageing; others may seek medical advice. The use of hypnotics or tranquillisers for the aged is best avoided. They may actually make the condition worse by leaving the person feeling drowsy and making him sleep during the day so that he feels even less tired at night. Reassurance that it is normal to need less sleep as one gets older, and simple measures like learning to relax when lying awake, avoidance of drinks containing caffeine during the second half of the day, a hot drink at night, reading or listening to music if awake, or more exercise during the day may all help.

Feeling frustrated or angry during the day or anxious about some impending or uncompleted task may cause difficult in falling asleep at night or repeated waking. Sadness may have similar effects (Crisp 1980b). Having had a relaxed and satisfactory day may have the opposite effect, helping a person to fall asleep quickly and to have a full night's sleep. Crisp (1980a) has also shown that diet and weight changes have an effect on sleep. Loss of weight, for example in anorexic patients, can be associated with less sleep, including early waking, while restoration of normal weight and weight gain increase the duration of both non-REM and REM sleep, and thus the total duration of sleep. These influences of weight changes are more marked during the second half of the night.

In insomnia due to mood changes related to upsetting events it is again best to avoid the use of tranquillisers or hypnotics, except for brief periods during a crisis, to avoid dependency. If necessary, temazepam 10 mg for a few nights can be helpful.

The fact that disturbed sleep and early morning waking are common in anorexic patients has already been referred to. Other psychiatric conditions that lead to insomnia are the affective disorders, especially a severe depressive illness, giving rise to early morning waking. In manic patients the duration of sleep is much reduced but, unlike the depressed patient, the manic patient welcomes the fact that he needs so little sleep and thus has more time for his many activities. In the affective disorders the sleep disturbance will respond to treatment of the underlying condition. Nocturnal restlessness with reduced sleep can also be an early feature of a schizophrenic episode. Increased alcohol consumption can also lead to early morning waking, and alcohol withdrawal can cause severe insomnia, as in delirium tremens.

Physical illnesses, especially painful conditions and respiratory or cardiac disorders, often cause insomnia, as does anxiety about being ill and being in the unaccustomed environment of a hospital ward.

Lastly, some patients complain that they never get sufficient sleep, even that they get hardly any sleep at all. If no cause can be found this is sometimes referred to as *primary insomnia*. When these patients are observed carefully throughout the night or investigated in a sleep laboratory with EEG recordings they are almost always found to sleep a normal number of hours with a normal sleep pattern. It seems likely that their real problem is anxiety about not getting enough sleep rather than insomnia proper.

Sleep walking (somnambulism)

Some people, especially children, have episodes during the night when they are found wandering about while they are asleep. This is more common in boys than girls; most children stop sleep walking as they get older but it may persist into adult life. Some of these children also suffer from enuresis, and there may be a family history of sleep walking.

Contrary to popular belief, sleep walking is not associated with dreaming. Sleep walking starts during the deep slow-wave sleep stages 3 and 4 of non-REM sleep, usually early in the night. This is not surprising as in REM sleep the muscles required for maintaining an upright posture are paralysed so that walking during REM sleep would not be possible.

The episodes of sleep walking usually only last a few minutes but sometimes longer. The person walks about as if in a trance, but sometimes more purposeful activities are carried out. When talked to, the person may either not respond at all or give only a few vague utterances. When the episode of sleep walking comes to an end the person usually goes back to bed and continues normal sleep but has no recollection of the event when he wakes up in the morning.

It is sometimes claimed that sleep walking is not associated with psychological disturbance, especially in children. However, like enuresis which may occur in the same child, emotional conflicts, family tension or traumatic life events may be present. When sleep walking persists into or starts in adolescence or adulthood, traumatic events, disturbed family relationships and personality disorders or anxiety states are often present (Sours *et al.* 1963). Calogeras (1982) has described a patient who had sleep-walked as a child and whose sleep walking returned when he was in psychoanalysis as an adult. He then remembered a traumatic event from his childhood which had preceded his sleep walking. When these memories had been worked through in his analysis his sleep walking ceased.

Treatment

Although sleep walkers do not usually injure themselves it is safer to prevent possible accidents by keeping doors and windows locked and anything potentially dangerous out of reach. Diazepam has occasionally reduced the frequency of sleep walking, but this is not usually necessary.

Night terror

These dramatic episodes, sometimes called *incubus attacks*, arise during stages 3 or 4 of non-REM sleep, like sleep walking. They may in fact occur in the same individual, in children or in adults. They usually start during the first or second non-REM period and the EEG shows sudden arousal from deep slow-wave sleep (Broughton 1970). The individual, fast asleep at one moment, and without having dreamt, suddenly experiences extreme terror, a sense of choking or of being crushed. He may suddenly sit up or even jump out of bed and scream loudly. Usually the attack only lasts a few seconds, but it sometimes leads to a brief period of sleep walking and the individual may, on very rare occasions, attack another person, say his spouse, while still asleep. The intense fear and sudden motor activity are accompanied by marked tachycardia and fast or irregular breathing. There may be no or only partial memory of the event in the morning.

Attacks of night terror must be clearly distinguished from nightmares. These are dreams with a frightening content so that the person suddenly wakes up from the dream in a state of fear. Unlike attacks of night terror, which are not preceded by dreaming, nightmares occur during REM sleep. Nightmares do not lead to sleep walking, and although the fear on waking is accompanied by autonomic arousal, the tachycardia and changes in respiration are usually less marked than during night terror.

A few cases have been reported where an individual attacked and injured or even killed another person during an episode of night terror or sleep walking. When there was sufficient evidence that the person carried out the attack while asleep, he has been acquitted.

As in sleep walking, diazepam can sometimes reduce the frequency or prevent attacks of night terror.

Narcolepsy

This disorder is characterised by attacks of sudden drowsiness several times during the day, each followed by an episode of irresistible sleep lasting 10-15 minutes or longer. These patients often also develop attacks of *cataplexy*, either at the time of onset of the attacks of narcolepsy or months or years later. These consist of sudden loss of muscle tone, the patient falling to the ground, unable to speak but fully awake. Cataplectic attacks are almost always precipitated by sudden emotional stimuli, usually laughter, but anger or being taken by surprise may have the same effect. They usually only last a minute or less.

Hypnagogic hallucinations when falling asleep at night or during the day are also common in association with narcolepsy. Rarely the patient also experiences brief moments of paralysis, so-called *sleep paralysis*, just before going to sleep or on waking.

Aetiology

A family history of narcolepsy has been found in several studies and has suggested a *genetic basis* for the disorder. This has found support in the recent discovery of an abnormal gene on the short arm of chromosome 6 (Langdon *et al*. 1984). There is no evidence of a structural abnormality in the brain, but the genetic abnormality may be responsible for biochemical changes leading to the disturbed sleep pattern.

While in normal individuals the first episode of REM sleep usually follows a period of 1-1½ hours of non-REM slow-wave sleep, patients with narcolepsy enter REM sleep almost immediately on going to sleep at night. This usually also applies during the narcoleptic episodes during the day. During the cataplectic attacks the EEG also has the characteristics of the REM phase but the patient remains awake. Abnormalities of regulation of the alternating non-REM and REM phases seem to be responsible for narcolepsy, and may be the result of the genetic abnormality.

Differential diagnosis

Once cataplexy, hypnagogic hallucinations or sleep paralysis have developed in addition to narcoleptic attacks the diagnosis is usually easy to make. If narcolepsy is the only symptom the attacks of drowsiness or sleep during the day may be mistaken for a functional disorder, e.g.

neurasthenia, neurotic depression or hysterical symptoms. Careful history taking and the absence of precipitating emotional factors should lead to the correct diagnosis.

Treatment

The narcoleptic episodes can often be controlled by maintenance treatment with amphetamines, e.g. dextro-amphetamine or amphetamine sulphate. However, the large doses that may be needed can cause insomnia at night, restlessness during the day, or even a paranoid psychosis. Clomipramine (50-100 mg daily) may control the attacks of cataplexy, if present. In milder cases drugs may not be needed. Taking brief naps regularly at planned times during the day may prevent the attacks of narcolepsy; avoiding occupations in which falling asleep could be dangerous, e.g. driving a car or operating machines, may be necessary.

Other causes of hypersomnia

Apart from the characteristic episodic attacks of narcolepsy, hypersomnia can result from other disorders.

The tendency to sleep longer in patients who have put on weight and are obese has already been mentioned. Patients with neurotic depression often tend to sleep well into the morning and have difficulty in waking (see p. 172). In others the tendency to sleep for many hours during the day can be due to psychological stress, sometimes in association with hysterical symptoms. Hypersomnia has been described in schizophrenia, but catatonic stupor may be mistaken for somnolence or sleep.

Prolonged sleep or drowsiness can also result from organic cerebral lesions, usually in the hypothalamus or midbrain. They may be due to tumour or vascular or degenerative lesions in the midbrain. Head injuries or encephalitis may also result in prolonged sleep sometimes lasting days or weeks. If the hypersomnia is associated with excessive hunger and weight gain the possibility of a hypothalamic lesion should be considered. Occasionally hypersomnia may be due to myxoedema.

A very rare condition, the *Kleine-Levin syndrome*, consists of recurrent periods of severe somnolence and deep sleep over a period of days or weeks at a time, associated with gross overeating when awake. When the patient wakes up he may greedily consume any food in sight, but he does not usually complain of feeling hungry if food is not available. If forcibly woken he may be irritable, aggressive and confused, with vivid fantasies, and he may have auditory or visual hallucinations.

The condition usually occurs in men, in adolescence or early adult life. Each episode lasts days or weeks, with normal periods of months or years in between. The mental state usually returns to normal in between the periods of somnolence and overeating. The episodes tend to disappear after several years. Lithium has helped to prevent the recurrent attacks in some cases.

In spite of the association of hypersomnia and voracious eating, suggesting an abnormality of diencephalic function, no local cerebral lesion has been found, nor is there any clear evidence of precipitating events or psychological abnormalities. Critchley (1962) has described several cases in detail and has suggested the term *megaphagia* for the abnormal eating behaviour.

FURTHER READING

General

Lishman, W.A. (1987). *Organic Psychiatry: the psychological consequences of cerebral disorder*, 2nd ed. Blackwell Scientific Publications, Oxford.

On AIDS

Fenton, T.W. (1987). 'AIDS-related psychiatric disorder: review article'. *Brit. J. Psychiat*. 151, 579-588.
Miller, D. (1987). *Living with AIDS and HIV*. Macmillan, London.
Miller, D., Weber, J. and Green, J. (1986). *The Management of AIDS Patients*. Macmillan, London.
Price, R.W. *et al*. (1988). 'The brain in AIDS: central nervous system HIV-1 infection and AIDS dementia complex', *Science* 239, 586-592.

On Parkinsonism

Sacks, O. (1982). *Awakenings*, revised ed. Picador, Pan Books, London.

On sleep disorders

Hartman, E. (ed.) (1970). *Sleep and Dreaming*. Churchill, London.
Parkes, J.D. (1985). *Sleep and its Disorders*. Saunders, London.

24

Psychiatric Aspects of Epilepsy

Between 2 and 6 per cent of the population will have non-febrile epileptic seizures at some point in their lives. In the majority, the epilepsy remits after a limited period of time. 'Active' epilepsy, defined as the occurrence of at least one recurrent non-febrile seizure in the last two years, has a prevalence of about 1 in 200, or 0.5 per cent of the population. In a general practitioner's average list of 2,100 patients, there will be 1-2 new cases of epilepsy each year, 1-2 patients with severe intractable epilepsy and 12-15 taking anti-epileptic drugs.

These figures, quoted from Oxley *et al.* (1987), emphasise that epilepsy is a common medical problem. An association between mental disorder and epilepsy has been recognised since antiquity but ideas about the nature of the disorder have changed over time. Old notions that personality deterioration and dementia are common or even inevitable outcomes for the epileptic are now known to be mistaken. Early studies of patients in mental institutions fostered such views, but more recent studies of patients attending neurology clinics or identified by general practitioners have shown that the majority of people with epilepsy do not suffer from conspicuous psychiatric disorder; among those that do neurotic disorders of depression and anxiety are the most common. An important study by Pond and Bidwell (1959) in fourteen general practices showed an increased prevalence of psychiatric disorder among epileptics; 29 per cent had sought or received psychiatric treatment. In a more recent survey, also of fourteen general practices but limited to South London, Edeh and Toone (1987) identified 48 per cent of a sample of adult epileptic patients as psychiatric 'cases' by means of research techniques more rigorous than those available to Pond and Bidwell; 31 per cent of epileptic patients had had a psychiatric referral.

PSYCHIATRIC DISORDERS AND EPILEPSY

In some patients both epilepsy and psychiatric disorder can be seen as the product of an underlying common cause, such as brain diseases including those causing severe mental handicap, dementia, tumours, and damage from alcoholism, trauma and other factors.

Sometimes the symptoms and behavioural changes induced by the epileptic discharge itself may present as a psychiatric disorder, usually with characteristic features of confusion, which differentiate these 'peri-ictal' disorders from the psychiatric disorders observed between fits, which occur with clear consciousness.

More problematical are questions about the extent to which, and in what way, epilepsy (or associated factors such as social disadvantage and drug therapy) predispose towards other disorders including neurosis, psychosis, personality deviation and antisocial behaviour. Of particular interest has been the observation that schizophrenic symptoms occur more often than by chance in people with temporal lobe and other types of epilepsy with a focal origin.

The interplay and overlap between the two types of diagnosis, epilepsy and psychiatric disorder, may present a challenging clinical problem in the individual case, requiring the skills and techniques of both neurology and psychiatry. The relationship between the two is also of great theoretical interest since it may yield important clues about how a physically demonstrable disturbance of brain physiology can be causally related to 'functional' disorder of the mind.

Study of the two kinds of disorder drew apart during the nineteenth century with the increasing differentiation of neurology and psychiatry. The congregation of patients with epileptic disorders in the old mental hospital is no longer seen in the psychiatric units of today. Hunter and Macalpine (1974) record, for instance, that in 1855 about 1 in 4 of the male patients in Friern Hospital had between one and two fits daily, and 1 in 5 of the women had an average of two fits a day. In a more recent survey of the hospital in 1983, epilepsy was reported in only 4.5 per cent of the 839 inpatients and was considered the primary diagnosis in only five patients.

Today there are improved methods of examining the electrical activity of the brain (such as prolonged EEG recordings using conventional leads, telemetry or ambulatory monitoring with a portable recorder) and imaging techniques to study the brain's structure and chemical activity: CT scanning, NMR (nuclear magnetic resonance) and PET (positron emission tomography). There is also much greater refinement in delineating psychiatric symptoms, e.g. by the Present State Examination (Wing *et al.* 1974). These developments give new vigour to the specialty of neuropsychiatry, and promise further clarification of the relationship between psychiatric illness and epilepsy.

CLASSIFICATION

Mental disturbances in patients with epilepsy are commonly classified according to their timing in relation to the *ictus* or fit, as *pre-ictal, ictal and post-ictal*, together comprising *peri-ictal* disturbances closely associated in time with a fit or fits, and *interictal*, occurring in the intervals between fits.

The classification of epilepsy itself can be confusing, with several different methods of categorisation, e.g. the clinical manifestations of the fit, the focus of origin, or the underlying cause, being used at the same time. A classification of epileptic seizures which combines clinical and EEG consideration has been proposed by the International League Against Epilepsy (Gastaut 1969). This makes a major distinction between *partial* seizures, in which a focal origin in the brain is indicated by clinical and EEG evidence, and *generalised* seizures, which are bilaterally synchronous without a focal origin. The latter group includes those forms of epilepsy manifest solely as *grand mal* tonic-clonic convulsions, together with some other non-convulsive forms without localising features. The partial group, in which a focal discharge may or may not spread to become generalised, is further subdivided according to the variety of symptoms into *elementary* and *complex*. The partial group with complex seizures includes those forms previously called 'temporal lobe' or 'psychomotor' epilepsy, and it is in these forms of *focal* epilepsy that peri-ictal and inter-ictal mental disturbances are most striking and common. Temporal lobe-type manifestations have been estimated to occur in between 30 and 80 per cent of epileptic patients.

Pre-ictal phenomena

Changes in mood and behaviour, such as increasing tension or irritability, sometimes precede the occurrence of fits by hours or even days, and are recognised by the patient or his relatives as the prelude to an attack. These are called *prodromata*, which must be distinguished from the much briefer aura described below. In some patients it appears that fatigue and emotion can precipitate attacks. Rare types of epilepsy are precipitated by specific stimuli, e.g. musicogenic epilepsy.

Peri-ictal phenomena of complex partial seizures

In this type of seizure pattern, foci are most common in the temporal lobe but may be localised elsewhere, usually in other parts of the limbic system, which has a central role in the neural basis of emotion. A variety of lesions in the temporal lobe have been identified in temporal lobes ablated by surgical operation. The most common lesion is *mesial temporal sclerosis*, attributed possibly to the occurrence of febrile convulsions in early childhood (Falconer and Taylor 1970). Attacks commonly start in childhood or early adolescence and may take a variety of forms, which include the following elements, alone or in combination: *auras, absences, psychomotor attacks, falling attacks* and *grand mal convulsions*. The pattern may vary in the same patient but is often fairly constant.

Auras are premonitory symptoms of focal origin lasting a few seconds, and derived directly from the abnormal electrical discharge. The most common are visceral sensations, such as a characteristic unpleasant and variously described sensation arising in the epigastrium and moving upwards into the throat. There may be odd feelings in the head, or in the genitals or rectum. Other symptoms include tinnitus and vertigo, alterations in taste, smell and hearing, emotional changes of intense anxiety or pleasure, an altered sense of perception (including a sense of strangeness or familiarity, micropsia and macropsia, déja vu or depersonalisation), and a variety of complex hallucinatory experiences which may range in emotional tone from the ecstatic to the terrifying and may be beyond words to describe. If the attack progresses, the patient may appear only briefly dazed, or there may be a fall, or a grand mal convulsion. Motor activity may take the form of *automatisms*, snatches of apparently purposeful behaviour such as drinking, searching or undressing, followed by a period of confusion or amnesia for the attack. Sometimes there may be a period of dysphasia.

Post-ictal phenomena and status epilepticus

The actual duration of epileptic attacks is very brief and does not extend beyond a minute or two. Attacks of both focal and generalised origin may, however, be followed by a more enduring period of confusion (sometimes manifest as a fugue or 'twilight state') or odd behaviour, particularly if repeated fits occur one after the other. Aggression may occur, especially if attempts are made to interfere with the patient before full recovery from the attack. Rarely *status epilepticus* from repetitive complex partial seizures or petit mal and other types of non-convulsive seizures may present as *confusional disorders* which may be prolonged for days or more; an EEG will reveal the diagnosis. Of particular medico-legal significance is the question of whether criminal acts may occur as *epileptic automatisms*: they can, but extremely rarely. The diagnosis requires particularly careful and expert assessment.

Interictal psychiatric disorders

Several interacting factors are likely to be involved in causing the association of psychiatric disorder with epilepsy, including the following:

(1) *The psychosocial consequences of having epilepsy.* The effect on a person of being 'epileptic' will depend on many variables in the social environment and in the genetic constitution and personal development of the individual. Public attitudes may still be ignorant and stigmatising, and there may be very real limitations on what the sufferer can do or on what is permitted by those around him. As with other kinds of disability, the sufferer may triumph over adversity, as shown by the careers of many famous epileptics in history, such as Julius Caesar.

(2) *The age of development.* Children with epilepsy appear to have a statistically increased risk of intellectual retardation, conduct disorders and psychosis. In the studies of children aged between five and fourteen in the Isle of Wright by Rutter *et al.* (1970), children with uncomplicated epilepsy had four times the frequency of psychiatric disorder found in

children without epilepsy, and the rate was doubled again when there was evidence of brain damage as well. Studies by Ounsted and colleagues in Oxford on an unselected population of children with temporal lobe epilepsy showed psychiatric difficulty of some form in 85 per cent at the original assessment in 1964. The follow-up report in 1977 indicated that the presence of disordered homes bore no relationship to the development of adult disorder, but failure of remission of fits, frequent seizures, male sex and left-sided lesions did (Ounsted and Lindsay 1981).

(3) *The focus of origin of the fits, type and frequency of seizure, and presence of identifiable brain lesion.* There is a general impression that people with temporal lobe and other forms of focal epilepsy have an increased risk of developing psychiatric disorder, particularly if there is an identifiable brain lesion. Poor seizure control and multiple drug treatment tend also to be commoner in this group than in patients with primary generalised epilepsy. In a series of 100 patients coming to temporal lobectomy for intractable epilepsy, only 13 per cent were considered psychiatrically normal before operation; psychopathic and neurotic disorders were most common (Falconer and Taylor 1970).

(4) *Genetic factors and inherited and acquired brain diseases.* Genetic factors can predispose to psychiatric disorder or epilepsy or to both together, as is found in inherited brain diseases such as tuberous sclerosis (see p. 524). Acquired brain disease, e.g. head injury (see p. 274), may cause both disorders. The incidence of epilepsy increases with severity of mental handicap.

(5) *Anticonvulsant and other drugs, including alcohol.* Adverse effects of drug therapy have received greater emphasis in recent debate on the psychiatric complications of epilepsy (Brown *et al.* 1986).

Types of psychiatric disorders

It does not seem possible to link the occurrence of epilepsy with a distinctive form of psychiatric disorder, other than schizophrenia (see below) and possibly characteristic personality features in some patients with temporal lobe epilepsy. Depression, anxiety and stress reactions have been most commonly identified in recent surveys. The 'epileptic personality', described in such terms as 'sticky' or 'viscous' and slow, hyperreligious, suspicious, irritable, pedantic and circumstantial, has been said in recent years to be a phenomenon of the old mental institution rather than characteristic of epilepsy in the general population, but there is some evidence for a statistical association of such features with temporal lobe epilepsy. Hypergraphia, a tendency to indulge in excessive writing, has been included in the features associated with a specific interictal syndrome of temporal lobe epilepsy by Geschwind (1979), together with hyposexuality and religiosity. Aggressiveness, crime and sexual disorder have been considered common in epileptics, but the association does not appear strong. Epilepsy was found to be significantly commoner among male prisoners than in the general population by Gunn

(1969), often associated with psychiatric problems, but there was no special association with violent crime. Hyposexuality seems more prevalent than rare cases of hypersexuality and fetishism, and may in part be due to drugs. Progressive cognitive decline due to a variety of causal factors is seen rarely. Suicide rates appear to be increased in epileptics.

Epilepsy and schizophrenia

An association between epilepsy and the occurrence of schizophrenia and other paranoid psychoses has long been recognised. It was also held by some authors, quoting the introduction by Meduna (1937) of convulsive therapy as a treatment of psychosis, that there were arguments in favour of an antagonism rather than an affinity between the two types of disorder, i.e. that the presence of one disorder decreased the likelihood of the other. Landolt (1958) named states in which the appearance of psychiatric disorder coincided with temporary remission of epilepsy and of EEG abnormalities as examples of 'forced normalisation'. The topic has been clarified by Wolf and Trimble (1985) who showed that the 'antagonism' hypothesis is likely to be a misunderstanding of Meduna's recognition that in some patients the occurrence of seizures was associated with a brief alleviation of psychotic symptoms; this observation does not contradict Meduna's familiarity with the association between epilepsy and psychosis.

In 1963 Slater and Beard reported on 69 patients with predominantly *temporal lobe epilepsy* who after many years developed a schizophrenic illness; they observed that the association was commoner than could be expected by chance and argued for characteristic features such as the absence of a family history of schizophrenia, good pre-morbid personality and a preservation of affect. Other studies, with some exceptions, have tended to support the general association with schizophrenia but have not always supported the more specific features. In some patients schizophrenia may develop earlier, perhaps preceding the epilepsy. There also appears to be an association between temporal lobe epilepsy and affective psychosis. Flor-Henry (1969) proposed that foci in the dominant temporal lobe might be particularly associated with schizophrenia, and in the non-dominant lobe with affective psychosis. Further evidence has been found in support of the association between schizophrenic symptoms and left-sided foci (Perez *et al.* 1985), but the suggested association between affective psychosis and non-dominant foci has not been confirmed.

Effects of anticonvulsant medication

In the assessment of psychiatric disorder in patients with epilepsy it is important to consider the possible adverse effects of anticonvulsant drugs. Modern practice favours optimal usage of one drug, but polypharmacy is common, and surveys have shown that drug treatment for epilepsy is often poorly managed. In children phenobarbitone may have adverse effects on mood, behaviour and learning. In adults, too, drugs like phenytoin may contribute to such sensations as fatigue, irritability, slowing-up and impairment of concentration. More severe idiosyncratic mental reactions to anticonvulsants have been described. Conversely, the anticonvulsant drug carbamazepine, initially introduced as a treatment for trigeminal neuralgia, was found to have beneficial effects on behaviour and mental state in some patients with epilepsy.

Psychotropic drugs and epilepsy

In general the physical treatment of psychiatric disorders in patients with epilepsy follows standard lines, including, if necessary, the use of ECT and antipsychotic drugs. In the latter group phenothiazines, particularly those with an aliphatic side-chain, lower the seizure threshold and may induce fits. Some antidepressant drugs, including imipramine, amitriptyline and mianserin, may also precipitate fits. It may be wise to choose a drug with relatively less risk, particularly if higher doses are required.

DIFFERENTIAL DIAGNOSIS OF 'ATTACKS'

The differential diagnosis of brief episodic disturbances of behaviour or consciousness involves four main groups of causes: epileptic, vascular (such as syncopal attacks and transient ischaemic episodes), biochemical (such as hyperventilation, hypoglycaemia, and the toxic effects of alcohol and drugs) and psychogenic. Anxiety attacks or panic disorder may not be recognised as such by the patient, but the symptoms and time-scale are usually characteristic.

In all types of epilepsy, diagnosis depends primarily on very detailed clinical observation, which will include not only the patient's account but the reports of witnesses to an attack of the patient's behaviour before, during and after the seizure. EEGs can support a diagnosis of epilepsy but cannot exclude it. The characteristic features of epileptic phenomena, compared to other disturbances of behaviour, mood or consciousness, are that they are usually very brief, sudden, out of character and irregularly recurrent.

Particular features to be recorded by the observer in the assessment of any 'attack' include:

(1) The circumstances of the attack; its timing, the emotional and interpersonal setting and what the patient was doing immediately beforehand.

(2) The initial changes and the chronological development of the attack, including evidence of premonitory symptoms or aura, lateralising movements in the face or one arm or leg, and the exact nature and

duration of subsequent movements.

(3) Evidence of automatic changes, such as flushing, pallor, sweating, pupil size, and of tongue-biting or incontinence.

(4) Evidence of change in consciousness and ability to speak, respond to painful stimuli, questions or commands or to describe the sensations experienced.

(5) The occurrence of any after-effects, such as confusion, dysphasia, sleepiness, automatisms, and the patient's subsequent behaviour.

Special difficulties may arise in the assessment of attacks which seem to be psychologically determined, perhaps as a response to emotional upheaval or frustration (Fenton 1986). 'Pseudoepileptic' attacks of this kind are often atypical in form, with a dramatic fall or collapse and perhaps grossly abnormal movements in the presence or hearing of other people, sometimes visibly increasing in severity when observers intervene. There are a number of pitfalls in diagnosis, and great care may be needed to avoid oversimple adherence to rules, such as that patients without true epilepsy do not injure themselves. Sometimes they do. There are also accounts of patients without epilepsy apparently feigning all the features of a true epileptic attack, including clonic convulsions, incontinence and even a Babinski plantar response, and perhaps functioning in society for many years as 'epileptics'. Patients with true epilepsy may in addition be subject to emotionally precipitated fits or 'pseudoepileptic' attacks (Fenton 1986) and may sometimes know how to induce a true convulsion. Trimble's (1978) observation that prolactin secretion is often elevated after a true convulsion has been used as a diagnostic test, but is not reliable. Videotaped records of attacks may help in the diagnosis, assisting the clinical and EEG assessments which are described in detail by Fenton (1986).

FURTHER READING

Fenton, G.W. (1986). 'Epilepsy and hysteria'. *Brit. J. Psychiat.*, 149, 28-37.

Laidlaw, J. and Richens, A. (eds) (1982). *A Textbook of Epilepsy.* Churchill Livingstone, Edinburgh.

Lishman, W.A. (1987). *Organic Psychiatry*, 2nd ed., ch. 7. Blackwell Scientific Publications, Oxford.

Riley, T.L. and Roy, A. (eds) (1982). *Pseudoseizures.* Williams & Wilkins, Baltimore/London.

Trimble, M.R. (ed.) (1985). *The Psychopharmacology of Epilepsy.* John Wiley & Sons, Chichester.

25

Psychiatric Illness in Old Age

People technically become 'elderly' at the age of sixty-five, but people of that age and over are not a separate race, and many of their psychiatric symptoms and their treatment are much the same as in younger people. Further, it is unusual for someone's basic personality and behaviour to alter greatly in old age. For example, a tendency to anxiety or depression, or to be suspicious or quarrelsome, is likely to be a continuation or worsening of patterns that were evident many years earlier. But certain categories of illness do have particular importance where the elderly are concerned, both because they are more common and because their consequences are likely to be more severe.

DEPRESSION

Depressive illness in the elderly does not differ greatly from depressive illness in other age-groups, but it should be remembered that the most common cause of depression in old people is physical illness, though loneliness and bereavement also play an important part. In the elderly it is not usually helpful to try to distinguish between reactive and endogenous depression.

Following careful history-taking and physical examination, it is next essential to assess the depressed patient in two broad areas. First, the mood alteration. This may range from mild pessimism to severe depression with suicidal ruminations. Depressive delusions are common and are likely either to be somatic in nature, such as a conviction that the patient has cancer, or to involve guilt and self-blame relating to past events, real or imagined, such as sexual or financial misdemeanours.

Secondly, there are likely to be biological changes, such as psychomotor retardation, constipation, disruption of sleep and loss of appetite. As a result an elderly person can slide rapidly into a dangerous state of self-neglect; the depressed elderly are a prey to starvation, dehydration, hypothermia and all the consequences of immobility, such as pressure sores, contractures and venous stasis. All the conditions in this sorry catalogue are common, so that in management the ever-present risk of physical deterioration has to be considered. The incidence of suicide also rises steeply in the elderly.

The first step in *management* is to protect the patient from the consequences of his illness. These include the risk of suicide and the physical effects specified above. Severe depression will therefore generally require that the patient be treated in hospital where both medical and psychiatric care can be provided. Otherwise, management does not differ in its essentials from that of depression in younger patients. Most antidepressants are effective, though the tricyclics are best avoided in favour of the tetracyclics, e.g. mianserin, since drugs in the latter group are less liable to cause postural hypotension, with the risk of ataxia and falls.

ECT (see p. 617) can be highly effective in the treatment of the depressed elderly, provided the patient is fit for an anaesthetic. There tends to be a remarkably low incidence of side-effects, even in the elderly.

PARANOID ILLNESS

It is very common for pathological suspiciousness or delusions of persecution to emerge strongly in old age. Common precipitating factors are loneliness, deafness, and visual impairment, especially due to cataract. The memory loss of early dementia often first declares itself in the form of paranoid delusions; an old person whose memory is failing tends to lose or misplace objects and then angrily accuses others of having moved or stolen them. In many instances there are auditory or even visual hallucinations.

At times the patient experiences and causes great distress; at other times the delusions of an elderly person are fairly innocuous rather than persecutory. For example, it is touchingly common for elderly ladies living alone to believe that they hear or see children.

In making an assessment, it should first be borne in mind that some organic disorders such as alcohol abuse or hypothyroidism may present with paranoid symptoms. A physical examination is always required, including assessment of vision and hearing. A full social assessment is equally important; isolation or loneliness may emerge as the main causative factors.

In *management* it is essential to try to do something about such isolation. Some form of day care or residential care may be indicated; alternatively the patient can be visited and supported at home, sometimes by members of voluntary bodies, but more often by Social Services or community nurses. Sometimes a sympathetic home help protects the elderly against isolation more effectively than staff in any other category. The doctor is usually accepted as a confidant even by a paranoid patient, provided he can adopt a neutral though concerned attitude towards the patient's beliefs, and the patient may benefit greatly from the sense of alliance that develops.

Clearly any underlying physical cause needs treatment in its own right. Where psychotropic medication is necessary, chlorpromazine tends to be the most effective drug, commencing usually at a dosage of 25 mg three times daily. Chlorpromazine may cause extrapyramidal side-effects (see p. 245) or, much less common, obstructive jaundice; thioridazine 25 mg three times a day is an alternative. It has a lower incidence of unwanted side-effects, but is marginally less effective in the treatment of paranoid symptoms. Whatever drug is used, it must be remembered that the elderly are particularly sensitive to medication; e.g. a relatively low dose of phenothiazines may produce confusion and drowsiness.

ACUTE CONFUSIONAL STATES

Acute confusional states are common in the elderly. They have been described on pp. 30 and 262. They usually present with clouding of consciousness and confusion of relatively recent onset. Table 25.1 gives a list of likely causes in the elderly, more or less in order of frequency. The conditions listed in the table can only be diagnosed by means of careful physical examination and investigations. Appropriate treatment of the cause may bring about dramatic improvement in the mental state, sometimes in a patient who has been thought to be suffering from dementia. It must also be remembered that even in a patient who has been suffering from dementia for some time a sudden worsening in his mental condition may represent an acute-on-chronic confusion resulting from a superimposed physical illness.

Table 25.1. Causes of acute organic confusional states in the elderly

Chest infection.
Cardiovascular disease, e.g. coronary thrombosis, heart failure.
Cerebrovascular accident, e.g. cerebral thrombosis.
Urinary tract infection, often presenting as incontinence.
Carcinoma, especially of the bronchus.
Clinically prescribed drugs, e.g. tranquillisers or hypnotics, diuretics.
Alcohol abuse.
Vitamin deficiencies and anaemia, e.g. due to self-neglect.
Dehydration.
Faecal impaction.
Hypokalaemia, e.g. dietary or the result of vomiting, diarrhoea, or the use of
    diuretics.
Hypothermia, e.g. due to lack of heating, infection, or cardiac failure.

DEMENTIA

Dementia may be broadly defined as acquired brain disease which is both diffuse and chronic, giving rise to widespread impairment of higher intellectual functions, especially memory, language and personality (see also p. 268). It is usual to refer to 'the dementias', since there are a number of sub-types, but the great majority of the dementing illnesses in patients over sixty-five fall into one of only two categories: *Alzheimer-type dementia*, also called Alzheimer's disease or senile dementia of the Alzheimer type, and *multi-infarct dementia*. These two conditions account for about 90 per cent of all dementias in the elderly, either separately or in combination.

The prevalence of these two forms of dementia is usually quoted as 12-15 per cent in those over sixty-five, and 20 per cent in those aged eighty and over. The true figures may be somewhat lower than this, since the major studies have been carried out in urban areas; there is now evidence that in such areas there is a somewhat higher than average prevalence of dementia.

Alzheimer-type dementia

Alzheimer's disease was first described in 1907. For many years it was believed to be a relatively uncommon form of presenile dementia, with onset before the age of sixty-five (see p. 278). It is now known that the morphological changes in the brain described by Alzheimer in presenile dementia are identical to those found in senile dementia. Therefore the term Alzheimer's disease is now widely used to describe the most common form of dementia, regardless of age of onset. It accounts for about 55 per cent of all presenile and senile dementias, and a further 20 per cent of dementias have an Alzheimer component.

Pathology

The cerebral changes in Alzheimer's disease are extensive atrophy of the brain with loss of cells from the cerebral cortex, amyloid or senile plaques, and deposits of fibrils in the neuronal bodies. The latter are the most characteristic features of Alzheimer's disease and mark an Alzheimer disease brain out most sharply from that of a normal elderly person; they are called *neurofibrillary tangles*; on electron microscopy they appear as paired helical filaments made up of two kinds of protein. They are particularly common in the cerebral cortex and hippocampal region.

Aetiology

The cause of Alzheimer's disease is unknown. There is, however, evidence for a *genetic component*; transmission may be by means of a single autosomal dominant gene with high penetrance by the age of ninety. There are no known factors which influence gene expression other than advancing age. Other theories of causation, e.g. that a transmissible agent may be responsible, have been put forward, but there is no evidence that this applies to Alzheimer's disease. It does, however, appear that, regardless of the primary cause, neurotransmitter abnormalities are responsible for at least some of the symptoms of Alzheimer's disease, the most widely recognised being a selective *failure of cholinergic transmission*. There is evidence that levels of choline acetyltransferase, responsible for the synthesis of acetylcholine, are reduced in the frontal cortex and hippocampal regions. There is no evidence so far that attempts to correct these abnormalities are of clinical value.

Clinical features

The clinical features of Alzheimer's disease or senile dementia (Alzheimer type) are described in detail on p. 268. In essence Alzheimer's disease is of insidious onset. It usually starts with memory loss and personality change, followed by progressive intellectual deterioration, ultimately leading to severe global dementia, accompanied by neurological deficits, general physical decline and death within a few years.

It must be diagnosed on the basis of positive signs of memory and intellectual impairment and personality change, usually associated with evidence of regional affiliations, as described in Chapter 3. In particular, evidence of disordered language function or of dyspraxia in an elderly patient will help to distinguish dementia from an affective disorder. If Alzheimer's disease is diagnosed too readily other often treatable psychiatric disorders, such as depression, acute confusional states, or paranoid states, may be overlooked. It is equally important not to miss such rare but occasionally treatable causes of dementia as cerebral tumour (p. 277), normal pressure hydrocephalus (p. 282), neurosyphilis (p. 284) or vitamin B12 deficiency (p. 302).

Multi-infarct dementia

This is the vascular type of dementia and accounts for 15-20 per cent of dementias in the elderly. It used to be referred to as 'arteriosclerotic dementia', but it is now generally recognised that emboli from the heart and great vessels are responsible for most of the damage. The morphological changes in the brain are characteristic in that damage is patchy, with areas of cell loss and gliosis clustered around damaged blood vessels. The clinical changes, as one might expect, mirror this pattern; the disease progresses in a stepwise fashion. An abrupt deterioration tends to be followed by a clinical plateau, or by partial recovery. Cognitive loss is also inconsistent; there may be severe dysphasia or severe memory loss, with relative preservation of other functions. There is likely to be other evidence of vascular disease both in the central nervous system and elsewhere – most commonly transient ischaemic attacks, stroke, hypertension, cardiac, renal or peripheral vascular disease. Course and survival are much less predictable than in Alzheimer's disease, since they tend to be determined largely by such conditions as coronary artery disease, renal involvement or cerebrovascular accidents.

Treatment of dementia

Dementia, especially Alzheimer's disease, is often said to be 'untreatable', and it is true that so far there is no medication that will arrest or reverse the process of brain cell degeneration. Yet there are many ways in which the condition of demented people can be greatly improved. These fall into four broad categories: the management of 'excess disability'; drug treatments; symptomatic treatment; and supportive therapy.

Management of 'excess disability'

Demented people are usually brought to the attention of a doctor because of some crisis or difficulty that has become superimposed on the dementia, rather than because of the cognitive impairment itself. Such crises tend to be either the result of a superimposed medical condition, or due to social problems, or both.

The common medical conditions have been listed in Table 25.1. Infections are particularly common, as are conditions like anaemia or dehydration due to self-neglect. Identification of the superimposed illness and its treatment can make for a considerable enhancement of the patient's overall functioning and he may well be able to go on living at home, usually with some community services and supervision, even though his underlying cognitive state is not greatly different.

On the other hand, the excess disability can result from social problems. These may be due to increasing isolation or difficulties on the part of those who look after the patient. Here a precise assessment of the patient's practical needs and the home conditions has to be made. Fortunately there is now a rapidly expanding range of locally based services that can enable demented people to live at home for as long as possible. There are too many to be listed, but major assistance comes from day centres, social workers, home helps, meals-on-wheels, district nurses, geriatric health visitors and community psychiatric nurses, many of whom now specialise in the elderly. Most Health Districts have consultants with special responsibility for the elderly mentally ill. Part of the task of such a consultant is to be familiar with local support services and to be able to advise on what would help a particular patient. In general, it is helpful whenever possible for him to assess the patient at his home as this provides the necessary information on his home conditions, and presence or absence of support from friends or relatives.

Drugs

There is very little that can be achieved by way of treating the cognitive impairment of dementia. Vasodilators are not helpful, and drugs that might correct neurotransmitter defects, e.g. by means of precursor loading, are still being evaluated. Hydergine, an ergot derivative, sometimes brings about slight improvement in alertness and overall functioning, and may be worth a trial in early cases of Alzheimer's disease. Multi-infarct dementia is managed by treating the underlying vascular disease, especially by control of hypertension.

Symptomatic treatment

Some of the more troublesome symptoms of dementia can be brought under control or ameliorated.

Especially in its early stages, dementia is often accompanied by sadness and apathy or anxiety and apprehension. Appropriate medication, especially for depression, can bring about a substantial overall improvement, but it is best to start with a low dose in view of the increased sensitivity of elderly patients to antidepressants and tranquillisers.

Old people often suffer from insomnia. They may be restless at night because they are inactive and lack stimulation during the day. Reorganising the daily programme, e.g. by arranging day centre attendance, often helps. Otherwise chlormethiazole or a short-acting benzodiazepine such as temazepam may be effective.

Incontinence is a common symptom in dementia, but it should not be dismissed as an inevitable feature; there is usually a separate cause for it. The patient should be screened for urinary tract infection, diabetes, prostatism, faecal impaction or some other bowel condition. Depression may cause incontinence, or it may be the result of immobility, when the problem can often be resolved by means of regular toileting. Unstable sphincter function often contributes to urinary incontinence in the elderly, and it is sometimes successfully treated with a small dose of imipramine.

Behaviour disorders are common. Wandering is best dealt with not by means of drugs or restraint, but by creating an environment in which the elderly person can walk about without risk to himself, e.g. in a home, sheltered accommodation, or a ward with an enclosed open space. Where this is impractical or if the patient is aggressive, thioridazine 10-25 mg three times daily is usually the drug of first choice. Sometimes an anticonvulsant, e.g. carbamazepine, may stabilise behaviour in restless or aggressive demented patients.

Supportive therapy

Supportive therapy, including personal interest in the individual patient's needs, is essential. Equally important is the need to support the patient's family, who may find it a great strain to look after a close relative whose behaviour is disturbed by his mental and physical disability.

Finally, although there are many forms of local residential care for demented people who can no longer live alone, a few patients are so severely demented that they will need continuing care in hospital. However, the pattern of care for such patients is changing. The 'dementia ward' in a mental hospital, a long way from the patient's home and family, should soon become a thing of the past. New patterns are beginning to take its place. These include:

(1) Locally based nursing homes, domestic in scale, where it is easy for families and friends to visit.
(2) Specialised old people's homes incorporating nursing, medical, occupational and other forms of care for the demented.
(3) Joint geriatric/psychogeriatric continuing care units in a general hospital for patients suffering from both dementia and chronic physical illness or incapacity.

FURTHER READING

Fraser, M. (1987). *Dementia: its nature and management*. John Wiley, Chichester.

Health Advisory Service (1982). *The Rising Tide: developing services for mental illness in old age*. Health Advisory Service, Sutton, Surrey.

Miller, E. (1977). *Abnormal Ageing*. John Wiley, Chichester.

Murphy, E. (ed.) (1986). *Affective Disorders in the Elderly*. Churchill Livingstone, Edinburgh and London.

Pearce, J.M.S. (1984). *Dementia: a clinical approach*. Blackwell, Oxford.

Pitt, B. (1974). *Psychogeriatrics*. Churchill Livingstone, Edinburgh.

Roberts, P.J. (ed.) (1980). *Biochemistry of Dementia*. John Wiley, Chichester.

Royal College of Physicians (1981). *Organic Mental Impairment in the Elderly*. J. Royal College of Physicians, London, 15, 141-167.

Wheatley, D. (ed.) (1982). *Psychopharmacology of Old Age*. OUP, Oxford.

26

Personality Disorders

Patients with a disorder of personality are commonly seen in medical and psychiatric practice and may be some of the most challenging and difficult patients to treat. Unfortunately the diagnosis is often arrived at by excluding other psychiatric disorders such as neurotic or psychotic illnesses rather than by eliciting positive features of the disorder itself. The term is also used as a pejorative label attached to difficult and uncooperative patients as a means of 'explaining' their behaviour. In this chapter the term personality disorder will be used to describe a group of patients who show persistent disordered behaviour, problems with interpersonal relationships and abnormal psychological development as a result of difficulties during their childhood.

DEFINITION

According to the International Classification of Diseases (ICD-9), personality disorders are defined as follows:

> Deeply ingrained maladaptive patterns of behaviour generally recognisable by the time of adolescence or earlier and continuing throughout most of adult life, although often becoming less obvious in middle or old age. The personality is abnormal either in the balance of its components, their quality and expression or in its total aspect. As a result either the patient or society suffers or both.

This definition concentrates on the behavioural aspects of personality and is thus descriptive in nature. Fundamental to this concept of personality disorder is the duration of the maladaptive behaviour. If the behaviour has been persistent over many years it is said to be due to personality disorder. Conversely, if an individual undergoes a sudden behavioural change it is likely to be part of an illness. This simple differentiation between personality disorder and illness is not as clear-cut as it may seem. For example, some illnesses such as schizophrenia may lead to behavioural changes which develop over a period of years. Furthermore, patients with abnormal personalities are vulnerable to psychiatric illness when under stress and it may be difficult to distinguish which aspects of behaviour are due to the illness and which arise out of the underlying personality disorder.

In the above definition the personality is described as being made up of components which are abnormally balanced or expressed. The term 'personality components' corresponds to the term *personality traits*, which are enduring patterns of perceiving, relating to, and thinking about the environment and oneself. The essence of this definition and the definition supplied by DSM-III in the USA, is that personality disorder exists when certain aspects of the personality predominate in a variety of disparate situations resulting in maladaptive behaviour detrimental to the individual's interpersonal relationships. Other more healthy components of the personality are concealed.

CLASSIFICATION

The approach to the classification of the different personality disorders is similar to that of other psychiatric disorders. Personality disorders may be classified according to descriptive or aetiological criteria. The approach adopted in the International Classification of Diseases is largely based on descriptive psychopathology. It therefore provides little understanding of the causation of personality disorders. The psychodynamic approach, on the other hand, provides a conceptual framework for classification based on psychodynamic principles which offers an understanding of the development of these disorders. This approach is less amenable to scientific evaluation and has thus fallen into disfavour with some psychiatrists, but in terms of understanding and helping patients it is often more useful in clinical practice.

The classification adopted here combines both descriptive and psychodynamic aspects in order to provide a comprehensive account of each personality disorder. The main types of personality disorder will be considered in turn, followed by a general discussion of aetiology and management. Psychopathic personality disorder, sometimes called sociopathic or antisocial personality disorder, will be considered separately (see p. 336) as more research into the aetiology of this most severe of personality disorders has been carried out. In addition psychopathic personality disorder differs from the others in that it is society rather than the patient who suffers as a result of the disorder and legal considerations are often involved. Borderline personality disorder is discussed in Chapter 27.

INDIVIDUAL DISORDERS

The following are the four main and most widely recognised types of personality disorder:

paranoid
schizoid
hysterical
obsessional

Paranoid personality

The essential feature of this disorder is a pervasive and unwarranted suspicousness and mistrust of other people (DSM-III). There is a tendency to distort experiences by misconstruing the actions of others as hostile. A combative and tenacious sense of personal rights predominates, resulting in an aggressive and insistent response when the person feels put upon. Excessive jealousy and self-importance are often evident. In severe cases the paranoid patient's behaviour may affect all his relationships, causing suffering both to himself and to those around him. Projection (see p. 56) is the defence mechanism most commonly associated with paranoid personality disorders. Unacceptable emotions such as jealousy and hatred are frequently projected by the paranoid personality, who then perceives the world as hostile and threatening. Men tend to be diagnosed as paranoid personalities more commonly than women. A.J.A. Symons (1934) has described such a personality in *The Quest for Corvo*.

Schizoid personality

This disorder is characterised by a defect in the capacity to form close personal relationships. Schizoid individuals have a wish for close relationships but once they become involved with another person they feel threatened by the other person's closeness and demands; when their own needs are not fulfilled they become angry and frightened of losing control. As a result the relationship breaks up, they withdraw and feel lonely and isolated. They often oscillate between brief close relationships and long periods of withdrawal and loneliness. Rey (1979) has described the behaviour and psychodynamic processes observed in schizoid personalities in a paper on 'the schizoid mode of being'. Ultimately they may retreat from social involvement altogether and become loners, with few, if any, close friends. They pursue solitary interests such as philosophy, mathematics, computer sciences, etc. Some are creative and original and become university dons, the university atmosphere giving them the security they need. They often have a rich fantasy life and day-dreaming is common. This increases their apparent detachment and aloofness. The novel *Steppenwolf* by Hermann Hesse gives a unique account of a schizoid personality.

Hysterical personality

Individuals with this disorder crave appreciation and attention. They are lively and histrionic, prone to exaggeration and seem to be acting out a role rather than revealing their true self. They seek novelty, stimulation and excitement and quickly become bored with normal routines. They are unable to tolerate frustration, and when their demands are not fulfilled they make a scene, develop temper tantrums or make suicidal and other threats. Their interpersonal relationships suffer in that they are often perceived as shallow and lacking genuineness, though superficially charming and appealing. They are often quick to form friendships but just as quickly they may become demanding, egocentric and inconsiderate. Their sexual behaviour is characterised by excessive seductiveness but with an inability to form a lasting sexual relationship. Promiscuity or sexual unresponsiveness may occur. This disorder tends to be diagnosed much more frequently in women than men. This may be due to the fact that some psychiatrists are reluctant to attach the label hysterical personality to men.

Obsessional personality

This is also known as the *anankastic personality*. People with this disorder are characterised by over-conscientiousness, perfectionism and a tendency to be inflexible in their behaviour and rigid in their attitudes. They often find it hard to decide between right and wrong, are troubled by doubts, and have difficulty in making decisions. They may be preoccupied with cleanliness and tidiness, and some of them are mean with their personal possessions and with money. These personality traits may prevent the person from being spontaneous, and they often appear rigid, cold and judgmental. If these traits are not too pronounced the person may be highly efficient at work, e.g. as housewives, secretaries or doctors; and some of them are creative and highly successful, being driven by their need for accuracy and perfectionism. Martin Luther (Erikson 1958) is an example of such a creative person with obsessional characteristics. It is in the obsessional personality in particular that the dividing line between obsessional characteristics in an otherwise normal person and a fully developed personality disorder where the whole personality is affected, is very difficult to define. It is important to note that if one or both parents have strong obsessional traits their children, having been brought up to be excessively well behaved, obedient, and perfectionist, are themselves likely to grow up with an overdeveloped conscience, obsessional characteristics and problems in their development.

In the obsessional personality intellectualisation and rationalisation (see p. 58) are used as defences against unacceptable emotions. The defence of reaction formation (see p. 59) may also be operative; this involves dealing with unacceptable feelings or desires by emphasising the opposite. For example, a woman who has desires to be messy and untidy may keep her home exceptionally clean and neat. In general, many of the obsessional character traits express the person's need to maintain tight control over unacceptable feelings and impulses.

*

Both the International Classification of Diseases (ICD-9) and the Diagnostic and Statistical Manual (DSM-III) list several other categories of personality disorder. Some of these are referred to next.

Affective personality

These individuals are either habitually gloomy and miserable (*depressive personality*) persistently cheerful and optimistic (*hyperthymic personality*) or oscillating between the two (*cyclothymic personality*) so that their lives are characterised by marked mood swings. Tasks taken up with enthusiasm during a period of activity and optimism tend to become a burden during a phase of despondency. It used to be thought that the cyclothymic personality predisposed to manic-depressive psychosis, but the evidence for this is unconvincing.

Narcissistic personality

In Greek myth Narcissus was a beautiful boy who fell in love with his own reflection. In psychiatric practice the term narcissistic personality is used to describe a group of patients whose central problem is a disturbance of self-esteem and self-regard. They are excessively self-centred and grandiose and require praise and appreciation from others. If this is not forthcoming they become dismissive and contemptuous of the very people whose admiration they crave and quickly find others who admire them in the way they need. Inevitably their relationships are short-lived and emotionally shallow; the narcissistic personality craves affection but is unable to give in return. Beneath the charming façade there is an inability to empathise and care for others. The inner world of the narcissist is full of fantasies of power and success, but beneath there are inner fears of emptiness, insecurity and inferiority. The defence mechanisms of denial, splitting and projective identification (see p. 55) keep these painful feelings at bay. Only when these defences fail does the narcissistic personality seek help or, in a final act of despair, attempt to kill himself. This description has many similarities to that of the hysterical personality, but narcissistic personalities are more severely disturbed in that their lack of self-esteem and their difficulty in caring for others are more profound.

Inadequate personality

This term does not appear in the ICD-9 or DSM-III. The corresponding terms in these classifications are *asthenic personality disorder* and *dependent personality disorder* respectively. The term inadequate personality is used here in view of its widespread use in general psychiatric practice. Inadequate personalities cannot lead a satisfactory domestic, social and working life even though they are of normal intelligence. They have an inner sense of helplessness and cannot rely on themselves. As a result they are dependent on others and only find security in supportive relationships, for example a marriage, or a work situation in which they are cared for and have little personal responsibility, e.g. residential employment. If their brittle security is threatened in any way, for example by a minor emotional upset, they fall back on others for support; doctors, social workers, nurses, and clergymen may become involved, often providing long-term support. Encouraging self-reliance is bound to fail.

AETIOLOGY

The determinants of the adult personality are found in early and later childhood influences and experiences (see Chapter 7). As such, the development of personality disorder is also rooted in childhood and is shaped by an interplay of genetic and developmental factors.

Genetic factors

Most genetic research into personality disorder has concentrated on psychopathic personalities and is considered later (see p. 339). There is little reliable evidence that genetic factors are involved in the other personality disorders, though some twin and adoption studies suggest that they may play a part (Shields 1962).

Psychodynamic factors

Chapter 7 described the way in which early and later childhood experiences influence the child's development into an adult and referred to the fact that some adverse experiences can lead to later disturbances of personality function and behaviour. There is no simple or specific developmental factor that can be held responsible for the development of any one of the personality disorders so far described and even less for personality disorders in general. However, some developmental factors appear to play a significant role and will be considered next. All these involve problems in the interaction between the child and its parents, especially the mother, early in development, as well as later influences and experiences in relation to other significant people.

There are four main areas of psychological development which need to be considered: *object relationships, instinctual development, superego formation and defence organisation.* These have been described in Chapters 5, 6 and 7. Pathological development during infancy or childhood in one or more of these areas leads to personality disorder in adult life. Such pathological development can occur at an early or primitive stage of an infant's psychological development, at an intermediate or at a later stage. It is therefore useful to divide personality disorders according to these three stages, as suggested by Kernberg (1970).

Personalities who function at an *early or primitive stage* of development, sometimes called the paranoid-schizoid position (see pp. 49, 70), tend to split people into either good or bad. They are unable to relate to others as whole persons or to experience a mixture of good and bad feelings towards them. Their inner world is characterised by either good or bad images of others, and similarly their view of themselves is determined by contradictory aspects; they see themselves as totally bad and hateful at one moment and as perfect or ideal at the next. This splitting of their inner world into either good or bad and their subsequent distortion of reality, i.e. constantly denigrating or idealising themselves and others, is all-pervasive.

These difficulties in relating to people as whole individuals limit the primitive personality's capacity to tolerate dissatisfaction. Intolerable frustration develops as soon as their needs are not met. They become aggressive and require instant 'solutions' to the pain in a desperate attempt to satisfy their unfulfilled needs. As a result drug addiction, sexual perversion, impulsive self-damaging acts and violent outbursts are common.

This splitting of the self and the world into polar opposites such as good or bad, right or wrong also impairs the primitive personality's capacity to experience guilt or show appropriate concern towards others, and their conscience or superego is poorly developed. After all, there is nothing to feel guilty about if the other person is totally bad and oneself totally good. Thus the primitive personality structure is characterised by the excessive use of the defence mechanisms of splitting, projection and projective identification (see pp. 49, 56).

The personality disorders which are best understood in terms of disturbance at this primitive level of development are the psychopathic, the borderline, the severely narcissistic, the schizoid and the paranoid personalities.

The *intermediate* level of personality disorder shows better integration. Their object relations are more stable and they are able to recognise that they and others have both good and bad aspects. As a result they have a capacity to form lasting and emotionally satisfying relationships with others. However, they develop excessive guilt if they experience aggressive or unacceptable wishes and feelings towards another person, especially a loved one, i.e. their capacity to tolerate ambivalence towards others is limited. For example, following a bereavement or break-up of a relationship they may feel their own destructive impulses and wishes were responsible for the death or separation and they become prone to self-punishment and depression. In other words, they have an excessively punitive conscience or superego. In an attempt to avoid depression and self-punishment these personalities either repress their aggressive and other unacceptable wishes or react against them by being exceptionally solicitous and loving. The defence mechanisms of repression, reaction formation, intellectualisation and rationalisation are therefore common. The more severe hysterical personality disorders, the affective, inadequate and some of the better functioning narcissistic personalities belong to this group.

Individuals with *higher* level personality disorders are relatively well-integrated and have reached a stable self-image. Object relations are fully developed and there is a capacity to experience a wide range of emotions and to tolerate guilt and loss. Social adaptation and the ability to form long-lasting relationships are not seriously impaired, hence these individuals function relatively normally and are able to develop caring sexual relationships. However, there is an excessive need to control themselves and others and an extreme degree of perfectionism leading to high personal expectations. The need to control others may become manifest in these high-level personality disorders only when a partner does not satisfy their needs and expectations. Jealous outbursts may then become common. Obsessional personality disorders and some of the better functioning hysterical personality disorders belong to this group.

This attempt to understand personality disorders in terms of development has several advantages. It is often difficult to fit a particular personality into one or other of the specific types described earlier in this chapter. The developmental approach allows a greater degree of flexibility and therefore complements the descriptive approach. Any individual with a personality disorder may show evidence of disturbed development at each of the three stages of development. For example, an hysterical personality disorder, most of whose disturbance can be understood in terms of high or intermediate levels of functioning, may also show evidence of narcissistic problems arising from a more primitive level of development.

In fact the developmental approach minimises the need to 'categorise' these disorders into specific personality types. What is required is a psychological understanding of how an individual experiences himself and the outside world. This may vary over time and in different circumstances and even from moment to moment. Understanding personality in terms of individual development is also helpful during the treatment of patients in psychotherapy, especially when attempting to understand the complexity and diversity of the individual.

PSYCHIATRIC ILLNESS AND PERSONALITY DISORDER

The relationship between mental illness and personality disorder is twofold. First, individuals with personality disorders are more likely to develop psychiatric illness than individuals with relatively stable personalities. It used to be thought that patients with particular personality disorders were prone to develop specific illnesses. For example, schizoid personalities were considered to be associated with schizophrenia, obsessional personalities with obsessive-compulsive neurosis, and so on. The evidence for this is unconvincing. It is now recognised that if a patient with a particular personality disorder develops a psychiatric disorder its nature is not necessarily or, if at all, only in part determined by his previous personality.

Secondly, the impact of psychiatric illness on the individual can profoundly affect his underlying personality. Thus a patient with a relatively normal personality may develop schizophrenia, which may cause an insidious deterioration in the patient's personality, particularly if the psychosis pursues a chronic course. This may become evident during periods of remission when the patient may be unable to cope with relationships, appear lacking in motivation, and be passively compliant. Other schizophrenic patients may exhibit antisocial behaviour unconnected with their psychotic symptoms.

ASSESSMENT

Patients with personality disorders tend to present for treatment when they are experiencing distress in their lives and relationships. Assessment involves first ascertaining whether the patient has developed neurotic or psychotic symptoms. If these can be excluded then a detailed profile of the patient's personality is required; this should include a full enquiry into his personal development. It also involves assessing his strengths as well as his weaknesses. The aim is to assess the severity of the personality disorder and the likelihood of bringing about any lasting change in the patient's intrapsychic structure and interpersonal relationships by psychotherapeutic means.

TREATMENT

The following comments apply to personality disorders other than the psychopathic or sociopathic, which is considered below.

The most radical treatment for personality disorder is psychoanalysis or analytical psychotherapy, individual or group. These aim to bring about major changes in the patient's personality and his way of understanding himself (see Chapter 44). However, only a small proportion of patients with personality disorders are sufficiently motivated to benefit from these approaches. Patients who are socially inadequate may be helped by social skills training to improve their social handicaps. This approach is not likely to be helpful in the more severe personality disorders, such as the paranoid, schizoid or narcissistic personality. The majority of patients, however, can make use of support with the emphasis on current problems. Support may be provided in either an individual or a group setting, often by social workers rather than medical staff. Drugs have virtually no part to play in the management of personality disorders.

PSYCHOPATHIC PERSONALITY DISORDER
(sociopathic or antisocial personality)

Psychiatrists in particular and society in general have found great difficulty in understanding individuals with psychopathic or antisocial personality disorders (Lewis 1974). One reason for this is that psychopaths often come into contact with the law and courts have to establish their criminal responsibility (see p. 697); this often boils down to a consideration of whether the offender is 'bad' or 'mad'. This is unfortunate because badness and madness are not mutually exclusive attributes and the offender may be both or neither (Bowden 1983). This preoccupation with the psychopath's responsibility for his actions has tended to cloud the issue when management is considered.

In 1801 Pinel coined the term *manie sans délire* to describe people who were prone to outbursts of violence and rage but were not mad, i.e. the disturbance was emotional and volitional in origin. This definition would include some patients now called psychopaths. The terms moral derangement and moral insanity were used in England (Prichard 1835) and were mistakenly assumed to convey a sense of moral depravity, thus attaching a judgmental aspect to the disorder. Others began to consider the effects of the individual's disorder on society. The American viewpoint has particularly emphasised this aspect, hence the terms *sociopath* or *antisocial personality*. The three terms psychopath, antisocial personality and sociopath are now often used interchangeably. The Mental Health Act of 1983 uses the term psychopathic disorder and gives the following legal definition:

> a persistent disorder or disability of mind whether or not including significant impairment of intelligence which results in abnormally aggressive or seriously irresponsible conduct on the part of the person concerned.

The term psychopathic personality will be used in this chapter in view of its continuing widespread use.

Clinical features

The types of personality disorder mentioned earlier in this chapter describe a number of characteristics which tend to predominate in and shape an individual's actions and interactions. There is an implication that the whole personality has not been described and that there are other healthy aspects which have been obscured and are potentially redeemable. This sense of optimism is usually lacking in the case of psychopathic personality. Here the personality is considered to be disordered in all its aspects. Thus there is a pervasive disregard for social obligations, a lack of feelings for others, impetuous violence and callous unconcern. The 'charm' of the psychopath is illusory as can be seen by his sudden change to aggression if frustrated. He is unable to learn from experience and blames others when his behaviour brings him into conflict with society.

All areas of the psychopath's life are affected by this disorder. His lifestyle tends to be itinerant with numerous casual jobs and relationships. There may in addition be excessive gambling, drug and alcohol abuse and problems with the law. This may result in many years of institutionalisation, more commonly penal than medical.

Seriously disturbed behaviour is often already manifest in childhood, when lying, stealing, truancy, excessive fighting and delinquency may occur. The work of Robins (1966) has shown that children who displayed such behaviour and were diagnosed as having a disorder of conduct were likely to become psychopaths in later life.

Although the capacity of the psychopath to cause suffering to others tends to be stressed, there are frequently signs of personal distress such as complaints of tension, depression, inability to tolerate boredom and paranoid ideas. Cleckley (1976) divides psychopathic personalities into primary and secondary. The *primary psychopath* tends to be affectively cold and aggressive and does not seem to be subjectively distressed by his disorder. In contrast, the *secondary psychopath* conveys a greater sense of personal suffering. Cleckley postulates that his behaviour is secondary to neurotic features. The secondary psychopath shows much higher levels of anxiety and tension, with low self-esteem and hidden guilt and regret, features lacking in the primary psychopath. This distinction, however, is often difficult to make.

Case illustration

A twenty-eight-year-old lorry driver was referred for psychiatric assessment during a period of remand in prison following a charge of causing grievous bodily harm to his common-law wife. He had stabbed her following an argument in which he had accused her of flirting with the milkman. He had a history of repeated criminal offences, some for theft and others for violence, and had spent a number of years at first in approved school and borstal and latterly in prison. He had also had one short psychiatric admission for treatment of alcohol abuse but had been discharged early after bringing alcohol on to the ward. He had been working in his present employment for three months, having persuaded his employers of his intention to 'go straight' despite his prison record and his history of erratic work.

In his childhood the patient had been beaten regularly by his alcoholic, violent father. He was the middle child of five, his mother spending little time with him as she needed to work to support the family. He had been referred to a child health centre at the age of ten following poor academic performance and truancy from school. He attended again a year later after setting fire to a disused factory. During adolescence he developed a consistent pattern of antisocial behaviour such as joy-riding and stealing. He had few friends and although sexually active he had no lasting relationships with women.

At interview he was cooperative and composed, yet appeared cold and threatening to the interviewer. He had a clear disregard for the psychiatrist and offered various rationalisations for the present and previous offences. There was no remorse. There were no disturbances in thinking and perception and his mood was characterised by a lack of emotional response rather than signs of anxiety or depression.

Aetiology

Genetic factors

The main criticism of genetic research on psychopathy is that it has tended to be carried out on populations drawn from criminal groups, thus providing data on the genetics of delinquency rather than psychopathy. Adoption studies in Denmark have shown that the adopted child grows up to resemble his biological rather than adoptive parents in terms of his liability to develop a psychopathic personality disorder. Robins (1966) in the USA has found an increased incidence of psychopathic behaviour and alcoholism in the fathers of individuals with psychopathic personality disorder. Chromosomal studies (Jacobs *et al.* 1965) suggested that men with the XYY karyotype were over represented in special hospitals and that this was a cause of abnormally aggressive behaviour. It is probable that the true incidence of XYY in the community had been underestimated, however, and there is no evidence that an extra Y chromosome is related to psychopathy.

Physiological factors

It has been postulated that in some cases psychopathy might result from delayed maturation of the brain. This idea has been supported by EEG studies which have shown excessive slow-wave activity in the posterior temporal region of the brains of aggressive psychopaths (Williams 1969). The term 'immature EEG' is sometimes used, as the slow-wave activity resembles that found in the EEGs of children. These abnormalities are present in patients even when conditions such as epilepsy, mental impairment or head injury are excluded. It is likely that cerebral pathology predisposes to psychopathic behaviour in some patients, but they are probably a minority.

Psychological and psychodynamic factors

The child's attachments and emotional experiences are of paramount importance in the aetiology of psychopathy. Bowlby (1951) first drew attention to the lasting damage that can result from early emotional deprivation and failure of *bond formation* between the child and its mother. Further research has been reviewed by Rutter (1981). It appears that failure of bond formation rather than its disruption is the main factor. Although the lack of bonding to the mother is particularly important it can be compensated for by the formation of bonds to significant others such as the father, and this may prevent serious consequences later in life. Children brought up in affectionless institutions without a close emotional attachment to any member of staff seem to be at particular risk. Later on other forms of disturbance in the family, e.g. the presence of an aggressive, uncaring father with whom the child may identify, a lack of affection towards the child, or hostility, violence and lack of affection between the parents, and absence of social stimulation, can all contribute to the development of psychopathy (Rutter and Madge 1976).

It has been suggested that psychopaths are more difficult to condition than normal people and therefore less able to learn from experience and develop socially acceptable behaviour. Again this may be true for some patients, but generally a multitude of factors contribute to psychopathy.

Management

Often the psychopath is referred for psychiatric assessment and possible treatment against his will, making the establishment of a therapeutic relationship almost impossible. This is particularly the case with the primary psychopath. Treatment should probably be reserved for those who are motivated to seek help. Those who show the capacity to become anxious and depressed are more amenable to a psychotherapeutic approach.

The treatment approach is also influenced by the setting; it may be in prison or hospital, in conditions of maximum security or with no restrictions. Generally individual psychotherapy is unsuccessful and a group approach appears to have better results. Within the prison service, Grendon Underwood Prison offers group-oriented psychotherapy for motivated psychopaths already serving a prison sentence. It tends to restrict itself to the less violent, more articulate psychopath. The most well-known therapeutic community within the NHS for psychopathic patients is the Henderson Hospital. Here patients live together and meet daily for group discussions which focus on the emotional and behavioural problems of each resident. The patients themselves share responsibility for the running of the hospital and the admission of new patients. For some patients the experience can provide an opportunity to learn how to relate to and develop concern for others; this helps them to control their antisocial behaviour and learn new ways of dealing with stressful situations and personal relationships (Whiteley 1986).

There is some evidence that sociopathic behaviour diminishes from middle age onwards, although problems in interpersonal relationships remain and the incidence of suicide and alcoholism is high.

FURTHER READING

Hare R.D. and Schalling, D. (1978). *Psychopathic Behaviour: approaches to research*. John Wiley, Chichester.

Kernberg, O. (1984). *Severe Personality Disorders: psychotherapeutic strategies*. Yale University Press, New Haven and London.

Lewis, A. (1974). 'Psychopathic personality: a most elusive category'. *Psychological Medicine* 4, 133-140.

Vaillant, G.E. and Perry, J.C. (1985). 'Personality disorders' in Kaplan, H.I. and Sadock, B.J., *Comprehensive Textbook of Psychiatry*, 4th ed., vol. 1, 883-894. Williams & Wilkins, Baltimore and London.

27

Borderline States

The concept of borderline states is controversial and confusing. The term borderline has limited acceptance amongst British psychiatrists, although it is widely used in the USA in a variety of ways, e.g. borderline personality disorder, borderline personality organisation and borderline schizophrenia. The meaning of these terms is discussed below.

BORDERLINE PERSONALITY DISORDER

The term borderline was first used by Stern (1938) in the USA. At that time patients were diagnosed as borderline if their symptoms appeared neurotic but their behaviour was suggestive of an underlying psychosis. These ideas were later developed by Kernberg (1975), an American psychoanalyst, and others who now suggest that borderline patients are not on the 'borderline' of psychosis and neurosis but have a specific pathological personality characterised by a tendency to regress under stress and to use primitive mental mechanisms, such as splitting, idealisation, projection and projective identification (see Chapter 6). Psychotic and neurotic symptoms may occur but they are not the focus of the disorder and only become prominent under stressful circumstances, e.g. in intimate personal relationships. Kernberg uses the term *borderline personality organisation*, but many psychiatrists prefer the term borderline personality disorder.

Instead of defining patients with a borderline personality in terms of mental mechanisms and intrapsychic disturbance as Kernberg does, Kolb and Gunderson (1980) have put forward easily observable characteristic criteria. These relate to five areas of functioning: social adaptation, impulse action patterns, affective symptoms, psychotic symptoms and interpersonal relations.

The *social abilities* of patients with borderline personality disorder may be reasonably good when they are not under stress; they may be normal in appearance and behave appropriately in social interaction. Unfortunately this outer appearance crumbles repeatedly over months and years when under stress and their behaviour becomes *impulsive* and *self-destructive*. This may be episodic, e.g. cutting themselves, taking overdoses, or breaking windows; or it may become chronic and part of a lifestyle leading, for example, to drug dependence, sexual perversion and promiscuity. This interferes with their social function and may lead to loss of employment or failure in academic achievements.

Two *affects* dominate the clinical picture, namely anger and depression. Anxiety may also be present. The depression is different from the typical guilt-laden, hopeless, remorseful type seen in depressive illness. Instead it takes the form of a sense of emptiness, isolation and loneliness with an inability to experience pleasure or satisfaction. This is occasionally described as 'existential despair'.

The tendency of patients with borderline personality disorders to develop *psychotic symptoms* is common. However, when psychoses do occur they are clearly stress-related, transient, lasting a few hours or days only, and unsystematised. Stable delusions or hallucinations are not a feature. The question arises as to whether all patients with borderline personality disorder develop psychotic symptoms at some point in their life. There is general agreement that only a sub-group of patients actually develop psychotic symptoms, but all patients with the disorder show impairment of reality testing under stressful circumstances.

Interpersonal relationships are often superficial and transient. Closer relationships tend to become clinging and demanding and are marred by manipulation, devaluation and destructive behaviour. This is in contrast to neurotic patients who are able to develop stable close relationships, and schizoid personalities who are withdrawn.

The concept of borderline personality disorder as described above is gradually being accepted in this country especially by psychiatrists with a psychodynamic approach. It is a useful term to describe patients seen in clinical practice who conform with the above criteria and who clearly differ from other personality disorders.

Aetiology

The aetiology of borderline personality is best understood in terms of personality development (see Chapter 7). A common finding is a history of disturbed early mother-infant interaction with extreme frustrations and intense aggression during the first few years of life. The result is a pathological developmental process which leads to excessive use of primitive mental mechanisms, distortion of object relationships and an inability to negotiate normal sexual development (Rey 1979). Adult, including sexual, relationships are then experienced as dangerous and imbued with aggression. Borderline personality is therefore classified as a primitive form of personality disorder, as described on p. 333 (Kernberg 1977a).

Treatment

The treatment of patients with a borderline personality disorder is difficult. Drugs, e.g. antidepressants or low-dose phenothiazines, may be used to help the patient tolerate increasing tension, but the treatment of choice is psychoanalytic psychotherapy, if available. Modifications to the psychotherapeutic setting and technique may be necessary to reduce the likelihood of psychotic episodes by emphasising reality testing and to prevent or control aggressive and self-destructive behaviour. The patient's environment must be carefully structured by using hospitals or hostels, especially at times of crises. Collaboration between the therapist and other professionals, such as social workers, general practitioners and nurses, is essential. Therapy may last a long time, and the therapist has to be prepared for crises to arise during treatment. He is likely to experience feelings of frustration, failure, anger or despair, but if he can keep these under control and maintain an attitude of reliable concern based on careful understanding of the patient's problems the possibility of a successful outcome is much improved. This can be a rewarding experience for both patient and therapist.

SCHIZOTYPAL PERSONALITY DISORDER

It is clear that the patients with borderline personality disorder described above are not schizophrenic. However, in the USA the term borderline has in the past been associated with schizophrenia, and this led to the concept of borderline schizophrenia (Kety *et al.* 1971), a term not used in the UK. In the USA the term schizotypal personality disorder has now been adopted; this is used in the DSM-III to describe those patients formerly diagnosed as having borderline schizophrenia (Spitzer *et al.* 1977). This personality disorder is characterised by odd speech patterns such as over-elaborate, circumstantial or metaphorical speech; by magical thinking such as marked superstition; and by poor rapport in personal interaction as a result of aloofness, coldness, superficiality and suspiciousness. Undue social anxiety is common and social contact may be limited to essential everyday tasks. There are none of the diagnostic criteria of schizophrenia. The term is of doubtful value and not used in the UK.

FURTHER READING

Dahl, A.A. (1985). 'Borderline disorders – the validity of the diagnostic concepts'. *Psychiatric Developments* 2, 109-152.

Kernberg, O. (1975). *Borderline Conditions and Pathological Narcissism.* Jason Aronson, New York.

Rosenfeld, H. (1978). 'Notes on the psychopathology and psychoanalytic treatment of some borderline patients'. *Int. J. Psychoanal.* 59, 215-222.

Steiner. J. (1979). 'The border between the paranoid-schizoid and depressive positions in borderline patients'. *Brit. J. Med. Psychol.* 52, 385-391.

Stone, M.H. (ed.) (1986). *Essential Papers on Borderline Disorders.* New York University Press, New York.

28

Psychosexual Problems

Psychosexual problems may be divided into two distinct groups, the *sexual dysfunctions* and the *sexual perversions*. In this chapter they will be discussed separately; occasionally a sexual dysfunction, such as erectile impotence, may arise as a result of an unexpressed perversion, but this is rare. Homosexuality, a psychosexual problem, is discussed separately (see Chapter 29), as it is common and often regarded as an acceptable alternative to heterosexual genital intercourse in a way in which the sexual perversions are not.

The term psychosexual is used here as the vast majority of sexual difficulties are of psychological origin; physical causes are rare.

SEXUAL DYSFUNCTION

Sexual dysfunction may be defined as the continual inability to achieve satisfactory sexual intercourse with a willing partner of similar maturity. The vast majority of couples or individuals who present with a sexual dysfunction are heterosexual. Occasionally homosexual couples seek help after failing to have a satisfactory sexual relationship.

Exactly what constitutes satisfactory sexual intercourse should be left to the couple seeking help. The doctor may have his own opinion and values, but these should not interfere with the treatment of his patients. It is best to find out how the individuals view their own problems and work within that framework.

A further point to remember is that sexual dysfunctions occur within the context of a relationship, and problems in the relationship may be the most important factor. For example, a couple may have severe interpersonal difficulties and share few interests. Their sexual relationship may deteriorate as a result and unless the marital problems are treated in their own right no improvement can be expected.

Classification

Sexual dysfunction may be primary or secondary. Individuals who have never been able to have a satisfactory sexual relationship are said to suffer from a primary dysfunction; those who have previously had a satisfactory sexual relationship but now have problems are said to have a secondary dysfunction.

Traditionally, sexual dysfunctions have been further subdivided according to the physiology of the human sexual responses (Masters and Johnson 1966) and divided into disorders of sexual desire, impaired sexual arousal, problems affecting orgasm, and others such as vaginismus, dyspareunia and sexual phobia. This classification is not particularly useful clinically as it fails to emphasise the importance of non-physiological factors in the aetiology of sexual dysfunction. Moreover the achievement of satisfactory sexual relationships, in both men and women, requires emotional responsiveness as well as physiological factors. Unfortunately there is no satisfactory classification which takes all these factors into account.

Mode of presentation

Men and women differ in the manner in which they present to the doctor with sexual problems. Women tend to view their sexual responsiveness in a subjective manner and within the context of their relationship. Bancroft and Coles (1976) found that women attending a clinic for sexual problems over a period of three years most commonly complained of a generalised feeling of unresponsiveness. Only about 18 per cent of women complained primarily about not being able to reach orgasm. Men, on the other hand, more often judged their sexual abilities in physical terms, probably because an erection is necessary for sexual intercourse. Thus men tend to complain of erectile or ejaculatory problems rather than lack of interest or emotional dissatisfaction. However a few complain of a lack of enjoyment of sexual intercourse despite achieving an erection followed by ejaculation.

Prevalence

There is little reliable information on the prevalence of sexual problems within the community as a whole. Information based on clinic attenders is likely to be unrepresentative, and surveys of a larger population are difficult and unreliable. Overall, dissatisfaction with sexual intercourse is probably extremely common and most couples will experience difficulties at some time in their lives, often as a result of emotional changes associated with events such as illness, a death in the family, childbirth, marriage, children leaving home, etc. Such sexual difficulties are usually only temporary.

Recent population surveys suggest that women show greater dissatisfaction with their sexual life than men. For example a study in Holland (Frenken 1976) reported that 28 per cent of men and 43 per cent of women felt that there were problems of enjoyment and arousal in their sexual relationships; a further 9 per cent of women expressed aversion to sexual intercourse. In a recent community survey in Oxford, Osborn *et al.*

(1988) found that one third of women between the ages of thirty-five and fifty-nine had sexual dysfunction, including impaired sexual interest, infrequency of orgasm and dyspareunia. Only a small proportion of these had asked for help.

The prevalence of each sexual dysfunction is equally difficult to obtain. Kinsey (1948) suggested that erectile impotence increases with age. Thus only 2 per cent of men under forty-five complain of permanent impotence, but this increases to nearly 30 per cent by the age of seventy. In women (Kinsey *et al*. 1953) more attention has been given to the attainment of orgasm, and reports on the prevalence of orgasmic difficulty have suggested that between 5 and 20 per cent of all women complain of such difficulties. Despite the wide variation in these figures there is general agreement that only a very small proportion of individuals with sexual problems actually seek treatment.

Sexual dysfunction in men

Impotence

Impotence, sometimes known as erectile failure or erectile impotence, is either the inability to achieve an erection or difficulty in sustaining it long enough for mutually satisfying sexual intercourse to take place. It may be primary, i.e. when a man has never had an erection when attempting intercourse, or secondary. Primary impotence is rare. Secondary impotence is more common and may be situational or global. For example, a man may be unable to have an erection with his wife but have successful intercourse with a girlfriend or with prostitutes, or be able to masturbate. In cases of impotence the ability to masturbate or the experience of an erection early in the morning indicate that the problem has a psychological basis rather than an organic cause. Organic factors may play a part, however, especially in the second half of life.

Premature ejaculation

In this condition ejaculation takes place either before penetration or shortly afterwards. As a result neither partner feels satisfied. It is this which determines whether ejaculation is premature or not, as the time lapse between erection and ejaculation required for mutual satisfaction will vary from couple to couple. The incidence of premature ejaculation is highest in younger men, probably as a result of their anxiety, inexperience or excessive excitement on first attempting to have intercourse.

Retarded ejaculation and painful ejaculation

Retarded ejaculation is said to occur when there is a long delay between a state of arousal and the onset of ejaculation. It is usually associated with sexual intercourse rather than masturbation. Painful ejaculation is rare and its cause unknown.

Sexual dysfunction in women

Vaginismus

This is characterised by spasms of the muscles surrounding the entrance to the vagina whenever sexual intercourse is attempted. It is independent of the woman's desire and not under her control. For example, a woman may feel deeply for her partner, enjoy being held and caressed by him but be overwhelmed by fear of being penetrated by his penis. Some of these women may not even be able to introduce a finger or tampon into their vagina. Guilt and fear of sexuality with ignorance about sexual function are usually found to be the major cause.

Anxiety and inexperience on the part of the woman's partner may exacerbate the problem, for example he may attempt penetration before adequate stimulation and vaginal lubrication have occurred. In some cases experience, tenderness and love on the part of the partner do not overcome the spasm and he may give up attempting intercourse and become impotent. In fact a woman with these sexual fears may choose a husband or partner who is himself not highly sexed and hesitant about approaching her sexually. For example, a woman whose marriage had remained unconsummated for five years said she had married her husband because 'he had never tried anything on'.

In fact *non-consummated marriage* commonly presents with the complaint of vaginismus but surprisingly sometimes with infertility. Some couples do not ask for help for several years after their marriage (Friedman 1962).

Dyspareunia

Pain on intercourse, or dyspareunia, occurs in both men and women. It is included here as it affects women far more often than men. Dyspareunia is often secondary to vaginismus, but in all cases organic causes such as episiotomy scars, infection, endometriosis or other pelvic pathology should be ruled out. Overall approximately 30 per cent of women with dyspareunia have pelvic disease. Post-menopausal women may develop dyspareunia as a result of atrophy of the vaginal mucosa and a reduction in vaginal secretions.

Orgasmic dysfunction (frigidity)

Women who persistently fail to achieve orgasm despite becoming sexually excited are said to have an orgasmic dysfunction. Whether or not this is a sexual problem depends very much on the individual's attitude and expectations. Even nowadays some women do not expect to enjoy sexual relationships or reach orgasm. Some women are able to achieve orgasm if their partner stimulates them manually or when they masturbate themselves but not during penetration. Others pretend to have reached orgasm in order not to disappoint their partner.

Primary orgasmic dysfunction is said to exist when a woman has never experienced an orgasm by any means of stimulation. In secondary orgasmic dysfunction the woman has previously experienced orgasm either by sexual intercourse or by masturbation. The achievement of orgasm in women increases with age, perhaps as a result of a decrease in sexual anxieties, choice of a new partner and greater sexual experience. Psychological factors which may be associated with difficulty in achieving orgasm include fear of pregnancy, worries about rejection, fear of damage to the vagina, hostility towards men, a disturbed relationship with her partner, and feelings of guilt about sexual wishes and fantasies. A history of child sexual abuse or an incestuous relationship may also play a part. Of course in some cases unresponsiveness in a woman may be to some extent due to her partner's poor technique.

Sexual dysfunction in both sexes

Sexual desire

The determining factor in defining a high or low sexual drive depends on the individual's estimate of his own sexual feelings. Low sexual desire often indicates difficulties within a relationship, perhaps due to a lack of attraction for the partner rather than a specific sexual problem. Occasionally individuals appear to have a long-standing low sexual drive with inhibition of sexual fantasies, infrequent or absent masturbation during and since adolescence, and few attempts at approaching the opposite sex. Women more often complain of a low sexual drive than men. Excessive sexual desire is a rare complaint, but occasionally couples experience difficulties if their sexual needs do not complement each other.

Sexual phobia

In a sexual phobia there is an avoidance of sexual experiences as a result of some specific anxiety. As in the other phobias, the fear is recognised by the individual as being excessive. The anxiety may be confined to a specific aspect of sexual intercourse such as kissing, seeing the partner naked or being seen naked, smell of sexual secretions, etc., or more generalised in which case sex is avoided altogether (Kaplan *et al.* 1982). Sexual phobia is rare but when present in one of the partners it seriously interferes with the development of an exciting sex life and may be responsible for unconsummated marriages or marital breakdown.

Aetiology

The causes of sexual dysfunction are best divided into organic, psychological and social factors. The three groups are not mutually exclusive. For example a diabetic may have minor problems with sustaining an erection as a result of peripheral vascular disease. This may lead to performance anxiety which further exacerbates the problem. If a poor marital relationship is superimposed, impotence may result. Thus it is essential to assess every sexual problem in the context of the individual's personality, physical health, and the relationship in which the dysfunction occurs.

Organic factors

Nearly 90 per cent of sexual problems have a psychological basis, and impotence in young men is almost always emotional in origin. It may rarely be associated with an organic disorder such as an endocrine abnormality, e.g. hypopituitarism or diabetes; a neurological disorder, e.g. multiple sclerosis, Parkinsonism, paraplegia; or any severe systemic disease. It also occurs as a complication of treatment with such drugs as hypotensive agents, beta-adrenoceptor antagonists, antidepressants, phenothiazines, benzodiazepines and alcohol. Similar factors may lead to low sexual desire or other sexual problems such as orgasmic dysfunction in women.

Psychological and social factois

Sexual dysfunction may be an early feature of mental illness such as depression or schizophrenia, but these causes are rare.

The commonest psychological state associated with sexual problems is anxiety. Anxiety may develop after the first attempt at sexual intercourse when excessive sexual excitement or anxiety about the unknown may lead to failure; this then causes additional anxiety about possible failure at subsequent attempts and sets up a repetitive cycle of failures. This is especially common in men who are impotent. It may also occur in women and lead to an inability to achieve orgasm. Common anxieties in men include fear of failure, of contracting venereal disease such as AIDS, of being too aggressive, of hurting their partner, and of ridicule. Feelings of excessive respect for the female may also lead to failure. For example, if a boy grows up with an image of his mother as a pure and idealised woman he may later be impotent with a woman who reminds him of his mother. In contrast he may be sexually aroused and potent with a woman for whom he has no respect, e.g. a prostitute.

Women may have similar fears, but worries about the penis, especially its size, are common. Such fears, if excessive, may lead to vaginismus. In many societies, including our own, the view used to be held, mainly by men, that sexual pleasure was not an essential experience for women; it was even thought that it was improper for respectable women to enjoy sex. Thus girls were made to feel guilty and denied or dissembled their sexual desires and feelings with the result that they developed sexual problems when they became sexually mature. Only in relatively recent years has the attitude of society begun to change; it is now recognised that orgasmic difficulty in women is as much a symptom that can be treated as is impotence in men. Women who have accepted their sexual function as a normal aspect of adult life are at least as capable as men of enjoying intercourse and reaching orgasm and often more capable.

Early childhood experiences are often important in the causation of sexual dysfunction in both men and women. For example, a puritanical upbringing, guilt about sexual activities including masturbation, fear of punishment, child sexual abuse and incest can all lay the foundation for disturbed psychosexual development (see pp. 70-5) and hence sexual dysfunction in adulthood. A very strict religious upbringing may reinforce such problems.

Apart from these general psychological and social considerations and misconceptions, there are a number of individual factors which may lead to a woman having sexual problems such as vaginismus or orgasmic difficulties. For example, her partner may be wrong for her physically or emotionally, or the circumstances may be unfavourable to allow her fully to relax during intercourse. Moreover a woman usually needs to be sexually aroused by her partner to reach a sufficient state of excitement. If the man's sexual technique and awareness of his partner's needs are defective this state will not be reached and orgasm will not occur. When this happens repeatedly and the woman remains disappointed and frustrated this may not only lead to more persistent sexual difficulties but also to marital disharmony.

Other factors common to both men and women include ignorance of sexual matters and problems associated with sexual orientation such as underlying homosexuality. Inevitably, problems in one of the partners may lead to difficulties for the other. For example, conflicts about sexual intercourse and anorgasmia in the woman may affect her partner who then becomes impotent.

Assessment

The assessment of a patient with a sexual problem may be difficult due to the embarrassment and shame felt by the patient. The doctor's initial task is to help the patient overcome this. This is best done by interviewing the patient and partner separately and only later seeing them together. Once the diagnosis of a sexual dysfunction has been established and major psychiatric disorders such as schizophrenia and depression ruled out the clinician must decide whether the likely cause of the dysfunction is organic or psychogenic. The most important differentiating feature is whether the dysfunction is situational or global. If the problem is situational, e.g. a man complaining of impotence with his wife but able to masturbate, then organic factors are virtually ruled out. The assessment should then aim to achieve a detailed account of the individual's psychological development and attitude to sexuality, and the state of the relationship between the partners. The nature of the disorder may also serve as a further guide. For example, premature ejaculation, retarded ejaculation and anorgasmia are rarely associated with physical causes even if they are global. On the other hand dyspareunia in both men and women often has an organic cause, especially when the pain only occurs in certain positions.

Treatment

Each individual or couple needs a tailor-made treatment programme. The assumption that the well-known techniques pioneered by Masters and Johnson (1970) and described below are useful to all patients with sexual problems is erroneous. Some patients may have severe underlying neurotic conflicts such as uncertainty about intimacy and commitment which manifest themselves as sexual problems within a relationship. These individuals will need psychoanalytic psychotherapy before their problems are likely to be resolved. In other cases the sexual difficulties may be the focus of apparently irreconcilable marital difficulties, in which case marital therapy (see p. 575) is the most appropriate treatment. Furthermore, those individuals who have a sexual problem but no partner are usually best treated in individual or group psychotherapy as both their single status and sexual disorder may be the result of personality problems.

Nevertheless, *sex therapy*, widely practised in the USA and increasingly in the UK, is useful in the treatment of some sexual dysfunctions such as impotence and orgasmic difficulties, especially if treatment takes place with the full cooperation of a caring partner. The couple can be treated by one therapist, but it is sometimes helpful for male and female therapists to treat the couple jointly.

Sex therapy was first introduced by Masters and Johnson (1970) in the USA and has been modified since. It requires flexibility from the therapist or therapists, as there are important educational, technical and psychotherapeutic components. Initially, ignorance and misunderstandings about the anatomy and physiology of sexual intercourse need to be corrected. Following this, open communication is encouraged and feelings such as anxiety, anger or guilt concerning the couple's sexual relationship have to be explored. Next, more specific sexual tasks are given to the couple to practise at home. This is best done in stages. In order to reduce anxiety about possible failure of either partner, e.g. failure to get an erection or failure to reach orgasm, in the early stages of treatment penetration and actual intercourse are not allowed. Instead the couple are instructed to touch and caress each other in areas which are pleasurable, so-called *sensate focus*, but without any genital contact. When the couples are able to relax and enjoy mutual caressing, genital contact is gradually introduced, sometimes involving mutual masturbation. Finally the couple are allowed to have sexual intercourse. Not infrequently the couple will have had intercourse successfully before having been instructed by the therapist to do so.

In the course of these progressive stages further anxieties and misconceptions may come to light. These need to be fully discussed with the therapist and dispelled if possible. It is particularly important to encourage each partner to pay attention to what would please and excite the other rather than concentrate only on personal gratification. If the original problem, e.g. impotence, premature ejaculation, vaginismus, or orgasmic difficulty has been treated successfully, any remaining non-sexual problems in the relationship between the partners may require attention, e.g. by a psychotherapeutic approach.

Certain specific techniques have been used in combination with the more general principles outlined above. For example, in the case of premature ejaculation the 'squeeze technique' is used, the woman being asked to adopt the superior position during intercourse and squeeze the man's penis with her hand if he is about to ejaculate.

The success rate with these techniques is good in well-motivated couples and those without serious marital, emotional or psychiatric disorders. There are obvious difficulties in treating patients who do not have a sexual partner and the introduction of a surrogate partner is now thought to be contraindicated as it raises serious ethical and legal problems.

SEXUAL PERVERSION

Sexual practices vary over time and differ from culture to culture, and Western society has increasingly accepted different forms of sexual expression and identity over the last century. As a result of these variations many people consider the terms perversion and deviation to be outdated, value-laden, unnecessarily pejorative, smacking of prim morality and likely to be abused in order to justify inappropriate repressive action against minority groups. Attempts have therefore been made to discard these terms altogether, and many psychiatrists avoid them. It is true that the use of the terms perversion or deviation to degrade and diminish an individual or to justify social repression is both dehumanising and dangerous. Furthermore to retain the concepts merely to preserve an out-dated social morality is equally unacceptable. In fact the use of the terms sexual deviation or perversion in a judgmental fashion is totally unjustifiable. In this chapter they are used quite specifically to define in an objective and descriptive manner certain sexual problems for which no other appropriate terms are available. No moral judgment is implied.

There are no clear or universally accepted definitions of sexual perversion and sexual deviation, and the terms are often used synonymously. Here they will be considered as distinct entities, and their definition follows the principles put forward by Robert Stoller (1979), an American psychoanalyst.

Sexual perversion is a form of sexual behaviour in which a habitual and compulsive sexual fantasy plays a central role. The fantasy is necessary for full sexual satisfaction and interferes, to a greater or lesser degree, with genital intercourse with a willing partner of the opposite sex and similar maturity. In the fantasy, sexual and aggressive impulses tend to be intimately linked. The fantasy is acted out either with another person, e.g. in sadomasochism or paedophilia, or with the self, as in transvestism. Occasionally the perversion exists in fantasy alone when it is either self-produced or stimulated by an outside source, as in pornography, and is accompanied by masturbation. The greatest excitement and satisfaction often depends on an element of risk-taking, for example in exhibitionism.

In contrast a *deviation* is not the result of an unconscious conflict concerning forbidden sexual desires, nor is it motivated by the compulsion to act out a particular sexual fantasy. Deviation merely implies a statistical variation from the norm and is therefore a term best reserved for the differences in sexual styles between cultures or the changes in sexual practices observed over time either within a culture or in an individual during his development. A common example of sexual deviation is the homosexual behaviour which occurs out of necessity in restrictive circumstances such as those found in prisons or single-sex institutions. As soon as circumstances change the behaviour ceases.

The importance of the definition of sexual perversion given above is that it does not require a particular behaviour to be present, nor does it need a 'moral norm' as a yardstick. Furthermore there is no necessity to find out how many people are engaged in a particular behaviour to decide if it is perverse or not. All that is required is a knowledge of the personality, fantasy and motivation of the individual, and the meaning the behaviour has for that person. As a result heterosexual genital intercourse is not by itself the epitome of normality and may in fact form part of a perversion if accompanied by a perverse fantasy. For example, a husband may have a habitual and compulsive fantasy of hurting his wife during sexual intercourse.

A sexual perversion forms an intrinsic part of an individual's personality and may therefore be associated with severe personality disorder and neurotic difficulties. However, it can be compatible with successful social functioning, high achievement and a heterosexual lifestyle. For example, many transvestites have successful careers, are married and have children (Prince and Bentler 1972). Despite this, sexual perversion is more commonly associated with an impairment of mutually satisfying relationships with adults of the opposite sex. Furthermore, the retention of child-like patterns in relating to others may be marked.

There is no universally agreed classification of the sexual perversions. However, it is useful to group together those conditions in which the nature of the object chosen to achieve sexual gratification is abnormal, e.g. paedophilia, bestiality, fetishism, necrophilia and some forms of homosexuality (see p. 371), and those in which the behaviour in relation to the object is abnormal, e.g. exhibitionism, voyeurism and sadomasochism. These may then be contrasted with the perversions in which there is a disorder of gender identity. *Gender identity* consists of the self-concept of being masculine or feminine (Stoller 1968) and the resulting attitudes and behaviour of the individual. Problems arise when an individual's self-concept is at variance with his biological sex, as happens in transvestism and transsexualism (Bancroft 1983). This classification is summarised in Table 28.1.

Table 28.1. Sexual perversion

Disorders of object choice and behaviour	*Disorders of gender identity*
Exhibitionism	Transvestism
Fetishism	Transsexualism
Voyeurism	
Sadomasochism	
Paedophilia	
Rape	
Others: necrophilia, bestiality	
Homosexuality	

Aetiology

Biological factors

Genetic factors have little importance in the development of sexual perversion, with the possible exception of homosexuality. Some genetic studies have demonstrated a higher concordance rate for homosexuality in monozygotic than dyzygotic twins (Heston and Shields 1968), while others have found no clear differences. No firm conclusion can be drawn from these studies, as it is likely that environmental factors, such as strong identification between twins, are responsible for the findings rather than genetic factors. In some cases genetic factors may sensitise the individual to later environmental influences.

Neuroendocrine factors have also been implicated in the development of adult male homosexuality. However, findings such as abnormal testosterone profiles have not been replicated (Pillard *et al.* 1974). Other studies have focused on the prenatal period (Dorner *et al.* 1975). It is known that hormones at critical times can have a marked influence on the later anatomical structure of the genitalia and on brain function responsible for future sexual behaviour. For example, if androgens are administered to animals such as rats and rhesus monkeys at certain critical periods during pregnancy, female offspring will be born with masculinised external genitalia, and will, as they mature, behave more like males than females. Conversely, if an anti-androgen is given to the pregnant female her male offspring will be born with feminised external genitalia and behave like females rather than males. However, the evidence that this is relevant to humans is limited. In fact, in human infants whose sex is uncertain or misdiagnosed at birth, e.g. in pseudohermaphroditism due to the adrenogenital syndrome where female infants are born with masculinised external genitalia, their future sexual behaviour and their subjective sense of gender identity is determined by whether they are brought up as boys or girls (Money and Ehrhardt 1968).

Interestingly, both temporal lobe epilepsy and chromosomal abnormalities such as Klinefelter's syndrome have been associated with fetishism (Epstein 1961), but their role in the sexual perversions in general is probably minimal. Overall, the evidence that sexual perversion is a result of physical factors rather than psychological forces is limited and unconvincing. Individuals who show aberrant sexual behaviour as a result of, for example, brain disease, temporal lobe epilepsy or testosterone abnormalities are unlikely to show the characteristics of sexual perversion defined earlier in which case they should not be diagnosed as suffering from a sexual perversion.

Social learning factors

Social learning theories suggest that sexual orientation and gender identity are formed by reinforcement and imitation. For example, boy-like behaviour in boys is reinforced by parental praise while girl-like behaviour is discouraged, and vice versa for girls. It is also suggested that children identify with the parent of the same sex and imitate or use that parent as a role model to shape their own behaviour. However, all small children identify with their mothers during the first few years of life, and children develop normal sexual orientation and identity in the absence of a same-sex parent. Despite these limitations of social learning theory, behavioural interactions between parents and their children are likely to play a part in the later development of sexual perversion.

Psychodynamic factors

Psychoanalytic theory views sexual perversion as arising out of early infantile and childhood experiences (Rosen 1979a). However, it is important to remember that a perversion is not a simple continuation of one aspect of infantile sexuality into adult life. In fact infantile sexuality has a polymorphous variable quality (Freud 1905), while perversions are specific, highly specialised, compulsive and organised. Thus the formation of the specific psychological organisation which forms a perversion must depend on the interaction of a host of factors occurring throughout childhood development, and no single factor can be isolated as the cause. Moreover, the different forms of perversion are determined by a constellation of different psychodynamic factors. However, psychoanalytic treatment of individuals with perversions has shown that there are a number of factors which are common to the perversions. These will be briefly described here.

Sexual perversions arise from unconscious conflicts between sexual desires, which are associated with guilt and anxiety, and various defences against these forbidden impulses; the perverse fantasies and behaviour then serve as a compromise which allows sexual satisfaction to be obtained. In this sense the origin of the perversions resembles that of neurotic symptoms (Gillespie 1964). An example of such a compromise would be a homosexual man who suffers from severe castration anxiety when faced with female genitals. Only by choosing another male as his sexual partner can he achieve sexual gratification without having to experience the fear of castration. This example also serves as an illustration of a perverse form of homosexuality as compared with homosexual behaviour as a deviation; in the latter a heterosexual man, free from castration anxiety, may have a homosexual relationship when he is confined to an all-male institution without access to women, but he can at other times enjoy heterosexual intercourse without accompanying homosexual fantasies. There may, of course, be an overlap between homosexuality as a deviation and a perversion.

In several of the perversions sexual impulses are found to be closely linked with aggressive impulses. It is important to recognise the difference between aggressive behaviour, which aims at the destruction and elimination of the other person, and sadism, which requires their preservation but in which the aim is to inflict pain and suffering, pleasure being derived from seeing the other person suffer (Glasser 1979, 1986). Sadism is, as it were, a sexualised form of aggression, and it is the latter which plays such an important part, not only in sadomasochism itself but also in the aetiology of many of the other perversions.

The sadist's compulsion to hurt or beat the partner during intercourse is an obvious example. Exhibitionism is another example, the exhibitionist deriving sexual satisfaction from frightening and shocking his victim by exhibiting his penis to her.

In masochism the sadistic wishes are entirely repressed and sexual satisfaction can only be obtained by becoming the victim of the partner's aggression instead, either in fantasy or by asking to be hurt, beaten, punished and made to suffer.

The question then arises why in the perversions sexual impulses are so often associated with aggressive impulses instead of with love and affection. During psychoanalytic psychotherapy or psychoanalysis of adults with a perversion it often comes to light that during the very early developmental stage when the infant had the experience of being merged in a symbiotic union with his mother (see p. 65) she, the mother, wished to prolong and maintain this state of being merged so that she failed to allow the child to become a separate autonomous individual. As a result the child feels engulfed, controlled and humiliated by his possessive and overprotective mother who, he feels, insists on his fulfilling all her needs while disapproving of any independent attitudes or forms of behaviour.

This leads the growing child to feel threatened, frustrated and hence aggressive towards her. At the same time he still needs her continuing love and protection so that he dare not express his anger or rebel. If this conflict remains unresolved it will subsequently interfere with his sexual development in so far as this conflict is re-experienced in relation to every woman he desires. He longs for a blissful sexual union with the woman but at the same time feels angry with her for having such power over him. He also fears closeness and sexual intimacy with her because this would once more make him feel engulfed and annihilated.

This basic conflict between loving and hating the woman, between wanting to be close and to be distant from her, has been called the *core complex* of the perversions by Glasser (1986). This aspect has also been discussed by Stoller (1977), who regards hatred, originally directed towards the mother and later towards sexual partners, as the core of the perversions. He suggests that the hatred 'takes form in a fantasy of revenge which is hidden in the actions that make up the perversion and serve to convert childhood trauma to adult triumph'. According to Stoller, the early trauma has been experienced as a severe threat to the developing sense of gender, i.e. to the person's inner sense of masculinity or femininity. This early trauma becomes converted by the adult into an active, aggressive and revengeful act directed towards the partner and is expressed in the perversion, for example in sadomasochism. But as the aggression has been made less destructive by being turned into sadism, its later acting out in a perversion results in a sense of triumph and mastery. This enactment involves the risk of the original trauma re-emerging into consciousness, but if this does not happen intense pleasure is realised via the perversion.

Fetishism serves as another example. Here the male partner controls and devalues the woman by insisting on her wearing a fetishistic object which is more important for his sexual gratification than the partner herself and her own body. Thus instead of being controlled and devalued by her he makes her feel inferior, unwanted in her own right, and under his control. Commonly the fetishistic object chosen symbolises a penis, as in this way any castration anxiety can be avoided and the woman's female role is denied.

Although these early problems in the infant-mother relationship are now recognised as significant factors in the aetiology of many of the perversions, other factors arising later in childhood also play an important role.

For example, a boy who feels rejected by his mother in his masculine gender role and treated like a girl may later as an adult feel sexually inadequate. He therefore resents and fears women, who represent his original mother. In his aggressive and perverse fantasies and behaviour, e.g. by exposing himself, he triumphs over the woman and temporarily regains his self-esteem and sense of masculinity.

Transvestism illustrates this further. If a boy has been treated by his mother as if he were a girl and his masculinity was devalued by her, he can as an adult triumph over her by dressing up in female clothes, thus making himself feel like a woman, but now being dressed as a woman has become a pleasure and allows him to feel sexually aroused and potent. At the moment of reaching orgasm he removes his clothes and triumphantly reveals his erect penis and masculinity. Thus in an omnipotent manner he is both man and woman but he has complete control over both.

Individual disorders

Exhibitionism

An exhibitionist is someone who exposes his genitals to a person of the opposite sex, usually a stranger, in order to obtain sexual pleasure without wishing to have sexual intercourse. Legally this offence is known as indecent exposure. It usually occurs in a public place and often leads to discovery and prosecution.

Exhibitionism is one of the commonest sexual perversions and is almost exclusively a masculine activity. It occurs in all age groups, although the incidence is highest in men under the age of thirty. Simple exposure of the genitals may occur, but this often does not provide enough satisfaction and masturbation follows. The penis may be erect or flaccid during the actual act of exposure. Occasionally, attempts are made to touch the victim but more often she is tormented by whistling, shouting or by obscene talk. Full satisfaction is often only achieved if the victim appears shocked and frightened.

Exhibitionists may be classified into two main groups – a simple type and an impulsive type (Rosen 1979b). The *simple type* of exhibitionist is a shy withdrawn individual whose exhibitionism follows on obvious disappointment such as a loss or sexual failure. He is usually a reasonably well-adjusted individual in many respects, as evidenced by his social relationships and work record. The exhibitionism appears to be an anomalous form of sexual advance. It may be repetitive and rarely involves any actual physical harm to the victim although it may cause psychological distress, especially if the victim is a child.

The *impulsive exhibitionist* is more severely disordered. The behaviour forms part of a severe personality disorder such as a psychopathic personality and has no obvious precipitants. It may lead to physical violence. Recurrence is common and other sexual perversions such as voyeurism may also be present.

Fetishism

In fetishism a non-genital object is required during a sexual act if full sexual pleasure and orgasm is to be achieved. Common fetishistic objects include articles of clothing such as fur, leather or a woman's shoe. The objects are usually touched during the sexual act or worn by the partner, but looking at or smelling the item occasionally suffices. In accordance with the definition of sexual perversion given earlier, a fantasy alone may serve as a fetish. For example, some individuals use a repetitive, stereotyped fantasy to enhance sexual pleasure, and this may become a requirement of full sexual satisfaction. Thus there is a broad range of fetishistic manifestations, some being more pathological than others.

The use of an actual object to enhance sexual intercourse is more frequent in men, but fetishistic fantasies may be equally common in men and women. The fetishist rarely presents to a psychiatrist as a result of his fetish. More commonly the fetish is an incidental finding during treatment for other problems such as anxiety, depression or marital difficulties. Occasionally a man seeks treatment for his fetish when his wife refuses to act out his fantasies and he becomes impotent or she becomes depressed.

Voyeurism

The voyeur obtains sexual gratification from looking at others engaged in a private activity such as undressing, courting, or preparing for or engaging in sexual intercourse. Voyeurism usually involves risk-taking and may be accompanied by masturbation. The voyeur rarely, if ever, proceeds to attack or rape his victim, and she may never know the interest taken in her. The habitual voyeur prefers peeping at female genitals, and the activity surpasses any other of his sexual activities. Other voyeurs may be married and have normal heterosexual relations alongside their voyeuristic behaviour. The wish to look at someone's genitals is the counterpart of the desire to be looked at, and in this way voyeurism and exhibitionism are often associated activities either in reality or fantasy.

Sadomasochism

In sadism, named after the Marquis De Sade (1740-1814), himself a sadist, sexual pleasure is obtained either from the fantasised infliction of pain upon another person or from actual acts of cruelty, e.g. whipping or caning; in masochism, named after the Austrian novelist Von Sacher-Masoch (1836-1895), himself a masochist, the excitement is obtained from having a punishment or actual pain inflicted on oneself either in fantasy or reality, i.e. being the willing subject of the acts of cruelty perpetrated by a sadist. It is common to find evidence of both traits in the same individual with one predominating.

Sadism is commoner in men and may be a normal variant in its mild forms. For example, erotic arousal from biting, or fantasised power during coitus is quite common. Sadistic acts may take the form of a general approach to another person, such as exerting power or humiliating the partner, or be very specific, such as acting out a particular ritual, e.g. bondage. Occasionally the sadistic act aims to produce a cherished end point such as the drawing of blood, at which point orgasm occurs. Whatever the form of the act, sadism may either accompany or precede sexual intercourse or even takes its place completely. Extreme acts of sadism may accidentally lead to murder.

Masochism is also common in mild forms, for example, obtaining pleasure from love-bites or from fantasies of being dominated may form part of normal sexual enjoyment (Kinsey *et al.* 1953). However, in its extreme forms masochism may lead to severe physical pain or even death. As the sexual excitement increases, awareness of the reality of what is happening diminishes, and death may result when the sadomasochistic ritual gets out of control.

Paedophilia

Paedophilia is a pathological sexual interest in pre-pubertal children, either in fantasy only, e.g. looking at pornographic pictures of children, or in reality. A paedophile is therefore someone in whom this sexual interest is the preferred and often the only means of obtaining sexual gratification. Actual or attempted intercourse is rare; genital touching, kissing or exhibition of the genitals is much more common. The condition is virtually confined to men and the child may be a young girl or boy aged between around eight years and puberty.

Occasionally adults who engage in paedophilia are of subnormal intelligence, alcoholic or suffering from dementia. Sometimes adolescent boys engage in sexual activities with pre-pubertal girls as they do not yet feel ready to have sexual relations with sexually mature girls of their own age or older. However, the vast majority of paedophiles are married although divorce and remarriage are common (Gebhard *et al.* 1965). Some may have children themselves and have obtained a position of responsibility working with children, e.g. a youth leader. Their family background often shows evidence of poor parental relationships characterised by an absence of emotional warmth. Consequently as adults they describe strong feelings of having missed out on love and tenderness, especially from their mother. They may attempt to make up for this by believing they are giving a child the love and tenderness that they themselves missed out on. Many find sexual relationships with adults threatening and turn to children to avoid feelings of inadequacy. Paedophiles have also been reported to view relationships primarily in terms of power. Such difficulties are easily diminished by turning to children, in which case the balance of power is obvious (Howells 1979).

Paedophilia differs from incest in that the sexual activities are carried out with children who are not close members of the family. The child may, however, be well known to the man, for example teacher and pupil, church worker and choirboy. Incest and child sexual abuse are discussed further in Chapter 43.

Paedophilia is probably more common than is often recognised. Overall approximately 25 per cent of children report pre-pubertal sexual experiences with post-pubertal partners (Kinsey *et al.* 1953; Landis

1956). The true figure of pre-pubertal sexual experiences is likely to be much higher, as many incidents go unreported. However, only a few of these sexual experiences between an adult and child continue over a prolonged period of time; those that do, e.g. between teacher and pupil, may seriously affect the child's psychological development and lead to anxiety and depression. Behavioural problems such as truancy, bedwetting and conduct disorder may also occur. However, the child's psychological development may already be disturbed as a result of inadequate parenting, a broken home or emotional neglect. In these cases the child may actively participate in what is to him a genuinely loving relationship.

Rape

Rape is defined in the Sexual Offences Act of 1976. A man is said to have committed rape if he has unlawful sexual intercourse with a woman who at the time of intercourse does not consent to it and at that time he knows that she does not consent to it or he is reckless as to whether she consents or not. Husbands cannot rape their wives as, in law at least, consent is deemed to be implicit within their marriage; boys under fourteen are also not considered capable of rape even though they may be capable of vaginal penetration.

The number of cases of forcible rape has increased dramatically both in this country and the USA over the last decade. This may to some extent reflect an increase in the rate of reporting of rape, but it seems likely that there has also been a true increase in the frequency of the crime. As a result of this increase, rape is being taken more seriously by the police and others, special examination centres are being set up, and specific procedures are carefully followed such as allowing the victim only to be examined by a female doctor.

The victim and the offender

Von Hentig (1948) proposed that some victims of crime were partly responsible for their plight, and this idea has been applied to rape victims both in the media and in legal circles. In fact there is little evidence for its validity and most women clearly do not encourage men to rape them. Most studies of rape victims, e.g. by Burgess and Holmstrom (1974) and Katz and Mazur (1979), have found only a small percentage of women whose behaviour before the rape was clearly related to the actual act; even if 'victim responsibility' is defined as any contact between the rapist and victim before the rape, the figure is less than 20 per cent (Amir 1971). However, there is some suggestion that certain women are prone to being raped, and 20 per cent of all rape victims have been the victims of at least one prior sexual assault. Rape victims are also more likely to be socially disadvantaged, known to the psychiatric services and to have had an incestuous relationship as a child.

The majority of victims are probably raped by strangers, although the figures for 'stranger rape' vary from 20 to 90 per cent. If the rapist and victim know each other before the act the rapist may believe that he has been encouraged to make sexual advances. However, it seems likely that most offenders know that their victim does not truly consent to the act.

Rapists are driven by a mixture of anger and desire for power as expressed through violent sexuality (Groth 1979), and have severe difficulties in forming close intimate relationships. They show little capacity to trust or empathise with others and can only deal with emotional distress or frustration through some physical act; they are not usually suffering from a psychiatric illness.

Psychological consequences

In many ways, the psychological consequences of being raped are similar to those found following any acute distressing event. However, rape involves both an intrusion of a sexual nature and a violent attack on the body. These factors make the psychological consequences profound and long-lasting. Burgess and Holstrom (1974) called the psychological reactions of the victim the *rape trauma syndrome*. This is characterised by three phases. Initially the victim is shocked and cannot cope with her normal everyday activities. After a few days feelings of guilt, self-blame and remorse occur, and these are often accompanied by various somatic complaints such as headache, abdominal pain, general weakness and palpitations. At this time anxiety becomes obvious and the victim may be frightened to go out, panic in the dark and avoid even trusted male friends. Later symptoms of depression emerge, and sleep disturbance, sexual difficulties and phobias of travelling alone may become severe. Normal sexual activity may not be resumed for three to six months. The husband or partner of the victim may suffer from similar difficulties, undergo marked emotional changes and become overprotective of his wife or girlfriend and even refuse to let her go out alone (Bateman 1986).

Treatment

Psychological help is often requested by rape victims. The commonest form of treatment available in the UK is counselling. This is offered by various voluntary support organisations and aims to help the victim return to a normal life and to alleviate feelings of guilt and unrealistic fears. On some occasions the reaction of the victim may be so severe that a psychiatric assessment is required followed by more intensive treatment, such as individual psychotherapy for the severe emotional difficulties, or a behavioural programme for any phobic symptoms. Counselling for families may also be required, especially if the victim has a partner or lives at home with her family.

Transvestism

Transvestism is the wearing of clothes appropriate to the opposite sex in order to obtain sexual excitement. It is almost exclusively a male activity, although a few cases of female transvestism have been reported. Some transvestites require only one garment, such as a piece of underwear, for their sexual satisfaction; others desire to be fully clothed in garments of the opposite sex. Occasionally a transvestite may wish to pass off as a member of the opposite sex over a period of time, but this is rare and probably indicates transsexual tendencies.

The male transvestite does not wish to become a woman; on the contrary his gender identity is predominantly as a man. He only wears women's clothes for full sexual excitement and almost always chooses a woman as his sexual partner. Thus most male transvestites are heterosexual and arouse themselves autoerotically by wearing a female garment. Female transvestites are almost always homosexual.

Transvestism is often known as fetishistic cross-dressing, as the female clothing is a specific fetish which is required for full sexual excitement and orgasm (Stoller 1971). However, cross-dressing initially used as a private and secret means of sexual arousal may later develop into a more overt activity and become linked to a sub-culture. In these cases gender identity may be more severely disturbed although, unlike the transsexual, the true transvestite never wishes to become a woman.

Cross-dressing is associated with the relief of anxiety as well as the stimulation of sexual pleasure. These different emotional responses to cross-dressing are sometimes used to identify different types of transvestism. Those patients who obtain sexual pleasures from cross-dressing are known as *symptomatic transvestites*, while those who primarily obtain relief from anxiety are known as *simple transvestites*. A simple transvestite may develop transsexual tendencies and wish to become a woman later in life. This differentiation is unhelpful as those individuals who obtain sexual pleasure from fetishistic cross-dressing, i.e. symptomatic transvestites, also obtain relief from anxiety if the act is compulsive and obligatory.

Transsexualism

A transsexual is an anatomically normal person who experiences himself as a member of the opposite sex. Transsexualism is rare. It is three times more common in men than women. The male transsexual believes he is a woman imprisoned in an anatomically masculine body.

There are two types of transsexualism. The *primary transsexual* has always experienced himself as a woman both in his early fantasy life and during his preferred childhood activities. His later interpersonal relationships and his social activities merely confirm his earlier beliefs. *Secondary transsexualism* arises out of some other condition such as homosexuality or transvestism. The secondary transsexual experiences urges to be feminine only later in life, usually during adolescence; before this he engaged in ordinary male behaviour. The feminine urges gradually develop into the wish to be a woman. The primary transsexual does not regard himself as homosexual nor does he have homosexual fantasies, whereas the secondary transsexual may do so. Both types of transsexuals seek surgical correction of their anatomy. In general terms the primary transsexual is likely to do better following surgical reassignment of his sex than the secondary transsexual. This and other aspects of treatment are discussed later in this chapter.

Treatment of the perversions

Treatment of patients with a sexual perversion is difficult. The patient may not wish to change, as his psychological state is the best possible adaptation under the circumstances. Change involves the risk of the release of aggression, violence and possible psychotic breakdown. Furthermore, many patients who present for treatment may not come under their own volition but as a result of social pressures, at their partner's insistence or sent by the courts. However, some patients do show a genuine wish to change and others a desire to feel better adjusted to their problems; it is probably these patients who benefit most from any treatment offered. Once the motivation of the patient and his aims have been established various treatments are available: psychoanalysis, psychotherapy, behaviour therapy and various physical treatments.

Psychoanalysis and psychotherapy

It is difficult to decide which patients with a perversion are suitable for psychoanalysis or psychotherapy. Those patients who show conflict about their perversion, i.e. on the one hand they experience depression and anxiety as a result of it and on the other they recognise the excitement contained within it, are probably the most suitable. Those patients who boast arrogantly of their perversion and are contemptuous of other normal activities are probably the least suitable. However, if these individuals are clearly aware that beneath this attitude of defiance lies an unthinkable pain they may be amenable to treatment. Primary transsexuals and patients who rely on severe sadomasochistic enactments to achieve orgasm rarely respond to psychotherapy.

The difficulties encountered by the therapist during treatment may be considerable. He is often treated in a manner similar to the way in which the patient treats his sexual object. For example, a masochist may provoke the therapist into attacking him verbally and enjoys being submissive, or a sadist may relentlessly attack the therapist verbally, trying, as it were, to get right inside him. This may become so frightening for the patient that he leaves therapy. In view of these intense anxieties, some patients are better treated in once-a-week psychotherapy rather than psychoanalysis. The treatment of patients with a perversion should only be considered by an experienced therapist.

In some cases it may have to be accepted that the perversion cannot be resolved; instead patients may be helped to reduce their need to act out their perversion and to lead a more contented life with less guilt and self-condemnation.

Behaviour therapy

Various behavioural treatments have been tried in the treatment of sexual perversions such as exhibitionism, fetishism, transvestism and some forms of homosexuality. Originally, the main emphasis was placed on the removal of behaviour of which the patient asked to be relieved. *Aversion therapy* was the method used to achieve this aim (McConaghy and Barr 1973). Mild electric shocks were administered either when the individual became aroused by the perverse stimulus, e.g. being shown a photograph of a naked young man in the case of a homosexual, or when he started to engage in his perverse activity, e.g. putting on female clothing in the case of a transvestite. Results of these early methods of using aversion therapy were very variable. The effect was often only short-lived and some patients became socially isolated and depressed because they had no alternative sexual outlet to replace their perverse form of gratification. Aversion therapy to decrease unwanted sexual behaviour has therefore been abandoned; instead increasing emphasis has been placed on using behavioural methods to increase more desirable forms of sexual behaviour (Bancroft 1983).

These methods include systematic desensitisation and positive conditioning. *Systematic desensitisation* is directed at the removal of anxiety experienced by the patient when confronted by a heterosexual stimulus. For example, some men experience severe anxiety when seeing female genitalia, or when conjuring them up in imagination, so that their perverse behaviour, e.g. use of a fetish or homosexuality, is at least in part due to the need to avoid heterosexual intercourse. If by means of graded desensitisation the patient's anxiety can gradually be reduced and ultimately extinguished, it is hoped that normal heterosexual desire and behaviour will increase.

In *positive conditioning* attempts are made to increase heterosexual desire by linking or pairing heterosexual stimuli or fantasies with sexual arousal. For example, when a homosexual has become aroused by a homosexual stimulus, say showing him a picture of, or asking him to fantasise about, some homosexual activity, he is presented with a heterosexual stimulus instead. Alternatively, he is told increasingly to conjure up heterosexual fantasies alongside his homosexual ones during masturbation. In this form of treatment the patient is instructed regularly to practise at home ways of linking sexual arousal with heterosexual images while masturbating or during sexual activity.

So far evidence about the effectiveness of these forms of behavioural therapy in the treatment of sexual perversion is limited, but in general long-term improvement is only seen in a small proportion of cases and adverse effects such as depression or breakdown of existing relationships are not uncommon. This is not surprising as sexual behaviour is intimately linked with many wider aspects of intrapsychic, interpersonal and social functioning. The patient's attitude to sexuality has to change as well as his overt sexual behaviour. Moreover, there is always a risk that a change in sexual behaviour may lead to the appearance of other forms of psychological or psychiatric disturbance, especially if, as is sometimes the case, the perverse behaviour served as a defence against a psychotic breakdown.

Ethical aspects must also be considered. Behavioural methods should only be used with the patient's own full agreement, and not under pressure from others, e.g. the courts, or at the request of a wife who insists that her husband gives up, say, his fetishistic behaviour or cross-dressing.

These various considerations, which are well known from psychoanalytic and psychotherapeutic work with patients with sexual perversions and deviations, are increasingly being taken into account by some behaviour therapists.

Drugs

Drugs are only used for those patients who show impulsive, repetitive and severely antisocial sexual behaviour which has been unresponsive to other treatments.

The anti-androgen cyproterone acetate suppresses hormonally determined sexual behaviour in men without inducing bodily feminisation. An initial dose of 100 mg daily is used to suppress sexual desire and a lower maintenance dose of 25 mg daily is then instituted. It is used more often on the Continent than in the UK. Other drugs such as benperidol, a butyrophenone, are also said to suppress sexual desire.

Surgical reassignment of sex

Most transsexuals refuse any treatment other than surgical reassignment of their sex. The treatment is contentious and only available in a few centres (Meyer and Reter 1979). Before a final decision is taken about surgery the transsexual is usually asked to live as a member of the opposite sex for up to two years. If this trial period is successful surgery may be offered. Some patients decline the offer, preferring to continue to cross-dress or to find satisfactory adjustment as a homosexual. Most of these patients are probably secondary transsexuals.

Only primary transsexuals should be offered surgery. The male transsexual requests removal of the penis and testes, the formation of a vagina, the development of breasts either by implants or by hormones, and the softening of body shape and removal of body hair by the use of oestrogens and electrolysis. The female transsexual seeks bilateral mastectomy, hysterectomy and on occasions the creation of an artificial penis. Secondary sexual characteristics of the male may be developed by testosterone.

Both before and after surgery the transsexual and his family will require a great deal of support and counselling (Money and Walker 1977). The difficult problem of the treatment of transsexuals has been discussed fully by Bancroft (1983).

FURTHER READING

Bancroft, J. (1983). *Human Sexuality and its Problems*. Churchill Livingstone, Edinburgh.

Freud, S, (1905). 'Three essays on the theory of sexuality', *Standard Edition*, vol. 7. Hogarth, London.

Kaplan, H.S. (1983). *The Evaluation of Sexual Disorders: psychological and medical aspects*. Brunner/Mazel, New York.

Mezey, G.C. (1985). 'Rape – victimological and psychiatric aspects'. *Brit. J. Hosp. Med.* 33, 152-158.

Rosen, I. (ed.) (1979). *Sexual Deviation*, 2nd ed. OUP, Oxford.

Stoller, R.J. (1975). *Perversion: the erotic form of hatred*. Harvester Press, Suffolk; reissued 1986 by Maresfield Library, Karnac, London.

29

Homosexuality

In recent years homosexuality has come to be regarded as a socially acceptable form of behaviour. It is common and has existed in many societies to a greater or lesser degree. Both male and female homosexuality were widely accepted in ancient Greece; Sappho, the poetess who expressed homosexual longings in her poetry, lived on the Aegean island of Lesbos, from which the term lesbianism is derived. Dover (1978) has discussed the nature and role of both male and female homosexuality in ancient Greece with special reference to its influence on society, literature and art.

In this country homosexuality used to be not only socially unacceptable but also a criminal offence, and although the Wolfenden Report of 1957 recommended changes in the law these were not enacted until 1967. The Sexual Offences Act of 1967 allows homosexual behaviour to take place in private between consenting males who are both over the age of twenty-one. This is in contrast to the age of sixteen in the case of heterosexual relations. Attempting to procure a male partner or actually engaging in homosexual behaviour in public remains a criminal offence, as does homosexual intercourse under the age of twenty-one. Homosexual behaviour by members of the Armed Forces and Merchant Seamen also remains illegal (Freeman 1979). There is no law governing homosexual behaviour between women.

The label of homosexuality is used in our society in many different ways. It may be used pejoratively or to justify social repression or even to humiliate an individual. There is no place for these attitudes, least of all in medical practice, and doctors should treat patients who present with problems connected with their homosexuality just as they would any other patient, i.e. with understanding and frankness and without condemnation or disapproval. The purpose of this chapter is to offer guidelines for understanding homosexuality and not to condemn it.

One way of defining homosexuality is in terms of behaviour, a homosexual being a person who repeatedly or episodically engages in sexual relations with a member of the same sex. If the individual engages in sexual relations with a member of the opposite sex little or no pleasure or satisfaction occurs. Those individuals who wish to have sexual relationships with a member of the same sex but do not do so are often said to show latent homosexuality. In many ways this definition of homosexuality is an umbrella term which says little, if anything, about the individual's personality, motivation or intent.

In fact homosexuality is a syndrome and not a unitary condition. Not all homosexuals are the same, and in clinical practice it is better to recognise that there are several different types of homosexuality. These are discussed below.

PREVALENCE

Kinsey and his co-workers (1948, 1953) reported on the sexual activity of a cross-section of the white American population. In a sample of 4,000 males it was estimated that 4 per cent were exclusively homosexual throughout their lives and that 37 per cent had had some adult homosexual experience leading to orgasm; the majority of these had occurred during adolescence. Available figures for women are probably less reliable but are consistently lower than for men. Kenyon (1968) estimates that about 1 in 45 of the adult female population, just under 2 per cent, is exclusively homosexual, about half as many as male homosexuals. Furthermore only 6 per cent of women, as compared with 30 per cent of men, had had some homosexual experience at some time in their lives. More recent studies by Gagnon and Simon (1973) have reached broadly similar conclusions.

Some reports, especially those from the homosexual community, have suggested that the figures for male homosexuality given above are far too low and that up to the two-thirds of the twenty to forty-year-old group have had some homosexual experience. It may well be that anxiety about AIDS (see p. 286) deters some people from experimenting with homosexuality who might otherwise be interested.

CLINICAL TYPES

The question is often asked whether all homosexuality should be considered to be a perversion. This depends on the definition of a perversion, which is discussed fully on p. 354. Following that definition, only that sub-group of homosexuals in whom a compulsive sexual fantasy dominates their sexual behaviour, and in whom sexual impulses are associated with aggressive rather than affectionate feelings, fall into the category of perversion. Other forms of homosexuality do not fall clearly under this category. The different clinical types will be considered next.

Many individuals, especially young people, have homosexual fantasies which cause them suffering, discomfort and guilt. They begin to believe themselves to be homosexual and become anxious, depressed or even suicidal. It is important not to assume that these individuals are necessarily homosexual. The presence of distress and guilt suggests this may not be the case. The fantasies may in fact be a way of coping with anxiety about heterosexual activity and feelings of inadequacy in relation to the opposite sex. Some may have a brief homosexual affair and, when it breaks up, experience great distress. Once again the homosexual affair does not confirm that the person is a homosexual, and a knowledge of the individual's motivation and underlying anxieties and wishes is essential. Some members of this group may find it difficult to choose between a person of the same or opposite sex and are often labelled bisexual. Careful interviewing usually reveals the nature of the underlying fantasies, and they may indicate, for example, that the homosexuality is a defence against anxiety associated with heterosexual intimacy. In some people, especially late adolescents and young adults, a period during which homosexual fantasies and relationships are prominent, homosexuality may be a passing phase on the way to heterosexuality. Sometimes the individual's anxiety about being homosexual may be so severe that it can only be relieved by 'coming out'. This enables the individual to feel accepted as a homosexual and thereby at ease with what he erroneously believes is his homosexuality. Later experiences may cause the individual to reconsider his or her sexual identity (Blumstein and Schwartz 1976).

In contrast to the group described above, other individuals may feel fully adjusted to their homosexuality and form stable and long-lasting relationships similar in strength and affection to happily married heterosexual couples. Their personalities are well-integrated and their social adaptation is good. Some of these couples may have a more open relationship in which casual affairs are tacitly permitted though not allowed to interfere with the primary relationship. These individuals rarely, if ever, attend psychiatric clinics for problems related to their homosexuality, and any problems that may arise are satisfactorily overcome just as in heterosexuals who have problems in their relationships.

It is within a third group that true homosexual perversion is found. In this group the homosexual fantasies are compulsively acted out and always contain a wish to control, dominate or hurt the partner. Sometimes these wishes may be reversed and lead to the wish to be dominated, beaten or used. Hence the mistaken belief that homosexuals are either active or passive. This is not the case, as the majority of homosexuals are flexible about their activities – although full gratification may only be obtained if one particular fantasy is acted out. In the more perverse group failure to establish a lasting relationship, promiscuity, sadomasochistic relationships, brief, purely sexual encounters, e.g. in public lavatories, and marked identification with the opposite sex are common. Distress concerning these activities is often absent, but some may experience loneliness, depression, low self-esteem and suicidal ideas, and present to the psychiatrist, perhaps after a court appearance. In some the disorganisation in lifestyle and personality may be so great as to suggest an underlying tendency to psychotic breakdown. At interview paranoid ideas may be marked and the individual may view the whole world as a threatening hostile place. Others protect themselves from these fears and paranoid feelings by becoming aggressive to others, especially their superiors, or by having violent rows with their sexual partners. In this perverse group of homosexuals an underlying personality disorder is always present, usually characterised by an inability to form meaningful and lasting relationships with another person.

The existence of these different clinical types of homosexuality serves to emphasise that homosexuality is not a unitary condition. However, to classify individuals in this way has its limitations and the three groups described may overlap. The categories should not therefore be used rigidly.

AETIOLOGY

The possible role of genetic and neuroendocrine factors in the origin of homosexuality is discussed on p. 355. Whatever the contribution of these factors to homosexuality, it is largely the relationship of the child to his parents and social influences which are important in the genesis of sexual orientation. Thus homosexuality has multiple determinants and no single factor can be put forward as its cause. Furthermore the origins of male and female homosexuality are likely to be different. However, certain early childhood difficulties can be discerned, especially in male homosexuality.

The background of male homosexuals commonly reveals an over-intimate mother who psychologically envelops the child and prevents him from developing autonomy. The child then becomes caught between his early state of symbiotic closeness to his mother and his attempts to separate. This inner conflict results in excessive anger and frustration so that aggressive wishes towards the mother begin to predominate. An absent, weak or rejecting father may compound this problem as the son is unable to model himself on and identify with his father. This constellation becomes fixed in the child's psychological development and distorts the later development of sexual identity by preventing the development of a sense of maleness (Bieber 1965; Zuger 1978). Later in life the conflict is resolved by running away from women, as only then can the intolerable anxiety, anger and frustration be avoided. Brief affairs with women may occur, but they inevitably rekindle these earlier feelings of being trapped by the mother or of feeling angry with her. These are then experienced in relation to the female partner and lead to a retreat from heterosexual relationships. However, the need for closeness remains and can only be found safely by choosing a man as a sexual partner instead.

Other psychological factors can be delineated in homosexuality. A sense of maleness, mentioned above, may be poorly developed in some homosexuals and only strengthened by identifying with the masculinity of the partner. Some homosexuals therefore choose a male partner whose masculine attributes and physical appearance are well-developed. These individuals feel strengthened during sexual activity by temporarily fusing and identifying with their partner.

Some of these factors are also found to be important in the genesis of homosexuality in women, though in reverse. For example, Wolf (1979) considered that the mothers of homosexual women were rejecting or distant. Homosexual women may therefore look for love and physical closeness from their partners to make up for what they missed out on in relation to their own mothers earlier in life. Moreover, just as the homosexual male may feel threatened by close physical contact with a woman, the homosexual woman may feel frightened of men, especially if the penis is felt to be a frightening and dangerous object. Sometimes these fears may arise out of the belief that their own fathers were sadistic, powerful and dominating individuals. These ideas have received some confirmation from Bene (1965), who made a systematic comparison between a group of lesbians and a group of married women. The lesbians were more often hostile towards and afraid of their fathers than the married women and felt little affection towards their mothers, whom they perceived and as cold and unemotional.

Whatever the causes of male and female homosexuality, each individual who comes for help should be assessed in his or her own right and not from a preconceived viewpoint; a company director, a doctor, a clergyman, and a psychopathic criminal may all be homosexual, but the factors which have moulded them may be radically different.

PSYCHIATRIC SYMPTOMS

Depression and attempted suicide are more common among men with a homosexual problem than among heterosexual men (Bell and Weinberg 1978). There are several reasons which make homosexuals seek help from a psychiatrist. These include a strong sense of guilt which often accompanies their sexual feelings and activities. Some of this guilt arises from earlier unresolved conflicts and becomes compounded by society's rejecting attitude. Occasionally the attitude of society is misperceived and exaggerated to justify self-condemnation and explain an over-whelming sense of shame. The doctor's task is to help such an individual to overcome this self-punitive attitude and ease his sense of shame. It should then become easier for him to accept his homosexuality.

Most homosexuals overcome their sense of guilt and are then able to develop more stable and intimate relationships. Some may have to rely on alcohol or drugs to diminish their guilt, though more often a greater sense of assurance is developed by mixing within a homosexual sub-culture, and some individuals choose an occupation in which they believe their sexuality will not be condemned. Homosexual affairs rarely last a lifetime, and older homosexuals may become increasingly isolated and lonely. Others may become depressed when facing the fact that as homosexuals they may never have a family of their own.

The problems of homosexuals have been exacerbated by the growing incidence of AIDS. Not only has this increased the prejudice against homosexuality held by some members of society, but some homosexuals have understandably become more anxious about contracting or passing on the disease and guilty about promiscuity (see p. 287).

Any of these problems may lead the homosexual to wish that his sexual orientation was different or could be changed. Thus an inner struggle may result leading to anxiety, depression or psychosomatic complaints, but a doctor should not assume that all the problems or symptoms of a homosexual are necessarily due to his homosexuality.

TREATMENT

Homosexuals are unlikely to consult their doctors unless they are in some way dissatisfied with their sexual orientation or it has led to symptoms such as depression or anxiety. Occasionally they may be referred by a court, e.g. for soliciting in a public lavatory or engaging in homosexual activities with a person under the age of twenty-one. A few male homosexuals ask for help with a sexual dysfunction such as impotence. They can sometimes be helped by sex therapy similar to that used for heterosexuals (Masters and Johnson 1979).

In many cases the aim of treatment will be to help the person to come to terms with his homosexual orientation and to help him overcome his feelings of guilt. If this is achieved he may be able to establish more stable and satisfying relationships. Occasionally a homosexual may wish to achieve a heterosexual orientation, but this is difficult to accomplish, especially if an individual has lived exclusively as a homosexual for many years. Attempts to alter sexual orientation are more likely to succeed if the person has at least some heterosexual desire and shows a sincere wish to change. He must also be prepared to accept that prolonged therapy may be needed.

The two main forms of treatment are psychotherapy or psychoanalysis, and behaviour therapy.

Psychotherapy

The form of psychotherapy chosen depends to a large extent on the wishes and aims of the patient. Some patients will need supportive psychotherapy to help them overcome short-term difficulties associated with their homosexuality such as the break-up of a relationship, while others may benefit from analytically-orientated psychotherapy, individually or in a group, to come to terms with feelings of shame and guilt. Those who genuinely seek a change in sexual orientation probably do best in psychoanalysis, although it may become clear during treatment that their true aim is to feel better adjusted to their homosexuality.

Behaviour therapy

The behavioural treatments to alter sexual orientation are described in

Chapter 28 (see p. 366). Earlier attempts to use aversion therapy have not proved successful in the long term. Nowadays behavioural methods are mainly used to reduce any anxiety the individual may have about heterosexual activity and to encourage heterosexual fantasies and behaviour (Bancroft 1983).

FURTHER READING

Dover, K.J. (1978). *Greek Homosexuality*. Duckworth, London.

Friedman, R.C. (1988). *Male Homosexuality: a contemporary psychoanalytic perspective*. Yale University Press, Newhaven and London.

Limentani, A. (1979). 'Clinical types of homosexuality' in *Sexual Deviation*, 2nd ed. (Rosen, I., ed.). OUP, Oxford.

Stein, T.S. and Cohen, C. (eds) (1986). *Contemporary Perspectives on Psychotherapy with Lesbians and Gay Men*. Plenum Press, New York.

The following novels are also of interest:

Baldwin, J. (1965). *Another Country*. Corgi, London.

Hall, R. (1987). *The Well of Loneliness*. Virago, London.

30

Alcoholism

Alcohol damages the physical, psychological and social well-being of an individual when drunk in excess or over long periods of time. Doctors tend to focus on the severe physical damage that occurs with excess alcohol consumption, but the psychological and social effects are equally serious and occur earlier in an alcoholic's decline. For example, depression, irritability, marital disharmony, accidents and disruption of employment may occur as soon as a drinking pattern becomes established, whereas serious physical damage may take many years to develop.

There is no fixed level of alcohol intake which determines whether an individual is alcohol-dependent or not. This is because the same amount of alcohol affects individuals differently. For example, women are more likely than men to suffer liver damage and progress to cirrhosis; some individuals are prone to aggressive outbursts due to the disinhibiting action of alcohol, while others may become depressed and suicidal.

DEFINITION

There is no satisfactory definition of alcoholism, but the most widely quoted criteria are those put forward by the World Health Organisation in 1952 and those found in the ICD-9 and DSM-III. Rather than quote each definition in turn, it is worthwhile examining the features which are common to all three definitions. First, there is the question whether the individual can control his alcohol consumption. He may be unable to either because of the need to experience the psychological effects of alcohol or because of the need to stave off physical withdrawal symptoms. This compulsion to drink or *alcohol dependence syndrome* (Edwards and Gross 1976) is one aspect of recent definitions. The second aspect focuses on the consequences of the compulsion; this is expressed in terms of physical, psychological and social function. Impairment of function in one or more of these areas is required to fulfil the criteria. The severity of an individual's alcohol dependence therefore depends on the strength of his compulsion to drink and the degree of damage caused by his drinking, both to himself and others.

EPIDEMIOLOGY

There is no accurate assessment of the number of alcoholics in the UK although figures of 250,000–500,000 in England and Wales are widely quoted, with a higher prevalence in men than women. These figures are less than in other countries such as the USA and France. Estimates are based on either field surveys or indirect methods. Examples of the former include general practice surveys. Thus Wilkins (1974) examined a practice in Manchester and concluded that out of a population of 12,000 registered patients, 155 were alcoholics and a further 250 were abnormal drinkers. Indirect estimates involve studying some alcohol-related factor, such as convictions for drunken driving, hospital admissions for alcoholism or the frequency of cirrhosis of the liver. It is assumed that an increase in these factors over time reflects an increase in the prevalence of alcoholism. These methods suggest a prevalence of alcoholism of 11 per 1000 in England and Wales. The prevalence of alcoholism increases as the per capita consumption of alcohol in the population increases. In the majority of countries surveyed over the last decade the per capita consumption has increased, and in the UK alcohol consumption has almost doubled in the past thirty years with a corresponding increase in alcoholism and cirrhosis. In contrast the prevalence of cirrhosis of the liver fell markedly during Prohibition in the USA.

Although alcohol abuse is found in all walks of life, certain groups are at greater risk. Men aged between forty and fifty-five who are divorced or separated and work in such occupations as journalism, the arts or medicine run the greater risk. Publicans, actors, printers, seamen and executives are also at risk (Murray 1975). The greatest increase in alcoholism is currently being seen in women and young adults under the age of twenty-five.

AETIOLOGY

There is no single reason why certain individuals abuse alcohol to the extent that they become physically and psychologically addicted to the detriment of their general well-being. Certainly the amount of alcohol available is important. However, genetic, personality and environmental factors are also of importance.

Genetic factors

Genetic studies of twins and adoptees show that there is an important genetic component to alcoholism. Concordance rates are higher in monozygotic than dizygotic twins (Kaij 1960), and the sons of alcoholic fathers adopted at birth have higher rates of alcoholism than adopted sons of non-alcoholic fathers (Goodwin *et al.* 1973). Attention has also been focussed on genetically determined biochemical factors (Ewing *et al.* 1974). For example, the enzyme alcohol dehydrogenase affects the rate of metabolism of alcohol, and minor variations in its activity may influence an individual's subjective experience of having taken alcohol, leading some people to find it more pleasurable than others.

Personality factors

Certain personality characteristics are commonly observed in alcoholics but there is no specific personality type regularly associated with alcohol abuse (Kessel and Walton 1969). However, Hesselbrock *et al.* (1985) found an antisocial personality disorder in nearly 50 per cent of hospitalised male alcoholics. It is important to remember that alcohol can profoundly affect an individual's personality, making it difficult to distinguish cause from effect. Alcoholics tend to react badly to frustrations, have low self-esteem and require continual appreciation. Whenever frustration looms they may become ingratiating, manipulative, demanding and persuasive; aggressive and violent tendencies are not far beneath the surface and are manifested as soon as any desires are thwarted. For example an alcoholic who feels the need for hospital admission may flatter the doctor, express sincere desire to reform and promise to abide by an inpatient contract. As soon as craving for alcohol becomes overwhelming, often after physical withdrawal has taken place, the promises are forgotten and the more the doctors and nurses impose sanctions the more the desire for alcohol increases. At this point anger may become overt, but more often the attack on the 'helpers' is covert and takes the form of secret drinking while appearing to abide by the original contract. Many of these characteristics are also found in other forms of drug abuse and are not specific to alcoholics. The history of some alcoholics suggests that as children they were already abnormally aggressive and antisocial; these characteristics continue into adult life and mask feelings of inadequacy, inferiority and sometimes homosexuality.

Learning factors

Learning theory stresses the effect of parental modelling on the development of alcohol abuse. Once a drinking pattern is established from modelling it becomes reinforced by the pleasurable feelings experienced with alcohol consumption.

Environmental factors

Cultural factors influence the individual's attitude to alcohol. For example, alcohol consumption is often considered to be a mark of masculinity in Western culture. This is reinforced by advertising. Individuals with a poor self-image, feelings of inferiority and sexual problems may need to adopt a façade of masculinity of which excessive drinking may form a part. Some occupations, e.g. being a barman or journalist, increase the risk of excessive drinking.

Psychiatric factors

Alcohol can also be a symptom of other psychiatric conditions. For example, individuals who suffer from an anxiety neurosis, depression, or social inadequacy or a social phobia may resort to alcohol as a form of self-medication. Alcohol abuse may also occur in the major psychoses. In fact, any physical pain or psychological distress may lead to alcohol abuse.

CLINICAL FEATURES

Alcohol has a number of pleasurable effects. It induces relaxation, relieves tension and gives a general sense of well-being. Initially only small amounts of alcohol are needed, but tolerance occurs and increasing amounts are required to achieve the same effect. This *pre-alcoholic phase* may last many years, but if underlying problems remain unresolved drinking continues and becomes a regular activity which takes precedence over everything else, including the family and work. As tolerance increases the drinker experiences a craving for alcohol and believes he can 'hold his drink'. He may continue to perform skilled tasks such as operating machinery or driving a car while drinking and denies he has any difficulties or is running a serious risk. His family and employers may notice a change in his personality and a decline in his abilities, but attempts to discuss the problems and to control his drinking only lead to increasing irritability, arguments and denial. Secret drinking may then become established and persist for many years.

Ultimately drinking starts early in the morning in an attempt to stave off withdrawal symptoms such as tremor, nausea, sweating and anxiety. The first drink alleviates these symptoms, calm returns and an *alcohol dependence syndrome* has become established. Ethical standards deteriorate, lying is common, accidents are frequent and cider and 'Special Brew' are drunk to obtain the most alcohol for the least money. At this point tolerance may fall and even small amounts of alcohol induce severe incapacity.

The damage caused by alcohol to an individual's physical, psychological and social functioning may be severe even if an alcohol dependence syndrome is not fully established. For example, marital disharmony may result from only moderate drinking and loss of employment from occasional drunkenness. Nevertheless, the features described below are usually more severe if excessive drinking has been prolonged.

Alcohol affects every system of the body, either due to a direct toxic effect or as a result of associated dietary deficiencies. The general medical consequences of excess alcohol consumption are too varied to discuss here. However, alcohol abuse should be suspected in any patient presenting with gastritis, peptic ulcers, pancreatitis, cirrhosis or peripheral neuropathy. Infections, including tuberculosis, are also common.

NEUROPSYCHIATRIC DISORDERS

These may be divided into three groups: intoxication phenomena, withdrawal phenomena, and disorders due to nutritional deficiencies.

Intoxication phenomena

Occasionally a heavy drinking bout can lead to an acute psychotic episode in which the patient becomes maniacal, violent and destructive. This is referred to as *pathological intoxication*. It is rare.

Memory blackouts are more common and indicate persistent heavy drinking if they occur regularly. Characteristically, there is amnesia for events that occurred during a drinking bout even though no gross change in the level of consciousness may have been noticed by others.

Withdrawal phenomena

Simple withdrawal symptoms occur in individuals who have been drinking heavily for some months or years. Symptoms usually occur early in the morning when the alcohol level is falling. They usually begin 3-12 hours after the last drink. Marked tremor is associated with sweating, nausea, restlessness and irritability. Misinterpretation of the environment may occur, leading to fearfulness and panic. All these symptoms are quickly relieved by alcohol.

Delirium tremens

Delirium tremens is the most serious of the withdrawal phenomena. It occurs in patients who have been drinking heavily for many years, usually when they drink less or stop drinking. The symptoms are conveniently divided into two groups: mental and somatic. They are invariably associated with clouding of consciousness and disorientation in time and place.

The *mental symptoms* include severe restlessness and agitation, fearfulness, and perceptual disturbances such as visual, tactile and auditory hallucinations. Visual hallucinations are the most common and may be very vivid. Misinterpretations of sensations or tactile hallucinations may lead to the belief that insects are crawling over the body so that the patient frantically tries to remove them.

Somatic symptoms include severe tremor, sweating, ataxia and epileptic fits. Complete insomnia may last for days. Examination usually reveals a tachycardia, raised blood pressure and dilated pupils. A head injury and chest infection should be excluded. Electrolyte disturbances, including hypokalaemia, hypomagnesaemia, alkalosis and dehydration are common. Liver function tests may be impaired, and hypoglycaemia can occur. There is a mortality of about 15 per cent unless the condition is rapidly controlled with intravenous diazepam or chlormethiazole, and all physical complications are treated, including the correction of dehydration and electrolyte disturbances. Intravenous parentrovite may be given (Victor 1983).

Alcoholic hallucinosis

This condition usually arises within the context of a changing alcohol level. It may, therefore, be associated with an increase or a decrease in consumption. Characteristically the patient suffers from persistent, threatening, fully-formed *auditory hallucinations* with no change in the level of consciousness. The patient is usually frightened and may develop paranoid delusions secondary to the hallucinations. The clinical picture may be difficult to distinguish from schizophrenia, but the history of alcoholism should assist in the diagnosis. Alcoholic hallucinosis usually clears within a few days or weeks after stopping drinking, but it may become chronic.

Nutritional disorders

These include Wernicke's encephalopathy and Korsakoff's psychosis, the combination of the two now being known as the Wernicke-Korsakoff syndrome, and alcoholic dementia.

Wernicke-Korsakoff syndrome

Wernicke's encephalopathy is the acute precursor of Korsakoff's psychosis and results from *thiamine deficiency*. It is characterised by sudden onset of ataxia, paralysis of external ocular movements, nystagmus and a confusional state. A peripheral neuropathy is common. Death may result unless prompt treatment with intravenous thiamine is given. Even with early treatment the majority of patients develop the chronic syndrome of Korsakoff's psychosis. Strictly speaking this is not a psychosis but consists of an *amnesic syndrome* (see also p. 34). The cardinal symptom is severe impairment of recent memory so that new learning becomes impossible and the patient is grossly disorientated. Immediate memory is preserved so that the patient can repeat a few digits or a name immediately after having been told them but will have forgotten them a few seconds later. Remote memory may be partly preserved but past memories may be used inappropriately to answer questions about current events; or patients produce answers which are completely false, so-called confabulations. Treatment consists of parenteral administration of vitamin B1.

After recovery from the acute stage the amnesic syndrome and a retrograde amnesia, often covering a long period before the onset of the illness, persist in about 50 per cent of patients; in the remainder there may be partial recovery.

The same histopathological changes are seen in Wernicke's encephalopathy and in Korsakoff's psychosis, namely petechial haemorrhages in the mamillary bodies, the periaqueductal grey matter and some thalamic nuclei. This is why the two conditions, originally described separately by Wernicke and Korsakoff respectively, are now grouped together as the Wernicke-Korsakoff syndrome.

Alcoholic dementia

Intellectual and personality deterioration probably occur in all heavy drinkers. However, older patients and patients who drink heavily without respite are at risk of developing alcoholic dementia. Nutritional deficiency may play a part, but so may a toxic effect of alcohol on brain cells. Alzheimer's dementia may be an associated disorder.

The clinical picture of alcoholic dementia is similar to that of other dementias (see p. 268). CT scanning shows enlarged ventricles and diffuse cortical atrophy. Abstinence may lead to improvement on the CT scan (Ron 1983).

PSYCHOLOGICAL EFFECTS

Alcohol has a profound effect on mood and may induce bouts of *depression*. However, the inter-relationship between alcohol and mood is complex as some depressed patients drink to alleviate their depression.

Initially alcohol may induce a state of fatuous euphoria, but prolonged drinking leads to bouts of depression and low self-esteem. However much an alcoholic initially deceives himself and others, in particular doctors, there are times when he is well aware of his alcohol problem and feels helpless and depressed. In addition he is aware of society's stigmatising and punitive attitude to alchoholism and sees himself as deserving punishment. His family, social and financial position may markedly deteriorate and the inevitable consequence is a further loss of self-esteem and a deepening of the depression. As a result *suicide* and *acts of self-harm* are common. Between 10-15 per cent of alcoholics end their lives by suicide. Alcohol is frequently consumed before acts of self-harm, and alcoholism is diagnosed in approximately 20 per cent of men and 15 per cent of women who harm themselves.

Another consequence of alcohol abuse is impairment of *sexual function*. There is an impairment of both sexual desire and sexual arousal, leading to erectile impotence in men and lack of sexual response in women. Of course sexual problems may themselves lead to alcohol abuse. Another condition associated with alcoholism is *morbid jealousy*, described in Chapter 21 (see p. 256).

SOCIAL DAMAGE

The social consequences of alcoholism either result from the physical and psychological consequences discussed above or arise independently. This can be the result of the alcoholic misperceiving his environment and misinterpreting verbal and non-verbal cues from other people. This is not necessarily related to an alcohol-induced psychosis or to being drunk. Thus the alcoholic, especially when in the company of other alcoholics, may suddenly become aggressive in response to a look or an innocuous remark which he misinterprets as hostile, or he may misperceive a person's behaviour as amorous and respond to it only to be rejected. It is unclear whether this process is due to the disinhibiting effects of alcohol on the personality or whether it results from the direct effect of alcohol on cognitive function; whatever the cause, the inability of the alcoholic to interpret correctly the cues other people give him may have profound adverse effects on his personal and social relationships.

Family disruption

The serious effects of alcoholism on family life have already been mentioned. There is also an association between domestic violence and alcoholism. Wife battering and child abuse are often perpetrated by alcoholic men.

Problems at work

The ability to work efficiently is impaired by alcoholism. Absenteeism is twice as frequent in alcoholics than non-alcoholics, and may be due to both physical and psychological factors. Eventual loss of employment will increase the financial burden on the alcoholic who is already spending large amounts of money on alcohol (Tether and Robinson 1988).

Crime

Approximately a third of the prison population are alcoholics. Alcohol problems are particularly common in those prisoners who commit petty crimes. It is often not clear whether alcohol causes the criminal behaviour or is an associated finding (see p. 697).

Vagrancy

'Skid Row' is the final destination for the chronic alcoholic if he loses his job, family, money, health and reason. Occasionally the adoption of a vagrant lifestyle results from a deliberate decision by the alcoholic to give up his previous social position in the hope that he may be able to return at a later date. This phenomenon is increasingly seen in the young homeless unemployed alcoholics who gravitate to the centre of large cities.

DETECTION AND ASSESSMENT

Among health professionals, the general practitioner is often best placed to detect alcoholism, but his success in so doing depends on his alertness. He should be particularly suspicious of high-risk groups such as psychiatric patients, patients who work in high-risk occupations, and those who have marital problems, a family history of alcoholism and, of course, those who smell of drink.

The next step is to take a detailed history followed by a physical examination and laboratory investigations. The presence of abnormal liver function tests, especially of raised glutamyl transferase, a macrocytosis and a decreased folate level are useful physical indicators of alcohol abuse.

Once alcoholism is suspected, assessment needs to be made of the severity of the problem in terms of the amount consumed and the individual's psychological, social and physical health. In addition any perpetuating factors need to be identified. To achieve these aims it is often useful to get an hour-by-hour account of what the patient does on a heavy drinking day. This should include how he feels on waking, when and why he takes his first drink, what makes him drink again during the day, how much and what he drinks, the effect of drinking on him and others, and so on in detail throughout the day. This provides a much better and usually more honest and accurate picture of his drinking habits than a general question such as 'How much on average do you drink per day?', which usually only leads to evasive or dishonest replies. Such a detailed and sympathetic enquiry is also more likely to make the patient feel that the doctor is on his side and wanting to help rather than criticise.

TREATMENT

The first step in the treatment of alcoholism is for the doctor to be sympathetic and supportive and not critical and condemning. He needs to be firm but not punitive, to avoid capitulating to unreasonable demands, and to treat the patient with understanding and hope. Many alcoholics are ambivalent about seeking treatment and will use any negative response from the doctor as an excuse for refusing or breaking off treatment.

Treatment of alcoholism consists of withdrawal from alcohol followed by maintenance of abstinence or controlled drinking. Treatment methods have recently been reviewed by Edwards (1988).

Withdrawal

This is often known as *detoxification* and is best done as an inpatient in a general hospital or in a specialised alcohol unit. However, outpatient withdrawal may be safe in well motivated patients. The aim is to avoid or minimise the development of delirium tremens and epileptic fits. This is achieved by the use of sedation either orally or parenterally. The drugs of choice are either chlormethiazole or chlordiazepoxide. For example, a dose of 20 mg four times a day is used initially and reduced over a period of about 7-10 days. A longer period increases the risk of dependence. High potency vitamins such as parentrovite are also given and fluid and electrolyte balance carefully monitored.

After successful withdrawal the use of other drugs is limited. It is best to avoid prescribing drugs such as benzodiazepines to patients who have withdrawn from alcohol as there is a danger of substituting one drug of dependence for another. However, certain drugs are occasionally used as adjuncts to other treatments. The most commonly used are deterrent drugs which sensitise the body to alcohol, such as *disulfiram* (Antabuse) and *citrated calcium carbimide* (Abstem); these are given daily. They inhibit the enzyme which carries alcohol metabolism beyond the acetaldehyde stage thus causing an accumulation of acetaldehyde in the blood if alcohol is taken. This results in very unpleasant and sometimes dangerous symptoms such as vasodilatation with flushing, throbbing headache, nausea and vomiting, and a fall in blood pressure. The patient must be strongly warned of the dangerous consequences of drinking while taking these drugs. On no account should they be prescribed without the patient being given full information about their use and effects. They are used less often than they used to be because of their possible dangers.

Maintenance of abstinence

The most important factor in maintaining abstinence is the patient's own motivation. Motivation changes over time and an alcoholic may quite suddenly lose all motivation, e.g. following a minor set-back in life. A carefully arranged support network is therefore essential if abstinence is to be maintained. Self-help groups such as Alcoholics Anonymous should form part of the support system as they can be contacted quickly in a crisis. Treatments which help patients remain abstinent are discussed below.

Supportive psychotherapy

This is vital in the treatment of alcoholics and in maintaining abstinence. Alcohol abuse is a symptom of some underlying psychological distress and this usually becomes evident when the patient has withdrawn from alcohol. In particular group therapy can help the patient understand the nature of his distress and prevent relapse. Such therapy is usually carried out in special groups for alcoholics and the mutual support is particularly valuable.

Self-help groups

The best-known self-help organisation is *Alcoholics Anonymous* (AA) which was started 50 years ago in the USA by two ex-alcoholics. The organisation holds regular group meetings and has branches all over the UK and elsewhere. Members may attend as many meetings as they wish but twice weekly attendance is recommended. The group activities are varied and include self-revelation and the discussion of the dangers of alcohol. Some people find the attitude of AA too moralistic, but others greatly value its continuing support and help at times of threatened relapse. The aim is to encourage total abstinence rather than a return to social drinking.

Two related organisations are Alanon and Alateen, which provide support for the spouses and children of alcoholics respectively.

Social support

The provision of after-care in terms of accommodation and financial assistance is important. There is no point in providing intensive treatment in a hospital setting or specialised alcohol unit if the patient is discharged to a life of homelessness or bed and breakfast accommodation. Hostels or therapeutic communities specialising in the care of alcoholics are very useful. The majority insist on abstinence as a condition of entry and continuing residence, and they offer long-term care and counselling.

Controlled drinking

The maintenance of abstinence used to be the goal in the treatment of alcoholism, but it is now becoming recognised that this may be unrealistic for some patients and that for them an attempt to establish a pattern of controlled drinking may be more appropriate (Sobell and Sobell 1974). Controlled drinking refers to the establishment of a normal drinking pattern. This means a drinking pattern which is characterised by periods of total abstinence, interspersed with social drinking. The individual should be able to revert to total abstinence when desired.

Attempts are made to modify drinking behaviour by identifying cues which lead the alcoholic to drink, e.g. passing a pub, and helping him resist the compulsion. In addition goals are set and worked towards in a graded fashion so that eventually the ex-alcoholic may even be able to sit in a pub and drink socially without the danger of relapse into alcoholism. This approach is of particular benefit for those patients who may find that total abstinence leads to social isolation because any attempt to socialise with friends risks relapse. It is estimated that less than 2 per cent of alcoholics are able to benefit from this approach (Helzer *et al.* 1985), and the use of controlled drinking as an alternative to abstinence has recently been questioned (Hore 1987).

PROGNOSIS

At least 50 per cent of alcoholics die from an alcohol-related disorder. In a 10-15 year follow-up study the death rate for male alcoholics was twice as high and that for female alcoholics three times as high when compared with the death rate in the general population (Nicholls *et al.* 1974). This gloomy outcome is little affected by treatment. However, the remainder benefit from treatment and either gain control of their drinking or are abstinent for long periods. Outcome is more dependent on factors within the patient than on the treatment method. Good motivation, the presence of a supportive family, high social class and the ability to form long-lasting relationships favour a good outcome.

FURTHER READING

Edwards, G. (1983). 'Alcoholism' in *Handbook of Psychiatry*, vol. 4, ch. 10.3 (Russell, G.F.M. and Hersov, L., eds). CUP, Cambridge.

Edwards, G. (1987). *The Treatment of Drinking Problems: a guide for the helping professions*. Blackwell, Oxford.

Royal College of General Practitioners (1986). *Alcohol: a balanced view* (Report from general practice, vol. 24). RCGP, Exeter.

Tether, P. and Robinson, D. (1986). *Preventing Alcohol Problems: a guide to local action*. Tavistock, London.

Victor, M. (1983). 'Mental disorders due to alcoholism' in *Handbook of Psychiatry*, vol. 2, ch. 14 (Lader, M.H., ed.). CUP, Cambridge.

31

Drug Dependence

The problem of drug dependence has increasingly become a focus of concern in the UK and many other countries. A recent government report described the misuse of drugs as 'one of the most worrying problems facing our society today'. However, there are conflicting attitudes to the problem of drug misuse among both the public and medical practitioners. On the one hand, drug dependence is seen as an illness requiring treatment; on the other, drug 'addicts' are regarded as people who are responsible for their own problem and so deserve punishment rather than special treatment. This conflict in attitudes is sometimes reconciled by portraying the drug 'addict' as the helpless victim of wealthy drug dealers. Yet this ignores the fact that a great number of drug misusers also deal in drugs, primarily to finance their own habit.

The medical practitioner needs to reconcile these conflicting attitudes in his own mind if he is to provide support and treatment for drug misusers. It is also important not to stereotype drug addicts as young adults who inject heroin; nowadays people taking benzodiazepines account for the largest group of drug misusers, and young adults are becoming dependent on a number of different drugs – a phenomenon known as polydrug misuse.

When the problem of drug dependence is viewed in an historical context or compared to alcohol dependence, the present concern may be considered an over-reaction. However, there has been an alarming increase in the number of drug misusers notified to the Home Office. In 1983 the total number of drug misusers known to the Home Office was 10,720, of whom 80 per cent used heroin alone or in combination with other drugs and 40 per cent were new notifications. This represents a 50 per cent increase of new notifications compared with the previous year. Furthermore the total number of misusers probably represents only a third to a fifth of those dependent on opioids because many do not seek medical help. Thus an estimate for 1983 of the number of misusers of opioids such as heroin and methadone is 30,000-50,000, of whom 40 per cent commenced drug misuse in that year. When compared to the 500,000 alcoholics in England and Wales the numbers appear small, but it is the rate of increase that causes concern.

DEFINITION

Nowadays the term *drug dependence* is preferred to drug addiction and *drug misuse* to drug abuse. The World Health Organisation (1969) defined drug dependence in similar terms to alcohol dependence, namely 'a state, psychic and sometimes also physical, resulting from taking a drug, characterised by behavioural and other responses that always include a compulsion to take a drug on a continuous or periodic basis in order to experience its psychic effects, and sometimes to avoid the discomfort of its absence. Tolerance may or may not be present. A person may be dependent on more than one drug'.

The severity of a person's dependence on drugs is related to the amount of physical and psychological distress associated with the drug's absence and the amount of effort required to resist the compulsion to take it.

AETIOLOGY

It is important to recognise that the factors which initiate drug taking are different from those responsible for maintaining dependence.

Initiating factors

Perhaps the most important initiating factor is the availability of drugs. Before the 1960s nearly all opiate addicts had been exposed to drugs either professionally or therapeutically. This is no longer the case. The availability and relatively low price of drugs now dictates the extent of drug dependence. This has been recognised to some extent and greater effort is being made to prevent the entry of large quantities of illegal drugs, especially heroin, into the UK. However, the question arises as to why some individuals succumb to the temptation to try drugs and others do not. Of course not everybody who experiments with drugs necessarily becomes dependent on them, but the ease with which dependence can become established is underestimated by many who try drugs out of curiosity.

The temptation to experiment with drugs is related to a number of factors. One important factor concerns the level of knowledge an individual has about the dangers of drug taking. A recent survey of fourteen and fifteen-year-olds (Wright and Pearl 1986) showed an alarming level of ignorance and misunderstanding, thus stressing the greater need for education about and demystification of drugs. For example, only 16 per cent of these teenagers thought heroin could cause addiction or dependence; in contrast 19 per cent thought LSD could. The level of ignorance was similar to that shown in an identical survey ten years earlier, yet the increase in public debate and media coverage has been considerable. Presumably those teenagers who are unaware of the dangers of dependence on heroin are more likely to experiment with the drug.

According to drug takers themselves the main reason that they start misusing drugs is the influence of social and peer group pressures. If they are part of a social group or culture which considers drug taking to be a high status activity then those individuals within the group seeking to boost their self-esteem may be at risk. It follows from this that most young people who start to take drugs are first offered them by friends rather than strangers. Other reasons given for starting drugs are curiosity, a search for an enlightening or spiritual experience and 'for kicks'. Less commonly, reasons are cited which reflect inherent factors within the individual such as feelings of inadequacy or tension which are removed by drug taking. This may be because drug misusers are more likely to attribute their drug taking to environmental or social factors than acknowledge emotional factors within themselves. However, although availability of drugs and peer group pressure are vitally important, factors within the individual must be acknowledged in order to try to establish why some people within a group are able to decline the offer of drugs and others are not.

There is no specific drug-dependent personality, but there is some evidence that drug misusers tend to show more features of anxiety and depression in their personality. In addition they may be poor at forming close emotional relationships, show low self-esteem and have problems of sexual identity. Thus the use of drugs may be a symptom of underlying personality problems which need treatment in their own right.

The families of drug misusers show higher rates of marital disharmony and alcoholism than average. Approximately 50 per cent of opiate users have been separated from their parents for more than one year before the age of sixteen.

To sum up, drug dependence is initiated by an interplay of social and individual factors. The availability of drugs and the sub-culture within which an individual lives are important. The socially anxious individual who has a poor self-image and is seeking to boost his confidence and standing within a group is particularly vulnerable.

Maintaining factors

Although the availability of drugs is also of importance in maintaining dependence the situation is complicated by the drug taker either seeking the pleasurable effect of drugs repeatedly, or avoiding the unpleasant effects of their absence. Some heroin users state that every subsequent injection of heroin is an attempt to re-live the pleasurable sensation of their first injection. They talk fondly of the 'buzz' of their first 'fix' and their desire to recapture that moment.

The lifestyle of the drug taker changes to accommodate and maintain his dependence. Thus he is likely to move within a social network of other drug takers where drugs are freely available and often the focus of his friendships. Obtaining money to buy drugs becomes paramount, to the extent that the drug taker's life revolves entirely around the need for the next 'fix'. This inevitably leads to criminal behaviour and increasing conflict with the law, reinforcing the delinquent, anti-authoritarian sub-culture of the drug misuser; this in turn may maintain the dependence, making therapeutic intervention even more difficult.

INDIVIDUAL DRUGS

Opiates

This class of drugs comprises both naturally occurring and synthetic substances. Examples are heroin, morphine, opium, methadone, pethidine and dipipanone. Dependence is characterised by marked psychological and physical craving for the drug.

The mode of taking the drug is by mouth, smoking, or injection, either subcutaneously (skin-popping) or intravenously (main-lining). Another popular method is known as 'chasing the dragon', in which the opiate, usually heroin, is heated on silver paper and the smoke inhaled.

Intoxication is characterised by an intensely pleasurable feeling, the onset of which may be dramatic if it is injected intravenously. Physical accompaniments include flushing and itching of the skin due to histamine release. Decreased respiratory rate and body temperature with hypotension and bradycardia occur, followed by drowsiness and sleep. Loss of appetite and libido are common.

Tolerance and physical dependence develop rapidly. For example, therapeutic doses given for a week can lead to withdrawal symptoms when discontinued. It has been estimated that 50 per cent of those who misuse opiates become dependent. The development of tolerance means that the dosage must continually be increased in order to obtain the desired effect or to avoid withdrawal symptoms. Accidental death due to an overdose may occur.

Chronic dependence leads to pinpoint pupils, tremor, malaise and physical weakness, although some long-term users suffer remarkably little physical deterioration. Many of the physical complications associated with opiate dependence result from the injection procedure. Serum hepatitis may be transmitted via contaminated needles as may sexually transmitted diseases, notably AIDS (see p. 286). Thrombophlebitis, cellulitis, abscess formation and lymphangitis result from the use of contaminated needles or impurities in the opiates. Bacterial endocarditis may also occur. Pregnant opiate users risk damage to the foetus and present considerable problems to obstetricians and paediatricians. Generally speaking women seen early in pregnancy should be encouraged to undergo detoxification but those seen in the third trimester should remain on opiates until term as death of the foetus may occur in utero if withdrawal is attempted. The newborn infant shows withdrawal symptoms with restlessness, tremor and failure to thrive.

The *withdrawal syndrome* is characterised by the onset of symptoms a few hours after the last dose; they reach a peak after approximately 36 to

72 hours. Craving and restlessness occur first and are followed by yawning, perspiration, lachrymation and rhinorrhoea. The next stage produces muscle twitching, tremors, aching limbs and piloerection, hence the term *cold turkey*. Blood pressure, pulse, temperature and respiratory rate all rise, and fever, vomiting and diarrhoea occur. This may be seen especially in enforced withdrawal and the sufferer may lie curled up in a foetal position waiting for the symptoms to subside. This usually occurs after a week to ten days. Grand mal seizures are rare in opiate withdrawal and although symptoms are extremely unpleasant, death is uncommon. The withdrawal symptoms following methadone misuse develop more slowly and last longer (see also p. 399).

Barbiturates

These are central nervous system (CNS) depressants causing both physical and psychological dependence. Examples are amylobarbitone (Amytal), pentobarbitone (Nembutal) and quinalbarbitone (Seconal). Tuinal is a combination of two different barbiturates, quinalbarbitone and amylobarbitone. Methaqualone (Mandrax) is no longer legally available in the UK. The short-acting barbiturates such as amylobarbitone and pentobarbitone are the most popular.

Some barbiturate abusers also use other non-barbiturate CNS depressants such as chlormethiazole, glutethamide, meprobamate and chloral hydrate, often in combination with alcohol.

Iatrogenic dependence used to occur following the prescription of barbiturates for insomnia, but doctors are nowadays more aware of the dangers of prescribing these drugs. Thus the number of people dependent on barbiturates is decreasing, but they are still used in association with other drugs, e.g. in polydrug misuse. In particular they are used to diminish the severity of the 'come down' phase following the use of amphetamine.

Barbiturates may be taken by mouth or injection. They produce relaxation and drowsiness, although in some people they release aggressive behaviour, especially if consumed with alcohol. Physical intoxication is characterised by ataxia, slurred speech, nystagmus and sedation which progresses with increasing dosage to respiratory depression and death.

Tolerance occurs rapidly, partly due to liver enzyme induction and neuronal adaptation. Cross tolerance may develop to alcohol and other sedatives including benzodiazepines, but not to opiates.

The *withdrawal syndrome* is potentially life-threatening. This is in contrast to opiate withdrawal but similar to delirium tremens. The risk of convulsions is high. Anxiety, restlessness, insomnia, nightmares and clouding of consciousness occur. Consequently withdrawal should only be undertaken under medical supervision and preferably as an inpatient. The daily dose of barbiturate taken by the patient is assessed and an equivalent amount of pentobarbitone elixir substituted. Approximately

200 mg of pentobarbitone given 4-6 hourly is needed to control withdrawal. It should be reduced slowly to prevent convulsions. Sometimes an anticonvulsant such as phenytoin is also given.

Benzodiazepines

Benzodiazepines have superceded barbiturates as the drugs of choice in the management of anxiety and insomnia. They are also used as anticonvulsants, muscle relaxants and amnesic agents for minor surgery. They are at present the most commonly prescribed drugs in the Western world. Benzodiazepines are safe and effective drugs for short-term administration only. Long-term use leads to psychological and physical dependence and loss of efficacy due to the development of tolerance.

Benzodiazepine dependence has become a problem of increasing concern to doctors and patients (Lader and Higgitt 1986). It develops quickly and is common. Psychological dependence develops rapidly and physical dependence may occur after only a few weeks' use. Over a third of patients taking benzodiazepines for six months become dependent.

Withdrawal symptoms usually occur as the dose is being reduced or on drug withdrawal, but they may develop as a result of steady chronic usage. The *withdrawal syndrome* is characterised by an initial period of acute anxiety and occasionally by psychotic symptoms; this is followed by a prolonged period of psychological and somatic symptoms. *Psychological symptoms* include anxiety, panic attacks, phobic symptoms, obsessional thoughts, perceptual distortions, feelings of depersonalisation and mood changes characterised by paranoid ideas, irritability and rage. Behavioural changes such as restlessness, insomnia and aggression are common.

Somatic symptoms are diverse. Cardiovascular symptoms such as palpitations, flushing and chest pain are often associated with distressing gastrointestinal symptoms such as nausea, vomiting, abdominal pain and diarrhoea. Neurological symptoms include parasthesia, tremor, ataxia and hypersensitivity to sound. Seizures may occur on abrupt withdrawal. Recovery may take six months or longer.

The withdrawal of benzodiazepines is best done by slow dosage reduction combined with symptomatic treatment (Lader 1986). Fortunately, withdrawal symptoms are rare if the drugs have been used for less than one month; benzodiazepine usage should therefore be restricted to a few weeks only and prescribed with great care. Medical concern about the dangers of benzodiazepines has led to modifications to the laws governing drug misuse. Benzodiazepines are now controlled by criminal law and it is an offence to deal in them in their raw form without a prescription. Unauthorised possession may lead to a maximum of two years in jail and suppliers face up to five years.

Cocaine

This is a stimulant drug with sympathomimetic activity. It may be injected or 'snorted', or the coca leaf may be chewed.

The psychological effects are highly esteemed but short-lasting. Euphoria, hyper-stimulation, over-alertness and feelings of heightened power occur but usually wane within twenty minutes, often leading to a post-cocaine 'crash' of depression and lethargy.

Physical dependence and tolerance do not occur, but psychological dependence may be extreme. Excessive use can cause visual hallucinations, tactile hallucinations of insects crawling over the body, a symptom known as *formication*, and possibly a paranoid psychosis. Excessive nasal inhalation may lead to ulceration of the nasal septum. There is no characteristic abstinence syndrome on withdrawal, but psychological craving may be marked.

Recently a relatively pure preparation of cocaine, known as 'crack' has appeared on the market. It is prepared by cooking cocaine hydrochloride powder with baking soda and water and dry heating the residue. When smoked and inhaled it induces a feeling of well-being within minutes, but this is short-lived. Its rapid action and pleasurable effect make it highly esteemed among drug takers. However it induces both psychological and physical dependence and may lead to death as a result of excessive sympathomimetic activity. Cocaine abuse has recently been reviewed by Spitz and Rosecan (1987).

Amphetamines

Amphetamines are stimulant sympathomimetics and used to be prescribed for depression, fatigue and obesity. They were widely used by soldiers during World War II. The only clinical indications for prescribing amphetamines nowadays are narcolepsy and the hyperkinetic syndrome in children in which they may be effective. Examples are dexamphetamine (Dexedrine) and methylamphetamine (Methedrine). Methylphenidate (Ritalin) is related to amphetamine and has similar effects. 'Purple hearts' were especially popular among drug misusers of the 1960s; they contained a mixture of amphetamine and barbiturate. Amphetamines may be taken by mouth, injected or 'snorted' if in sulphate form. They elevate mood and induce a feeling of well-being. They increase energy, drive and concentration, although the ability to learn new material while under the influence of the drug may be impaired. The pupils dilate and blood pressure rises.

Although physical dependence is not a feature, marked tolerance can occur and chronic users may require massive doses to achieve the desired effect of well-being and euphoria. Long-term use may result in a paranoid psychosis, sometimes indistinguishable from paranoid schizophrenia, but detection of amphetamine in the urine should assist in the diagnosis. As the drug wears off profound fatigue, depression and sometimes suicidal ideation occurs. Some amphetamine users seek to avoid this phase by taking barbiturates to induce sleep.

MDMA (3,4-methylenedioxymethamphetamine), also known as 'ecstasy', is an amphetamine analogue. It is a 'designer drug', so-called because it was tailor-made for specific selected effects and originally went through a process of chemical engineering to create a substance that was not illegal at the time. Ecstasy is, however, now an illegal drug. Effects generally appear within one hour of taking the drug. The user experiences a 'rush', usually described as mild but euphoric. This levels off to a plateau, usually lasting two to three hours, followed by a 'coming down' sensation. Some users become less inhibited psychologically and report a feeling of increased empathy for others. Strong amphetamine-like effects on the body can occur, such as dilated pupils, dry mouth, erectile difficulties in men and inhibition of orgasm in both men and women. Heavy use can be associated with extreme anxiety, confusion and depression.

Hallucinogens

This class of drugs includes lysergic acid diethylamide (LSD), mescaline and psilocybin. More recently phencyclidine (PCP or 'Angel Dust') has become available in the UK. This is an alarming trend, as it can cause hypertensive crises, hyperthermia, delirium and death in relatively small doses.

The best known hallucinogen is LSD, sometimes referred to as 'acid'; it can cause hallucinatory experiences in as small a dose as 50 micrograms. LSD was synthesised in the 1940s (see p. 598) and used for a while in Western countries to produce spiritual experiences and to recall early memories as an adjunct to psychotherapy. This has been abandoned on account of its dangerous side-effects. Hallucinogens are found in plants and mushrooms and have been used in Mexico and South America for primitive religious ceremonies for at least 2000 years.

The drugs are taken by mouth. The effects or 'trips' start after about thirty minutes and may last for twelve hours with a peak at two hours. Visual and auditory perception can be greatly enhanced, giving rise to fascinating and exciting experiences, either highly pleasurable or extremely frightening, so-called 'bad trips'. The taker may be totally involved in what he is experiencing or so terrified that he needs to be taken care of by his friends. Elation or depression are common and visual hallucinations and a distortion of temporal and spatial sense can occur. Delusions may occur with potentially harmful consequences, e.g. a patient may think he can fly and hence step out of a window and fall to the ground. Blood pressure and temperature may rise and the pupils dilate.

There is no physical dependence but psychological dependence may occur. Prolonged use can lead to transient re-experiences without taking the drug; these are known as flashbacks. Some patients may develop a psychotic illness. This may either be a result of intoxication and therefore short-lived or due to the drug precipitating a psychosis in an individual already vulnerable to the illness.

Cannabis

Cannabis is obtained from the flowering tops and leaves of the Indian Hemp plant. It grows extensively in temperate zones and its cultivation is widespread. The dried leaves (marijuana) and the resin (hashish) are usually smoked or mixed with food. The active constituent is tetrahydrocannabinol (THC).

Cannabis induces relaxation and a subjective feeling of well-being. Vivid dreams or visual hallucinations may occur, often associated with a distortion of the passage of time, which may seem to have slowed. Short-lived psychotic reactions characterised by marked anxiety, paranoid ideas and depersonalisation have been reported. An *amotivation syndrome* has been described in chronic users, characterised by apathy, lethargy and lack of drive or ambition.

Physical dependence does not occur, although psychological dependence may be marked. Recently an increased incidence of foetal abnormalities has been described in pregnant cannabis users (Albengres and Tillement 1983).

Cannabis usage does not necessarily lead to other drug abuse, and there are many times more cannabis than heroin users, but the majority of heroin or other opiate users have smoked cannabis.

Solvents

A variety of chemicals which contain acetone or toluene as a base substance cause depression of the central nervous system when inhaled. This is often described as *glue sniffing* because contact adhesives are the most commonly used solvents. However a variety of other solvents are inhaled, including paint thinner, nail varnish remover, gas lighter fluid and dry cleaning fluid.

Glue sniffing has been known in the UK since the 1960s and there has been a worrying increase in inner city areas among children, sometimes as young as eight, and in groups of adolescents. An association with delinquent behaviour and disrupted family background is common.

The solvent is inhaled either directly from a bottle or tube, via a handkerchief saturated with the substance, or from a small bag containing the solvent. Glue sniffers can often be recognised by the smell of glue and the reddened area around their mouth and nose. The effects are similar to those caused by inhaling other anaesthetics, namely an initial period of excitement and euphoria followed by drowsiness, slurred speech and ataxia. High doses will lead to unconsciousness and coma. Perceptual disturbances such as visual hallucinations may occur. Partial or complete memory loss for the experience is not uncommon.

Toxic effects include liver, renal, bone marrow and cerebral damage. Death may result from suffocation, inhalation of vomit or cardiac arrhythmias.

Physical dependence does not occur but psychological dependence is common. Management is directed towards the underlying problems facing the adolescent rather than focussing on the glue-sniffing itself.

Amyl nitrite

This causes relaxation of involuntary smooth muscles, including blood vessel muscles, and is used to relieve the pain of angina pectoris. It is prepared in glass ampoules which are crushed in a handkerchief, the user then inhaling the vapour. The principal appeal to drug takers lies in its reputation for enhancing sexual performance and orgasm, an effect thought to be caused by its vasodilator properties. The main side-effects are transient headache, increased heart rate, drop in blood pressure and dizziness. Large doses can cause nausea, vomiting and fainting.

ASSESSMENT OF DRUG MISUSE

Various misconceptions have arisen in the past about the assessment of the severity of an individual's drug misuse. First, drugs were divided into *hard*, e.g. opioids, and *soft*, e.g. cannabis, amphetamines and LSD, the notion being that the latter were less harmful but could lead on to the former. Secondly, those individuals who injected drugs were considered to be more dependent or disturbed than those who ingested or inhaled them. Indeed some of the early drug rehabilitation units adopted a policy of separating injecters from non-injecters to lessen the risk of 'contamination'.

Nowadays these distinctions are considered to be less important. Perhaps the main reason for this is the trend towards polydrug misuse, in which a variety of drugs are used at different times, some injected and others not. Emphasis is placed instead on the meaning and purpose of the particular pattern of drug use to each individual. Drug misusers are a heterogeneous group, but three main categories of user may be identified:

(1) Experimental or recreational users, often adolescents, who take drugs intermittently, who may not, at the time of referral, be dependent, but who are at risk of increasing the frequency of their use with ensuing dependence.

(2) Compulsive drug users who are psychologically or physically dependent and whose lives centre around drugs. They are often members of a drug sub-culture and may have many other problems, not necessarily drug related.

(3) Stable drug users who are often long-term users, and both psychologically and physically dependent. The drugs may initially have been prescribed for physical disorders or as part of a previous policy of

treatment for drug dependence. This group may have achieved a stability in their social and working lives which might be threatened if their drug supply were to cease.

The essential feature in assessing the severity of drug misuse in any individual is the degree of control which that individual exerts over his drug use. This is more important than the pharmacological characteristics of the drug itself. For example, a recreational user who initially takes drugs intermittently in pursuit of pleasurable effect, but begins to find that his use is for relief of symptoms such as physical withdrawal or psychological distress, may find that he is beginning to lose control over his drug use and is starting to take them more frequently. Although less physically dependent than a stable drug user, he is more out of control.

There is no inevitable association between regular drug use and social and physical deterioration. Furthermore the length of drug use is not necessarily a guide to the severity. Some long-term users are relatively unimpaired by their drug use, whereas others develop severe physical and social complications relatively soon after getting involved in drugs, perhaps even before they have become physically or psychologically dependent. For example, some individuals may accidentally overdose or come into contact with the law for possession of drugs early in their abuse. Thus assessment must be made of how a drug affects an individual's life and how much control he has over his drug use rather than focussing on what drug he takes and whether tolerance and physical dependence are present. However, the latter needs to be taken into account when considering management.

MANAGEMENT OF DRUG MISUSE

The management of drug misuse is relevant to all medical practitioners and presents special problems and challenges. All doctors in the UK are required to notify the Home Office of any suspected cocaine or opioid user they attend within seven days. For general practitioners the major difficulty may be coping with the demands of a drug misuser. The ability to withstand an unwarranted demand for drugs by being firm and yet not rejecting or dismissive and to engage a drug misuser in discussion about his problems requires tact, understanding and skill. The approach will fail many times, but the support offered by a general practitioner may reinforce the patient's motivation to become drug free and result in a request for help.

For casualty officers the challenge is to provide first-class medical treatment to somebody who may have damaged himself physically as a consequence of drug misuse. Thus patients suffering from abscesses, septicaemia or an overdose of drugs, even if they have no intention of giving up their drug use, need to be treated. This may lead to frustration on the part of the hospital doctor who may prefer to discharge the patient as early as possible rather than attempt to engage him in treatment and provide an opportunity for him to consider becoming drug free.

For all doctors the challenge is to overcome their own pessimism or anger with regard to drug misusers and to remember that even if drug users attempt to manipulate them they should try to provide a receptive and supportive approach and allow the patients' own motivation to give up drugs to become more fully formed and expressed.

No drug misuser will give up drugs until he is ready to. In fact any attempt to coerce a drug user to give up often has the reverse effect. However, motivation is often a fleeting changeable state of mind, and the doctor's response to a patient's request for help in coming off drugs may have a profound effect on an individual's motivation. A negative response may shatter the fragile good intentions of the drug misuser, providing him with an excuse to continue his drug taking by claiming that help was not available when requested.

Each individual drug misuser has a different reason for wanting to give up drugs, but each one may have reached the personal cross-roads in his life when he decides he must stop. The stimulus may be a prison sentence or ill-health or the realisation that drugs are no longer pleasurable but simply a way of staving off withdrawal symptoms. No reason is better than any other as long as the decision has been reached to give up drugs. Unfortunately a phase of good motivation may last only 24 to 48 hours and at present most drug treatment units have long waiting lists and are unable to respond quickly enough.

Thus the first step in the treatment of the drug misuser is for professionals, parents and family to be available and supportive when the decision to come off drugs has been reached. Treatment then falls into two phases – the achievement of a drug-free state, accompanied and followed by help in understanding and overcoming the problems underlying the individual's drug misuse.

Withdrawal from drugs is best managed as an inpatient and preferably in a drug treatment unit or other specialised therapeutic community. An assessment is made of the drug misuser's daily intake of drugs and a baseline daily dosage is agreed with him, from which he is then withdrawn. For opiate misusers, whether injecters or not, the drug of choice for withdrawal is oral methadone. Most patients will require between 20-60 mg of methadone per day initially and this dose is then gradually reduced over three weeks or less.

Individuals vary greatly in the ease with which they can successfully negotiate physical withdrawal. Outpatient withdrawal may take longer. In the past, drug units were prepared to maintain opiate misusers on large doses of methadone or even heroin. In some cases this created long-term stable drug dependence, but now the trend is towards withdrawal and only exceptionally should maintenance be offered. Withdrawal from barbiturates has been discussed earlier.

Physical withdrawal from drugs is much easier than maintaining a drug-free life. After stopping there is a continual temptation to restart, prompted by social situations, anxiety, depression or just boredom.

Successful rehabilitation requires the drug misuser to become more aware of the social and emotional factors which trigger a desire to take drugs. This is sometimes best achieved as an inpatient in a therapeutic community where the staff provide firm encouragement and groups are used to increase motivation and mutual support. Others may benefit from peer group support either as outpatients or in organisations such as Narcotics Anonymous. Individual psychodynamic psychotherapy is rarely of any use, but long-term supportive psychotherapy, preferably in groups, is essential. For some patients drug taking may serve as an attack on parents with the intention of making them suffer, and a family therapy approach may then be appropriate. In other words, drug misusers are individuals who have different needs and the services provided must be flexible enough to respond in a variety of different ways.

PROGNOSIS

Giving up drugs often means giving up a whole lifestyle. Staying off drugs may mean continually resisting the temptation to take them. Nevertheless the rather pessimistic view held by many that 'once a junkie always a junkie' is by no means accurate, and many drug misusers will achieve increased stability in their lives and ultimate abstinence.

A study by Stimpson *et al.* (1978) of 128 British heroin addicts who attended a drug dependence unit showed that at seven years follow-up 36 per cent had stopped taking drugs, 48 per cent continued their drug misuse and 12 per cent were dead; 4 per cent were not contacted. In contrast Robins *et al.* (1974) in a study of Vietnam war veterans who became dependent on opiates while in Vietnam showed that 95 per cent achieved abstinence on their return home, emphasising the importance of environmental factors in initiating and terminating drug abuse.

Thus the prognosis is better than for many other medical and psychiatric conditions. Drug misuse often occurs in young people and the challenge of helping them achieve a drug-free life is well worth accepting.

FURTHER READING

Edwards, G. and Bush, C. (eds) (1981). *Drug Problems in Britain: a review of ten years.* Academic Press, London.

Edwards. G., Russell, M. and Hawks, D. (eds) (1976). *Drugs and Drug Dependence.* Saxon House, Westmead.

Medical working group on drug dependence (1986). *Guidelines of Good Clinical Practice in the Treatment of Drug Misuse.* DHSS, London.

Royal College of Psychiatrists (1987). *Drug Scenes: a report on drugs and drug dependence.* Gaskell, London.

32

Disorders of Impulse Control

This chapter examines a few disorders of impulse control which have not yet been considered: shoplifting, pathological gambling and arson.

SHOPLIFTING

Shoplifting, which can be defined as theft from a shop by a customer or apparent customer, accounts for a significant loss of income for shopkeepers. About 5 per cent of all shoppers shoplift at some time or other. Many are 'professional' thieves who plan to steal. Shoplifting is a legal offence provided it is done with the intention to steal. This means that if the theft is carried out while the person's mental state and behaviour is disturbed for medical or psychiatric reasons this can serve as a defence, and may lead to the person being found not guilty (Craft and Spencer 1984).

The incidence of mental abnormality among shoplifters has been studied by Gibbens and Prince (1962), Gibbens *et al.* (1971) and Gibbens (1981) in London, and by Cameron (1964) in Chicago. The highest incidence for shoplifters is among middle-aged women, many of whom show evidence of depression at the time. There is also an increased incidence among adolescents, both boys and girls. Some adolescents shoplift in gangs, presumably as an expression of disturbed adolescent behaviour, not necessarily associated with psychiatric disturbance. Men who shoplift more often belong to older age groups; they often show signs of dementia with forgetfulness, memory impairment and disorientation. In others shoplifting is associated with mental handicap, and in a few there may be evidence of psychosis, schizophrenia or affective disorders, or of organic psychiatric disorder. Occasionally confusion due to alcohol, drugs, or physical ill-health plays a significant role.

Shoplifting can also occur as a transient reaction to severe emotional stress. Some shoplifters are motivated by the excitement of taking a risk and getting away with it without being caught. In this group the condition has a compulsive quality so that the person may shoplift repeatedly and collect a large number of items, many of which are of no use to him. It used to be thought that women are more liable to shoplift during the premenstrual period but this has not been confirmed.

Lastly, minor acts of stealing from shops can occur in children (see p. 501). They may steal sweets, stationery or small toys either for themselves or to give to others to gain popularity among their peers. Such behaviour is often seen in children from disturbed or broken families who are emotionally deprived and feel unloved. Their stealing may represent an attempt to comfort themselves or to gain attention and friendship from other children as compensation for what they are missing at home.

Assessment

Psychiatrists are sometimes asked for reports on patients caught shoplifting, either before the trial, perhaps by a solicitor or general practitioner, or at the time of the trial. It is not the task of the psychiatrist to comment on whether or not the person is guilty but on whether there are any psychiatric or emotional factors or stressful situations which should be taken into consideration. The report may have to comment on whether the accused is fit to plead, on the influence of psychological factors on his behaviour, on any treatment required for psychiatric or emotional disorder, and on the risk of further offences. In the latter context it should be noted that repeat offences are more common in men than women, and a history of previous shoplifting is the best indicator of likely further offences.

If there is clear evidence of psychiatric disorder, e.g. depression in a middle-aged woman caught shoplifting, or early dementia, or confusion due to drugs or alcohol, appropriate treatment should be recommended; this also applies to a first offender who has shoplifted at a time of severe emotional stress.

Treatment

Any psychiatric illness, if present, should be treated. When emotional problems, say in an adolescent, or stress factors are involved psychotherapy is required, and marital or family therapy may be helpful. In the case of children referral to a child guidance clinic and family therapy, or psychotherapy for the child and counselling for the parents may be indicated.

PATHOLOGICAL GAMBLING

Pathological gambling is a chronic and progressive disorder characterised by an irresistible urge to gamble. Its compulsive nature leads the individuals to take ever-increasing risks, gambling excessively, sometimes with borrowed money, and often running into serious debt or illegal activities. The pathological gambler may conceal his gambling from others and lie about it when asked by relatives or friends. As a result his professional, personal and family life are likely to become seriously disrupted.

Pathological gambling must be distinguished from the widespread tendency to enjoy gambling occasionally, often on special occasions or in the company of others, but without running the risk of losing large sums of money. Such occasional social gambling is associated with pleasure in risk-taking and excitement but it does not lead to any of the serious consequences associated with pathological gambling, nor is it uncontrolled or irresistible.

There are no reliable statistics on the incidence of pathological gambling in this country, although surveys of bookmakers for horse racing and greyhound racing suggest that there are more than 80,000 pathological gamblers in the UK. There is a high incidence of pathological gamblers among prisoners; a report from the Royal College of Psychiatrists (1977) found an incidence of 10 per cent among the population in British prisons and reception centres. The condition is more common in men than in women.

Moran (1970a) has described several varieties of pathological gambling and has investigated some of the clinical and social aspects of risk-taking (Moran 1970b). In one group social pressure and ready access to opportunities for gambling predominate; in others underlying psychoneurotic disorders play a major role; pathological gambling may be symptomatic of depression; and in about 25 per cent of cases the gambling is an aspect of a psychopathic personality disorder. Depression and anxiety can also be a consequence of pathological gambling, partly due to guilt and partly due to the serious personal and financial consequences.

The disorder often starts in adolescence or early adulthood and gets progressively worse. There is a tendency for sons of fathers who are pathological gamblers to become gamblers, presumably due to modelling and identification. A disturbed family background is common, and in some cases it is associated with alcoholism.

Treatment

Treatment of pathological gambling is difficult, as is the treatment of other addictive disorders. The patient may lack the motivation to stop gambling, even when he is in serious financial trouble and has lost his job or the support of his family and friends. In part this is due to the patient's desperate hope to win large sums of money to remedy the situation, usually with the result that he loses even more money and his situation deteriorates further.

The first step is to try to increase his motivation. Treatment usually involves a period of forced abstinence coupled with counselling, group therapy and behaviour modification. Social help for the patient and his family are also needed. The organisation Gamblers Anonymous (GA) has had some success and provides an opportunity to share the problem with other gamblers and to give mutual support. A recent retrospective study of attenders at GA by Stewart and Brown (1988) has shown that 22 per cent of attenders dropped out after only one attendance, and another 47 per cent dropped out after having attended between one and ten meetings. Total abstinence for two years or longer was attained by only 7 per cent of all comers. However, some patients attended for two years or longer and were able to reduce their gambling or only relapsed occasionally.

ARSON

Arson or firesetting is legally defined as the destruction of property belonging to another by fire, without lawful excuse. It is a criminal offence under the Criminal Damage Act 1971. The majority of offenders are motivated by financial gain and do not suffer from a mental disorder.

There is however a particular group of arsonists with psychiatric implications. These individuals have an irresistible desire to set fire which is then followed by intense fascination when they see the fire burn. The act is usually preceded by a build-up of tension, followed by making preparations to start the fire. The disorder is sometimes called pyromania, e.g. in the DSM-III. This impulsive activity is extremely dangerous as it can cause serious destruction of property, though not for financial gain, and loss of lives.

Historical background

In the early nineteenth century the term pyromania was used, particularly by French and German psychiatrists, for a form of insanity in which there was an uncontrollable urge to set fires. This classification resulted in laws being passed which protected such individuals from the death penalty. Stekel (1924) published a study of 90 firesetters and suggested the notion of an underlying sexual basis for the condition, the fire being associated with sexual arousal.

Nowadays arson is viewed as one of a number of expressions of disturbed behaviour perpetrated by individuals who, more often than not, are severely damaged psychologically.

Classification

Arsonists who are not motivated by criminal or political reasons or by profit, e.g. to claim insurance, can be classified into two main groups:

(1) Those suffering from overt mental illness.
(2) Those suffering from a disorder of personality.

A Polish study (Fleszar-Szumigajowa 1969) which investigated 311 arsonists in psychiatric hospitals over a ten-year period, found that 25 per cent were schizophrenic, 20 per cent mentally handicapped, 15 per cent alcoholic and 15 per cent had organic psychoses or epilepsy. In the schizophrenic patients the firesetting was often committed in response to auditory hallucinations or delusions.

Many adolescent arsonists do not suffer from mental illness. When asked their reasons for firesetting, they often claim to do so out of boredom or desire for excitement. In the absence of other behavioural or emotional disturbance, one should be wary of applying the term personality disorder to explain this behaviour. However, some individuals who raise multiple fires show evidence of severe psychopathology and personality disorder.

A large study of 1,145 firesetters was published in the USA by Lewis and Yarnell (1951). They estimated that 50 per cent of their sample could be described as 'motiveless' firesetters. Generally these people were adolescent or young adults, more likely to be male, and they described a fascination with fire itself. They were enthralled by their power to create such potency by the trivial act of striking a match. Others described an irresistible desire to set fires not unlike a compulsive phenomenon, while some experienced intense sexual arousal and would masturbate while watching the flames.

Developmental factors

Firesetting may be carried out in childhood; in some child guidance clinics 15 per cent of the children had set fires (Vandersall and Weiner 1970). There are often serious disturbances in family relationships and marked social maladjustment. Several studies have noted the association with an absent father (Macht and Mack 1968). Most of the children set fires in their own homes and demonstrated other disturbed behaviour such as temper tantrums, bed-wetting and difficulty in forming relationships with their peers.

In contrast, adolescents tend to set fires away from home, often with a partner. They often display other features of conduct disorder, such as delinquency and truancy. In adolescent girls there may be an association between arson and self-injury, both of which seem to provide a release of tension.

Management

If the arsonist is mentally ill, treatment will be directed at the underlying disorder. However, because arson is such a serious offence and can lead to loss of life and property, such patients may require treatment in conditions of special security, perhaps with a restriction order under the Mental Health Act 1983 (see p. 702).

Children and adolescents who set fires are generally treated in the same way as others suffering from conduct disorder (see p. 500). Behavioural approaches specifically aimed at the firesetting, combined with positive reinforcement when the child resists the temptation to strike matches, have been successful in some cases.

Many adult firesetters are sent to prison, where psychological help is limited. However, Grendon Prison can offer group and individual psychotherapy to selected prisoners. Unfortunately, many arsonists tend to be silent and withdrawn in therapeutic groups, and less motivated to seek help than other prisoners (Hurley and Monahan 1969).

Prognosis

This largely depends on the underlying psychiatric disorder. One of the best predictors of future behaviour is past behaviour. Thus those arsonists who have set multiple fires are those at most risk of re-offending.

One important question is whether children who set fires become adult firesetters. A study from Scotland by Strachan (1981) concluded that only 9 per cent of children referred for firesetting continued to set fires over a one to five year follow-up period. In contrast a follow-up study in the USA showed that 23 per cent of children were still fire-setting one to five years after the initial referral (Stewart and Culver 1982).

FURTHER READING

Shoplifting

Craft, M. and Spencer, M. (1984). 'Shoplifting' in *Mentally Abnormal Offenders* (Craft, M. and E., eds). Baillière Tindall, London.

Fisher, C. (1984). 'Psychiatric aspects of shoplifting'. *Brit. J. Hosp. Med.* 31, 209-212.

Pathological gambling

Cornish, D.B. (1978). *Gambling: a review of the literature and its implications for policy and research*, Home Office Research Study no. 42. HMSO, London.

Arson

Faulk, M. (1988). 'Destructive offences' in *Basic Forensic Psychiatry* (Faulk, M., ed.). Blackwell, Oxford.

Part V

Pregnancy, the Puerperium and Gynaecological Disorders

33

Pregnancy and the Puerperium

It has long been known that during the puerperium women are liable to abnormal mood changes, especially depression. In this chapter we shall consider first some of the psychodynamic aspects of normal pregnancy and the puerperium; secondly, the common but brief period of only a few hours or days when women may be mildly depressed shortly after delivery, the so-called maternity blues; thirdly, the development of puerperal (postnatal) depression; and lastly the rare complication of a puerperal psychosis.

Being pregnant and having a baby are two important events in a woman's life, each with its own psychological significance. It is therefore essential for anyone looking after a woman at such times to obtain as full an understanding as possible of how she feels about being pregnant and having a child. Her attitude may also be affected by her relationship to her husband or partner and any existing children, and by her social circumstances, including, perhaps, her work or career. These factors are especially important in women suffering from psychiatric complications.

PSYCHODYNAMIC ASPECTS

We consider these first as they provide a basis for understanding why some mothers develop a puerperal depression or become depressed during pregnancy, while others enjoy their pregnancy and the puerperium and do not encounter any major problems. What follows is largely derived from the study of pregnant women who have been seen in analytical psychotherapy or psychoanalysis.

There is perhaps no branch of psychoanalysis that has undergone such major changes as the understanding of femininity and female sexual and reproductive function. Freud considered female sexuality largely from the masculine standpoint prevalent in his time. For example, he considered that a woman's wish to have a baby arose, at least in part, from her supposed wish to compensate for not having a penis. Since then psychoanalysts, especially Helen Deutsch (1945), Benedek (1959) and Bibring *et al.* (1961) have helped to replace this outdated concept by the realisation, now generally accepted, that the wish to become pregnant and to have a baby is an integral part of femininity, to a large extent influenced by the girl's ability to identify with her own mother and her sexual and maternal functions. Bibring *et al.* (1961) have pointed out that a woman's psychological readiness for pregnancy and motherhood by the time she has reached early adulthood depends on her earlier personality development. Many conflicts which are only partly resolved are often stirred up by a woman's first pregnancy. This may therefore present the woman with a psychological crisis, but it may also provide her with the opportunity for further growth and maturation. This has since been amply confirmed by many psychoanalysts, including Raphael-Leff (1980) and Pines (1972, 1982).

Pines has particularly stressed the important distinction between the wish to become pregnant and the wish to have and to look after a baby. A woman may wish to become pregnant and enjoy the sense of symbiosis with her baby still inside, but she may feel emotionally far from ready to give birth and look after the baby as a separate, demanding and controlling individual.

Briefly, a healthy and relatively conflict-free attitude to pregnancy and motherhood depends on the woman having had, as an infant and young girl, a 'good enough' relationship with her own mother (see p. 64). This will have enabled her to identify with her mother so that she in turn can look forward to becoming a mother and enjoy looking after her own baby. She also needs to have developed a sense of her own separate individuality and independence, and to have established a satisfying adult sexual relationship with her husband or partner. She must have learnt to cope with ambivalent feelings of love and hatred which are bound to be stirred up, particularly when she is responsible for and looking after her baby.

Pines (1972) has described how conflicts related to earlier stages of development may be revived during pregnancy or after delivery. These may include a woman's unresolved ambivalent feelings towards her mother, and problems of sexual identity which may lead to difficulties in her sexual and emotional relationship with her husband. Further, feelings of jealousy she may have experienced in childhood following the birth of a younger sibling may now be re-experienced after the birth of her own baby and directed against it.

However, as mentioned earlier, for some women the first pregnancy and the experience of looking after the baby can be a period of further maturation and resolution of such earlier conflicts. The support provided by a caring husband or partner and, perhaps, now also by her mother or women friends can help greatly in this process. The widely accepted practice of the husband being present during the delivery and the greater readiness of most fathers to be fully involved in the care of the baby can be of considerable help in this process.

MATERNITY BLUES

About a half to two-thirds of women become mildly depressed, anxious, tearful and easily upset between the third and seventh day after delivery.

The blues clear up within a few hours or a day or two but are distressing to the mother and her husband or other relatives while they last. Reassurance and sensitive handling and support by doctors, nurses and the husband are needed at the time. The subject has recently been reviewed by Stein (1982).

The cause of the blues remains uncertain. Search for hormonal abnormalities has been unsuccessful, although it has been suggested that the sudden fall in progesterone level after delivery may play a part.

Psychological factors probably play a major role. These include the change from being pregnant, with the baby still inside, to being responsible for and having to care for a separate person who needs to be fed, changed and comforted. Lack of sleep and perhaps exhaustion following the delivery may be contributory factors. Obstetric complications do not play a significant role in causing the blues, nor are the blues related to hospitalisation; they occur just as often after home deliveries.

PUERPERAL DEPRESSION

Puerperal (postnatal) depression, unlike the maternity blues, is a serious disorder. It causes considerable distress to the mother and to her husband or partner, and it may have adverse effects on the psychological development of the baby. In its moderately severe form the *incidence* varies from 10 to 15 per cent of women following delivery, but milder forms may be more common (Pitt 1968, 1985; Kumar and Robson 1984; Watson *et al*. 1984).

The condition resembles other forms of neurotic depression but, not surprisingly, both its aetiology and its clinical features are largely determined by the fact that the woman has recently had a baby. This has been clearly shown by the detailed study of Kumar and Robson (1984); the earlier views of Brown and Harris (1978) that childbirth only acts as a non-specific life event cannot be maintained.

Clinical features

Puerperal depression usually starts gradually within a few weeks of delivery. Anxiety about the baby is an early symptom. It usually takes the form of worrying about the baby's health, feeding the baby, its weight, its stools, its appearance. An early sign of postnatal depression is that the worried mother keeps bringing her baby to her general practitioner or health visitor with these anxieties. At the same time she complains of feeling exhausted and being unable to cope with the baby and her other children, and blames herself for being a bad mother. In fact during postnatal depression the mother's capacity to form an emotional attachment or bond with her baby is often impaired.

Gradually the mother becomes more obviously depressed and hopeless, tearful and irritable, especially with her husband and other children but often also with her baby. When she feels frustrated with her screaming baby and cannot fathom what it wants, she feels angry or even tempted to hit it, and she may fear losing control of her aggressive feelings. This further increases her lack of self-esteem as a mother, her guilt, self-hatred and depression. In practice mothers with puerperal depression rarely give way to these impulses, but non-accidental injuries occur occasionally. Other mothers may become over-protective. Sleep disturbance, loss of appetite and loss of libido are common, and lack of interest in making love may lead to problems in the marriage. Suicidal thoughts may occur but suicide attempts are rare.

It is significant that mothers with postnatal depression often fail to recognise that they are suffering from depression and feel ashamed of feeling as they do. Only about 50 per cent of these depressed mothers ask for help from their general practitioner on their own account. Often it falls to the general practitioner or health visitor to recognise the mother's depression, perhaps because she is constantly asking for advice about the baby, or because her husband asks for help because he cannot cope with his wife's misery, irritability and failure to look after the family and the baby.

If unrecognised or untreated the condition may persist for several months, up to a year or so after delivery. However, in just under half of these mothers emotional problems may persist for several years and lead to difficulties in relation to the husband, the baby and other children so that psychiatric and psychotherapeutic help may still be needed (Pitt 1968; Kumar and Robson 1984). Unfortunately these long-term aspects of puerperal depression are often missed and the necessary help is not provided.

Aetiology

Psychodynamic factors

In comparison with the psychodynamic aspects of normal pregnancy and the puerperium, women who develop puerperal depression are often found to have more serious unresolved emotional conflicts. Their relationship to their own mother in infancy and childhood has often been marked by rejection, separation or death. As a result aggressive feelings and fantasies directed towards their mother have remained unresolved. This is also likely to happen if their own mother was depressed and unable to provide good enough mothering when they were little. Instead of having been able to identify with a 'good enough' mother (see p. 64) they have identified with a bad, rejecting mother. As a result, when their own baby is born they feel incapable of loving it, and the more demanding the baby becomes the greater will be their anger and hatred and their fear of losing control. Their guilt and self-hatred is often exacerbated by the conflict between how they feel towards their baby in reality and their idealised concept that they should feel nothing but maternal love (Breen 1975). The sense of having to give all the love and affection to the baby which they themselves never received in infancy and childhood, often makes them feel envious of the baby. The baby may be felt to be too greedy and demanding so that the mother experiences it as threatening and persecutory. The mother's ambivalent feelings may also be displaced from the baby on to her husband. This may lead to marital conflicts and deprive her of the care and affection she especially needs from her partner, now that she has the baby to look after.

If some of these conflicts enter consciousness while the woman is still pregnant, she may become depressed even before giving birth. Kumar and Robson (1984) and Watson *et al.* (1984) have found that between 6 and 10 per cent of pregnant women develop neurotic depression in the first three months of pregnancy. Such *depression during pregnancy* is more common in women who also have marital conflicts and in those who have had serious doubts about continuing the pregnancy. Antenatal depression is also significantly more common in women who have had one or more previous abortions, but not in those who have had a miscarriage. This suggests that dormant guilt feelings, unresolved grief and fear of retribution, e.g. that the baby they are now carrying may be deformed, are being revived now that they are pregnant again (Kumar and Robson 1978).

Other psychological and social factors

Epidemiological studies, including those by Pitt (1968), Frommer and O'Shea (1973), Watson *et al.* (1984) and Kumar and Robson (1984) have shown significant association between postnatal depression and certain psychological and social factors. Several of their findings are in keeping with the psychodynamic considerations described above. These include separation from or loss of a parent in childhood, present-day problems in relation to the mother, marital conflicts, infrequent sexual intercourse, difficulty in conceiving, and serious doubts whether to go through with the pregnancy. In some, but not all, studies women over thirty were found to be more prone to postnatal depression than younger women, as were women whose husbands had a history of psychiatric problems (Kumar and Robson 1984). The latter findings may have been due to the fact that these husbands were less able to give their wives or partners the support they needed. Other life events like bereavements or loss of the baby may precipitate the onset, and so may severe social deprivation.

Obstetric complications, other than premature birth, do not increase the likelihood of postnatal depression. Watson *et al.* (1984) have found an association between depression and previous psychiatric illness; previous consultations for emotional problems are also more common in women who later develop postnatal depression.

Biological factors

Attempts have been made to ascertain whether endocrine changes, e.g. the rapid fall in progesterone after delivery, play a part in the causation of puerperal depression. However, no consistent results have been obtained and there is no convincing evidence that endocrine or other physical changes are responsible.

Prevention and management

If during pregnancy there is evidence of emotional problems, anxiety, depression, serious marital conflict, doubt about continuing the pregnancy or a history of previous psychiatric illness, psychotherapy may sometimes help to prevent the development of postnatal depression.

Once a diagnosis of puerperal depression has been made it is important to establish how severe it is. The condition must be distinguished from psychotic depression (to be described below). Neurotic depression in the puerperium can almost always be managed at home. Practical help with the baby, support and in some cases psychotherapy usually suffice, but if the depression fails to respond to these measures tricyclic antidepressants may be needed in addition. As they do not enter the breast milk the mother can continue to breast feed her baby. Benzodiazepines and phenothiazines do enter the breast milk and should be avoided.

If anxiety and depressive symptoms persist and the mother is willing to get help with her problems, more long-term analytical psychotherapy should be considered. This is particularly important as persistent depression in the mother may affect her child's emotional development and lead to disturbance later in life. Cognitive development may also be affected, as shown by Cogill *et al.* (1986) who found that when children's cognitive ability was tested when they were four years old it was impaired if their mother had suffered from postnatal depression during the first year of their life.

PUERPERAL PSYCHOSIS

Incidence

While neurotic depression occurs in 10 to 15 per cent of women in the first few weeks after delivery, the incidence of a puerperal psychosis following childbirth varies from 0.1 to 0.2 per cent, or 1:1000 to 1:5000 women. Figures vary according to the diagnostic criteria used and the length of time regarded as constituting the puerperium, e.g. the first three weeks or the first three months after delivery.

The risk of developing a puerperal psychosis is higher in primiparae (Kendell *et al.* 1981; Kendell *et al.* 1987); for a woman who has had one puerperal psychosis the risk of developing a psychotic illness after further pregnancies is greatly increased, almost a hundred fold (Kendell 1985).

Clinical features

The majority of puerperal psychoses show the features of an affective disorder, either psychotic depression or mania; a schizophrenic picture is much less common. Kendell *et al.* (1987) have stressed that most puerperal psychoses resemble a depressive or manic psychosis. The onset is usually acute. During the first few days up to a week or two following delivery the woman may appear normal, the so-called lucid interval; in some cases this may extend to four weeks. She then becomes irritable, with mood changes, disturbed behaviour, especially in relation to her baby, and marked sleep disturbance. Delusions, often paranoid in nature, and hallucinations become apparent, and if the picture is that of psychotic depression suicidal thoughts and attempts are common. Her delusions often involve the baby and she may direct her aggressive and destructive feelings and impulses towards it; or she may feel that both she and the baby are being persecuted. Her mental state and bizarre behaviour make it impossible for her to be trusted with the care of her baby unless she is being carefully supervised.

The picture described so far is based on that seen in women who had to be admitted to a psychiatric unit. Less severe cases may be seen in obstetric units or in the community. In such cases the evidence of a psychosis may be less clear; frank delusions and hallucinations may be absent and their behaviour less severely disturbed. This may make it difficult to distinguish between severe neurotic postnatal depression and a puerperal psychosis. The degree of disturbance of the mother's relationship to her baby may be a useful diagnostic indicator.

Aetiology

Several factors interact in the origin of a puerperal psychosis. The first is the influence of *genetic factors*. Family histories show an increased incidence of functional psychoses, mainly manic-depressive psychosis, in the relatives of women who develop a puerperal psychosis. A previous history of psychotic, depressive or manic episodes greatly increases the risk of puerperal psychosis. This has been confirmed in a recent epidemiological study by Kendell *et al.* (1987); this study also showed that while a past history of manic-depressive psychosis or unipolar depression was associated with a greatly increased risk, there was no such association with a past history of schizophrenia. This gives support to the view that puerperal psychosis may be a form of manic-depressive psychosis precipitated by childbirth and that a genetic predisposition to manic-depressive psychosis rather than schizophrenia plays a significant role. It should be noted, however, that a puerperal psychosis can develop in the absence of past psychotic episodes and that further psychotic episodes may be restricted to the puerperal period.

This raises the question why childbirth can act as a *precipitating factor* of a psychotic illness, especially in women with a genetic predisposition to manic-depressive psychosis. Metabolic factors have been suggested but have not so far been demonstrated. *Emotional stress* at the time of childbirth plays an important role. Kendell *et al.* (1987) have shown that the incidence of puerperal psychosis is greater in women who are unmarried and have no partner when the baby is born, and also if the baby dies in the perinatal period. Other less obvious stresses may be involved. The *psychodynamic factors* discussed earlier in this chapter are also likely to play a significant role, especially what it means to the woman to have become a mother and to be responsible for her baby. Past emotional deprivation in relation to her own mother, uncertainty about her maternal role and ambivalent feelings towards the baby could all act as predisposing or precipitating factors.

Management

This includes both the treatment of the mother's mental illness and careful consideration of her relationship to the baby. Every effort should be made to encourage and maintain close contact between mother and baby in order to maintain or foster the mother's attachment to the baby. In most cases admission to a psychiatric unit is essential, and whenever possible mother and baby should be admitted together (Douglas 1956; Margison and Brockington 1982). Skilled nursing care and supervision are needed by staff who are experienced in the care of severely ill psychiatric patients and in looking after babies, especially if there is a risk of the mother damaging or killing the baby. During the acute stage a nurse may have to be present and assist and supervise the mother whenever she feeds or is with her baby. Admission to a specialised mother-baby unit therefore has many advantages. If this is not possible, special arrangements may have to be made in a local psychiatric unit (Kumar *et al.* 1986).

The initial treatment of the psychotic illness is essentially the same as that of any other functional psychotic illness. As the phenothiazines, haloperidol and lithium all enter the breast milk, breast feeding should be discontinued when these drugs are used. Tricyclic antidepressants do not enter the breast milk in significant amounts so that breast feeding can be continued. ECT is needed occasionally if the condition fails to respond to psychotropic drugs. These physical treatments must be combined with a supportive and psychotherapeutic approach with special emphasis on the mother's relationship to her baby.

Most women make a good recovery from the acute episode within two to three months, but there is a high risk of recurrence: 20 per cent of these women will develop a puerperal psychosis if they have another baby. Moreover, the mother's relationship to her child and hence its emotional development may remain impaired if psychiatric symptoms or emotional problems persist. After recovery from the acute symptoms long-term support and counselling are therefore needed. Consideration should also be given to the use of dynamic psychotherapy to help the mother to accept her maternal role and provide the emotional care essential for her child's psychological development. In some women this may also help to prevent a recurrence if they become pregnant again.

FURTHER READING

Brockington, I.F. and Kumar, R. (eds.) (1982). *Motherhood and Mental Illness*. Academic Press, London.

Kumar, R. (1983). 'Reproduction and psychiatric disorders in women' in *Handbook of Psychiatry*, vol. 2: *Mental Disorders and Somatic Illness* (Lader, M.H., ed). CUP, Cambridge.

Kumar, R. and Brockington, I.F. (1988). *Motherhood and Mental Illness – 2: causes and consequences*. Butterworths, London.

Pitt, B. (1985). 'The puerperium' in *Psychological Disorders in Obstetrics and Gynaecology* (Priest, R.G., ed.). Butterworths, London.

34

Termination of Pregnancy

SOCIAL AND LEGAL CONSIDERATIONS

Both attitudes to the termination of pregnancy and legal provisions for it vary widely in different countries and are liable to change over time as social attitudes change. In some countries termination is prohibited whatever the circumstances, while in others it is allowed whenever a pregnant woman asks for it – so-called abortion on demand. In other countries, such as the UK, it is allowed under certain specified circumstances, e.g. if continuation of the pregnancy constitutes a threat to the woman's life or to her physical or mental health.

Different groups hold strong, often contradictory, views on the subject. There are those who object to termination on moral and religious grounds. These objections are often supported by arguments concerning the sanctity of life and the right of every foetus, whatever its stage of development, to reach maturity. At the opposite extreme are those who consider that every woman should have the right to decide for herself whether or not she wishes to go through with the pregnancy. A pregnant woman may, however, have conflicting feelings about whether or not she wishes to have the baby, so that she may need help to sort out her ambivalent feelings before she reaches a decision.

Doctors are likely to have their own personal views on this controversial issue. However, they should not let their prejudices interfere with trying, as objectively as possible, to understand each woman's personal reaction to being pregnant. The doctor must consider the woman's health, personality, wishes and fears, and her social and marital circumstances, so that he can advise her as best he can within the limitations of the law.

The Abortion Act (1967)

Since the introduction of the Act it has become considerably easier for a pregnant woman in the UK to obtain a legal termination of pregnancy. The Act applies to England, Scotland and Wales but not to Northern Ireland. In essence it states that termination is permissible if two registered medical practitioners are of the opinion, formed in good faith, that

(1) the continuance of the pregnancy would involve risk to the life of the pregnant woman or risk of injury to her physical or mental health greater than if the pregnancy were terminated, or

(2) risk of injury to the physical or mental health of any existing children of her family, is greater than if the pregnancy were terminated, or

(3) there is a substantial risk that if the child were born it would suffer from such physical or mental abnormalities as to be seriously handicapped.

The Act also includes what is called a 'social clause', which states that, when assessing the risks mentioned under (1) and (2) above, account may be taken of the pregnant woman's actual or reasonably forseeable environment.

Any two medical practitioners can make a legally valid recommendation. Neither has to be a psychiatrist, nor does the gynaecologist who carries out the termination have to be one of the two doctors, although this is often the case. One of them is often the patient's general practitioner. If one or other doctor or the gynaecologist approached by the patient objects to abortions on religious, moral or other conscientious grounds he should refer the patient to another doctor. The two doctors recommending the termination have to sign a standard form, and the Health Authorities have to be informed within seven days of the termination. In an emergency one doctor can recommend a termination if he considers that the woman's life or mental health is in immediate danger. The Act also lays down that the termination has to be carried out in an NHS hospital or, if carried out elsewhere, e.g. in a private hospital or clinic, the institution must be approved by the Minister of Health.

The upper time limit for a termination laid down by law is 28 weeks, but with increasing facilities for keeping foetuses at earlier stages of development alive, several attempts have been made to lower the limit. From both the gynaecological and psychological point of view, if an abortion is indicated it is certainly best done within the first 12 weeks.

Before the Abortion Act (1967) there were few psychiatric and virtually no social grounds for a legal termination in England and Wales (the legal situation in Scotland was less restrictive even before the Act). The severe restrictions often caused a great deal of distress not only to women with unwanted pregnancies but also to doctors who considered there to be strong psychological and social indications but who were prevented by law from advising a termination. As a result many women sought illegal 'back-street abortions' which caused a great deal of anxiety and often serious financial problems to women in poor economic circumstances. Back-street abortions also carried a high morbidity, mainly due to sepsis or haemorrhage, and hence involved considerable risk to the woman's life.

Since the Act came into force the number of legal terminations has approximately trebled. At present over 100,000 are carried out annually on women resident in England and Wales. Most are performed for psychiatric, including social, reasons.

ASSESSMENT

When the Act was first introduced women with unwanted pregnancies were often referred for a psychiatric opinion. Over the years many general practitioners and gynaecologists have learnt to form their own opinion, and few such women are seen by a psychiatrist nowadays. In fact, the patient's own general practitioner may sometimes be better able to assess the psychological and social aspects, provided he has known the woman and her family for some time.

However, psychiatrists are asked for their opinion if the situation is complicated, e.g. if the woman is suffering or has previously suffered from a serious mental illness, or if she has conflicting feelings or is suffering from a personality disorder. In some obstetric departments a psychiatrist attached to the department may be consulted, sometimes in conjunction with a psychiatric social worker or a counsellor with special experience in this field. One advantage of this procedure is that in difficult cases the psychiatrist or social worker whom the woman has got to know during the initial assessment may be able to help her after the termination by providing the necessary support.

There is no simple solution to the problem whether or not to advise a termination. Each woman has to be assessed in the light of her individual circumstances. The doctor should throughout respect the patient's wishes while remembering his obligation to the law. From the outset he should make it clear to her that his primary concern is to advise and help her, and that this makes it necessary for him to get to know her present circumstances, hopes and fears as fully as possible.

In many cases there will be no readily definable psychiatric illness. A variety of emotional problems, symptoms of anxiety, mild depression or other neurotic symptoms, as well as emotional immaturity may come to light. Special attention will have to be paid to the woman's and her family's social circumstances and to her relation to her partner or husband. In many cases it will be helpful to interview the partner before coming to a decision, bearing in mind that time is limited as the termination is best carried out before the 13th week if at all possible.

It is important to give the woman every opportunity to talk about any regrets she might have if she had a termination, and how she might feel if she had the baby after all. It is especially important to find out whether she herself wants the termination or whether she is asking for it under pressure from her partner or, in the case of a young unmarried girl, her parents. A few women may change their minds in the course of the interview, but most of them will insist on having the pregnancy terminated.

After having thus formed as full an opinion of the woman's mental state, attitude and personal and social circumstances as possible, the doctor has to give consideration to the likely consequences of recommending or refusing a termination.

PSYCHOLOGICAL CONSEQUENCES OF TERMINATION

Contrary to earlier views, it is now established that serious psychiatric complications following a termination are rare and considerably less common than after childbirth, provided the termination was carried out at the woman's own request. Psychotic illness after termination hardly ever occurs unless the woman has already suffered from schizophrenic or manic-depressive episodes in the past. Nor does such a history by itself necessarily constitute an indication for termination if the woman insists on having the child, as with support and maintenance treatment, if required, relapses during the remainder of the pregnancy can usually be treated or prevented. In view of possible adverse effects on the foetus, the administration of lithium during the pregnancy should however be avoided. The use of antipsychotic drugs during pregnancy is still controversial. Their possible teratogenic effects, especially in early pregnancy, have to be balanced against the risk of relapse of schizophrenia (Loudon 1987). Severe disability, e.g. due to chronic schizophrenia, may however seriously interfere with a woman's ability to look after her home and children, and this may be a strong point in favour of a termination. These issues should be disussed fully with the woman and her partner.

Depressive illnesses are also rare after a termination, and certainly less frequent than in the puerperium. In fact, the majority of women feel greatly relieved immediately after the termination, and any depressive and anxiety symptoms they had beforehand rapidly improve. This applies particularly to young women with an unwanted pregnancy who are unmarried or have no stable partner, and to older women who already have several children and do not want another child.

At the same time it must be remembered that some women experience regret and guilt feelings after a termination. This is to be expected as a termination, whatever the conscious and realistic arguments in its favour, involves destroying a baby the woman could otherwise have had. In most women these guilt feelings clear up within a few weeks. In others, especially women with long-standing emotional problems, they may persist and be associated with a fear of not being able to have another baby or of having a deformed baby. Such fears may be reawakened if the woman becomes pregnant again and may lead to neurotic depression in the early months of pregnancy (Kumar and Robson 1978). The disturbing memory of an abortion continues to trouble some women for several years, and they may recall, on each anniversary of the day the baby might have been born, how old the child would now be. This is particularly likely if the woman has only agreed to the abortion under pressure from others, e.g. her partner, husband or parents. This also applies if the woman was persuaded by her doctor to have a termination on medical grounds when she would have been prepared to take a risk and have the baby (Ashton 1980).

PSYCHOLOGICAL CONSEQUENCES OF REFUSAL

In some women with unwanted pregnancies there will not be sufficient legal grounds for doctors to recommend a termination. The question therefore arises what the consequences of refusing a termination are likely to be.

First, it should be noted that about a third of women who are initially refused a termination ultimately succeed in persuading two other doctors to recommend it. Some of these terminations are probably carried out in the private sector, and if the delay has led to the termination being carried out after the first three months there is increased risk of physical complications.

McCance *et al.* (1973) followed up a group of women whose pregnancy continued after a termination had been refused, for a period of 18 months following their original request for termination. At follow-up 20 per cent of the unmarried, and 10 per cent of the married women in this group still had severe regrets at having had to continue the pregnancy, but 60 per cent of all the women (both unmarried and married), were by then glad to have had their baby. Some women who give birth to a baby they did not want may continue to reject the child with resultant adverse effects on the child's development in years to come.

MANAGEMENT AFTER TERMINATION

Two main problems have to be dealt with after the termination. One is the prevention of further unwanted pregnancies; the other is the provision of support and treatment for untoward psychological sequelae. The former requires expert advice on contraception. Sterilisation may be indicated in some women, especially older married women who do not want further children, but this decision should only be made some time after the termination when the acute crisis is over (see p. 428).

From the psychological point of view, follow-up and support during the first few months should always be offered to help the woman cope with early feelings of regret, guilt or depression, even though some women may refuse it or fail to attend. Those who have more long-standing problems or personality disorders should be assessed as to their suitability for psychotherapy. Some may benefit from joint therapy with their husband or partner.

FURTHER READING

Olley, P.C. (1985). 'Termination of pregnancy' in *Psychological Disorders in Obstetrics and Gynaecology* (Priest, R.G., ed.). Butterworths, London.

35

Menstrual Disorders

There is ample evidence that some menstrual disorders are associated with emotional and psychiatric disorders. These include secondary amenorrhoea, some cases of dysmenorrhoea, menorrhagia, premenstrual tension and some menopausal symptoms.

SECONDARY AMENORRHOEA

This is best defined as amenorrhoea for more than three months in a woman who has previously had menstrual periods. It must be distinguished from primary amenorrhoea, usually of organic origin, which is defined as failure to have started menstruating by the time an adolescent girl has reached the age of sixteen. Amenorrhoea is accompanied by anovulation, and the same usually applies to oligomenorrhoea, characterised by menstrual periods only occurring at intervals of more than six weeks.

It is not surprising that secondary amenorrhoea can be of psychological origin. The regular menstrual cycle depends on the secretion by the hypothalmus, itself under higher cerebral control, of gonadotrophin releasing hormone. This is a decapeptide hormone which passes down the hypothalamic-hypophyseal portal venous system and acts on the anterior pituitary gland. In response the gonadotrophs of the pituitary secrete follicle stimulating hormone (FSH) and lutein stimulating hormone (LH). These in turn act on the ovaries and lead to folliculogenesis and steroidogenesis. These result in ovulation and secretion of 17-beta oestradiol, the predominant oestrogen secreted by the ovary, and the development of the corpus luteum with the production of progesterone. These processes are controlled by feedback mechanisms which operate at all levels of the hypothalamic-pituitary-gonadal axis.

The organic causes of secondary amenorrhoea will not be considered here, except to say that amenorrhoea can, of course, be due to an unsuspected pregnancy which should be excluded first.

Secondary amenorrhoea of psychological origin is a common complaint in women under stress. Its causes include emotional conflict, the break-up of a relationship, marital discord, bereavement, moving from one country or home to another, internment, problems at work,

examinations, and other anxiety-producing situations. Several psychiatric disorders are also associated with secondary amenorrhoea. These
include affective disorders, especially depression, anxiety states,
anorexia nervosa, pseudocyesis, acute schizophrenia and some organic
psychiatric disorders. Chronic alcoholism and drug dependency can also
cause amenorrhoea. The therapeutic administration of phenothiazines
can lead to hyperprolactinaemia with galactorrhoea and amenorrhoea.

Other conditions that need to be considered are weight loss of any
cause, such as any chronic debilitating illness or malnutrition, including,
of course, anorexia nervosa. Excessive physical exercise, e.g. in girls
heavily engaged in athletics, is another cause.

MENORRHAGIA

This is usually of organic origin but there is some evidence that
menorrhagia can be associated with emotional stress. For example,
Greenberg (1983) found a significant association between depression and
menorrhagia, and Ballinger (1977) and Gath et al. (1987) found an
association between emotional stress and menorrhagia in women
approaching the menopause. Menorrhagia can also cause emotional
stress, making it difficult to decide which is the cause and which the
effect. Hypothyroidism, itself a cause of depression, can also lead to
menorrhagia.

DYSMENORRHOEA

Psychological factors can play a significant role in the causation of
dysmenorrhoea, although here too it may be difficult to decide to what
extent emotional stress causes the symptoms or is the result of the
painful periods. It is likely that a vicious circle, involving both physical
and psychological factors, plays a part. Gath et al. (1987), using
standardised psychiatric interviews and questionnaires, showed in a
community survey of women aged between thirty-five and fifty-nine that
in the premenopausal women of this group psychiatric morbidity and
vulnerability were associated with dysmenorrhoea, as well as with
menorrhagia and with premenstrual tension.

PREMENSTRUAL SYNDROME

Opinions differ widely with regard to the nature, prevalence and
aetiology of the premenstrual syndrome or premenstrual tension, as it is
often called (Clare 1983). There are many women who complain of feeling
tense, irritable, anxious and depressed for a few days or a week or more
before their periods, the symptoms clearing up rapidly with the onset of
menstruation. In addition there may be physical symptoms, especially
complaints of feeling bloated, with swelling of fingers or legs and painful
swelling of the breasts. There may also be behavioural disturbance,

including tearfulness, aggressiveness and quarrelsome behaviour.

Attempts at establishing the prevalence of the premenstrual syndrome have given variable results depending on the definition used, the time of occurrence of symptoms and the population studied. For example, Rees (1953) reported a prevalence of 21 per cent in normal women and 62 per cent in women attending various outpatient clinics. Clare (1983) found that 75 per cent of women attending their general practitioners with complaints other than premenstrual tension had at least one premenstrual symptom, and those who had a psychiatric illness had more premenstrual psychological symptoms than those who were not psychiatrically ill.

Aetiology

There is as yet no agreement as to the aetiology of the premenstrual syndrome, but a combination of physical and psychological factors is the most likely cause. Dalton (1977) advocated the view that it was due to a fall in progesterone levels. Alternative views involving the role of sex hormones included an increase in the ratio of oestradiol over progesterone. A raised level of prolactin has also been suggested, but none of these hormonal causes have been confirmed. Other workers have suggested that sodium and water retention have an important role.

Psychological factors undoubtedly play a significant part (Clare 1983; Gath *et al.* 1987). In the study by Gath and his colleagues there was a strong association between premenstrual tension and the mental state, which in turn was correlated with recent life events. This is in keeping with the clinical finding that such stresses as marital and sexual disharmony, family crises, losses and bereavements all tend to increase the liability to premenstrual tension. More long-standing personality problems, including attitudes to sexuality and menstruation, also play a part in some women.

MENOPAUSAL SYMPTOMS

The menopause has in the past been thought to be responsible for a large number of somatic and psychological symptoms. More recent community studies, including the study by Gath *et al.* (1987) have confirmed that vasomotor symptoms, i.e. hot flushes and bouts of excessive sweating, are significantly more common during the pre-menopausal period and in the first few years after the menopause, but there is no evidence that psychological symptoms and psychiatric morbidity, e.g. depression, anxiety and irritability, are specifically related to the menopause.

The view widely held nowadays is that the common occurrence of somatic symptoms, i.e. of hot flushes, excessive sweating and also of vaginal atrophy in the pre- and post-menopausal years is directly due to low oestrogen levels. The fact that these symptoms are also common in women following bilateral oophorectomy and that they respond to oestrogen therapy is in keeping with this explanation.

There is, however, no evidence that when emotional symptoms, especially depression and anxiety, develop in the perimenopausal years this is due to hormonal changes or due to the menopause as such. It is far more likely that these symptoms are the result of changes in the woman's personal and social circumstances at this time of life. Such changes may include an awareness of getting older and sexually less attractive, dissatisfaction in the relationship with her husband, or children leaving home. The realisation by a childless woman that she can no longer conceive, or the lack of a fulfilling occupation outside the home may also play a part.

The emotional reaction of some women to the development of hot flushes or the much rarer development of dyspareunia due to vaginal atrophy may contribute to anxiety and depression. There is also some evidence that with increasing age, and hence at the time of the menopause, there is some decrease in sexual desire and responsiveness (Priest and Crisp 1972) although this may be determined by the woman's relationship to her husband rather than by age as such.

In general, it is now accepted that depression at the time of the menopause does not differ from depression at other times of life. The earlier concept of so-called 'involutional melancholia' has therefore now been abandoned.

FURTHER READING

Clare, A.W. (1983). 'Psychiatric and social aspects of premenstrual complaint'. *Psychol. Med. Monograph Suppl.* 4.

Drummond, L.M. and Tonks, C.M. (1985). 'The premenstrual syndrome' in *Psychological Disorders in Obstetrics and Gynaecology* (Priest, R.G., ed.). Butterworths, London.

36

Gynaecological Surgery

Until the early 1970s the view was widely held that gynaecological operations, especially hysterectomy and sterilisation, were often followed by psychiatric complications, mainly depression. This was thought to be largely determined by the effect of such operations on a woman's view of herself as a woman and her sexual and reproductive functions. Since then more careful, prospective epidemiological studies have been carried out (Gath and Cooper 1982; Gath and Rose 1985). In general, recent studies have shown that depression after these operations is less common than used to be thought and that women who were not emotionally disturbed and free from psychiatric illness before the operation are unlikely to become psychiatrically ill afterwards.

HYSTERECTOMY

The uterus has several functions, especially childbearing and menstruation, but it may also be felt by some women to be essential for the maintenance of youth and sexual attractiveness; in their view of themselves it may therefore be intimately related to their sense of femininity and sexual functioning.

Early studies, e.g. by Lindemann (1941) and Barker (1968), suggested that after hysterectomy major problems of emotional adjustment occurred. These were thought to happen more often after hysterectomy than after other surgical procedures, and depression was thought to be the commonest psychological complication of hysterectomy. However, these and other early studies were based on samples that were either too small or mixed in their composition of gynaecological indications; e.g. some of the hysterectomies were performed for dysfunctional uterine bleeding, others for major physical pathology of the uterus, and a distinction was often not made between hysterectomies carried out for benign or malignant disease. The psychiatric state was often not assessed pre-operatively or only retrospectively, nor were quantitative measures used to assess psychiatric morbidity.

Gath *et al.* (1982a, 1982b) have published studies in which they examined their patients for psychological disorders, first before and then at intervals of six and eighteen months after the hysterectomy. They used standardised psychiatric measures, and studied a sample of 156 women of varying age and social status. All the women had dysfunctional menorrhagia or menorrhagia of benign origin; those with malignant conditions were excluded. They found that of the 90 women who were psychiatrically disturbed as detected by the Present State Examination (PSE) (Wing *et al.* 1974) before the hysterectomy, 51 were no longer disturbed eighteen months after the operation. Of the 66 women who were psychiatrically normal before the operation, only 9 were found to be psychiatrically disturbed eighteen months later. They concluded that 'hysterectomy seldom leads to psychiatric morbidity and in many cases alleviates psychiatric disorder'. Pre-operative psychiatric morbidity and a history of previous psychiatric illness were the main predictors of post-operative depression. These findings by Gath and his colleagues at Oxford were similar to those obtained at St Louis in the USA by Martin *et al.* (1980).

Gath and his colleagues also found that the frequency and enjoyment of sexual intercourse increased in a significant proportion of women following the operation. It is likely that psychiatric improvement and better sexual functioning in some women was due to relief from long-standing distressing menorrhagia. It should also be noted that if a hysterectomy is combined with bilateral oophorectomy this does not increase the risk of post-operative psychiatric complications, although the development of somatic menopausal symptoms, such as hot flushes and bouts of sweating, is likely to increase.

While these epidemiological studies have provided reliable statistical data about the psychiatric effects of hysterectomy and have refuted the earlier view that the operation carries with it a high risk of post-operative depression and emotional or sexual maladjustment, each individual woman needs to be assessed in her own right. Not only should this include a pre-operative assessment of her emotional and psychiatric state, but the woman's feelings about a possible hysterectomy, her psychosexual adjustment, her relationship to her partner and her life situation all need to be taken into account.

STERILISATION

In the past sterilisation was often performed for medical reasons, sometimes in young or childless women who regretted having to be sterilised, or as a contraceptive measure immediately after a termination. As in the case of hysterectomy, it was claimed that there was an increased risk of psychiatric morbidity and a higher incidence of sexual dysfunction after the operation. In some cases serious regret about the loss of fertility followed at a later date, e.g. if the woman remarried or following the death of a child.

In the last ten to twenty years there have been several important changes in the indications, timing and frequency of female sterilisation. Fewer operations are carried out for medical reasons, especially if the woman is reluctant to be sterilised, and far more sterilisations are done at the woman's own request for contraceptive reasons, even in young women. When performed for contraceptive purposes, the operation is usually done as an elective procedure some time after a delivery or termination to give the woman and her partner more time to consider carefully how she feels about being sterilised, bearing in mind that her circumstances might change and that the procedure is almost certainly irreversible. The frequency of sterilisation, now often performed by laparoscopic technique, has increased considerably, as much as ten times in some centres in the UK.

Recent prospective studies by P. Cooper *et al.* (1982) and by Bledin *et al.* (1984) have shown that elective tubal ligation does not lead to psychiatric disorder within eighteen months after the operation unless there was evidence of psychiatric and emotional disturbance beforehand. In some women sexual enjoyment increased after the operation, perhaps because there was no longer any fear of pregnancy. However, a small proportion of women experienced regret some time after having been sterilised, mainly because their circumstances had altered and they wanted another child.

As in the case of hysterectomy, it is now accepted that when a sterilisation is carried out as an elective contraceptive procedure at the woman's own request, there is no serious risk of psychiatric illness after the operation unless there is evidence of pre-operative or earlier psychiatric disturbance. It does, however, remain essential to explore carefully with each individual woman who is asking for a sterilisation why she prefers this contraceptive procedure, which in most cases will be irreversible. This is particularly important in young women and in those who have no children, or, perhaps, only one child, and in women whose marriage is unstable or in danger of breaking up. Both the surgeon and the patient may seriously regret having agreed to a sterilisation when her circumstances change later on, sometimes several years later.

Some young women with a personality disorder and conflicts about their sexual identity may ask to be sterilised because they reject their feminine and maternal role. Their psychosexual development may progress later, either spontaneously, or in response to new influences and experiences, or in the course of psychotherapy; they may then deeply regret having been sterilised earlier on. All these possibilities need to be explored and discussed with the woman and, if available, her partner or husband, before reaching a decision.

FURTHER READING

Gath, D. and Cooper, P.J. (1982). 'Psychiatric aspects of hysterectomy and female sterilisation' in *Recent Advances in Clinical Psychiatry*, vol. 4 (Granville-Grossman, K., ed.). Churchill Livingstone, London.

Part VI

Psychiatry and Medicine

37

Psychosomatic Medicine and the Psychosomatic Approach

The term 'psychosomatic' is being used nowadays in several different ways: psychosomatic medicine, psychosomatic symptoms, psychosomatic disorders and psychosomatic approach. In this chapter we clarify these different meanings and describe some of the factors involved in the causation of psychosomatic symptoms.

PSYCHOSOMATIC MEDICINE

Scientific advances in our understanding of the origin, course and manifestations of physical illnesses and their prevention or treatment have led to increasing specialisation within medicine. This has benefited innumerable patients suffering from organic diseases, but at the same time has resulted in a tendency for doctors to pay more attention to disease entities and technical considerations in diagnosis and treatment than to the person who has the disease. The concept of 'psychosomatic medicine' was originally used to counteract this tendency and to remind doctors of the need to treat not only the disease but also the patient, by paying equal attention to the psychological, social and biological aspects of illness and their interaction. General practitioners often see patients with physical symptoms that are not due to any known disease entity but may represent the patient's response to stress, usually in his family or social relationships or at work. General practitioners tend to be more aware of these aspects of medical practice than hospital specialists, but even in general practice these person-related aspects of medicine are often overlooked or dealt with inadequately.

If the term psychosomatic was used simply as a reminder to practise whole person or 'holistic' medicine, it would only have a somewhat vague, though important, educational significance. But if, as is now the case, psychosomatic medicine is recognised as that discipline which specifically concerns itself with the interaction of biological, psychological and social aspects of medicine, it covers a wide field, including research, clinical practice and medical education.

An important aspect of psychosomatic research is the study of the psycho-physiological mechanisms involved in the influence of emotional stress on physiological function. Closely related to this is research on the role that emotional stress might play in causing physiological dysfunction and possibly structural lesions and organic disease, usually if not always in conjunction with biological factors. These aspects are considered further in Chapter 38, e.g. in relation to gastric function and peptic ulcers (see p. 450), and skin disorders such as urticaria (see p. 463).

The influence of social and cultural factors on the development and course of a variety of disorders can be investigated by means of epidemiological studies. Studies of this kind usually have to be done on large groups of patients, while in clinical practice it is the individual patient, his life before the onset of his symptoms and his relationship to his doctor and others involved in looking after him which have to be the focus of attention. There is in fact some danger that the emphasis rightly placed on psycho-physiological and epidemiological studies in psychosomatic research could lead to relative neglect of the individual patient and his personal experience, aspects which psychosomatic medicine originally set out to emphasise. Individual case studies of patients followed up over a long period and the detailed study of patients in psychotherapy can be of considerable value in research and in clinical practice.

The clinical aspects of psychosomatic medicine will be dealt with further when we consider medical-psychiatric liaison work in hospitals (see Chapter 39) and the management of patients in general practice (see Chapter 55). Attention needs to be drawn here to the central importance of learning how to relate to and interview patients who are physically ill in order to gain an understanding of any relevant personal problems and of their anxieties associated with being unwell. The patient's relationships to his doctor, nurses, social workers and others helping to look after him are particularly important here.

PSYCHOSOMATIC DISORDERS

In the early days of psychosomatic medicine, in the 1940s and 1950s, the term psychosomatic came to be applied to a small group of diseases with structural abnormalities in whose origin specific psychological factors were thought to play a particularly important aetiological role. Franz Alexander (1950), a psychoanalyst in Chicago, called these the 'psychosomatic disorders' and included peptic ulcer, ulcerative colitis, bronchial asthma, thyrotoxicosis, rheumatoid arthritis, essential hypertension and neuro-dermatitis.

This concept of a small group of seven so-called psychosomatic disorders has since been questioned and has largely outgrown its usefulness. It is now recognised that multiple factors have to be taken into account when considering the aetiology of many diseases. These include genetic, biochemical, immunological and infective, as well as psychological and social aspects. In bronchial asthma, for example, all these factors play a part to varying degrees in different individuals (see

p. 459). Moreover, psychological factors influence the onset and course of many disorders other than the few mentioned above. Diabetes (see p. 295), the course of which is well known to be affected by emotional stress and by the patient's attitude to his disease and its control, is a good example. Coronary thrombosis (see p. 455) is another in as much as its onset may be precipitated by stressful life events especially losses such as bereavements or retirement.

THE PSYCHOSOMATIC APPROACH

The concept of a small group of specific psychosomatic disorders has now been superseded by what is called the psychosomatic approach to patients and their illnesses. It is no longer helpful to discuss whether or not a particular disease *is* psychosomatic. Instead the issue is whether psychological and social factors, alongside biological factors, may be playing some part in influencing the onset and course of any illness, and to what extent this might apply to any particular patient. In other words, psychological factors may be particularly important in the small group of disorders mentioned above, but there are many other conditions, including the eating disorders, diabetes, myasthenia gravis, possibly cancer, and so on, to which this may also apply. The term *psychosomatic approach* is therefore used to refer to that approach which pays attention to the possible interaction of psychological, social and biological aspects in all patients, whatever symptoms or disorder they may be suffering from.

It is important not to confuse psychosomatic symptoms with hysterical conversion symptoms (see p. 176). The latter are physical symptoms of psychological origin in which abnormal *mental* mechanisms, e.g. conversion and symbolisation, are responsible for the production of the symptom. A hysterically paralysed arm is a good example.

Psychosomatic symptoms, on the other hand, are physical symptoms due to either structural lesions, e.g. duodenal ulcer or ulcerative colitis, or physiological dysfunction; the latter are sometimes called functional psychosomatic symptoms or disorders. Tension headaches, palpitations, overbreathing and nervous dyspepsia are examples of psychosomatic symptoms due to physiological dysfunction. In these, emotional stress such as anxiety, losses or fear of loss has resulted in physiological dysfunction which in turn determines the nature of the symptom. For example, tension and anxiety can lead to spasm of the occipital muscles causing tension headaches; or anxiety before an examination may cause increased intestinal motility and functional diarrhoea.

Unlike hysterical conversion symptoms, functionally or structurally determined psychosomatic symptoms do *not* usually have any symbolic meaning. Earlier attempts to interpret all psychosomatic symptoms in symbolic terms (Groddeck 1923, 1925; Sperling 1960, 1978) have largely been abandoned. Instead the symptoms can usually be explained in terms of pathological lesions or physiological dysfunction associated with emotional stress. Of course, some patients may attribute symbolic meaning secondarily to a psychosomatic symptom; for example, severe tension headache may be seen as a punishment for forbidden actions and desires. Such secondary meaning attributed by a patient to his psychosomatic symptoms must not be confused with the pathological and physiological mechanisms involved in their aetiology.

Personality characteristics

The suggestion has been made that certain specific personality types predispose patients to the development of a particular disease. This hypothesis was put forward by Flanders Dunbar (1943) in the United States and is still being investigated. There is, for example, now some support for the view that persons with the so-called type A personality are liable to develop coronary heart disease (see p. 456). People with type A personality are ambitious, competitive, self-driving and aggressive, although they may try to conceal their aggressive tendencies. These personality traits are, however, not present in every patient who develops a myocardial infarct, and similar characteristics are found in many people who do not suffer from coronary heart disease. Other factors, such as coexistent hypertension, dietary habits and life events, play an important part as well.

Another example is ulcerative colitis which often occurs in people who are meticulous, obsessional, dependent and over-sensitive to being hurt or rejected. Here again, these personality traits are only found in a proportion of patients who subsequently develop colitis. Jackson (1977) has pointed out, however, that the psychopathology of patients with ulcerative colitis may only emerge during detailed psychodynamic interviews or psychoanalytic psychotherapy (see p. 452). In general it is essential to enquire into the personality characteristics of each individual patient with psychosomatic symptoms and to take these into account in diagnosis and treatment.

Alexithymia

Recently attention has been drawn to another characteristic of patients suffering from functional or structural psychosomatic symptoms or disorders. It has long been known in clinical practice that such patients often have difficulty in expressing what they feel, i.e. they 'bottle up' their feelings. French authors (Marty and de M'Uzan 1963) have called this *pensée opératoire* or operational thinking. Such patients describe their physical symptoms in great detail over and over again, but when talking about painful events, such as the recent death of a close relative, which occurred before the onset of their symptoms, they do so in a purely factual manner with no sign of any emotional upset.

Sifneos (1973) has coined the term *alexithymia* to describe this restriction of emotional and fantasy life. Essentially it consists of an inability to be in touch with and give expression to feelings and fantasies.

These characteristics are observed in many, though not all, patients with psychosomatic disorders. In interviewing such patients the interviewer is likely to feel bored and frustrated because he cannot get through to what the patient feels. Careful control of his counter-transference and repeated interviews over a long period of time or analytical psychotherapy may be needed before the patient can be helped to get in touch with his feelings and fantasy life (Wolff 1977; McDougall 1974).

Specific conflicts

Another hypothesis put forward by Alexander (1950) was that specific unconscious conflicts were correlated with certain disease entities; this corresponds to Freud's discovery of the close relation between unconscious conflicts and neurotic disorders. To give one example, Alexander put forward the view that patients with duodenal ulcers had strong unconscious dependency needs which were in conflict with the wish to appear self-reliant and independent. While such conflicts can be recognised in some patients with duodenal ulcers they are not always present, and identical conflicts can be demonstrated in normal people and in people with other conditions, including those with psychoneuroses but without structural organic disease. In general, there is no evidence to support the view that specific conflicts are necessarily associated with particular disease entities, even though this may apply to some disorders, e.g. anorexia nervosa (see p. 443).

Early object relationships

Dynamic psychotherapy and psychoanalysis place considerable emphasis on the importance of the relationship to parents, especially the mother, at early stages of development. This has led to the view that disturbance of these early object relationships (see p. 64) may play a particularly important role in making the child and future adult vulnerable to the later development of psychosomatic disorders (McDougall 1974; Taylor 1987). The infant's body is intimately involved in the early relationship to its mother; emotional deprivation and developmental failure at this stage may therefore leave a person with a strong tendency to react with bodily rather than mental symptoms to emotional upsets. Taylor (1987) considers that in psychotherapy of such patients special attention needs to be paid to early developmental aspects of their psychopathology rather than to emotional conflicts which arise at later stages of development and which may a play a more central role in psychoneurotic patients. However, present-day analytical psychotherapy is increasingly emphasising the influence of disturbed early object relationships in the origin of the neuroses as well.

Life events

The role that life events can play in precipitating the onset and relapses of both psychiatric and physical illnesses has been discussed in Chapter 4 (see p. 39). Losses such as bereavements and the break-up of close relationships commonly precede the onset of physical disorders or psychosomatic symptoms (Birley and Connolly 1976). In life-event studies it is essential to differentiate between the external life event and the individual's internal stress response to it. A life event such as a bereavement, separation, loss of employment or retirement, may be experienced as extremely stressful by one person but not by another. The fact that the internal stressful response to a bereavement partly depends on the nature of the relationship to the deceased before his death has already been described (see p. 24). It is the *meaning* the event has for the individual rather than the external event as such that determines the nature and intensity of the stressful response. The response will also be influenced by the person's previous life experience. For example, a person who has lost his mother early in childhood is known to be sensitised and hence more vulnerable to serious losses later in life (Brown and Harris 1978). The nature of the person's adult personality, especially his defence mechanisms, also affect his stress response to losses like bereavements. For example, a very independent, over-controlled person who habitually uses denial will be much less affected by a bereavement, at least initially, than an insecure, dependent person who is prone to excessive anxiety and finds it difficult to cope and adjust.

There is also a close correlation between the degree of stress a person is experiencing and his physiological, including endocrine, responses. Rise in heart rate and of the systolic and diastolic blood pressure, changes in gastric motility and secretion of hydrochloric acid are well-known examples. Similar relationships have been demonstrated between the degree of stress a person is experiencing and the amounts of 17-hydroxycorticosteroids and catecholamines produced. A study of parents of children dying of leukaemia has shown that urinary levels of 17-hydroxycorticosteroids were highest in those parents who found it hardest to cope with the anticipation of their child's death (C.T. Wolff *et al.* 1964); after the child had died the parents who remained acutely distressed continued to have high urinary levels which only fell in the course of a year or two if they were able to overcome their grief (Hofer *et al.* 1972).

There is, however, no evidence that individual disorders are related to *specific* life events. It seems that non-specific psychological stress and emotional arousal can initiate the onset or relapse of a variety of physical disorders, such as as asthma or ulcerative colitis, in individuals who are predisposed to the disease by genetic or acquired biological factors necessary for the development of the particular disorder. The same patient may also react to stressful life events in different ways at different times, developing, say, migraine at one time, asthma at another and a depressive illness at yet another.

In clinical practice the psychosomatic approach pays attention to the person as a whole and to the many factors that have been discussed. These include genetic vulnerability and other biological factors, the patient's present personal and social circumstances, including any recent life events and his reaction to them, his personality make-up and defence mechanisms and how these have developed in terms of early and later object relationships.

FURTHER READING

Taylor, G.J. (1987). *Psychosomatic Medicine and Contemporary Psychoanalysis.* Int. Univ. Press, Madison, Connecticut.
Weiner, H. (1977). *Psychobiology and Human Disease.* Elsevier, New York, Oxford and Amsterdam.

38

Psychosomatic Aspects of Individual Disorders

EATING DISORDERS

It is well known that emotional factors can have an effect on appetite in healthy individuals. In some conditions, often referred to as eating disorders, there is a serious disturbance of food intake. These include anorexia nervosa and bulimia, which are described below, followed by a brief account of obesity.

Anorexia nervosa

Anorexia nervosa presents a good example of a condition that is best understood in psychosomatic terms. It arises from psychological conflicts concerned with puberty and the move from childhood to adulthood; these conflicts lead to dieting, weight loss and physical complications and these, in turn, cause further emotional problems in the patient and her family.

Clear descriptions of cases of anorexia nervosa have been given since Richard Morton (1694) first described it as 'nervous consumption' in order to distinguish it from consumption due to tuberculosis. It was subsequently called anorexia nervosa by William Gull (1868, 1874) who considered a morbid mental state to be a factor in its causation. Lasègue (1874) also described the condition, calling it hysterical anorexia.

Anorexia nervosa is characterised by intense fear of fatness and gaining weight, associated with preoccupation with food and a disturbed body image; this leads to weight loss as a result of dieting, self-induced vomiting, purgation and exercising, and to amenorrhoea in females.

Incidence

The condition occurs mostly in emotionally disturbed girls after puberty but can occur in older women and occasionally in children before puberty. Between 5 and 10 per cent of cases occur in adolescent boys.

Cultural and social factors play a significant role in determining the incidence of the disorder. It is much more common among white than black populations, probably because of the different meaning of the onset of puberty and body shape for members of different cultures. The incidence is higher among girls from professional families and those training to be ballet dancers or models, and among girls from upper social classes. Crisp *et al.* (1976) found that in private or grant-aided schools there was one severe case of anorexia nervosa for every 100 girls aged sixteen to eighteen, while the corresponding figure in State schools was one in 300 (milder cases were not included). There is also some evidence that the incidence of anorexia nervosa is increasing in both lower and upper social classes.

Clinical features

The cardinal symptom is the fear of getting fat. This leads to constant preoccupation with weight, to dieting and hence to weight loss so that the weight may drop to dangerous levels, as low as 35 kg or less.

Dieting often starts in the teenage girl because she wishes to slim, especially as in Western society it is more acceptable for girls to be slim than fat; or she may have been teased for being too fat. Sometimes it follows a stressful life event, e.g. family discord, a serious loss or a threatening sexual encounter. After a while she cannot stop dieting and does not eat even when hungry. She is not in fact anorexic in the usual sense of having lost her appetite; she avoids eating because she is phobic of putting on weight.

Carbohydrate foods in particular are avoided, especially bread, potatoes and sweets of any kind. Ultimately the girl may only eat small amounts of salads, tomatoes, fruit and perhaps a little fish or chicken, often playing with her food on the plate rather than eating it. Some girls eat a little but then secretly make themselves vomit in the toilet or bathroom. There may be occasional bouts of bingeing as in bulimia (see p. 447), but this is followed by guilt, self-induced vomiting and a return to self-starvation. The girl may also take purgatives in order to lose more weight.

The girl's *body image* is distorted so that she considers herself to be too fat even when she is seriously emaciated. She may be especially afraid of developing large breasts, fat thighs or a large abdomen.

Amenorrhoea is an early symptom. Sometimes it precedes the weight loss but more often the periods stop after some weight has been lost. After recovery the periods only return several months or longer after normal weight has been restored. If the condition starts before puberty the development of secondary sexual characteristics and the onset of menstruation will be delayed (Russell 1983).

The girl usually denies that there is anything wrong with her. In fact anorexic girls are often restless and overactive, taking excessive exercise which further contributes to their weight loss. In severe untreated cases extreme emaciation may ultimately lead to hypotension, hypothermia, dehydration and intercurrent infection. This may lead to a fatal outcome, as may the hypokalaemia due to potassium loss, the result of purgation. Dilatation of the stomach is another serious complication, sometimes precipitated by bingeing or being made to eat a large meal.

The girl's behaviour, her progressive weight loss and emaciation naturally cause intense anxiety in her family. Her mother is likely to feel especially concerned, feeling that she is failing in her task as a mother. She therefore responds by pressing her daughter to eat more and to tempt her by providing special meals. This only serves to increase her daughter's fear of gaining weight so that a battle ensues between mother and daughter. The situation in the family is often made worse by the fact that the daughter may insist on cooking for the family and try to persuade her parents or siblings to eat more while she eats less and less and becomes more emaciated.

The clinical features in the small number of adolescent boys who are affected is very similar, except that instead of developing amenorrhoea they may lose sexual desire and become impotent.

Mental and physical state

This depends on the stage of the illness when the patient is first seen. In some milder cases girls who recognise that they are losing too much weight may agree to see a doctor before the weight loss is severe and, apart from amenorrhoea, there may be no evidence of physical complications. At the other extreme are the girls who are brought to a hospital after a long period of self-starvation in a serious state of physical collapse. They require urgent medical attention before their mental state can be properly assessed.

The majority fall in between these two extremes. They are usually brought to the doctor against their will by an anxious parent, and are emaciated with a weight well below the average for their age, sex and height. In addition, physical examination may reveal downy, so-called lanugo hair on the back, between the shoulder blades, and on the face. The limbs may be cold due to hypothermia; chilblains are common in cold weather. The blood pressure may be low and the pulse rate slow. Investigations may show a low serum potassium level, an alkalosis and evidence of dehydration. Hypoproteinaemia with oedema is another complication, and there may be evidence of reduced thyroid function.

The endocrine changes responsible for the amenorrhoea are due to disturbed hypothalamic-pituitary-gonadal functions. These are in part secondary to the weight loss and in part directly due to the effect of the patient's emotional state on the hypothalamus. The secretion of gonadotrophin releasing hormone by the hypothalamus falls so that the blood levels of follicle stimulating and luteinising hormones (FSH and LH) and hence of oestrogens fall below normal. In anorexic boys the plasma levels of gonadotrophins and testosterone similarly drop below normal levels.

The most prominent abnormality in the mental state is the patient's denial that she is too thin, that she is not eating enough, that her weight is too low and that she is ill. Any suggestion that she needs help in order to put on weight makes her acutely anxious, and hence angry, sullen and uncommunicative with anyone, parents, doctors or nurses included, who point this out to her. In fact anorexic patients hold on to the belief that they are going to be too fat if they eat more as an *over-valued idea*. As Crisp (1980a) has put it, they suffer from a severe phobia of increase in body weight.

There may be some evidence of depression and anxiety, but intellectual functioning remains good unless the girl is close to physical collapse. In fact, many anorexic girls and boys are excessively preoccupied with their studies and achievements at school.

Aetiology

There has been, in the past, a good deal of controversy as to whether the condition is of biological origin, perhaps due to primary hypothalamic dysfunction, or of psychological origin, the eating disturbance and other physical symptoms being secondary to the emotional disorder. It is now widely accepted that the psychological disturbance comes first and that the endocrine changes and clinical symptoms are the result of the psychological and consequent physical disturbances.

Genetic factors

It has been suggested that hereditary factors may predispose an individual to the development of anorexia nervosa. Holland *et al.* (1984) found a significantly higher concordance rate for anorexia nervosa amongst monozygotic than dizygotic twins. It is not yet clear to what extent these findings are genetically determined or at least partly the result of shared environmental factors and the psychological problems of having an identical twin.

Psychological factors

Many different aspects of psychological development have been thought to play an aetiological role. Early psychoanalytical views based on instinct theory emphasised the persistent unconscious identification of oral with sexual impulses. Thus fear of sexuality with the approach of puberty was thought to result in fear and avoidance of eating. These views have been largely replaced under the influence of present-day object relations theory, greater emphasis being placed on problems in the mother-child relationship, especially failure to achieve a sense of separateness and of personal autonomy (see p. 47). This results in a conflict between persistent dependency needs and the opposite wish to be independent. As food plays such an important part in the child's relationship to its mother refusal to eat could then serve as a rebellious act against her. Unfulfilled emotional needs can also result in a persistent desire for total gratification; fear of greedy impulses may then be defended against by denial which finds expression in the refusal to eat. The occasional breakthrough of these impulses then leads to bulimic episodes. These conscious and unconscious conflicts often contribute to the origin of anorexia nervosa but on their own they cannot account for all cases as such conflicts are common in many people who do not develop the disorder.

Hilde Bruch (1974, 1978) has stressed the frequent failure of anorexic girls to have achieved a sense of autonomy, often due to excessive parental pressure. Minuchin *et al.* (1978) and Selvini Palazzoli (1978) have stressed the role of family influences. Patients with anorexia nervosa often come from enmeshed families (see p. 578) in which the developing child's own views and personality are not properly acknowledged. Application of these findings has made important contributions to the use of family therapy in some cases of anorexia nervosa, as described below.

An important contribution to the understanding of anorexia nervosa has been made by Crisp (1980a). He postulates that as puberty approaches the girl develops an intense fear of the impending changes in the shape of her body, because these changes represent for her the development into a sexually mature adult, with which she feels quite unable to cope. Similar fear of the 'sexual body' in adolescents has also been described by Laufer and Laufer (1984). In order to prevent these changes occurring the girl is determined to lose weight and thus maintain her pre-pubertal state and body shape. This can only be achieved and maintained by controlling her eating. Her refusal to eat therefore represents a 'phobic avoidance' of any increase in body weight. At times this avoidance posture may break down, giving rise to an episode of bingeing, but this only increases the girl's fear of becoming fat and developing the body of a sexually mature woman so that vomiting is the only way out and avoidance of eating is resumed. The resulting weight loss then leads to the inhibition of hypothalamic-pituitary-gonadal activity normally responsible for pubertal and post-pubertal sexual functioning. In this way the girl has successfully – from her point of view – regressed to a pre-pubertal stage, not only in psychological but now also in biological terms. The question remains why these girls are so frightened of adult sexuality and the bodily changes that go with it. Some of the underlying psychological conflicts have already been discussed. Guilt and misconceptions about sexuality and serious conflicts in relation to the mother undoubtedly play an important part and usually have their origin in disturbance of personality development earlier in childhood (see Chapter 7).

This account of the psychopathology of anorexia nervosa applies mainly to girls, as they constitute 90 per cent of patients with anorexia nervosa. Much less is known about the psychopathology of anorexia nervosa in boys. However, several of the factors mentioned earlier apply equally to boys. These include fear of becoming too fat, especially if one of his parents is overweight; feelings of inadequacy about sexual relations with girls, leading to the wish to remain pre-pubertal and not yet ready to engage in sexual relations; fear of being too greedy; rebellion against parents, especially in enmeshed families in which the boy has problems in establishing his independence. In some cases problems of sexual identity and identification with girls may also play a part in the origin of anorexia nervosa in boys.

Treatment

The treatment of patients with anorexia nervosa has two main objectives. First, to help the patient accept that she needs medical help and to eat and put on weight. To achieve this it is necessary to treat her in an environment, be it at home or in hospital, in which she can gradually overcome her fear of fatness. Only then will she be able to eat normally and regain and maintain a weight appropriate to her age and height. At the early stages of treatment any serious or life-threatening physical complications will require medical attention, e.g. correction of electrolyte disturbances, dehydration or hypoproteinaemia.

Secondly, there is the more long-term aim of helping her outgrow her conflicts concerning puberty and sexuality and promoting psychological maturation so that in due course she can accept herself as an independent adult, able to establish satisfactory relationships.

These two aims are closely inter-related. While initially priority has to be given to her physical recovery and to the prevention of relapses, the psychological changes and personal development require long-term treatment, often over a period of two or three years or longer, involving both the patient and often also her family.

The majority of patients are brought to the doctor at a relatively advanced stage with a weight between 30 and 35 kg or even less. They require urgent admission to hospital, but may, even at this stage, protest against admission. It is usually possible to persuade the patient to accept admission, even if reluctantly, by explaining firmly and clearly the serious physical dangers involved. Compulsory admission is hardly ever required. Those whose weight loss is less advanced when first seen are usually even less willing to accept admission. A period of preliminary work with the patient and her family is often needed.

The patient is best admitted to a special unit for the treatment of anorexic patients, if available. Initially she is given a diet of 1500-2000 calories with normal carbohydrate content, and this is gradually increased to 3000-4000 calories. No additional food, e.g. brought in by relatives, is allowed. At first the patient is confined to bed to ensure she takes the diet and to prevent secret vomiting or purgation. It is usually best to set as the initial target weight the weight appropriate for her age and height at the time when her illness first commenced (Crisp 1977). When this has been reached she is allowed to eat with the other anorexic patients on the ward so that they learn from each other to regain normal eating habits while being helped and supervised by the nursing staff. The nurses' relationship to the patients is of fundamental importance; it should be based on psychological understanding of the patients' underlying conflicts concerned with weight gain, body shape and fear of growing up. Firmness needs to be combined with explanation and encouragement, rather than threats or punishment. Occupational therapy and schooling are needed to divert attention from food and eating. The use of drugs such as tranquillisers or antidepressants hardly ever helps and should be avoided.

From the beginning the parents or family need to be involved in the treatment programme by explaining to them the immediate and longer-term aims. Social workers are often particularly skilful in helping parents not to interfere with the treatment procedure and in giving them the support they need.

As soon as the immediate physical dangers have been overcome individual *psychotherapy* should be commenced on a once or twice weekly basis. This should be continued by the same therapist, if possible, after discharge. The therapist should not be involved personally in the patient's physical treatment or weight control, which should be left to the medical and nursing staff. In many cases the parents also need continued psychotherapeutic help.

In some cases *family therapy* may be helpful. The patient and her family are seen together, either starting in hospital or at home (Minuchin *et al.* 1978). Dare (1986) has shown that young patients, less than seventeen years old, usually do better in family than in individual therapy, and Russell *et al.* (1988), in a detailed study comparing family therapy with individual supportive psychotherapy, have shown that better results, in terms of weight gain and psychological changes, were obtained with family therapy than with individual supportive therapy. This, however, only applied to younger patients who had not yet become chronic anorexics or suffered the frequent relapses so common in this disorder; moreover, these patients have so far only been followed up for one year. In older patients individual analytical psychotherapy is usually more helpful, especially in helping them to establish their separate sense of identity and resolve their sexual problems. Therapists working with anorexic patients often have to tolerate their refusal to get involved with them and to accept the understanding offered. This corresponds to their refusal to accept food from their mother, and is re-experienced in the transference.

Lastly, there is a group of anorexic patients in whom weight loss is slight and who may recover spontaneously or with support from their general practitioner. Some of these become sufficiently aware of their underlying psychological problems to benefit from psychoanalytic psychotherapy.

Course and prognosis

The most striking feature of moderate or severe cases of anorexia nervosa is the fact that in spite of intensive and successful initial inpatient treatment in terms of weight gain, relapses are common, requiring one or more readmissions, so that the condition may become chronic. Studies by Morgan and Russell (1975), Crisp (1977) and Hsu *et al.* (1979) have shown that on average at follow-up after four years or longer the outcome was good in 40-50 per cent of patients in terms of having regained and maintained normal weight and regular menstrual periods, and to some extent also in terms of social and sexual adjustment. In about 30 per cent of patients body weight and menstruation had not been fully restored to normal, relapses still occurred and psychosexual adjustment was impaired. In about 20 per cent the condition had become chronic. Between 2 and 5 per cent had died, either of inanition, or due to suicide in chronic and relapsing cases. Even among those in whom the outcome in physical terms is satisfactory further psychotherapy may be needed to achieve resolution of remaining psychological problems. There is some evidence that a poor prognosis is associated with onset at a relatively late age, persistent disturbance in family relationships, long duration of the illness before treatment was started, and possibly the presence of symptoms of bulimia.

Bulimia nervosa

This eating disorder may occur in girls with anorexia nervosa (Russell 1979), but it can also occur as a distinct entity independent of anorexia nervosa (Lacey *et al.* 1986). It occurs most frequently in women between the ages of fifteen and thirty, but about 10 per cent of patients are male. It is characterised by frequent episodes of uncontrolled eating of very large quantities of high calorie food, especially carbohydrates, over short periods of time, so-called *bingeing*. Binges are terminated by self-induced vomiting associated with feelings of guilt, depression and self-disgust. The patient knows that this pattern of eating is abnormal but cannot resist the temptation. She may induce vomiting by putting her fingers down her throat, and this may cause abrasions or scars on the backs of the hands. In addition, she may use purgatives to control her weight and this, together with vomiting, may cause hypokalaemia, fluid depletion and alkalosis.

Bingeing is usually solitary and kept secret from everyone. Many patients do not eat regular meals and find it difficult to recognise when they have had enough to eat. Fluctuations in weight do occur but, unless the patient has associated anorexia nervosa, these are not severe. The weight often remains close to or a little below the patient's normal weight for her age and height.

The underlying psychopathology often resembles that of anorexia nervosa. Fear of fatness is in conflict with an uncontrollable desire to eat excessively. Conflicts concerning sexuality and femininity, a disturbed body image and underlying depression, guilt and anxiety are common findings. The bingeing episodes bring about temporary relief but leave the patient feeling even more guilty and depressed afterwards. In fact when during therapy their bingeing ceases they often pass through a period of depression.

Treatment

Treatment may be short-term, as advocated by Lacey (1983), using a short initial behavioural approach to stop the episodes of bingeing, followed by dynamic group psychotherapy to deal with the emotional problems. Persistent emotional and family problems may require more long-term individual or family therapy. The various forms of psychotherapy used in bulimia and in anorexia nervosa are discussed by Garner and Garfinkel (1985).

Obesity

This condition is characterised by excessive accumulation of fat in the body. Although it is difficult to define exactly at what weight a person should be regarded as obese, an increase of 20 per cent above the expected weight for sex, age and height can be regarded as abnormal. In all cases the condition results from an imbalance between the energy intake, i.e. the amount of food and drink consumed, and the energy output, determined by the amount of physical activity. Primary disorders of the endocrine system, such as Cushing's disease, or of the locomotor system leading to immobility, such as severe muscular dystrophy, are rare causes.

In most patients with simple obesity several factors contribute to their condition. Although genetic and metabolic factors may play some part, psychological and environmental factors are of great importance. While in underdeveloped countries obesity occurs more commonly among the privileged classes, presumably because they can afford more food, in developed countries it is commoner among the lower socio-economic classes. It occurs more commonly in women than in men. Its peak incidence is between the ages of twenty and fifty, but it is quite common in children and adolescents, especially in girls.

Many psychological and familial factors affect eating patterns. In cultures and families in which a great deal of emphasis is placed on eating large meals, parents and children tend to become overweight. If a mother lacks confidence in her maternal role she may over-compensate for this by providing plenty of food for her children, expressing regret and concern if they do not eat everything she has offered them. In her mind love and food are equated, and this pattern of overfeeding may result in childhood obesity.

Eating often serves to allay anxiety and depression. The way in which oral gratification can be used to provide comfort at times of stress has already been described (see p. 71). Such stresses include losses like separations, the end of close relationships and bereavements, leading to loneliness and social isolation. For example, a widow may turn to eating large quantities of food when she returns to her lonely home after having spent the day at work, and thus puts on weight. She is unable to eat less because if she tries to do so she feels more miserable and depressed.

Compulsive overeating may also be a feature of depression, or serve as a defence against it. Episodes of bulimia (see p. 447) may occur in depressed women, and rarely obesity develops after recovery from anorexia nervosa.

Of at least equal importance are the psychological consequences of being overweight. Children who are fat are often teased at school or by their siblings; this makes them feel unloved and miserable and may make them eat even more, e.g. sweets and cakes between meals. In adolescent girls and young women obesity often causes serious distress as they consider themselves to be unattractive to men, especially as in our culture being slim is equated with being attractive.

Later in life, especially in middle-aged men, obesity is often accepted as a normal part of being confident and successful. Such men are often free from anxiety or depression. However, the knowledge that obesity may lead to such physical complications as hypertension or heart disease may cause anxiety.

Treatment

A pattern of overeating is notoriously difficult to break, and even those who are well motivated find it difficult to adhere to a reducing diet. Joining a self-help group like Weight Watchers may help. A few patients with associated psychological problems may undertake psychotherapy but this is rarely successful and personality changes have to precede any expectation of weight loss. In cases of gross obesity the strict dieting required may only be possible in hospital. There is little if any place for appetite suppressants as they can be addictive in the long term. Occasionally strict dieting may uncover underlying depression.

The place of surgery in the grossly overweight – 50 to 100 per cent above the expected weight for sex, age and height – is controversial. Operations such as a *jejuno-ileal bypass* my occasionally be helpful physically and psychologically in carefully selected cases. However, after the operation physical complications like persistent diarrhoea and malabsorption occur in almost half the cases, quite apart from the fact that the operation itself carries a mortality. Serious psychiatric complications are rare except in those patients who suffer from continued post-operative complications, when anxiety and depression are common (Castelnuovo-Tedesco *et al*. 1982).

GASTROINTESTINAL DISORDERS

Gastrointestinal symptoms are among the commonest psychosomatic disorders and may affect any part of the gastrointestinal tract. They can be either functional or structural. Difficulty in swallowing of functional origin (globus hystericus), air swallowing (aerophagia), functional vomiting, nervous dypepsia, abdominal pain, constipation, diarrhoea, and the irritable bowel syndrome, also known as functional bowel disease or spastic colon, are common functional disorders. Structural psycho-somatic disorders include peptic ulcer and ulcerative colitis.

Peptic ulcer

Clinical observations strongly suggest that psychological factors play a part in determining the onset and course of peptic ulceration, but research in this area comes up against considerable difficulties: gastric and duodenal ulcers, though similar in some respects, are not identical disorders; moreover the precise relationship between acid and pepsin secretion and peptic ulceration is still unknown.

Effects of emotion on gastric secretion

There is ample experimental evidence that gastric secretion and motility in healthy people are affected by emotional stimuli. As early as 1833, Beaumont demonstrated that anger and fear produced an increase in acid secretion in his subject Alexis St Martin, whose gastric function could be easily studied through a fistula following a gunshot wound. Harold Wolff and Stewart Wolf (1947) in studies on their laboratory assistant Tom, who also had a gastric fistula, described similar observations. Engel *et al.* (1956), who studied an infant called Monica with a gastric fistula, showed that not only the girl's emotional state but also her relationship to the experimenter and others, affected acid secretion. When she was actively involved, either happily or in anger, acid secretion was high; when she was inactive and withrawn it fell. It is now established that acid secretion is affected by the person's emotional state, by the nature and severity of conflict situations and by the degree of involvement with other people, but there are considerable differences from person to person and the exact relevance of these observations for the formation of peptic ulceration remains uncertain.

There is also some evidence in animals that stressful situations can produce increased acid secretion and peptic ulcers. For example, Brady *et al.* (1958) gave repeated electric shocks to two groups of monkeys. One group could avoid being shocked by pressing a lever. In this group of 'executive' monkeys there was a significantly higher incidence of peptic ulceration and of increased acid secretion than in the second group, who were not provided with a method of avoiding the shocks. It seems that the avoidance behaviour in the first group acted as a stress factor in the production of peptic ulceration.

Personality factors

It was Franz Alexander (1950) in Chicago who first put forward the hypothesis that alongside constitutional and other physical factors a specific unconscious conflict situation predisposed to the development of duodenal ulceration. He postulated that these patients had long-standing oral and passive dependency needs; some over-compensated for these wishes by outwardly appearing confident and independent, while others openly revealed their wish to be loved and cared for; some alternated between these two modes of behaviour. Alexander also suggested that in either case the frustrated dependency needs were responsible for gastric hyper-secretion and thus led to ulcer formation.

This hypothesis has gained only limited support. That there is some correlation between dependency needs and the development of duodenal ulcers in men has been confirmed in a predictive study on American servicemen by Weiner *et al.* (1957). In this study Weiner confirmed a hypothesis, originally proposed by Mirsky *et al.* (1952), that increased levels of serum pepsinogen, a measure of gastric secretion of pepsin, were correlated with the formation of duodenal ulcers; he also showed that there was some correlation between increase of pepsin secretion and oral dependency needs.

It seems therefore that, alongside genetic and other as yet unknown physical factors, frustrated dependency needs may predispose to duodenal ulceration. Anxiety in response to a variety of stressful situations appears to be responsible for actually precipitating the onset, exacerbation and relapses of the condition. Stress can also lead to excessive alcohol consumption and cigarette smoking, and these are further contributory factors.

Management

Attention must be paid to both physical and psychological aspects. The medical and surgical treatment will not be described here. Support and discussion of personal problems and their possible relation to the disorder should be combined with medical treatment. Discussion with relatives may be helpful if inter-personal conflict is an important factor, and working conditions may have to be reviewed or changed. Psychotherapy is not indicated on account of an ulcer alone but may be helpful in a few cases if the patient is aware of underlying conflicts and is asking for psychotherapeutic help.

Irritable bowel syndrome

In this disorder there are no structural lesions but there is an altered frequency of bowel movements or alternating episodes of constipation and diarrhoea. There are associated abdominal pains, and sometimes periods of abdominal distention and flatulence. Often the patient is unduly preoccupied with his bowel function. It is a common disorder that affects men and women equally, and about one third of patients attending gastroenterology clinics suffer from it (Harvey *et al.* 1983). It may present as an acute disturbance of bowel function. In its chronic, relapsing form it may have taken the patient from doctor to doctor in search of a cure, leading sometimes to a host of unnecessary physical investigations and even surgery.

Aetiology

Both physiological and psychological factors play a part in the aetiology of the syndrome. Recordings of muscle action potentials in the colon of these patients show increased slow wave, 3 cycle per minute activity (Snape *et al.* 1977). However, similar findings have been obtained in normal subjects at rest and during emotional arousal. The significance of the findings is therefore unclear. Whatever the nature of the underlying physiological abnormality, the characteristic symptoms can occur in response to either physical, e.g. dietary, factors, or in response to emotional stress and anxiety, or both. The latter are often responsible for relapses and aggravation of the disorder. Some patients show abnormal personality traits, e.g. obsessionality. As a group they find it difficult openly to express what they feel – the condition called alexithymia, so common in patients with psychosomatic symptoms in general (see p. 436).

Management

It is helpful if a physician who suspects that he is dealing with an irritable bowel syndrome warns his patient before he commences any physical investigations that these may reveal no abnormality and that anxiety and stress may be playing a part in causing the symptoms. This will help in the subsequent exploration of underlying emotional problems if no organic abnormality is detected. These patients need supportive psychotherapy in combination with attention to diet and symptomatic relief by means of antispasmodic drugs. Unless severe depression or anxiety are present there are no indications for antidepressant drugs or tranquillisers. Svedlund (1983) and Svedlund and Sjödin (1986) have shown that brief and flexible psychotherapy directed at ways of coping with stress and emotional conflicts, combined with medical treatment, produced better short-term and long-term symptomatic improvement than medical treatment alone. Some patients benefit from long-term psychotherapy, individual or group, especially to help them express what they feel and reduce their level of anxiety. Paulley (1984) has described the psychological management of patients with the irritable bowel syndrome.

Ulcerative colitis

The aetiology of ulcerative colitis is still obscure. Many factors, genetic, auto-immune, infective, social and psychological, have been considered.

Psychological factors

Murray (1930), while still a medical student, found that psychological factors played a significant part in its aetiology. No one now claims that psychological factors alone can cause the disease, but there is evidence that personality characteristics and life events can affect the onset, relapses and course of the disorder provided the necessary, though as yet uncertain, constitutional and physical factors are present as well. The condition can commence at any age; although the peak incidence is in the twenties and thirties, it can start early in childhood and in middle or old age so that different psychological factors may have to be considered depending on the person's age and personal relationships at the time.

That bowel function can be affected by anxiety in normal people, e.g. diarrhoea before an examination, is well known. Studies of colonic function, using the balloon technique, have confirmed that emotional stimuli and the relationship to the observer can affect both the motility of the colon and the appearance of the colonic mucosa in normal people as well as in patients with colitis (Grace *et al.* 1951; Groen and van der Valk 1956). These psychophysiological findings make it easier to understand how the symptoms of colitis can be influenced by emotional factors, but they do not account for the origin of the disorder.

Certain *life events* have been identified as being particularly likely to initiate the disorder or precipitate relapses (Engel 1958). These include bereavements and other losses or separations from people the patient is attached to and on whom he is dependent. A patient with colitis who has formed a strong, dependent relationship with his doctor can suffer an exacerbation or relapse if the relationship is suddenly ended or interrupted. Other significant events include humiliations, fear of failure and of not being able to live up to other people's expectations. It seems likely that this over-sensitivity of patients with ulcerative colitis to losses, humiliations and disappointments is the result of a disturbed mother-child relationship and other disturbances in the family during childhood, leaving them with unresolved dependency needs and fear of failure and rejection. They feel compelled to please others, are afraid of loss of control and often show evidence of obsessionality and perfectionism. Jackson (1977) has shown that in patients with ulcerative colitis these personality characteristics and their psychopathology may only come to light during dynamic psychotherapy. He therefore refers to their initial apparent normality or 'pseudo-normality'.

Quite apart from the personality characteristics and life events that predispose to or initiate the disorder, the experience of having colitis can have serious effects on the patient's psychological function and behaviour. Anxiety and depression due to the disabling symptoms of diarrhoea, often associated with fear of soiling and incontinence, pain and bleeding, are almost inevitable in this chronic or relapsing disorder. Some patients feel humiliated by their symptoms and consider themselves to be unacceptable to others. Fear of further relapses and, in chronic cases, the fear of developing cancer of the colon or of needing a colectomy and ileostomy are common features. If an ileostomy becomes inevitable they often, incorrectly, fear that this will interfere with their sex life and, in women, with being able to have children.

Management

Only the psychological aspects of the management of ulcerative colitis will be considered here. It is obvious that in such a serious and potentially life-threatening condition physical treatment, medical or surgical, has first priority. However, in view of the known and important influence of psychological factors on the onset and course of colitis it is essential to introduce a supportive psychotherapeutic approach from the start. The general practitioner or physician needs to establish himself as a person on whose medical expertise the patient can rely; at the same time he has to encourage the patient to talk about any stressful experiences which may have preceded and influenced the onset of the disease or its exacerbation and relapse. Acute symptoms may improve more rapidly if the patient feels understood and able to talk freely about whatever is troubling him. Such *supportive psychotherapy* needs to be maintained and, if symptoms recur, easy access to the doctor is essential; it has already been noted that absence of the doctor can cause a serious relapse in patients with this disorder.

If surgery is being considered it is essential to explain in detail to the patient what it is like to live with an ileostomy and to relieve any unrealistic anxieties, e.g. about sexual function and relationships. Talking to another patient who has had an ileostomy for some time or to a nurse who has special experience in dealing with ileostomy patients, the so-called stoma nurse, may be helpful.

There is some evidence (Karush *et al.* 1977) that patients who receive *dynamic psychotherapy* combined with physical treatment have a better prognosis than those receiving physical treatment and supportive therapy only, in respect of both the course of the illness and adjustment to their condition. This applies particularly to those patients who are severely emotionally disturbed. Karush's study also suggests that the effectiveness of dynamic psychotherapy in these patients is greater if the therapist is well trained, able to establish a good relationship with his patient and flexible enough to adapt his psychotherapeutic approach and the duration of therapy to the particular patient's needs. In general, dynamic psychotherapy for patients with colitis is best carried out by medically qualified psychotherapists, as they will be familiar with the physical aspects of the disorder. Close collaboration with the physician is essential. However, in the majority of cases such additional formal psychotherapy is not needed provided the clinician himself is sensitive to his patient's problems and able to provide the necessary support and understanding.

CARDIOVASCULAR DISORDERS

Functional cardiovascular symptoms are common manifestations of emotional distress. Anxiety causes an increased heart rate and a transient rise of systolic and diastolic blood pressure so that patients with anxiety states may present with physical rather than psychological symptoms. Anxiety may also precipitate attacks of paroxysmal tachycardia. The so-called effort syndrome or cardiac neurosis is a disorder of psychological origin, presenting with functional cardiac symptoms; it is described below. Psychological factors also play a part in the aetiology of some structural cardiovascular disorders, especially coronary disease. Their role in the aetiology of essential hypertension is less certain. Conversely, organic heart disease may lead to psychiatric disorders, including anxiety and depression; cardiac surgery may be followed by an acute organic confusional state. Bypass surgery for coronary artery disease may be followed by depression. Lastly, psychotropic drugs may cause cardiovascular complications; for example, tricyclic antidepressants can cause cardiac arrhythmias, and monoamine oxidase inhibitors, by causing an increase in blood pressure, may cause a subarachnoid haemorrhage. Conversely, some hypotensive agents like reserpine can cause depression (see also Chapter 49).

Cardiac neurosis

This condition has been variously called da Costa's syndrome, effort syndrome, soldier's heart, disordered action of the heart, neurocirculatory asthenia, and cardiac neurosis. The last is probably the most appropriate term as the condition is now known to be a form of anxiety neurosis; there is no structural cardiac abnormality.

The patient presents with palpitations, precordial pain or discomfort, dyspnoea and a sense of fatigue. This is accompanied by anxiety, usually a fear of heart disease, panic attacks and fear of dying. There is evidence (Salkovskis *et al.* 1986) that in some cases the anxiety can lead to hyperventilation, causing an alkalosis and lowering of pCO_2. This in turn can cause some of the physical symptoms listed above, and these evoke further anxiety thus establishing a vicious circle, so commonly seen in psychosomatic disorders.

Treatment

This includes reassurance after cardiac or respiratory disease have been excluded, followed by exploration of the underlying anxiety. When over-breathing plays a part in causing the disorder, it may be possible to interrupt the vicious circle by teaching the patient to control his breathing, especially when anxious or under stress. Patients who are aware of psychological problems and well motivated may benefit from psychotherapy.

Coronary artery disease

Coronary arteriosclerosis and hypertension are probably the two most important physical factors in the aetiology of myocardial infarction (MI);

dietary factors, being overweight and cigarette smoking also play a significant role. The precise contribution that psychological factors make to the causation of coronary artery disease is still under discussion.

Stress and life events

Stressful life events like bereavement or retirement often precede the onset of a MI, usually by a number of weeks or months (Connolly 1976). Sudden anger, fear or anxiety can act as immediate precipitants. In patients with angina the attacks are often brought on by sudden emotional distress. There is also some evidence that after the onset of a MI fear, pain and acute distress may cause ventricular arrhythmia, fibrillation and sudden death.

Personality characteristics

As early as 1910 the physician William Osler (1849-1919), in his Lumleian Lecture on angina pectoris, suggested that certain personalities were more prone to develop coronary disease than others; he described these as 'keen and ambitious men, the indicator of whose engine is always at full speed ahead' (Osler 1910, p. 849). This does not differ fundamentally from the view put forward more recently that patients with the so-called *type A personality* are predisposed to the development of coronary heart disease (Friedman and Rosenman 1974; Price 1982). These authors have described the type A personality as being characterised by an 'excessive competitive drive and an enhanced sense of time urgency'. Such people are driven by an intense desire to achieve success and gain recognition; they constantly take on new tasks and are pressed for time.

A prospective study by Rosenman *et al.* (1975) has given support to this hypothesis. They followed up a large group of healthy men, aged between thirty and fifty-nine, in California over a period of 8½ years. 1,589 of this group had type A and 1,565 type B personalities; the latter are much more relaxed and easy-going, although they may be equally successful in their lives. At 8½ years follow-up over twice as many of the type A personalities had developed coronary heart disease than those with type B personalities, and twice as many in the type A group had had a fatal MI. Another study, carried out by the Recurrent Coronary Prevention Project in the USA, suggests that counselling directed at modifying type A behaviour can reduce the recurrence rate in patients who have had a MI (Friedman *et al.* 1984; Price and Friedman 1986).

The precise role of the type A behaviour pattern in coronary artery disease is, however, still unclear and its significance should not be overestimated (Marmot 1980; Sensky 1987). Only about 15 per cent of type A personalities develop coronary artery disease, and similar personality characteristics occur in patients who develop conditions other than a MI, e.g. duodenal ulceration. It seems safe to conclude that the type A behaviour pattern may play a significant role in causing myocardial infarction in some patients predisposed by coronary arteriosclerosis or hypertension, and that this should be taken into consideration in prevention and management.

Management

Medical help should be sought as quickly as possible after the onset of chest pain as persistent pain and anxiety may contribute to sudden death within the first few hours of the onset. Unfortunately some patients take a long time to decide whether or not to get help and this may worsen their prognosis. The early use of painkillers and sedatives is essential.

As the patient is recovering the physician needs to reassure him that he will be able gradually to return to a normal life, although some limitations may have to be accepted. Early physical rehabilitation combined with encouragement and support plays an important role in allaying the patient's anxieties about his future (Cay *et al.* 1976). Depression and anxiety may follow a MI and need to be treated with supportive psychotherapy and in more severe and persistent cases with antidepressants or tranquillisers. The patient's lifestyle needs to be explored; if he does tend to drive himself excessively he should be encouraged to change this pattern. However, it is important to realise that for some patients who for years have been used to a life of constant striving and over-activity to be told to stop doing so may be a serious threat. This applies particularly to those whose lifestyle has been a defence against self-doubts and feelings of inadequacy. If they try to be less active they may become anxious and depressed. Simply to tell a patient to work less hard may be not only useless but counter-productive, leading to serious emotional conflict and distress. Occasionally more long-term supportive psychotherapy may be helpful, especially if emotional problems and difficulties in relationships persist.

Essential hypertension

Essential hypertension was classified as a psychosomatic disorder by Alexander (1950), who considered that conscious or unconscious conflicts concerning the expression of feelings of hostility and aggression were important aetiological factors. Since then a great deal of research on the physiological and psychological aspects of hypertension has been carried out and reviewed by Weiner (1977) and Steptoe (1986), but the role of psychological factors is still uncertain.

In both normotensive and hypertensive subjects a transient rise in systolic and diastolic blood pressure occurs in response to stressful stimuli like feelings of anxiety, anger or having to carry out difficult mental tasks. The cold pressor response, in which the blood pressure rises when a hand and arm are immersed in ice-cold water, has been shown to be due the pain induced during immersion of the limb (Wolff 1951). There is, however, no proof that frequent but transient elevation of the blood pressure can lead to a sustained increase and thus to established essential hypertension.

The high incidence of essential hypertension in some families supports the view that genetic factors play a significant role in its aetiology, although shared psychological and social stresses within the family may also play a part. In this context it is interesting that in some strains of mice and rats genetically predisposed to the development of high blood pressure, social stresses such as over-crowding, persistent exposure to noise or avoidance behaviour may lead to established hypertension.

Although it is unsafe to generalise from such laboratory experiments in animals to hypertension in man, the findings give some support to the view that in humans who are genetically predisposed to hypertension, social and psychological stresses may act as contributory factors. Such stresses include social disintegration, violence, unemployment, marital discord and separations. Separation experiences may also precede the change from benign to malignant hypertension. Anger or sudden fear may also precipitate a cerebrovascular accident in patients with established hypertension.

There is no firm evidence that *specific personality* traits or psychological conflicts predispose to the onset of esential hypertension (Mann 1984), although recently claims have been made that the type A personality traits found in some patients who develop coronary artery disease (see p. 456) may also play a part in the development of essential hypertension. The difficulty in carrying out reliable prospective studies on the influence of such predisposing factors is that the onset of hypertension is gradual and difficult to determine. It is therefore difficult to decide whether the common tendency of hypertensives to be easily moved to anger is an aspect of the pre-morbid personality, or the result of suffering from high blood pressure, or a mixture of the two.

When psychological or social factors affect the onset or course of hypertension this takes place partly through increased activity of the sympathetic nervous system and increased production of circulating catecholamines; how this interacts with the production of renin, angiotensin, the effect of an increased salt intake and other pathophysiological mechanisms that increase cardiac output and peripheral vasoconstriction is as yet uncertain.

Management

Medical treatment, including the use of hypotensive agents and dietary control, should be combined with attention to any relevant psychological and social aspects.

RESPIRATORY DISORDERS

Two disorders will be considered here: bronchial asthma and the hyperventilation syndrome.

Bronchial asthma

Epidemiology

Bronchial asthma is a common disorder in both children and adults. Its *prevalence* varies from country to country and in different populations studied, but in the UK the prevalence among children is about 2 per cent, among adults about 1 per cent. The prevalence in the USA appears to be higher, about 4 per cent in both children and adults. In about a third of patients it starts before the age of five, and in two-thirds before adolescence. Between 30 and 45 per cent of children with asthma outgrow it as they get older. Asthma is a potentially fatal condition and the death rate in this country is increasing.

In about two-thirds of children with asthma there is a significantly higher proportion of other allergic disorders, especially infantile eczema (see p. 467) and allergic rhinitis, than in control groups of children without asthma. About 25 per cent of children with infantile eczema develop asthma later on.

Aetiology

Genetic factors

A large proportion of patients with asthma have a positive family history, with figures varying from 20 to 80 per cent depending on the population studied. Relatives of patients with asthma also have a higher incidence of allergic disorders, especially eczema and vasomotor rhinitis, than relatives of non-asthmatics. Twin studies of asthmatics also suggest that heredity plays a part, the incidence of asthma among monozygotic twins being greater than among dizygotic twins. While these findings suggest a genetic basis, environmental factors such as parental attitudes, the family atmosphere and the parent-child relationship may also play a significant role.

Psychological factors

While allergic and infective factors have long been known to predispose to and initiate attacks of asthma, the role of psychological factors has also gained increasing recognition. All three factors and their interaction must be taken into account in each case. The final common pathway responsible for the attacks is widespread bronchoconstriction, accompanied by increased bronchial secretion and oedema. Several studies, including those by Rees (1956, 1964) have tried to determine the relative importance of these three interacting factors. Weiner (1977) and Groen (1976) have reviewed the literature.

The findings vary with age. In children psychological and infective factors are more often the dominant factors than allergic ones; in adolescents and young adults up to the age of thirty-five allergic factors predominate, while in middle and old age psychological and infective factors are once more of greater importance than allergic factors. In general, psychological factors play some part in about 70 per cent of patients, but their nature varies with age.

It is often difficult to decide whether psychological factors precede the onset or are the consequence of suffering from bronchial asthma. Only prospective studies could give a clear answer to this question, and these are difficult to carry out. Psychological factors can predispose to the disorder and precipitate attacks, but the frightening nature of the attack, whatever its cause, can in turn cause serious psychological distress, especially in children and their parents, so that a feedback effect is set up which can influence the course of the disorder and of individual attacks.

There is no one personality type associated with bronchial asthma. Many different psychological aspects seem to play a significant role. These include disturbance in relation to parents in childhood and to others later in life, problems in personality development, and conflicts related to closeness and dependency. Equally important are life events and stimuli that produce emotional arousal, often associated with difficulty in expressing feelings. These aspects will be considered next in relation to different age groups.

In children the relationship to the parents, especially the mother, plays a central role. Fear of separation from the mother, often associated with marital disharmony and a disturbed family atmosphere, are particularly important. Such children tend to be over-dependent and may develop an asthmatic attack when they feel unloved, unprotected or rejected. Feeling over-protected and engulfed may be equally threatening and can precipitate attacks. The attitude of the parents plays an important part here. Over-protective, perfectionist parents who are too controlling or ambitious in relation to their children may make it difficult for the child to develop a sense of freedom and independence, thus perpetuating an atmosphere that maintains the liability to further attacks. It must be stressed that the child's over-sensitivity to parental attitudes often plays an important role.

Equally important is the fact that having an asthmatic child is bound to influence parental attitudes, usually by making the parents even more anxious and over-protective, which may aggravate rather than relieve the tendency to attacks.

As the child gets older frequent attacks of asthma may also interfere with schooling and other activities outside the home; this, in turn, may make the child feel anxious, insecure and different from other children.

In adolescents some of these earlier problems may continue to be

operative, especially conflicts concerning the achievement of independence and separation from the parental home. Once such independence
has been achieved the asthma may improve, but the liability to further
attacks may return if conflicts of dependence versus independence are
re-awakened in relationships outside the original family. Sexual arousal,
over-excitement and feelings of anger may precipitate individual attacks,
especially if these feelings are not expressed. In some adolescents, as in
children or adults, physical exertion can also bring on attacks.

In adults any of these earlier psychological conflicts may be stirred up
by life events which can thus precipitate the onset or recurrence of
asthma, sometimes after many years of freedom. It is particularly in this
age group that the inability to express feelings of sadness in response to
losses or disappointments, or to express anger when feeling oppressed or
frustrated, can precipitate attacks. There is no evidence that either
neurotic or psychotic illness is more common in asthmatics than in
control groups.

Management

Here we concentrate on the psychological aspects of management; details
of medical treatment can be found in medical textbooks.

In each case the role of allergic, infective and psychological factors
must be assessed. The presence of infection is usually not difficult to
determine. Careful history-taking may give a clear indication of allergic
factors, e.g. seasonal incidence or sensitivity to such allergens as house
dust, pollens, moulds, animal hair, or feathers and certain foods. It is
important not to let too extensive or prolonged investigations for a
possible allergic basis prevent or delay adequate exploration of
psychological factors. Physical treatment must start at the earliest
opportunity, but at the same time possible psychological factors must be
looked for in every case.

In children it is essential to get to know the child and his parents in
order to assess the nature of family interaction, parental attitudes, the
child's feelings towards his parents, and their reaction to his attacks. If
significant psychological factors are identified, a number of talks with the
parents, offering support and explanation to modify their attitudes, are
needed. Talking to the child, either alone or with the parents, is equally
important. In severe intractable cases admission to hospital may break
the vicious circle by freeing the child from exposure to a disturbed family
atmosphere. This can be particularly effective if the mother is
over-protective or over-anxious, but unless work with the parents
changes their attitudes and improves the situation at home the child may
relapse soon after discharge. Psychotherapy for the family or the child
may be indicated if psychological factors predominate. In any case,
prolonged support and readiness to deal with new emotional problems as
they arise remain essential.

In adolescents a similar approach is indicated, but greater emphasis needs to be placed on helping the adolescent in his own right by offering supportive psychotherapy and discussion of emotional, including sexual, problems.

In adults it is essential to enquire into the patient's present family and other personal or social relationships. One of the problems in adults with asthma is that some avoid contact with their doctor, preferring to handle their own illness. They seem to fear over-involvement with their doctor, just as asthmatic children often feel threatened by over-involvement and excessive closeness to their parents (Lask 1966). It is important therefore for doctors treating asthmatics to avoid being too controlling or over-anxious. It is essential to respect the patient's independence, while being firm, supportive and easily available when needed.

Formal psychotherapy, individual or group, can help in a small proportion of patients if psychological problems turn out to be of major importance. Sometimes helping the patient to express feelings of sadness by crying or to release anger in an interview may be helpful. However, this requires skill and caution on the part of the doctor or therapist as cases have been reported in which, following an abreactive interview, the patient has developed a severe asthmatic attack.

In some cases relaxation techniques help patients to avoid or control their attacks, provided they also use any physical treatments that have been prescribed and found effective. Hypnosis and auto-hypnosis (Maher-Loughnan *et al.* 1962; Maher-Loughnan 1976) have also been shown to be effective in some cases.

Ultimately the skill of looking after patients with asthma lies in the doctor's ability to choose the appropriate forms of physical treatment and medication, and combine these with the psychological approach and treatment methods suitable for each individual patient, often over a long period of time.

Hyperventilation syndrome

This functional disorder consists of episodes of over-breathing, both the rate and depth of respiration being increased. It is almost always due to anxiety, sometimes associated with a hysterical personality disorder. The anxiety may lead to air hunger which may make the person take fast, deep breaths to relieve the sensation. Occasionally hyperventilation is the result of having been told to take deep breaths when feeling tense and under stress in order to relax.

It has long been known that hyperventilation, by lowering of pCO_2, can lead to tingling in hands and feet and ultimately to tetany. The role which hyperventilation may play in cardiac neurosis has been discussed earlier (see p. 455). Bass and Gardner (1986) have investigated respiratory function and the effect of hyperventilation on pCO_2 in this syndrome. They have confirmed that anxiety, especially phobic anxiety, is a common aetiological factor but consider that in some patients somatic factors, e.g. asthma and pulmonary embolism, may be responsible.

Treatment

In the acute episodes treatment consists of making the patient breathe more slowly, possibly into a bag to raise the pCO_2, combined with sedation if necessary. Thereafter relaxation and breathing exercises to correct faulty breathing habits may help prevent further attacks. At the same time the causes of the underlying anxiety state need to be explored and in some cases supportive or more formal psychotherapy will be needed.

SKIN DISORDERS

Psychological aspects are of particular importance in skin disorders for two reasons. First, emotional factors play an important part in the onset and maintenance of many common dermatological conditions. Secondly, having a skin disease can be very distressing to the patient, and sometimes also to people in his environment. There are several reasons for this. Skin lesions are often visible and unsightly, thus making the patient feel self-conscious and embarrassed; they arouse fears of looking sexually unattractive, e.g. in adolescents with acne; they may cause anxiety about having been infected or about infecting others, justifiably so in cases of veneral disease or scabies, but also when the condition is in fact not infectious. If there is itching the conflict between wanting to scratch at the expense of further damage to the skin and abstaining from scratching leads to tension and anxiety, and after a bout of violent scratching the patient may feel guilty and depressed. Itching also leads to mental irritation, insomnia and depression.

Some skin diseases become chronic and patients may become preoccupied with their appearance, constantly looking at themselves in the mirror and perhaps trying to cover up minor or even non-existent blemishes. They may also direct their feelings of frustration at not getting better on to their doctor and become angry with him. Whether or not psychological factors played a part in originally causing the disorder, a vicious circle is often set up as these emotional reactions may in turn aggravate or prolong the illness.

Psychophysiological aspects

Everyday experience shows that mood changes influence the function of the skin. Thus shame and embarrassment lead to vasodilatation, making people blush, while anxiety and fear may lead to vasoconstriction, causing pallor and increased sweating. In this sense the skin is sometimes said to be the 'mirror of the mind'.

It has been demonstrated experimentally by Graham and Wolf (1950) that the state of the blood vessels in the skin can be altered by emotional stress. Similarly the effect of stress on palmar sweating, which is controlled by the sympathetic nervous system, has been studied by

MacKinnon (1964). The changes in electrodermal activity (skin conductance) due to emotional tension are secondary to altered function of the sweat glands. Measurements of *electrodermal activity* have been widely used to study psychiatric disorders (Lader 1975). It has also been shown that the vascular component of the allergic skin response to the local injection of tuberculin can be prevented by suggestion under hypnosis (Black 1963; Black *et al.* 1963). Itching can also be reduced by relaxation or hypnosis and is increased by emotional stress.

There is thus plenty of evidence that skin function can be affected by psychological factors, but opinions still differ as to the relative importance of such factors in the origin of different skin conditions. It is likely that in the individual patient several factors, including constitutional, allergic, infectious and psychological influences play a combined role. However, in the conditions described below psychological aspects tend to be particularly important. Sensitive interviewing is needed to elicit the role of emotional conflict and stressful life situations, which may be missed if attention is focused mainly or entirely on a search for physical causes.

Pruritus (itching)

Itching is often due to physical causes, e.g. eczema and other skin diseases, or threadworms in pruritus ani, but sometimes psychological factors are contributory or indeed the only cause (Musaph 1964). Psychogenic itching may be generalised or localised, e.g. to the nape of the neck, the genital region, or the anus. The psychological factors may be concerned with conflicts concerning sexuality and aggression. For example, people who cannot express feelings of anger and frustration may develop itching and scratch themselves instead. Sometimes the irresistible bouts of scratching are accompanied by pleasurable autoerotic sensations. Scratching also occurs in the absence of itching and this has been referred to as *derived activity*, i.e. an activity through which feelings which cannot find direct expression find an outlet. For example, people often scratch themselves when they feel frustrated, e.g. when held up in a traffic jam. Severe and repeated scratching may in turn cause itching which may lead to further scratching and sometimes to lichenification and localised dermatitis. By explaining these processes to the patient and helping him to relax and express more openly how he feels, the itching and scratching may be considerably relieved.

Excessive blushing

Blushing normally accompanies feelings of embarrassment, but it may be widespread and excessive. This occurs more often in young women than in men and may itself lead to further embarrassment. It is usually a symptom of anxiety and may be associated with guilt about sexual or aggressive feelings.

Hyperhidrosis

Excessive sweating (hyperhidrosis), particularly of palms, soles and axillae, often starts in adolescence and may be due to underlying psychological conflicts and anxiety, but it can be the result of overactivity of sweat glands in normal people in response to heat or emotional stimuli. Occasionally it is associated with local skin disorders. Increased sweating may itself become a source of embarrassment and anxiety.

Urticaria

This common skin condition is characterised by the transient appearance of erythematous and oedematous swellings or 'weals' due to local vasodilatation and increased capillary permeability of the skin, usually the result of local release of histamine. It can be entirely allergic in origin. In some cases, however, it occurs in response to acute emotional stress and arousal, especially embarrassment, anxiety, frustration and suppressed anger. The following examples given by Musaph (1964) illustrate this further.

A recently married woman of nineteen developed attacks of urticaria whenever her mother-in-law called on her or was expected to visit. The mother-in-law was deeply attached to her son, the patient's husband; she had strongly disapproved of the marriage and was constantly criticising and belittling the patient. The latter felt completely unable to cope with her mother-in-law, assumed a submissive role and suppressed all her rage and resentment.

Another patient, a seamstress, had to prepare dresses for others to finish. When people came to collect the dresses while she was still working on them she made great efforts to finish them but inwardly felt annoyed with the people who were hurrying her and also with herself for keeping them waiting. As soon as they left, her skin would start to itch and she developed acute urticaria.

In patients with psychogenic urticaria a few interviews during which the patient can talk openly about underlying conflicts or precipitating events and in which he can express his previously suppressed feelings may help to alleviate or prevent further attacks. Sometimes more formal psychotherapy is needed. If the stressful situation involves other family members family therapy may be helpful (De Korte *et al.* 1986).

Atopic dermatitis (atopic eczema)

This common disorder occurs in infancy, when it is called infantile eczema (see p. 467), as well as later in childhood and in adulthood. Relapses are common and children who have recovered from infantile eczema may relapse later in childhood or as adults. Others make a complete recovery. The adult form used to be called neurodermatitis, a term rarely used nowadays. Infantile eczema is often associated with bronchial asthma. Severe itching and scratching are important features of the condition at all ages.

Aetiology

Genetic, allergic and psychological factors interact in causing the disorder. There is often a positive family history, and a higher incidence in monozygotic than in dizygotic twins supports a genetic basis.

Immunological factors play a significant role, but even positive skin tests to specific allergens and increased levels of IgG and IgE reagins do not necessarily signify that the patient's condition can be controlled by avoiding contact with an identifiable allergen. In infants with infantile eczema sensitivity to cow's milk or egg protein must be considered as a possible factor.

The role of *psychological factors* in patients with atopic dermatitis has been well established in clinical practice and supported by various studies. Denis Brown (1967, 1972) has reviewed the literature and studied the personality characteristics and the role of emotional stress in 82 adult patients with eczema, using patients attending a dental hospital as a control group. Brown (1972) stressed the importance of using clinical interviews in addition to questionnaires as many patients who had at first denied psychological conflicts or life stresses when asked to complete questionnaires, were later able to reveal such aspects during sensitive interviewing. This equally applies to many other psychosomatic conditions in which the role of psychological factors is being investigated.

Briefly, Brown's (1967) review of the literature showed that a high proportion of patients with atopic eczema have vulnerable personalities before the onset of the disorder, but there is no one personality type characteristic of atopic dermatitis. The only consistent finding is that these patients may suppress or inhibit expression of aggressive impulses, especially when their dependency needs are not being met.

In about two-thirds of his own patients Brown (1967) found that stress factors or evidence of personality disorder preceded the onset of the skin condition. He also found that his group of patients could be divided into two sub-groups. About two-thirds acknowledged that they were also suffering from psychological symptoms and had been under stress; he called this the psychologically 'unstable' group. One third initially denied such symptoms but were able to admit their presence and to get in touch with associated feelings in the course of detailed interviews; he called this the 'superstable' group. This corresponds to Jackson's (1977) observation of pseudo-normality in some patients with ulcerative colitis (see p. 453).

In his second paper Brown (1972) found that compared with a control group his patients had experienced significantly more stressful *life events*, such as separations, frustrated dependency needs, severe shock, worry and interpersonal difficulties, during the preceding six or twelve months before the onset of their eczema.

These findings confirm the clinical experience that personality factors and stress play an important role in determining the onset and course of atopic dermatitis (Musaph 1964). It is equally important to note that, once established, dermatitis greatly increases the patient's distress, often leading to further frustration, irritability, anxiety and depression.

Treatment

It is essential to combine physical treatment with detailed attention to the patient's present and past emotional conflicts and life situation. In order to achieve this the general practitioner or dematologist or, when available, psychiatrist or psychotherapist attached to the dermatological department needs to provide a setting in which the patient can talk freely about problems that may be related to the onset or relapse of his skin condition, as well as his reaction to the disorder. A few patients who are sufficiently motivated benefit from dynamic psychotherapy, and those whose conflicts are related to disturbance within the family may benefit from family therapy (De Korte *et al.* 1986). The use of self-help groups and group psychotherapy for a variety of patients with chronic skin disorders has been described by De Korte and Vintura (1986).

Infantile eczema

This needs to be considered separately from atopic eczema in adults. As in the latter, constitutional, including genetic, factors are important predisposing factors, and allergy, e.g. to cow's milk or eggs, may play a significant role.

The important psychological factors to be considered are problems in the infant-mother relationship. Psychological problems may both precede and follow the onset of the eczema. It used to be thought that infantile eczema occured more often in babies of mothers who had difficulty in accepting their maternal role, were emotionally unresponsive to their baby, and hence gave too little physical comfort, including skin contact, to the baby, thus making it feel frustrated and rejected. This has not been confirmed, however, as these observations have been made retrospectively on mothers whose babies had already developed infantile eczema. Once the baby has developed eczematous lesions, which are often exudative and unsightly, mothers as well as fathers may find it hard to touch and hold their baby. The child's crying and obvious distress may also lead to irritability and frustration in the parents, thus creating a vicious circle.

As a good mother-child relationship, including holding, touching and caressing, is essential for the child's emotional development, children who have had infantile eczema are often left with increased needs of dependency and fear of rejection. This may account for the fact that adults who had infantile eczema are often left with such characteristics later in life (Pines 1980). In treatment it is therefore essential to combine physical treatment of the child with support to both parents, especially the mother, in an attempt to establish and maintain a close physical and emotional relationship with the child.

Psoriasis

This is one of the most common chronic skin disorders of unknown aetiology. In some patients the unsightly scaly patches on exposed body surfaces or on the scalp, the itching, the shedding of scales in the bed or bathroom and the reaction of others to the condition may cause considerable distress and lead to disturbances in their personal, sexual and working lives. Emotional factors may also precipitate or aggravate psoriasis. Support and encouragement must always be combined with physical treatment. Counselling and self-help groups can be helpful for some patients (De Korte and Ventura 1986).

Alopecia areata

Alopecia areata, or patchy hair loss, is often precipitated by acute emotional stress in children and adults. In 10–20 per cent of cases there is a family history. The psychophysiological mechanism responsible is not known.

Trichotillomania

Trichotillomania is the compulsive pulling out of hair, which may lead to large patches of baldness. The patient sometimes swallows tufts of hair she has pulled out. It usually occurs in adolescent girls; among adults it is also more common in women. It is also common in mentally subnormal children. Many of the patients suffer from underlying emotional conflicts, sometimes associated with sexual problems, which may only come to light in dynamically oriented interviews or psychotherapy. Minor degrees of hair pulling may sometimes be regarded as a habit similar to other comforting habits of childhood, such as thumb-sucking and, unlike the more severe cases, may clear up spontaneously. Behaviour therapy has been tried in trichotillomania but usually without success.

Artefacts (dermatitis artefacta)

Quite apart from the fact that in many skin diseases the patient may scratch and make his skin condition worse by producing excoriated lesions, psychiatrically ill or emotionally disturbed patients may damage their normal skin, e.g. by burning or cutting themselves, by applying chemicals to their skin, or by injecting substances under the skin and so producing a variety of unusual lesions. The patients, women more often than men, may be unaware of what they are doing or conceal the truth. It is much more important to discover the underlying reasons than to make the patient confess what she is doing. A punitive attitude will make it impossible to establish a relationship with the patient in which the underlying personal problems can be explored. A personality disorder or depression is often found in these patients. In a study by Sneddon and Sneddon (1975) a high proportion were adolescent girls. Some recovered after psychotherapeutic interviews focused on underlying conflicts and stressful situations; others failed to recover until their life situation had improved, sometimes only several years later.

Psychiatric disorders focused on the skin

In the skin disorders described so far psychological factors have in varying degrees played a part in the causation and course of the condition. In addition, there are patients with psychiatric disorders who present with the belief that there is something wrong with their skin without this being the case; or they may become obsessionally preoccupied with minor blemishes of the skin that others would ignore. For example, patients with an anxiety state may watch their skin for the presence of blemishes, or depressed patients may become hypochondriacally preoccupied with the idea that they have a skin disease.

Other patients may present with the delusion that their skin is infested with parasites. This is now called *delusional parasitosis* (Batchelor and Reilly 1986) but used to be referred to as acarophobia. The delusion is accompanied by disturbed behaviour such as attempting to extract insects from the skin by picking or scratching, or constantly looking and examining the skin to check for parasites. This condition is more common in women than men. Sometimes there is an underlying functional or organic psychosis, but in other cases the delusional belief is not associated with any other psychiatric abnormalities, in which case it is referred to as a *monosymptomatic hypochondriacal psychosis* (Munro 1980). The condition is difficult to treat but may respond to antipsychotic medication, e.g. pimozide, combined with support and reassurance.

RHEUMATOID ARTHRITIS

There is considerable controversy about the role of psychological factors in rheumatoid arthritis (Weiner 1977). Alexander (1950) included it among the group of psychosomatic disorders (see p. 434). He suggested that in patients with rheumatoid arthritis there was a conflict between aggressive feelings and the opposing need to appease others and hence to repress these impulses. Since then a great deal of progress has been made in our knowledge of the biological, more specifically immunological, basis of rheumatoid arthritis, and further research on the psychological aspects has thrown considerable doubt on Alexander's claims. The following is a brief summary of the present position.

Immunological factors

It is now known that the presence of rheumatoid factor is essential for the development of rheumatoid arthritis. Rheumatoid factor is an autoantibody against the constant fraction of the patient's immunoglobulins. It is made by lymphoid tissue and may be of the IgM, IgG or IgA class. The reason for its production is unknown, but genetic factors may play a part. In rheumatoid arthritis there is infiltration of the synovial tissues in the affected joints by B-lymphocytes, plasma cells and macrophages. A few patients with rheumatoid arthritis, especially in the younger age groups, may not have rheumatoid factor in the serum at the onset of the disease, but it may appear later and is present in 90 per cent of cases at some stage. It is also present in about 6 per cent of normal individuals, especially in the older age groups, and in some conditions other than rheumatoid arthritis.

Psychological factors

It is now generally accepted that there is no specific personality type characteristic of· patients with rheumatoid arthritis. No reliable prospective studies of pre-morbid personality traits are available. A few retrospective studies suggest that among patients with rheumatoid arthritis some tend to repress aggressive impulses or fail to express anger; others dominate people they are close to, or behave in a submissive, masochistic manner towards them. Other patients show none of these characteristics.

There is, however, a good deal of evidence that life events can precipitate the onset of the disease or aggravate the disorder. The physician William Osler (1927) commented on the frequent association between rheumatoid arthritis, then called arthritis deformans, and anxiety, worry and severe strain. Separations, the loss of a person the patient used to dominate and control, bereavements and marital disharmony are among the circumstances that may initiate the disease. Rakola (1973) has studied the influence of family disharmony on its onset and course. However, none of these factors are specific to rheumatoid arthritis; they can play a similar role in many other acute and chronic diseases, both physical and psychiatric. It is also known that the onset or recurrence of rheumatoid arthritis can be precipitated by injuries, operations, infections and pregnancy.

At least as important from the psychological point of view is the fact that such a painful and disabling chronic disorder as rheumatoid arthritis often causes anxiety, despair and depression due to the problems it may create in personal and social relationships and at work. Some patients tend to become overwhelmed by their constant pain and physical limitations, while others continue to lead active lives, determined not to succumb to their disabilities.

Management

There is no convincing evidence that psychotherapy has a significant effect on the progress of rheumatoid arthritis. Physical treatment has first priority in all cases. Some patients benefit if those who look after them give them the opportunity to express how they feel about problems and stresses which have contributed to the onset or relapse of the disorder. In all patients every effort has to be made to relieve pain and give assistance with existing physical disabilities. Attention must be paid to the patient's reaction to his illness by letting him share his anxieties and despair while strengthening his resolve not to be defeated and to lead as normal a life as possible.

IMMUNITY AND PSYCHOLOGICAL PROCESSES

It is appropriate to consider here how psychological factors are related to immunological processes in general, and how this might affect the onset and course not only of rheumatoid arthritis but also of other illnesses such as asthma, hay-fever and atopic eczema in which allergic reactions are involved (Lancet 1985). The subject has recently been reviewed by Baker (1987).

The immune system has until recently been regarded as a 'closed', self-regulating or autonomous system. There is, however, increasing evidence that the brain can influence immunological processes and that these can in turn affect the brain by feedback mechanisms (Besedovsky *et al*. 1983).

Briefly, lymphocytes have receptors for a variety of hormones and neurotransmitters. These include corticosteroids, insulin, prolactin, growth hormones, oestradiol and testosterone, as well as beta-adrenergic agents, acetylcholine and neuropeptides. As the production of most hormones is under the control of the hypothalamus via the pituitary, it is not difficult to see that stress and associated emotional arousal could affect immune responses. In fact the immediate environment of the lymphocytes in the spleen and in the thymus gland contains these hormones as well as neurotransmitters and neuropeptides. In the spleen and thymus there are also many sympathetic nerve fibres surrounding the lymphocytes which could thus also be influenced directly by nervous impulses.

A feedback system has also been demonstrated. In rats during immune responses mediator substances are liberated by the lymphocytes which can in turn influence hypothalamic function, e.g. the rate of neuronal firing and release of catecholamines.

Turning to research on the influence of stress on immune processes (Marx 1985), there is evidence in rats that acute stress, e.g. electric shocks, can cause diminished production of the maturing T-cells in the thymus gland and reduce the immune response to known immunogens. Both the cellular and humoral immune response in rats can also be suppressed by classical conditioning (Ader and Cohen 1975).

In man there is evidence that widowers whose wives had recently died of breast cancer showed reduction of T-cells and impaired immune responses (Schleifer *et al.* 1983). Bartrop *et al.* (1977) have found similar changes after bereavement. Impaired lymphocyte function has also been demonstrated in patients with severe depression (Schleifer *et al.* 1984). There is some evidence that academic stress in students can cause suppression of immune responses, e.g. in dental students during the month preceding their final examinations (Jemmott *et al.* 1983).

In general, these findings concerning the interactions between the central nervous system, emotional states and the immune system make it easier to understand how life events could affect the onset and course of such physical diseases as rheumatoid arthritis, bronchial asthma, vasomotor rhinitis, atopic dermatitis, some infectious diseases and autoimmune diseases.

Psychological aspects of cancer and the immune system

It has been suggested that the onset and course of some forms of cancer could be influenced by psychological factors (Greer 1983; Cooper 1984; Greer and Silberfarb 1982). There is some evidence that neuro-immunological mechanisms might play a part in this process. For example, Greer *et al.* (1979) showed that women with breast cancer who, when told the diagnosis following mastectomy, showed either a fighting spirit or denial, had a significantly higher survival rate than women who reacted with hopelessness or depression. Greer and his colleagues (Pettingale *et al.* 1981) also showed that the women who showed denial and lived longer had higher serum levels of immunoglobulins than those who showed hopelessness or 'stoic acceptance'.

Similarly, the possible influence of personality factors and life events on the onset of cancer has been investigated. For example, Greer and Morris (1975) showed that women under fifty who could not express feelings of anger were more likely to develop breast cancer, and Kissen (1963) came to similar conclusions in men who developed lung cancer. The possibility that immune mechanisms may play a part in the influence of psychological factors on the onset and course of cancer is beginning to throw light on the physiological mechanisms that might be involved (Fox 1981).

MIGRAINE

In migraine psychosomatic considerations are particularly relevant as psychological factors play a major role in precipitating attacks and psychiatric features are common. Oliver Sacks (1981) has paid special attention to the subjective experience of patients with migraine. His study is based on 1,200 patients, and he starts by saying that 'a migraine is a physical event which may also be from the start, or later become, an emotional or symbolic event. A migraine expresses both physiological and emotional needs: it is the prototype of a psychophysiological reaction' (p. 30). It is a common disorder often associated with psychological features.

Between 5 and 10 per cent of the population are likely to develop migraine at some stage in their lives. If all forms of migraine, including the milder forms and migraine equivalents, are taken into account, the figure is nearer 20 per cent. Women are affected more often than men. In about two-thirds of patients there is a family history of migraine, indicating that genetic factors play a role in predisposing the individual to the disorder. It usually begins in childhood or early adult life. The liability to attacks persists throughout life, but there may be long free periods and in some the frequency and severity diminish with age.

Clinical features

Various forms of migrainous attacks have been described, of which the best known is *classical migraine*. This starts with an aura followed after 10 minutes to an hour by severe throbbing headache, usually but not always unilateral, and this in turn is followed by nausea and vomiting. The attacks usually last from several hours up to a day, but occasionally as long as two or three days. In about two-thirds of cases the headache is not preceded by an aura, in which case the condition is called *common migraine*. Conversely, some patients with classical migraine may at times experience the aura without subsequently developing headache or vomiting.

The *aura* can take several forms. By far the commonest are visual in nature. They often start with the appearance of bright, moving stars or other shapes, sometimes called fortification spectra, associated with or followed by scotomata which move around in one or both visual fields and often have bright edges, so-called scintillating scotomata. Less common are tactile auras where parasthesiae or areas of anaesthesia appear in the periphery of one or more limbs or in the face. Sometimes the aura affects higher neurological or mental functions, e.g. brief episodes of dysphasia or apraxia; body image disturbances; impairment of consciousness; of suddenly being two personalities; dreamy states; sensations of terror; strangeness; enlightenment or even mystical experiences. These disturbances of higher mental function may resemble the aura observed in temporal lobe epilepsy (see p. 314). In fact migraine and epilepsy may occur in the same individual. Usually these complex migraine auras are soon followed by the typical headache, but occasionally a migraine sufferer may experience the psychological disturbances without developing an attack of migraine, and rarely they may last for several hours or even a day or two, thus causing problems in diagnosis.

Next in frequency following the common and classical forms of migraine are the so-called *migraine equivalents*. These consist of brief periodic attacks, lasting from a few hours up to at most a day or two, during which the patient has no headache, or only a very mild one, but he complains of a variety of other physical or mental symptoms. These include attacks of vomiting ('cyclical vomiting' or 'bilious attacks') or epigastric pain ('abdominal migraine') and, less often, severe drowsiness or mood changes; they are more common in children than adults. The differential diagnosis from organic illnesses can be very difficult, especially if the symptoms are those of acute abdominal pain, vomiting or diarrhoea. The periodicity of the attacks and their short duration and spontaneous recovery may assist in making the correct diagnosis. There may be evidence of emotional stress or excitement preceding the attacks. In the long term the diagnosis may be confirmed by the fact that, say, a child who suffers from cyclical vomiting or abdominal migraine may cease to have these symptoms but develops classical migraine as he gets older. Adults, too, may suffer from migraine equivalents at some time in their lives and from classical migraine at others.

A few other rare varieties of migraine have been described, as follows:

(1) *Migrainous neuralgia* or *cluster headaches*. These consist of severe attacks of pain of acute onset, usually on waking or during the night. The pain is unilateral and may affect the head, face, temple, eye or ear. The eye on the affected side may discharge tears or the nostril may be blocked or discharge. Characteristically they occur in clusters over a period of days or weeks. The attacks usually only last a few minutes, at most one or two hours. Some patients who suffer from cluster headaches get classical or common migraine at other times.

(2) *Basilar artery migraine*. This rare form occurs especially in adolescent girls. A visual aura is followed by evidence of brain stem involvement, e.g. dysarthria, paraesthesiae in the periphery of arms or legs, tinnitus or vertigo; these are then followed by severe migrainous headache. Impairment or loss of consciousness lasting up to half an hour has been described.

(3) *Hemiplegic migraine*. Some patients with migraine develop unilateral motor or sensory disturbances either as part of the aura or accompanying the headache, sometimes persisting for a day or two after the attack.

(4) *Ophthalmoplegic migraine*. Here the attacks of migraine are accompanied by paralysis of external ocular movements, or sometimes by total ophthalmoplegia.

Mechanism of the attacks

There is some evidence that the migrainous headache is due to vasodilatation of extracranial arteries; the aura and the various neurological or mental symptoms that can precede or accompany the attack may be due to vasoconstriction and spasm of cerebral blood vessels. The various manifestations could then be explained by the particular blood vessels and regions of the brain that are affected in the attack.

The question remains as to the precipitating factors responsible for initiating the attacks. The role of emotional factors is undoubted and is discussed below. In addition, a few patients find that certain foods may precipitate their attacks, e.g. chocolate, cheese or alcohol, but there is no evidence that food allergies or other forms of allergy play a significant role. A small proportion of women find that their attacks are related to their menstrual periods, and the contraceptive pill is known to aggravate the condition. Migraine often improves during pregnancy.

Psychological aspects

Personality characteristics

Harold Wolff (1963) has claimed that migraine is associated with certain personality characteristics. These include driving, perfectionist personalities with obsessional tendencies, poor tolerance of frustration and the need to exert control over others. Paulley and Haskell (1975) have also stressed the perfectionist and self-driving characteristics of migraine patients and especially their inability to relax. These characteristics are common but not present in all patients.

Emotional stress

Equally important is the finding that the attacks are often brought on by tension and emotional stress. This is not necessarily related to major life events. Persistent emotional tension, situations in which the individual cannot express strong feelings, e.g. of anger or rage, sudden excitement, the anticipation of pleasurable events, e.g. meeting a friend or the beginning of a holiday, are among the many events known to initiate attacks. They can also occur at the beginning of a 'let down period', e.g. when a harassing day is over or at weekends. However, some attacks may not be preceded by any known precipitating event.

Psychiatric accompaniments

The psychological features associated with some of the more complex types of the aura have already been described.

The attacks themselves are usually accompanied by irritability, sensitivity to light or noise or any other form of interference, drowsiness and the wish to be left alone. An inability to think clearly or to concentrate, depression and anxiety are common. In more severe attacks there may be marked impairment, clouding or even brief loss of consciousness; or a confusional state with impaired memory, visual or auditory hallucinations and disturbance of body image. Some of the more severe mental abnormalities may outlast the attack by several days.

Some patients may develop unremitting or continually recurring severe attacks of migraine over a period of several weeks or longer. Such *chronic migrainous disability* may be associated with severe depression.

Treatment

The pharmacological aspects of treating the attacks will not be discussed here except to mention that ergotamine tartrate and analgesics like aspirin, codis or panadol taken at the earliest sign of a warning aura may abort the development of a full-blown attack. Clonidine or propranolol taken regularly sometimes help to prevent attacks.

It is equally important to spend time with the patient in order to discover factors which initiate the attacks, so that they can if possible be prevented or minimised. Attention to stressful circumstances in personal relationships or at work is particularly important, as are attempts to help the patient to stop driving himself and living under constant pressure. A supportive doctor-patient relationship may help the patient to learn how best to control or live with his attacks with the minimum of interference to his life. Paulley and Haskell (1975) emphasise the need to teach migraine patients how to relax.

Formal psychotherapy is hardly ever indicated for migraine as such, but patients who enter long-term therapy for other reasons may find that their attacks diminish or even clear up.

MUSCULOSKELETAL DISORDERS

Muscular and skeletal pains are common complaints. They can be of organic or emotional origin, or a combination of both. The most common examples are tension headache, pain and stiffness in the neck, backache, or pain in the limbs. Quite often the persistent discomfort causes anxiety, depression and irritability, which in turn increase muscle tension so that a vicious circle is set up. A few of these conditions will be discussed here, followed by a brief account of disorders of movement.

Tension headache

Here the headache is associated with persistent contraction of the muscles of the head and neck. It is almost always caused by emotional tension, anxiety or depression which leads to the painful muscular contraction. The headache is usually bilateral and starts in the occipital, frontal or cervical region. It may be a dull ache but can become more severe and throbbing in nature. Attacks often last all day and may occur daily for days or weeks and, in turn, cause further anxiety and tension. Unlike migraine there is no aura or other neurological disturbance. Nausea and vomiting are rare.

Emotional factors are always present, often associated with difficulties in personal and family relationships, pressure at work, or depression.

In treatment the use of mild analgesics should be combined with reassurance that the headache is not due to organic disease, and with supportive psychotherapy. This should be directed towards helping the patient to understand the cause of his headache, express his feelings and, if possible, find ways of resolving his problems. Relaxation exercises are sometimes helpful. Tranquillisers should be avoided because of the risk of dependency, and antidepressants should only be given if there is evidence of an underlying depressive illness.

Backache

Chronic or recurrent backache, especially low back pain, is an extremely common complaint. Pain in the back causes more time off work than any other single condition in the UK and USA. Barlow (1986) quotes a figure of 12 million working days lost per year in the UK. Only a small proportion of people who complain of backache consult their general practitioners, and they refer only 10 per cent of the patients they see to hospital. Of those actually seen in hospital only about 12 per cent have significant organic disease of the spine, such as arthritis, prolapsed intervertebral discs, ankylosing spondylitis, osteoporosis, or secondary carcinoma. In the great majority of patients with backache the pain is due to muscular tension, often caused by emotional stress and sometimes associated with faulty posture or muscular strain due to unusual or poorly coordinated movements. The persistent pain in turn causes further anxiety and depression.

The psychological aspects need to be considered in diagnosis and management. Provided there are no major organic abnormalities, the following considerations have to be taken into account. The presence of any significant emotional problems affecting the patient at the onset or relapse of his backache is particularly important. It also helps to discover why the patient who has had recurrent backache for a long time has decided to consult his doctor now. The question must also be considered whether his reaction to the pain is excessive and especially whether he is getting a significant amount of secondary gain which may be leading to his adopting a sick role. This is not uncommon, e.g. in patients following a laminectomy. Some patients with anxiety states or depression complain of and focus their attention on back pain, often developing hypchondriacal fears of, say, cancer or permanent invalidism.

It is equally important to pay attention to the patient's posture. Here an osteopath may be helpful both for diagnosis and treatment. In fact many patients with chronic backache seek help through osteopathy, acupuncture or homeopathy because they feel disappointed in what orthodox medicine has to offer them. Barlow (1973) has stressed the value of the Alexander Technique which teaches patients how to use their body correctly. In general, patients with chronic backache, be it due to physical or psychological causes or both, need an approach that pays equal attention to any physical and emotional factors.

Spasmodic torticollis

In this disorder of movement the head and neck are repeatedly pulled to one side by sustained spasmodic contraction of the neck muscles, especially the sternomastoid and trapezius. Sometimes the spasm becomes permanent, with hypertrophy of the sternomastoid muscle. It usually starts in adults and often becomes chronic, continuing for years on end, sometimes interrupted by periods of remission; a few milder cases recover spontaneously. The movements are characteristically made worse by emotional upset or excitement, and cease during sleep.

Aetiology

The exact aetiology remains unknown. Both physical and psychological factors probably play a part to varying degrees in different patients. There is hardly ever any evidence of associated neurological disorders although disorders of the extrapyramidal system may be involved. In some patients the condition commences after an emotional shock. In many there is evidence of sustained emotional tension, often associated with marital or other interpersonal conflicts.

Treatment

This is difficult and often unsuccessful. Earlier attempts using collars to immobilise the head and neck have been abandoned. Relaxation methods have largely failed. So has the use of drugs, although phenothiazines or haloperidol have helped a few patients temporarily. Various surgical procedures, including division of the accessory nerve or of the sternomastoid, have been only partially successful, or have led to serious complications; they have therefore been abandoned. Some patients have been helped by psychotherapy, and others by behavioural techniques. One or other of these two methods or a combination of both is probably worth a trial in patients who are motivated to try a psychological approach. Others will need long-term support.

Occupational cramps

The commonest of these is *writer's cramp*. Here the patient develops spasm in the small muscles of the fingers and hand as soon as he begins to write or soon after. This leads to considerable disability. The patient may attempt to circumvent the disorder by various means, including learning to write with the other hand, but the spasm may then develop in that hand as well.

Other occupational cramps include violinist's cramp, when the wrist goes into spasm when trying to use the bow, pianist's cramp, typist's cramp and so on. In all occupational cramps the spasm is limited to the group of small muscles the patient has learnt to use for skilled movements, often after many years of practice. As it often affects the person's professional skill, e.g. in musicians, it may lead to serious personal, financial and social disability.

Aetiology

There is no evidence that organic factors play a significant role. Psychological factors can often be identified by exploring the patient's personality and lifestyle. In particular, the patient may have highly ambivalent feelings about his occupation; for example, a violinist who has been forced to practise since early childhood may resent having to do so but at the same time may want to continue to play. Suppressed resentment, impatience and frustration, and associated conflicts can all play a part. Once any of these occupational cramps are established maladaptive conditioned responses often develop and maintain or reinforce the disorder.

Treatment

This is difficult and requires patience on the part of the doctor, therapist and patient. If emotional conflicts are prominent exploratory psychotherapy should be tried. Various behavioural methods, including desensitisation and deconditioning techniques may be helpful, especially if combined with psychotherapy. A retraining programme combined with learning how to relax is essential. Propranolol has helped some patients, while others have responded to acupuncture. Others fail to recover or relapse in spite of all efforts and may be forced to change their occupation.

Tics

Simple tics or habit spasms are common in children and usually start between the ages of five and ten, more often in boys than in girls. They consist of regular, rapid and involuntary contractions of isolated muscle groups, usually in the face, especially around the eyes, but sometimes in the limbs. The majority of children lose their tics within a few months. There is often evidence of disturbance in the family, and tics tend to appear at times of emotional stress and may be associated with other developmental disorders of childhood. They are made worse by anxiety, and when attention is paid to them by over-anxious parents.

Treatment

The parents should be encouraged to ignore the tics and any significant emotional problems in the family should be dealt with, if possible. In a few cases behaviour therapy, e.g. massed practice or relaxation techniques, has been tried but rarely with lasting effects.

Gilles de la Tourette syndrome

In a very small proportion of children with tics the condition fails to improve. Instead, as they approach adolescence their tics become multiple and more severe, spreading to the trunk and limbs. The rapid involuntary movements become more forceful, sometimes causing involuntary jerks affecting the whole body. In the course of a few years, but sometimes sooner, involuntary utterances are added to the picture in about 40 per cent of cases (Lees *et al.* 1984). These consist of grunting noises and expletives, often of an obscene, blasphemous and aggressive nature, referred to as *coprolalia*. In some patients the disorder is associated with *obsessional features* (Frankel *et al.* 1986). The syndrome is named after Gilles de la Tourette who first described it (De la Tourette 1885). Its relation to tics in childhood has been stressed by Corbett *et al.* (1969) and Corbett (1971). It is more common in males than females, and may persist for many years into adult life. The clinical findings have been studied by Lees *et al.* (1984) and Robertson *et al.* (1988). It is a very disabling condition, made worse by emotional stress and whenever the patient's attention is drawn to his abnormal movements and utterances. Both of these cease during sleep.

Aetiology

A psychological aetiology used to be considered but is unlikely in view of the severity and persistent nature of the involuntary movements. Organic factors probably play a major role. It has, for example, been claimed that abnormalities of neurotransmitters, brain damage and developmental factors may play a part. The fact that there is a higher than expected incidence of tics in close relatives of patients with Gilles de la Tourette syndrome suggests a genetic factor.

Treatment

Psychotherapy, behaviour therapy and stereotactic surgery have all been tried, but none has proved effective. More recently, however, it has been found that haloperidol in large doses and maintained over several years before the dose is slowly reduced, is successful in 80–90 per cent of cases. Pimozide or fluphenazine are also effective in some cases and have fewer extrapyramidal side-effects. The fact that dopamine blocking agents can control the symptoms further supports an organic basis for the disorder (Lawden 1986). In addition long-term support and rehabilitation are essential.

The condition has been fully reviewed by Robertson (1989).

PSYCHOSOMATIC ASPECTS OF PAIN

Pain is a common symptom in many medical and psychiatric disorders. A few of these have already been discussed in this chapter, e.g. migraine, tension headache, backache and rheumatoid arthritis. This section considers some issues central to the understanding of pain and its role in medicine and psychiatry. It also summarises some of the circumstances which can make patients experience pain and which may affect its nature and severity.

First, it needs to be stressed that pain is a subjective experience. It may arise from peripheral stimuli caused by local tissue damage, or it may be of psychological origin, i.e. due to mental and associated cerebral processes in the absence of a peripheral stimulus. This must be emphasised because patients and even doctors often find it difficult to accept that pain which is of psychological origin is as real an experience, and often at least as severe and disabling, as the experience of pain due to an identifiable organic cause. Patients also tend to feel that if they are told that their pain is not due to physical disease but of psychological origin, say, due to emotional stress, they are suspected of imagining the pain or are being accused of 'putting it on'.

The experience of pain also differs from one individual to the next, and it is influenced by the meaning of the pain to the individual, the circumstances under which it arises and his psychological state at the time (Merskey 1976). Relaxation, suggestion, treatment with placebos or hypnosis can all reduce pain, while fear, anxiety, anger and tension can increase it.

The remainder of this chapter consists of a brief summary of the main conditions responsible for pain and their psychological aspects.

Pain due to organic disease

Here the psychological aspects are largely concerned with the patient's reaction to pain due to some physical disorder, and how it affects his behaviour. Many patients' reaction is appropriate to the severity and duration of the pain. Others cope with it exceptionally well or even ignore or deny it, while others become depressed. Anxious patients may over-react or develop hypochondriacal fears, e.g. a fear of cancer or that they are about to die. If the pain is chronic or relapsing patients may consciously or unconsciously use it for secondary gain, e.g. in their personal relationships or in their attitude to work. This may lead to the adoption of a *sick role*, often leading to increased pain and disability. The term *abnormal illness behaviour* is sometimes used in such cases (Pilowsky 1983).

Some patients with chronic pain may use it as a form of communication. For example, a patient with frequent backache due to a prolapsed disc may come to see his doctor with pain he has had for a long time but on enquiry the general practitioner may discover that the patient actually wants to talk about some personal problems that worry him; he is using his pain, as it were, as a respectable excuse for seeking a consultation.

Pain due to major psychiatric illness

It is not unusual for pain, e.g. facial or abdominal, to be a major presenting symptom of a depressive illness. Here the differential diagnosis from organic disease may be difficult, especially if there are no other obvious symptoms of a depressive illness. In that case the pain is said to serve as a *depressive equivalent* (see p. 201). If pain due to a depressive illness is located in the face it is often called *atypical facial pain* because it lacks the characteristics of organic causes of facial pain such as trigeminal neuralgia or pain due to dental disease or sinusitis.

Treatment with antidepressants may confirm that the pain was due to depression if it responds, perhaps alongside any other depressive symptoms that may have been present as well.

Pain as an hysterical symptom

Pain is a common symptom of hysteria (see p. 176). It is often described by the patient in exaggerated, bizarre terms. Sometimes its meaning can be readily understood in psychodynamic terms; for example, a man whose father died of a myocardial infarct may develop acute chest pain due to identification with him in an unconscious attempt to deny the loss and to avoid having to mourn him. Such pain in turn is likely to lead to the fear of having a heart attack himself and of dying like his father. Sometimes a husband may identify with his wife and develop abdominal pain and other gastrointestinal symptoms while she is pregnant or goes into labour, the so-called *Couvade syndrome* (Trethowan and Conlon 1965; Enoch and Trethowan 1979).

Pain due to anxiety

Minor pains are common expressions of an *anxiety state*, e.g. precordial pain; this in turn may lead to the fear of having heart disease and by increasing the patient's anxiety may lead to the development of a cardiac neurosis (see p. 455).

Psychogenic pain

A variety of pains commonly develop at times of emotional stress and difficulties in personal relationships, in the absence of any clearly definable physical or psychiatric illness. Such pains are sometimes loosely referred to as 'psychosomatic'. Any part of the body may be involved; common examples are headache and backache. Occasionally the site of the pain will be determined by the site of a painful organic disease the patient has had in the past, e.g. right-sided upper abdominal pain may develop under stress in someone who has previously had biliary colic; or someone who has had a prolapsed disc in the past may develop backache at times of stress. The differential diagnosis from organic disease may then be very difficult. In many cases both psychological and organic factors and their interaction may play a part and equal attention needs to be paid to both aspects in diagnosis and treatment.

The term *psychogenic pain* is often used when psychological factors are clearly of major importance and are responsible for the onset of the pain. In fact the DSM-III (American Psychiatric Association 1980) provided a diagnostic category of *psychogenic pain disorder*. This has been changed to *somatoform pain disorder* in the revised edition, DSM-III-R (American Psychiatric Association 1987). In both editions the disorder is defined as pain which occurs in the absence of abnormal physical findings but with evidence for the aetiological role of psychological factors; the pain is not due to any other mental disorder nor is there any obvious psychological mechanism for it.

The term psychogenic pain will also be included in the forthcoming ICD-10 due to come into clinical use in 1991 or 1992 (Sartorius *et al.* 1988). In the ICD-10 the diagnosis of psychogenic pain will be subsumed under 'somatoform disorder', as it is in the DSM-III-R.

There are several reasons why, in general, the use of terms like psychogenic and psychogenesis has led to a good deal of controversy among psychiatrists (Lewis 1972; Campbell 1983). If the term psychogenic is used to imply no more than that pain or some other physical symptom, like vomiting, is of psychological *origin* it is fully acceptable and inclusion of the term psychogenic pain in the DSM-III and the ICD-10 is helpful. If, however, it is wrongly taken to indicate that physical mechanisms in the brain and in the periphery are not involved in the production of the somatic symptom – an out-of-date dualistic concept – it is misleading. Psychological processes are in fact always associated with cerebral processes at the level of brain function, as discussed in Chapter 2 (see p. 26). Moreover, in most cases psychological factors give rise to physical symptoms through intermediary neurophysiological mechanisms, e.g. spasm in muscles, blood vessels and visceral organs like the gut, even though in the individual case this may be difficult to demonstrate. Organic factors may also be responsible for the vulnerability of the part of the body or organ in which the pain is felt. Terms like psychosomatic or somatoform can be helpful, as they draw attention to the fact that interaction between psychological and somatic mechanisms is involved even when psychological factors are of primary aetiological importance.

In some cases of psychologically determined pain abnormal *mental* mechanisms can be identified, e.g. repression of emotional conflicts and conversion. The pain then has the characteristics of a hysterical conversion symptom, often with an exaggerated and bizarre response to the pain.

Malingering

In a few patients a complaint of pain may be the result of malingering. The circumstances, such as wanting to escape from an intolerable situation, may provide a clue, but often it is difficult to be sure of the diagnosis. Even then it is important to discover the reasons that led the patient to malinger. Munchhausen's syndrome (see p. 183) is a rare but important example.

FURTHER READING

General

Kaplan, H.I. and Sadock, B.J. (eds) (1985). *Comprehensive Textbook of Psychiatry*, 4th ed., ch. 25: 'Psychological factors affecting physical conditions (psychosomatic disorders)'. Williams & Wilkins, Baltimore and London.
Weiner, H. (1977). *Psychobiology of Human Disease*. Elsevier, New York, Oxford and Amsterdam.

Anorexia nervosa and bulimia

Bruch, H. (1978). *The Golden Cage: the enigma of anorexia nervosa*. Open Books, London.
Crisp, A.H. (1980). *Anorexia Nervosa: let me be*. Academic Press, London.
Garfinkel, P.E. and Garner, D.M. (eds) (1982). *Anorexia Nervosa: a multi-dimensional perspective*. Brunner/Mazel, New York.
Garner, D.M. and Garfinkel, P.E. (eds) (1985). *Handbook of Psychotherapy for Anorexia and Bulimia*. Guildford Press, New York and London.
Szmukler, G.I., Slade, P.D., Harris, P., Berton, D. and Russell, G.F.M. (eds) (1986). *Anorexia Nervosa and Bulimic Disorders: current perspectives*. Pergamon, Oxford.

Gastrointestinal disorders

Creed, F.H. and Lennard-Jones, J.E. (1982). 'Gastrointestinal symptoms' in *Medicine and Psychiatry: a practical approach* (Creed, F. and Pfeffer, J.M., eds). Pitman, London.

Skin disorders

Sneddon, J. and Sneddon, I.B. (1982). 'The psychiatrist's role in the skin clinic' in *Medicine and Psychiatry: a practical approach* (Creed, F. and Pfeffer, J.M., eds). Pitman, London.

Headache and migraine

Lance, J.W. (1982). *Mechanisms and Management of Headache*, 4th ed. Butterworths, London.
Sacks, O. (1981). *Migraine: the natural history of a common disorder*. Pan Books, London.
Wolff, H.G. (1963). *Headache and Other Head Pain*. OUP, New York.

39

Liaison Psychiatry

The growing interest among psychiatrists in the psychosomatic aspects of medicine and the establishment of departments of psychiatry in general hospitals has led to increasing collaboration or 'liaison work' between psychiatrists and their non-psychiatric hospital colleagues. In the US and Canada specialised medical-psychiatric liaison services or departments have been set up in several of the larger hospitals (Lipowski 1967a). In West Germany the first university department of psychosomatic medicine was established in Heidelberg by Alexander Mitscherlich in 1948, followed by several similar departments in other universities. In the UK liaison psychiatry has only recently begun to be recognised as an area of specialisation among psychiatrists. Although there are no separate departments of liaison psychiatry, some psychiatrists have developed a special interest in liaison work.

There are several areas covered by the term liaison psychiatry. These include:

(1) The influence of psychological and social factors on the origin and course of physical illness
(2) Psychological reactions to physical illness
(3) Somatic symptoms of psychological origin
(4) Organic psychiatric reactions due to physical illness
(5) Problems between patients and staff

There is a tendency to broaden the concept of liaison psychiatry, e.g. by also including the diagnosis and treatment of patients admitted following an act of self-harm. This important aspect of psychiatric work in general hospitals is considered in Chapters 19 and 54. Another area concerns consultations requested by non-psychiatric colleagues concerning patients admitted under their care for medical reasons but who may also be suffering from formal psychiatric illnesses such as schizophrenia or affective disorders. Such consultations constituted an important part of the psychiatrist's function in general hospitals long before the concept of liaison psychiatry became established. If the concept is used too widely its more specialised function, i.e. the care of patients suffering from physical disorders in which psychological aspects play a significant role, is in

485

danger of being lost.

In fact, if a psychiatrist who is asked by a non-psychiatric colleague to see a patient on a medical, surgical, obstetric or paediatric ward or as an outpatient restricts himself to deciding whether or not the patient has an identifiable psychiatric illness, he may miss the very purpose of the liaison consultation, namely to help his non-psychiatric colleagues to uncover relevant psychological or social aspects, and to identify and deal with the patient's reactions to his physical disorder. Lipowski (1967a, 1967b, 1968) has reviewed the clinical and theoretical aspects of liaison (consultation) psychiatry, basing his account on the practice in general hospitals in Canada and the USA. He also makes a useful distinction between the more usual patient-oriented consultations and consultations requested because of difficulties between the medical consultant and his patient (consultee-oriented consultations) and difficulties between ward staff and the patient (situation-oriented consultations).

Medical-psychiatric problems are at least as common or even more so in general practice and need careful attention from general practitioners (see Chapter 55). It is important for medical students and postgraduate psychiatric trainees to become acquainted with these aspects of patient care during their training; experience in liaison psychiatry in hospital and during general practice attachments can be used to prepare all doctors for these aspects of their future work, be it in hospital or in general practice. Guidelines for the training of psychiatrists in liaison psychiatry have been published by the Royal College of Psychiatrists (1988).

PSYCHOSOCIAL FACTORS IN PHYSICAL ILLNESS

Here the liaison psychiatrist's task is to decide whether any relevant life events, inter-personal problems, conflicts or personality characteristics may have played a significant part in determining the onset, course, or relapse of the patient's physical symptoms or illness. A useful question to ask oneself when carrying out such consultations is 'Why has this patient developed this particular disorder at this particular time in his life?' This applies to both organic diseases with structural abnormalities, e.g. ulcerative colitis, and to functional disorders due to physiological dysfunction, e.g. the irritable bowel syndrome. In practice many patients suffering from a wide variety of medical disorders may benefit from such a liaison-consultation.

The patient is more likely to cooperate with the liaison psychiatrist if the purpose of the consultation has already been explained to him by the medical and nursing staff. They in turn are in a better position to do so if they have worked with the same liaison psychiatrist for some time so that they are aware of the contribution he can make to the diagnosis and management of their patients.

It is particularly important for the psychiatrist to make it clear to the patient that his physical symptoms are being taken seriously, and certainly not thought to be imaginary; some patients fear this may be the case when they are referred to a psychiatrist. Taking a brief history of the patient's physical complaints, perhaps carrying out a brief physical examination and looking at the results of physical investigations may help to overcome this problem, quite apart from making the liaison psychiatrist recognise more fully the nature of the patient's medical condition. This can lead on to explaining to the patient that stress and personal problems are known sometimes to influence the physical disorder from which he is suffering. This should be followed by an unstructured interview – not a formal psychiatric interview – in which listening to the patient and constructive use of one's own emotional responses play a central role.

Some patients with a physical illness may be unaware of any relevant emotional problems and may be out of touch with their feelings. This attitude, described as alexithymia by Sifneos (1973) (see p. 436), makes it very difficult to get patients to talk meaningfully about themselves and what they feel. Some doctors may reinforce this behaviour if they, too, prefer to consider only the patient's physical symptoms or illness and to ignore his personal and social circumstances and how he feels about them. In liaison work the psychiatrist has to tolerate his own feelings of frustration when confronted with such alexithymic patients and help them slowly, if necessary in a series of interviews, to get in touch with their feelings and to express themselves openly. This in itself may serve as a relief to the patient, sometimes leading to diminution of his symptoms; however, as he may now be faced with painful feelings and conflicts he finds it hard to cope with, it is essential to see him again soon and to arrange regular follow-up and support. Occasionally this may lead to a period of psychotherapy if the patient is now sufficiently motivated to work on psychological problems related to his illness. This kind of liaison work is therefore best carried out by psychiatrists with experience in general medicine and in unstructured interviewing and psychotherapy.

PSYCHOLOGICAL REACTIONS TO PHYSICAL ILLNESS

The patient's reaction to his illness may take many forms. Any illness or physical symptom is likely to make him anxious, sometimes out of proportion to the real nature of his illness. The following may serve as examples. A young woman with ulcerative colitis may live in fear of having to have a colectomy and ileostomy because she is convinced that no man would then make love to and marry her, and that even if she did get married she could not have children as during pregnancy the ileostomy would burst open. A man who has had a myocardial infarct may fear that any physical exertion will cause another infarct. A woman who has had a hysterectomy may believe that this will leave her frigid or unable to have intercourse. The psychological effects of a mastectomy are particularly stressful and women need a great deal of help and support from doctors and nurses after the operation.

Ignorance almost always leads to exaggerated fears, and many patients feel too embarrassed to mention them. It is the doctor's, nurses' and, if necessary, the liaison psychiatrist's task to make it as easy as possible for patients to reveal their anxieties; for example, he may himself broach the topic – fear of cancer, of dying, of invalidism, of sexual inadequacy, etc. – and this often makes the patient respond by saying 'Well as a matter of fact I did wonder ...', and he will be relieved to have been understood and listened to and, when appropriate, reassured. Doctors vary greatly in their ability to talk to their patients about such problems; some physicians, surgeons and general practitioners are exceptionally skilled in doing so. Others may find it very difficult, especially when it comes to sexual anxieties or the many issues concerned with death and dying that affect the terminally ill. It may then become the task of the liaison psychiatrist, sometimes in conjunction with general practitioners or the medical and nursing staff.

Occasionally a patient with a serious, perhaps incurable illness will develop a reactive depression which requires support, possibly combined with antidepressant medication. Or a patient with an organic disease may develop superimposed hysterical conversion symptoms; for example a patient with mild symptoms due to multiple sclerosis became so frightened of becoming completely disabled that she developed an hysterical paralysis of her legs. At an unconscious level it was better to be paralysed already than to live in fear of losing the use of her legs.

SOMATIC SYMPTOMS OF PSYCHOLOGICAL ORIGIN

Another group of patients in whose diagnosis and management the opinion of a liaison psychiatrist may be needed are those with physical symptoms for which, in spite of numerous investigations, no organic cause has been found. Many of these patients have multiple symptoms and have been investigated in several departments with negative results, often over a period of years. They therefore often have thick medical folders and continue to look for further opinions and investigations.

Occasionally a psychiatric disorder may underlie their symptoms; e.g. a depressive illness may present with physical pain or anxiety about physical disease, such as cancerophobia. In others the physical symptom may be a conversion symptom due to hysteria (see p. 176). Lloyd (1986) has reviewed the somatic presentation of psychiatric disorders.

In the majority, however, no such psychiatric diagnosis can be made, and several interviews may be needed before the relation between stress factors and the patient's symptoms comes to light. Not infrequently careful enquiry into the patient's history and personality development may reveal serious emotional deprivation early in childhood (see p. 437). Sometimes, it becomes apparent that he comes from a family background where the parents, usually the mother, failed to respond adequately to his emotional needs, responding only, and often with excessive anxiety, to his physical needs and complaints. This then becomes the only way in which the child can get the mother's attention. It has been suggested (Wolff 1973, 1977) that such people, as they grow older, are conditioned to respond to stressful situations by developing physical symptoms rather than expressing their distress in emotional terms. Winnicott (1966) has drawn attention to this split between physical and mental functioning in some patients with psychosomatic symptoms and has emphasised the need to help them reintegrate physical and emotional experience. During interviews it may be possible to help the patient recognise the emotional distress underlying his physical complaints.

Unfortunately, the secondary gain associated with long-standing physical complaints may be so great that by the time the patient is seen as an adult and the underlying emotional disturbance is recognised, treatment, including psychotherapy, may fail. Long-term support by the patient's general practitioner, perhaps in conjunction with the liaison psychiatrist, may then be the only way of helping such patients.

ORGANIC PSYCHIATRIC REACTIONS TO PHYSICAL ILLNESS

The requests for consultation considered here are those which arise in relation to patients who develop psychiatric symptoms of organic origin as a result of primary medical or surgical conditions. These organic psychiatric reactions have been described elsewhere (see Chapters 22 and 23). The commonest types of organic psychiatric reactions seen on medical or surgical wards take the form of acute or chronic confusional states which have arisen as a complication of systemic illnesses. These include hypoxia due to acute or chronic respiratory disorders or cardiac failure, metabolic disorders due to renal or liver failure, and electrolyte disturbances, either due to medical conditions or occurring post-operatively. Infections causing prolonged fever, e.g. septicaemia, a carcinoma, e.g. of the bronchus, with cerebral secondaries, or systemic lupus erythematosus are further examples. The organic psychiatric complications of alcoholism may first present on medical wards, and are described in Chapter 30.

Other requests for liaison consultations may arise in patients with psychiatric complications due to medication, e.g. hypnotics, artane, levodopa, cimetidine, propranolol or digoxin. Organic reactions due to diseases of the brain itself include dementia, cerebrovascular accidents, cerebral tumour and infections like encephalitis or meningitis. The tables on pp. 263 and 267 list the causes of acute and chronic organic psychiatric reactions.

Many of these disorders will be dealt with by physicians or surgeons treating the primary condition without psychiatric assistance, but psychiatric advice may be needed in some cases.

PROBLEMS BETWEEN PATIENTS AND STAFF

Another area in which the help of liaison psychiatrists may be needed concerns problems in the relationship between the patient and his doctor (consultee-oriented consultations); or difficulties that arise between the patient or his relatives and members of the treatment team (situation-oriented consultations) (Lipowski 1967b).

Not surprisingly, doctors, nurses and others involved in looking after patients prefer those who are cooperative, who readily and without question accept whatever investigations and treatments, medical or surgical, are being advised and who do not make excessive demands. In reality few, if any, patients fall into this category. Terms like 'non-compliance' or 'abnormal illness behaviour' are sometimes used to describe such situations. A more helpful approach is to try to understand the patient's, sometimes also his relatives' and the staff's reactions and help them to handle these more appropriately. There are several factors to be considered.

Any physical symptom, illness, injury, operation or other treatment procedure, or investigation is likely to make the patient anxious and to affect his attitude to his doctor. However, the doctor's own attitude, be it the general practitioner or hospital doctor, and that of the nursing staff are equally important. Some doctors or nurses become hostile when faced with patients' difficult behaviour, e.g. when they become uncooperative and angry. If the doctor then becomes impatient and loses control the chances of establishing a better doctor-patient relationship are further undermined. It may at times become the task of the liaison psychiatrist to help the staff to understand and handle such situations. His awareness of his own similar reactions to patients should help him in this task.

Admission to hospital is a stressful event in itself, be it an emergency admission, or admission for investigation or for surgical treatment, especially after a long period on a waiting list. Perhaps the most stressful aspect is being uncertain about what is going to happen. For children separation from parents is particularly traumatic (see p. 68); elderly patients often become confused and disoriented in a strange hospital environment. Liaison psychiatrists may be asked by the ward staff to help in such situations.

During their stay in hospital severely ill patients often regress to a state of childlike helplessness and dependency. This may make them extremely demanding so that nurses and doctors resent their behaviour. For example, extreme regression made a seriously ill inpatient aged twenty-five refuse to take any food other than what his mother brought in for him, much to the annoyance of the nursing staff. In such a situation the liaison psychiatrist will have to explain to the nurses and doctors how the patient's behaviour can be understood. Occasionally a liaison psychiatrist can help the staff to understand why a patient unreasonably refuses a particular investigation. For example, a liaison psychiatrist working on a neurological ward was asked to see a patient who had refused to have a skull X-ray. She was on the point of discharging herself and the neurologist was about to let her go because she was so uncooperative. The psychiatrist, when talking to her, found out that she thought the X-ray photograph of her head would reveal to everyone all her most intimate thoughts of which she felt guilty and ashamed.

There are certain medical and surgical departments in which particularly difficult problems between patient and staff are likely to arise. On intensive care units the staff work under great pressure and carry responsibility for life and death. The seriously ill patients are likely to be equally anxious; being monitored and surrounded by technical equipment and seeing other patients die can all increase their fear and discomfort. The problem of whether or not to keep a patient on a respirator or to discontinue it causes much stress and anxiety to staff and relatives. A psychiatrist attached to an intensive care unit for liaison work is often able to help the staff, patients and their relatives in some of these highly stressful situations. The same applies to renal dialysis units and to transplant surgery where the problems of selection of patients and their fears and angry feelings, if rejected, can cause a great deal of stress to both patients and staff. Staff looking after patients with AIDS may benefit from support from a liaison psychiatrist. On obstetric wards the liaison psychiatrist may be able to help the staff to deal with patients with psychiatric problems in the puerperium.

Cosmetic surgery can present special problems that require cooperation between surgeon and liaison psychiatrist. Some patients with dysmorphophobia (see p. 258) may try to persuade the surgeon to operate on some part of their body, e.g. the nose, which they consider to be deformed, in spite of his advice against surgery; or the patient may become highly critical of the surgeon if, as is often the case, the patient is dissatisfied with the result of the operation. It may then become the task of the liaison psychiatrist to try to resolve the situation or take over the patient's care.

ORGANISATION

Liaison work demands a great deal of collaboration between the psychiatrist and the medical, nursing and social work staff. The best results are obtained if sufficient psychiatric staff are available for a particular psychiatrist to be allocated to individual wards or departments so that he and the ward staff can get to know each other and work together, sometimes in regular staff groups. Such attachments are particularly useful for research, and for teaching medical students, junior medical staff and psychiatric trainees in liaison work. This is considered further on p. 713.

Whatever form of organisation is used, personal contact between the psychiatrist and his colleagues is essential for good liaison work. The psychiatrist's conclusions should be expressed, both verbally and in written reports, in simple language that is easily understood, and any psychological jargon should be avoided. It is equally important that any advice given on the patient's management should be as practical and helpful as possible, and the psychiatrist must be prepared to visit the patient on the ward several times after the initial consultation, and if necessary follow him up as an outpatient after discharge.

FURTHER READING

Gomez, J. (1987). *Liaison Psychiatry: mental health problems in the general hospital*. Croom Helm, London.

Part VII

Child Psychiatry

40

Disorders of Childhood

A child is considered to be psychiatrically disordered when his behaviour or emotions are abnormal and he either experiences personal suffering or shows impaired personality development, or both. However, psychological problems in childhood often present as exaggerations of normal behaviour and feelings rather than distinct entities, making it difficult to define and classify child psychiatric disorders. Abnormalities of behaviour in childhood must be seen in the context of the child as a developing individual whose constitution and temperament may make him vulnerable to environmental influences. These may serve either to precipitate or to perpetuate abnormal patterns of behaviour.

Symptoms of psychiatric disorder in childhood must be considered in relation to the child's age. Behaviour which is normal at one stage of life may not be so at another. The sex of the child is also important: most psychiatric disorders in childhood, though not in adolescence, are commoner in boys. The severity, frequency and number of discrete symptoms and the context in which they appear must also be considered. Sudden and radical alterations in a child's behaviour are more ominous than an exacerbation of previous characteristics. The persistence of an unusual pattern of behaviour for an unduly long time may also connote serious disturbance, e.g. school refusal. The precise nature of the symptoms has less significance in childhood than in adult life, though some features such as disturbed relationships with peers almost always indicate psychiatric disturbance.

CLASSIFICATION

Several different systems are used to classify psychiatric disorders in childhood. The World Health Organisation has devised a system in which disorder on several axes is recorded, the *multi-axial system of classification* (Rutter et al. 1975b). The system as originally devised uses five axes (Rutter and Gould 1985):

(1) Clinical psychiatric syndrome, e.g. conduct disorder or hyperkinetic syndrome
(2) Specific delays in development, e.g. reading retardation

(3) Intellectual level, e.g. mildly retarded
(4) Medical (organic) conditions, e.g. asthma or epilepsy
(5) Abnormal psychosocial situations, e.g. family discord

Currently only three axes are often used:

(1) The psychiatric syndrome
(2) Intellectual level
(3) Associated organic factors

While the multi-axial classification has many advantages, especially for research, in everyday practice most child psychiatrists still use the system of categories of diagnoses based on the predominant clinical features. Both the ICD-9 and the DSM-III use this system although several diagnoses may be present in the same child, e.g. conduct disorder and eating disorders. The DSM-III differs from the ICD-9 in that it uses clearly defined operational criteria for the different diagnostic groups while the ICD-9 is more descriptive. The DSM-III also makes greater allowance than the ICD-9 for the co-existence of several psychiatric disorders in the same child by using five axes to record abnormal findings.

In this chapter psychiatric disorders in childhood will be considered under six headings:

(1) Emotional disorders
(2) Conduct disorders
(3) Developmental disorders
(4) Hyperkinetic syndrome
(5) Psychoses specific to childhood
(6) Miscellaneous disorders, e.g. enuresis, faecal soiling, encopresis, school refusal and truancy.

This is a purely descriptive classification which eschews aetiological implications. Reference will be made to the age of the child at which the disorders occur: infancy, early childhood, school age or adolescence.

In reaching a diagnosis the psychiatrist must always give due consideration to the interplay between developmental and historical factors, the family background, including the current interaction between various members of the child's family and the child's feelings as expressed through what he says, his behaviour, play and fantasy life.

EPIDEMIOLOGY

The most widely quoted study of the prevalence of psychiatric disorder in mid-childhood is known as the Isle of Wight Study, in which 2,193 children aged ten and eleven were screened for educational, intellectual, physical and psychiatric handicaps (Rutter and Graham 1966). The findings of all the studies of children on the Isle of Wight, including follow-up into adolescence, have been summarised by Rutter *et al.* (1976b). Questionnaires were completed by both parents and teachers. Those children thought to have psychiatric disturbance on the basis of the initial screening or because they were already under the care of relevant services were later given a psychiatric interview and psychological tests. It was established that 6.8 per cent of ten and eleven-year-olds were disturbed to the extent that either they or their families suffered; this suffering interfered with their everyday lives. The rate was twice as high in boys than in girls. The results suggested that there was no significant relationship between parental social class and psychiatric disorder in children. The prevalence of psychiatric disorder in the children increased as their IQ decreased. If a physical disorder such as asthma was present, psychiatric disorder was twice as common as in healthy children; if a brain disorder such as epilepsy was present, psychiatric disorder was four times as common. Furthermore the rate of psychiatric disorder increased if there was excessive family discord, psychiatric disorder in one or both parents and an absence of emotional warmth given to the child.

The rate of occurrence of psychiatric disorder throughout childhood is higher in urban than in rural areas (Rutter *et al.* 1975a). Nearly all problems in childhood are commoner in boys than in girls, a situation which gradually reverses during adolescence.

EMOTIONAL DISORDERS

Infancy and early childhood

Generally, the younger the child the more diffuse and non-specific are the symptoms of an emotional disorder, whereas older children tend to show features closer to those seen in adults.

Separation anxiety

The very young infant is completely dependent upon his parents, especially his mother or her surrogate. The gradual move towards independence does not occur smoothly. It is achieved through mastery of the fear of separation from familiar adults (see p. 66). The manifestation of this fear is referred to as separation anxiety. Although inferred in the first few month of life, it becomes clearly observable from the age of about six months, usually abating somewhere between the age of three-and-a-half and four. The child becomes distressed when separated from familiar adults, may cling to the adult and sometimes withdraws into a state of apathy and self-comfort derived from self-stimulation, e.g. thumb sucking, rocking and masturbation.

Separation anxiety is particularly noticeable and severe when affectional bonds are forcibly disrupted, as when a young child is admitted to hospital (Bowlby 1979) (see also p. 68). The reaction proceeds through a series of stages with initial protest, e.g. crying and clinging, followed by despair, e.g. withdrawal and misery. This gives way to detachment as evidenced by apparent indifference to the parents' presence. These stages are often reversed upon the child's return home. The older the child, the more he is likely to have internalised his attachment figures so that the manifestations of anxiety are less apparent. Children who have an insecure relationship with their parents, who have experienced previous repeated traumatic separations or who have been brought up in an overprotective and anxious environment are more prone to separation anxiety.

Separation anxiety is an important factor in the development of emotional problems later in life, e.g. school refusal and phobic anxiety states.

Sleep disturbance

Children vary considerably in terms of their regularity and placidity, and some small children are quite difficult to settle at night. This problem occurs more frequently with first-born children. Parents of small children can sometimes be helped to deal with the problem by keeping a sleep diary in which all features pertaining to the child's sleep pattern are systematically noted. The parents may then be better able to decide whether to allow the child to cry without paying attention or, if the child comes into their bedroom, whether promptly and firmly to return the child to bed. Parents can also introduce a graded programme by which they gradually increase their distance from the crying child, starting by lying down with the child, then sitting close to the child, and gradually moving further and further away. Bringing the child's bedtime forward by a few minutes each night can also be effective. Medication, e.g. trimeprazine tartrate 7.5 to 15 mg at night may occasionally be useful in children older than one year as a short-term expedient to allow exhausted parents some sleep. Children should never be locked into their rooms.

In some families sleep disturbance in an infant or child represents a reflection of disturbed family relationships or personal problems in one or both parents. Such parents sometimes respond to a series of psychotherapeutic interviews, especially when they are resistant to a more directive approach, with resulting improvement in the child.

Later childhood and adolescence

Feelings of sadness and anxiety, normal reactions to ordinary life stresses, sometimes become so persistent and intense in children that they interfere with their normal activities and therefore constitute an emotional disorder. Excessive feelings of fearfulness, shame and self-consciousness may also develop in childhood and adolescence and form part of an emotional disorder. In general, the older the child the more the symptoms resemble those of the adult neuroses. Children in middle childhood usually present with a more diffuse mixture of depression, anxiety and social withdrawal, but hysterical and obsessional features may be present.

The prevalence of emotional disorders is about 5 per cent, with boys and girls equally affected until adolescence when the proportion of girls increases. Emotional disorders are more likely to occur in children whose parents are emotionally disturbed themselves and in those who have experienced the threat or the reality of serious losses or other severely traumatic life events.

Adult-type depressive syndromes are rare before puberty but increase in frequency during adolescence. For many years it was argued that certain kinds of behaviour such as school refusal, stealing or enuresis were depressive equivalents. This is no longer thought to be the case, but young children who do not thrive, are fretful, anorexic and irritable may well be experiencing an early childhood equivalent of adult depressive illness. A *depressive syndrome* similar to that seen in adults may be identified in a small group of pre-pubertal children (Barrett and Kolvin 1985). These children show a depressed mood which is persistent and relatively independent of environmental changes. Features of sleep disturbance, excessive anxiety and suicidal ideas may be present. Such feelings as hopelessness, guilt and unworthiness are rarely openly expressed by pre-pubertal children although they may become apparent during psychotherapy; they become more frequent following puberty.

Completed suicide before the age of fifteen is very rare. Various explanations have been put forward for this. Shaffer and Fisher (1981), for example, suggest that children are unable to formulate concepts such as despair and hopelessness and cannot undertake the complicated planning necessary to complete suicide. Furthermore most children have sufficiently good psychological and social support either within the family or from their school. When suicide does occur the child tends to be male, aged over twelve, and of either very high or very low intelligence. There is often a family history of psychiatric disorder, and the child may have shown evidence of other disturbance such as conduct disorder and emotional problems.

A small number of children in their early school years develop a condition called *elective mutism*. This is usually classified as an emotional disorder although developmental defects such as speech delay and EEG immaturities may be present. The children may talk freely to close family members but are stubbornly mute in other situations, e.g. at school. Some show marked separation difficulties, while others appear to be caught in some sort of obsessive-compulsive disorder regarding their speech. Occasionally elective mutism may follow a severe trauma, but such cases are rare. While spontaneous recovery occurs in most cases, a few persist into adolescence.

Treatment of the condition should be based on careful formulation of the cause of the problem. Behavioural methods may be helpful, the child being rewarded for talking, and individual or family therapy may be needed.

Aetiology of emotional disorders

A comprehensive assessment of developmental and temperamental factors and family influences and of the child's internal world should be made. Several factors probably contribute to the development of emotional disorders in children. The significance of separation anxiety has already been discussed. Genetic factors may play a part, but disturbance in family relationships and the child's relationship to his parents probably have the major role. The fact that children and adolescents are traversing highly significant stages of emotional development is particularly important (see Chapters 7 and 8).

Prognosis and management

The prognosis for emotional disorder is good. Only a few children with such problems become psychiatrically disturbed as adults. None the less, because such disorders are responsible for considerable suffering in children and their families some therapeutic intervention is indicated unless there is rapid resolution of the problems.

Specific phobias are best treated by behavioural methods, while children with predominantly internalised conflicts require individual psychotherapy. Psychotherapy in early childhood usually involves the use of toys through which the child expresses his conflicts, feelings and fantasies. Such play therapy is usually practised by trained child psychotherapists (see p. 564). Descriptions of child psychotherapy are given by Winnicott (1977) and Axline (1971).

When disturbed family relationships perpetuate the symptoms of the child, family therapy may be indicated. Medication, especially minor tranquillisers, should be avoided. Occasionally, e.g. in severe depression, the use of an antidepressant such as imipramine or amitryptiline, in addition to counselling and psychotherapy, may be indicated.

CONDUCT DISORDERS

A child is said to have a conduct disorder if he exhibits antisocial behaviour, often involving acts against people or property, which is persistent and intense and evokes social disapproval. Other features include lying, stealing, disobedience, insolence, temper tantrums and verbal and physical aggression. Juvenile delinquency is also subsumed under this heading.

Conduct disorders have a prevalence varying between 5 and 15 per cent, depending on age, and are more common in boys than girls. There is a higher incidence of neurological disorders among these children, and academic failure due to learning disabilities is common.

The child with a conduct disorder may have a temperamental liability to abnormal behaviour. This is often observable from the earliest weeks of infancy, when the child may be relatively overactive, irregular in habits and somewhat more irritable and fractious than other children.

A lack of stability and consistency within the family is equally important; frequently there is a high degree of social disorganisation and criminality. Such families often lack reliable caring parental figures with whom the child can identify; this also exposes him to an atmosphere of rejection and lack of affection.

The child may indulge in antisocial behaviour in order to seek approval from his peers, and such approval can often act to reinforce his behaviour pattern. Emphasis has recently been placed upon the part played by the community, in particular the school which the child attends, as a factor predisposing towards conduct disorder. For instance, it has been observed that within the same locality there is a much higher incidence of conduct disorder among children attending particular schools, despite the similarity in the backgrounds and social class distribution of the pupils of the schools surveyed (Rutter *et al.* 1979).

Stealing is perhaps the commonest symptom. It is often carried out to gain peer approval and to compensate for lack of parental affection. Initially a child may steal sweets and share them with his friends. This activity may result from his belief that his parents do not care for him in the way that he believes his friends' parents care for them. Sometimes the object stolen helps one to understand the motivation behind the activity. For example, one boy only stole books about travel and far-away places; this represented his wish to get away from his parents who had severe marital problems. Such stealing may have a compulsive quality and is frequently done in a way which virtually ensures discovery and punishment.

When the behaviour of the child contravenes the law it is designated as *juvenile delinquency*. This frequently involves destructive acts against property. Delinquent acts may be carried out in the company of peers, when it is called socialised; or by an individual acting alone, when it is referred to as unsocialised. Of all the forms of delinquency arson is probably the most serious and usually connotes severe emotional disturbance (see p. 404). Another form of conduct disorder is truancy. This will be discussed further below (pp. 509-11).

Assessment and treatment

In the assessment of a child with conduct disorder, due attention must be paid to his social circumstances and family background as well as to psychological and temperamental factors. The attitude of the parents towards the child's behaviour is of particular importance, and those children who come from antisocial families which collude with their behaviour are difficult to treat. Conversely, the more stable and less disturbed the families are, the more likely it is that neurological or developmental factors are important in the aetiology of the conduct disorder.

Minor conduct disorders require little intervention other than counselling and advice to the parents. For those families in whom there is evidence of severe dysfunction, family therapy is probably the treatment of choice. During these sessions it may come to light that problems within the family are being expressed through the child and he has become the family scapegoat.

In those children in whom there is an association between conduct disorder and educational problems it is usually more beneficial to tackle the latter first through remedial education at school. Improvements in the child's learning and academic performance may result in raising his self-esteem and subsequently lead to improvement in his behaviour. The more severe forms of conduct disorder, which usually occur in children who have experienced profound emotional deprivation, may require institutional care. Children with severe forms of conduct disorder tend to have a very poor prognosis. They show a high incidence of psychiatric illness in adult life and many develop psychopathic or other personality disorders.

DEVELOPMENTAL DISORDERS

Most disorders of development, especially those with physical manifestations, come to the attention of paediatricians rather than child psychiatrists. Perhaps the commonest of the developmental problems to require psychiatric intervention is the group referred to collectively as specific learning disorders.

Specific learning disorders

Specific learning disorders are among the commonest of the developmental disorders to occur in children of normal intelligence. Between 4 and 10 per cent of ten-year-old children have a specific learning difficulty. The most common is a reading disability. This, in turn, is commonly associated with difficulties in writing and spelling. Other relatively common learning disorders are those related to language and speech. These include aphasia and stammer. Most cases of specific developmental learning retardation are associated with a disadvantaged background and are often accompanied by behaviour disturbance. The prevalence of specific learning disorders is higher in urban areas. For example, Berger *et al.* (1975) found that 10 per cent of ten and eleven-year-old children in inner London suffered from dyslexia compared with only 4 per cent on the Isle of Wight.

If learning disorders go unrecognised and uncorrected they can lead to educational failure, which in turn can cause psychiatric disorder, particularly disturbance in behaviour. In a small number of cases emotional factors may precede the learning difficulty, but the vast majority are examples of developmental delay.

The commonest form of reading retardation is often called *dyslexia*. This term is used to delineate a sub-group of children who have a specific reading retardation. However, children with dyslexia do not form a homogeneous group. Some can recognise letters but not whole words, some seem to be stuck at a particular point on the normal pathway of learning to read, e.g. they continue to muddle up *p* with *q* or *b* with *d*, and yet others cannot recognise patterns and shapes. None the less certain features seem to differentiate dyslexic children from those with a general backwardness in reading. For example, dyslexic children show a greater than expected number of neuropsychiatric symptoms such as poor right-left differentiation and developmental speech delay in infancy, and they often have a family history of reading disability. Their IQ is usually normal. This is important in diagnosis as children with handicapping cerebral disorders, one of the commonest causes of poor reading skills, have low intelligence. Social and biological factors may both be responsible for reading retardation to varying degrees.

Early recognition and diagnosis of learning disorders, often by means of specific psychological testing, is important especially for mild to moderate cases as children respond well to remedial education. Tizard *et al.* (1982) have shown that reading difficulties respond best if parents as well as teachers help the child to improve his reading. The outlook for the most severe cases is poor with at best slow and incomplete acquisition of the retarded skill.

HYPERKINETIC SYNDROME

Hyperkinetic syndrome, also known as *attention deficit disorder*, occurs predominantly in boys, usually presenting in the pre-school or early school years. It is characterised by restlessness, physical overactivity, disorganised behaviour, impulsiveness and lack of attentiveness. The children have often been difficult feeders and irregular sleepers in infancy, and when they begin walking they gradually become markedly overactive, highly distractable and lacking in concentration. The condition has been reviewed by E. Taylor (1985).

A child with the hyperkinetic syndrome is unable to continue with a constructive activity for as long as other children of the same age. Impulsiveness and disorganised behaviour may also lead to recurrent accidents. Overactivity should not be confused with a high level of energy and it should never be assumed that a report, either by a parent or a teacher, that a child is overactive necessarily means that the child has a hyperkinetic syndrome, especially if the overactivity is only present in one particular situation. A detailed account should be obtained about the child's behaviour during all his everyday activities, including looking at books, watching television or eating his meals, by interviewing all those involved with the child. In the hyperkinetic syndrome, especially if the hyperactivity is severe, it is usually noticeable in all these situations. There is a strong association of this syndrome with aggressive behaviour and developmental delays, e.g. specific learning difficulties.

There is a large discrepancy in the prevalence of this condition between the UK and the USA, the condition being diagnosed much more commonly in the USA. Different diagnostic criteria between the two countries and varied methods of investigation such as interviewing parents, giving questionnaires to school teachers, or studying clinic populations, probably account for these differences. In their Isle of Wight study Rutter *et al.* (1976b) found only two school children with the disorder, i.e. 0.1 per cent of all the ten and eleven-year-olds studied. This is in contrast to figures varying between 5 and 20 per cent of school children in various parts of the USA.

Aetiology

The aetiology of the hyperkinetic syndrome is unclear, but there are probably several interacting factors. Genetic factors may play a part, in that there is often a history of hyperkinesis in the childhood of parents of the affected children (Cantwell 1975). Environmental influences are also important: there is a high rate of family disharmony, social disadvantage and untoward early childhood experiences such as repeated separations. Parental mental illness is common. Some of the children show non-specific EEG abnormalities suggesting a neurological dysfunction.

Food allergy has been suggested as a possible cause, especially sensitivity to food additives, but its place in the aetiology of the hyperkinetic syndrome is controversial. Attempts to treat the disorder with strict diets have only been effective in a very small proportion of children. In general, the part played by food allergy in causing the syndrome is probably very small (E. Taylor 1984).

Treatment

Treatment is difficult. In general, the children should be under- rather than over-stimulated and may need special educational provisions so that what they are expected to achieve is compatible with their attention span and need for space. The principle of rewarding the child's appropriate behaviour with more attention and tending to ignore inappropriate behaviour can be usefully applied at school and at home. In severely affected children the use of stimulant medication may be considered, e.g. methylphenidate. However, because of the high incidence of side-effects, possible delay in response and need for prolonged treatment, this form of therapy should only be prescribed by a child psychiatrist or paediatrician.

Attempts to treat the hyperkinetic syndrome with strict dietary regimes have already been mentioned. These tend to be extremely troublesome for the family and may have marked adverse psychological effects both on the child and on his parents. Often it is the child's favourite food that needs to be cut out of the diet as most of the regimes avoid sweets, chocolate, soft drinks and ice cream. Overall, studies suggest that only a very small proportion of hyperactive children are helped by these diets. A trial of an appropriate dietary regime may very rarely be indicated when there is severe hyperactivity and there is a previous history of allergic reactions such as eczema.

Prognosis

The prognosis of the hyperkinetic syndrome varies considerably. Some children who are overactive in early childhood progress to conduct disorders in middle childhood. A few actually become lethargic and underactive in adolescence. When the condition is associated with conduct disorders, learning delays and aggressive behaviour the outcome is worse.

PSYCHOSES SPECIFIC TO CHILDHOOD

The most common form of childhood psychosis is infantile autism, which is discussed in detail in Chapter 42. However, another even rarer childhood psychosis, known as a *disintegrative psychosis*, at times may be difficult to distinguish from infantile autism. In this condition, unlike autism, a normally developing child may, at the age of three to four, undergo a massive regression in speech and language, often following a vague illness. This may be accompanied by severe overactivity, dementia, mannerisms and stereotypies. There are probably a number of different causes of the disintegrative psychoses of childhood. Some follow measles encephalitis; in some, post-mortem examination shows that the condition was the result of one of the lipoidoses or leucodystrophies affecting the brain; but in most the cause remains unknown. In some cases the child may end up severely mentally retarded but survive for many years without speech and language, often without any abnormal neurological findings. In others the illness progresses inexorably to premature death.

Schizophrenia in children is extremely rare and hardly ever occurs before the age of seven. When it does occur in childhood the symptoms are similar to those found in adult schizophrenia. Manic-depressive psychosis is even rarer and probably does not occur before puberty.

MISCELLANEOUS DISORDERS

Enuresis

Lack of bladder control after the age of five is called enuresis; it may be nocturnal, i.e. bed-wetting, or diurnal. If the child has never had a lasting period of bladder control, the enuresis is termed primary, whereas if there has been a prolonged dry period, after which the child loses control of his bladder, it is described as secondary.

By the age of five, 15 per cent of children are still wetting. This figure decreases to 7 per cent by the age of ten; by fifteen only 1 per cent of the population is so affected. Boys are far more frequently enuretic than girls, who tend to achieve bladder and bowel control earlier. Most children are dry at night by between the ages of three and four and achieve full bladder control irrespective of toilet training. Excessive emphasis placed by parents on toilet training can result in a battle between child and parents, and may occasionally delay or interfere with bladder control.

Aetiology

Among the important aetiological factors, the following are usually cited:

(1) Genetic factors. 70 per cent of bed-wetters have a first-degree relative who was wetting after the age of five, and monozygotic twins show a concordance rate twice as high as that found in dizygotic twins (Bakwin 1971).

(2) Intelligence. Enuresis is commoner in children of low IQ.

(3) Associated psychiatric disorder. This is found in 15–25 per cent of bedwetters and is slightly commoner in enuretic girls. No specific psychiatric disorder is associated with enuresis. The associated psychiatric disorder may be a response to the enuresis rather than its cause. Sometimes both may be attributable to common factors such as family disturbance.

(4) Small functional bladder capacity. Presumably as a result of immaturity of the bladder neck innervation, some children reflexly micturate in response to a small volume of urine. This too may be the result of enuresis rather than its cause.

(5) Urinary tract infection. This is a rare cause but should always be excluded. It is more frequent in girls.

(6) Stressful life events, including separations and hospitalisation. These are found more frequently in the first four years of the lives of enuretics (MacKeith 1968). Frequent causes of temporary secondary enuresis due to regression include the birth of a younger sibling, admission to hospital, change of home or starting school.

(7) Large families. Enuresis is commoner in later-born children.

(8) Institutional upbringing.

(9) Social disadvantage.

In general, children who are of average intelligence and biologically maturing at an appropriate rate will achieve dryness. Those who are genetically predisposed to a delay in achieving bladder control, who are unduly anxious or poor learners will fail to achieve control. This is specially so if their environmental circumstances lessen the chance of social approval.

After children have started school enuresis can become a source of considerable embarrassment, a focus for teasing and a cause of social isolation. The symptom may also lead to family tension and battles between the child and his parents.

Treatment

Initially urinary tract infection, to which enuretic children are predisposed, should be excluded. After this various procedures may be employed in the treatment of enuresis.

(1) Day-time training. This is most suitable for younger children who are coaxed by a parent to desist from passing urine for gradually increasing periods. This raises the volume of urine contained in the bladder before reflex micturition occurs. This training can be used in conjunction with a star chart.

(2) Star chart. This, like the preceding treatment, emphasises the child's successes rather than his failures. Whenever the child remains dry he is rewarded with a star to place on his specially prepared chart. A special reward may be given after a certain number of stars has been collected.

(3) Enuresis alarm (buzzer and pad). In well-motivated children this device, which probably works through a form of conditioning, can be highly effective (see p. 588). More than 80 per cent of children will obtain marked symptomatic improvement after 6-8 weeks and if a relapse occurs the success rate on reintroduction of the technique is even higher.

(4) Medication. Imipramine hydrochloride 25-50 mg at night will help between 50 and 75 per cent of enuretic children. The treatment should be discontinued if there is no response within three weeks; if effective, it should be continued for a few months. The relapse rate is high after it is discontinued, and reintroduction is less effective than initial therapy. It can be used in conjunction with a star chart. The mechanism by which the medication works is uncertain. It probably works neither through its antidepressant nor its anticholinergic properties, but possibly through its action on the brain stem or autonomic nervous system.

(5) Psychological treatment. In the course of treating a child with any of the above techniques various problems within the family or in the child or both may come to light. If the associated difficulties are seen to be intrapsychic he may benefit from individual psychotherapy, preferably after the enuresis has been controlled. Similarly, problems seen to derive from pathological family interactions may require family therapy.

Faecal soiling

There are three types of faecal soiling. The commonest type seen in psychiatric clinics is known as *encopresis*. This is the passage of normal stools in inappropriate places, e.g. clothing. It is virtually always of psychological origin and the child is able to control the physiological process of defaecation.

Secondly, soiling may result from excessively fluid faeces due to physical illness, e.g. ulcerative colitis, or be secondary to retention of faeces within the rectum leading to constipation with overflow. This may be due to an anal fissure or, very rarely, undiagnosed Hirschsprung's disease. These children are easy to differentiate from those with encopresis by their abnormal stools. Occasionally constipation with overflow is a consequence of the child's wish to retain his faeces. If this is the case it is sometimes classified with encopresis as an emotional disorder even though the stools are abnormal.

The third type of faecal soiling consists of true failure to gain bowel control. In these children stools are normal but defaecation occurs randomly both at home and at school. Children in this group may have associated physical handicap and be of below average intelligence, but some may have had poor or inconsistent toilet training and be of normal intelligence. Only encopresis will be considered further here.

Encopresis

Encopresis can be continuous, i.e. present from birth, or discontinuous, i.e. occurring after a period of bowel control. The discontinuous variety rarely commences after the age of seven. Bowel control is normally established by the age of three to four. The onset of encopresis or soiling in an older child, especially a girl, should raise the suspicion of sexual abuse.

The prevalence of encopresis in childhood is approximately 1 per cent, boys being affected about four times as often as girls. It is associated with indicators of social disadvantage, e.g. generally unkempt and dirty appearance, educational underachievement, enuresis and conduct disorder.

Aetiology

Encopresis is usually caused by problems in the relationship between the child and his parents, although continuous encopresis may result from faulty toilet training, more often laxity than excessive rigour. However, there is no specific pattern of relationship of the child and his parents which results in encopresis.

In some cases the child's psychological problems are important. At the age of three to four faeces often have a special meaning to the child. For example, he may view them as an important and valued part of himself; letting his faeces go and seeing them disappear may therefore lead to severe anxiety. Alternatively, the child may view his faeces as a dirty part of himself which he tries to hide inside himself resulting in faecal retention. The parents may become involved in these internal conflicts, and a power struggle may result between the child and, say, a demanding obsessional parent, leading to an exacerbation of the problem. Alternatively the child may develop difficulties in expressing aggressive feelings and start to use his faeces as a way of showing hostility and aggression towards his parents. For example, faeces may be smeared on the walls or even placed in the parents' bed.

In some children encopresis is due to regression. For example, it may occur as a response to increasing demands being made on the child to become more independent and mature, perhaps after the birth of a new sibling.

The commonest time for an encopretic child to defaecate is on the way home from school or shortly after arrival home. If he is embarrassed about this and ashamed of his problem he may well hide his underpants. Other encopretic children deny their problem and refuse to acknowledge that they smell or that their underwear is soiled. Encopresis may constitute a symptom which draws attention to tensions within the family. Parents of these children may be excessively punitive or obsessional about cleanliness, and dispute between the parents about the child's symptom may disguise other marital or family conflicts. The encopretic child may then become a scapegoat and a repetitive cycle follows whereby the child responds to this process by an exaggeration of his symptom.

Treatment

The management of encopresis and soiling partly depends on whether or not it is associated with constipation. A combination of physical treatment, behavioural treatment and psychotherapy is often used, and the choice of treatment should be determined by the major aetiological factors found in each individual child.

Constipated children may require drugs such as docusate sodium to soften their faeces. In cases of severe constipation with faecal impaction suppositories, an enema or a bowel wash-out may be necessary initially. When the constipation, if present, has been treated, a behaviour modification programme should be developed to encourage regular toilet habits; a star chart may be used to assist this process. Although most encopretic children can be successfully treated by their parents at home, the most recalcitrant cases may require inpatient treatment, either on a paediatric ward or in a child psychiatric unit. Wherever the treatment takes place, a punitive or critical attitude towards the child must be avoided. Family or intrapsychic problems should be treated by family therapy or individual psychotherapy respectively.

Encopresis almost always clears up by adolescence, but this should not discourage treatment at a much earlier age. If treatment is not undertaken emotional repercussions may be severe and long-lasting leading to emotional or conduct disorders which then have a worse prognosis. Interestingly, some children's aggressive behaviour is exacerbated by successful treatment of the encopresis.

School refusal and truancy

The term truancy was originally used to describe both these disorders, but nowadays the two terms denote different conditions, both characterised by the child being absent from school. In *school refusal*, the child is absent from school for long periods and stays at or near home but the parents know where he is. In *truancy* the child stays away from school on his own initiative and neither his parents nor his teachers know his whereabouts. The child may go to school in the morning but leave later in the day.

School refusal in which the child is afraid of attending school is sometimes referred to as *school phobia*. However, this term should only be used when the child shows unequivocally that he suffers from some specific anxiety about school or some aspect of attending school.

The distinction between school refusal and truancy is not absolute, but Hersov (1960a, 1960b) and Hersov and Berg (1980) have demonstrated clear differences between the two groups. School refusers are found in all social classes and their families are usually intact. The children are of average or high intelligence and are often high achievers at school. Evidence of antisocial behaviour is usually absent but some symptoms of emotional disturbance, e.g. depression, may be present. The children are often regarded by both parents and teachers as normal and are seen as compliant, if anything.

In contrast, school truants more often come from socially disadvantaged families, especially one-parent families or those with persistent, violent marital discord, criminality and poverty. The children are of lower intelligence, show academic under-achievement and a higher rate of conduct disorder. Truancy is usually a socialised activity and may lead to episodes of juvenile delinquency. The truant tries to hide his non-attendance at school whereas the school refuser is usually solitary and spends his time away from school at home, or, if prevented, on some site which is close to and symbolically representative of home, e.g. a local library. School truancy is much more common than school refusal.

Many children with school refusal suffer from marked separation anxiety. School refusal is commoner in boys and reaches its highest incidence at the age of eleven to twelve. This is a time of conspicuous physical development with the onset of puberty as well as social change, such as a move from primary to secondary education. Other peaks of incidence are at the age of five, i.e. the beginning of primary education, and at fifteen to sixteen, when compulsory education is drawing to a close and the impetus towards independent activity is heightening. The families of school refusers, ostensibly unremarkable, may show a characteristic constellation. The affected child may hold a special place in the feelings of one of the parents, usually the mother; her relationship to the child may represent a re-creation and idealisation of a close relationship which she either had or had wished for with one of her own parents. Anxiety about separation is shared by both child and mother but is more overtly expressed by the child. The father in these families is often a good, responsible breadwinner but distant from the emotional life of the family and unable to give enough emotional support to his wife.

The school refuser may also be troubled by problems with aggressive impulses, either his own or others'. For example, he may explain his non-attendance at school by complaining of being bullied but when this is investigated little firm evidence may be found. Alternatively he may become anxious about harm coming to his mother or the home, and thereby justify his reluctance to be separated from either. In each case the child's anxiety about school or home or both should be taken into account and explored.

The onset of school refusal may be acute and may follow an illness, e.g. influenza, a bereavement or other major life event. It may also occur after a long school holiday. A 'somatic disguise' is common, e.g. abdominal pain, nausea, headache or sore throat, and the symptom may well 'miraculously' vanish once non-attendance has been sanctioned. Of course school refusal and true physical illness may co-exist. Other children may suddenly and blatantly refuse to leave for school and exhibit uncharacteristic stubbornness and rage if an attempt is made to thwart their decision. Perhaps a commoner, though less dramatic, onset is seen when the child develops a pattern of frequent and increasingly long-lasting periods of absence from school. Some parents collude with this process and consciously withhold their child from school, but in other families the collusion is unconscious. Such families are often difficult to engage in treatment, hence the child has a worse prognosis.

Management

Initially school refusers and truants are mainly treated by educational psychologists or school welfare officers. The child should be returned to school at the earliest possible moment and any recommendations which could perpetuate the problem, e.g. home tuition or individual psychotherapy, must be delayed until the child returns to school. If this simple directive procedure is unsuccessful or if the problem becomes chronic, referral of the child or the family to a child psychiatric unit is indicated. Careful assessment is then required; this usually includes several family interviews and at least one interview with the child alone, as well as meetings with the staff of the school and the family's general practitioner. A plan of treatment is jointly drawn up to expedite the child's return to school and to deal with any family issues, problems at school or intrapsychic problems.

Various therapeutic techniques are used with school refusers. In family therapy, perhaps the most frequently employed, an attempt is made to relate the child's symptoms to other aspects of the family's function, to increase the father's involvement in the emotional life of the family and to disentangle the often enmeshed relationship between mother and the affected child (see p. 578).

Behaviour therapy may be useful, especially in clear cases of school phobia. When used in school refusal it is only an adjunct to individual or family-based treatment. The child is given a programme of graded return to school. He is gradually taken nearer and nearer to the school, then collects books from the school, enters the classroom and eventually stays at school for longer periods. The parents must be helped to cope with the child's anxiety and to maintain a firm but kindly stance if the child continues to attempt to remain at home.

Antidepressant medication, e.g. imipramine hydrochloride, has been suggested but should only be tried in those children with overt symptoms of depression. It can occasionally be used as an adjunct to family therapy, as can a short course of a minor tranquilliser taken to reduce the child's anxiety in the morning before going to school.

Individual psychotherapy is indicated for those children with anxieties arising from intrapsychic conflicts which persist after their return to school.

Children who do not respond to any of these therapies may require temporary placement in a tutorial class away from the school or in a residential treatment centre such as a child or adolescent inpatient unit. Apart from separating the child from his parents, these units have educational facilities on site and can accelerate the child's return to full-time education.

A small number of children with school refusal fail to respond to all forms of treatment. These children are usually recommended to attend a boarding school which caters for children with special educational needs.

Prognosis

The outlook for mild cases of school refusal is quite good, with the majority of children returning to school within 6-9 months. However, the chronic, intractable cases have a poor prognosis. A small but significant number go on to develop a variety of neurotic problems or personality disorders in adult life, e.g. work refusal or agoraphobia, especially if the onset of school refusal is in adolescence, or if there are severe personality or family problems. Nevertheless the majority of children with even severe school refusal do not have psychiatric disorders as adults (Berg *et al*. 1976).

PHYSICAL ILLNESS

Chronic physical illnesses

These occur in approximately 5–10 per cent of all children. Psychological and social factors often play a significant role in their course and prognosis and occasionally also in their aetiology, e.g. in bronchial asthma (see p. 460). In illnesses such as asthma and diabetes mellitus, psychological and social aspects make treatment difficult and must be carefully considered if the management of the ill child is to be successful. Child psychiatrists and related professions therefore often work with paediatricians and others in the management of children with such illnesses. The commonest conditions requiring a joint approach are bronchial asthma and neurological conditions such as epilepsy.

The impact on the parents of a child suffering from a chronic disabling illness, including physical or mental handicap, can be profound and diverse. Being presented with the diagnosis may lead to a state of shock in the parents and this is often followed by feelings of denial, anger, sadness and guilt. Most parents eventually adapt to the illness, and the presence of a disabled child in the family can act as unifying bond. However for some parents the presence of a disabled child can exacerbate existing differences and may result in marital breakdown. Normal siblings are also often affected, either because they feel neglected when the sick child gets all the attention or because they are subtly coerced into a caretaking and responsible role before they are ready for it. The ill child is often loved or over-protected but may be rejected.

The child may adapt to his disability, but some suffer serious distortions of body image and self-esteem during their development. This applies particularly to children with congenital deformities or chronic physical handicap and may lead to personality problems when they grow up. These children also have a higher rate of psychiatric disorder than normal children.

Recurrent abdominal pain

One of the less serious physical disorders frequently seen in childhood is recurrent abdominal pain. This occurs in about 15 per cent of school-aged children and is rarely due to an organic condition. However, on occasions an organic disease may cause abdominal pain which later becomes recurrent even though the causative disorder has resolved. There is a tendency to assume that if no organic aetiology can be found the cause must be psychological. However, a diagnosis of a psychogenic disorder should only be made on positive findings of emotional disturbance or stressful life events. In particular, features of anxiety or depression, including covert depressive symptoms, or a conduct disorder in the child and marital or family dysfunction should be looked for. Some children with recurrent abdominal pain come from families whose members tend to somatise their feelings rather than express them directly (see also p. 488).

In managing cases of recurrent abdominal pain it is important not to over-investigate the symptom but to concentrate on recent stressful life events. It is essential not to suggest that the pain is imagined. Pain of psychological origin is as painful as pain due to a physical disease. Careful explanation and reassurance is usually all that is required, but the more intractable cases or those in which there is clear evidence of associated psychiatric disturbance in the child or the family should either be seen jointly by a paediatrician and child psychiatrist or referred to a child psychiatric unit.

Hospitalisation

The effects of hospitalisation on young children have been described earlier (see p. 68). The adverse responses can be mitigated by preparing the child for hospitalisation, by daily visits from the parents or, even better, if a parent is able to stay in hospital with the child. The better the parent/child relationship the less intense is the distress likely to be. The attitude of doctors and nurses and the atmosphere on the ward also have an important influence on the response of children who are admitted.

The dying child

In recent years much attention has been paid to the emotional needs of dying children and their families. Nowadays death in childhood in developed countries is an uncommon event, occurring mostly because of congenital abnormalities in early infancy and, in later years of childhood, as a result of accidents or neoplasms. The reaction of children to a potentially fatal illness varies according to their age. Most children do not develop a sense of the true meaning of death in terms of its inevitability, finality and universality, until the age of four to seven. Until then the fears and anxieties of sick children are related to separation from their parents, especially the mother, and the painful medical procedures which may become associated with being ill. Some children deny the seriousness of their illness, others react to it with anger, often directed towards parents or staff on the ward. Yet others, perhaps sensing their parents' inability to face their impending death, act protectively towards them. Obviously the attitudes of the parents and the ward staff can have an important influence on the child's response to the vicissitudes of his illness.

Parents who are informed of their child's potentially fatal diagnosis often experience emotional responses similar to, but more intense than those they experience following the birth of a child with a physical or mental handicap (see also Chapters 9 and 41). While waiting for their child to die they may go through what is sometimes referred to as 'anticipatory mourning'. Following the death of their child, the parents undergo another mourning process; if they do not, they may subsequently develop a depressive illness or other emotional problems which may have adverse effects on the psychological development of other children in the family.

Families with a dying child need a great deal of professional support both during and after the illness (Dominica 1987; Buckman 1988). Although the decision whether to communicate the prognosis to the child rests in the last resort with the parents, they often appreciate medical advice. This should be sensitive, undogmatic and related both to the needs of the child, in terms of his age, developmental stage, mental state and physical condition, and to the needs of the parents and siblings. Some families require extended counselling after the death of a child.

CHILD ABUSE

There are four types of child abuse: physical abuse, sexual abuse, emotional abuse and neglect. All four may be present together. Sexual abuse is discussed separately in Chapter 43. The following account is mainly concerned with *physical abuse* or *non-accidental injury* (NAI).

When either parents or guardians commit a physical act which violates a generally accepted standard of child-care or fail to provide a level of care which ensures their child's well-being, physical abuse or non-accidental injury (NAI) is said to occur. The vagueness of this definition makes it difficult to establish the prevalence of actual physical abuse or *child-battering*, but approximately 0.5 per cent of children under three suffer serious physical abuse each year.

Abused children and abusing parents show certain characteristics. The children are often unattractive, the youngest in the family, and cry a great deal. There is often a history of separation from their mother in the neonatal period and prematurity is common. The responsible parent tends to be young and single, to have low self-esteem, and to have suffered from abuse herself as a child. Disturbed interaction between the child and his parents is very common; the mother may have suffered rejection, separation and emotional deprivation from her own parents in childhood and consequently have serious problems in accepting her maternal role, with marked feelings of aggression towards her own child (see also p. 410). Unemployment and social isolation are also associated with abuse.

Physical abuse may be accompanied by *emotional abuse*. This often takes the form of constant threats, excessive teasing, aggressive behaviour, e.g. whenever the child cries and cannot be comforted, malicious comments or overt rejection. When rejection leads to failure of the parent to provide for the child's safety, health and regular nourishment, *neglect* is said to occur. The child may then show retarded language development, fail to thrive, and become withdrawn and lethargic. These severe forms of emotional abuse are relatively easy to recognise, but milder forms are commonly overlooked.

Physical abuse should always be suspected whenever a child has an unusual injury, or the injury occurred in suspicious circumstances, even though the parents insist that it was in some way caused by an accident. Head or eye injuries, long bone or rib fractures, burns, especially circular burns from cigarettes, or localised burns due to contact with hot objects, stocking-glove burns from immersion in hot water, bite marks and finger and thumb grip marks should all arouse suspicion. A delay in reporting the injury, bizarre explanations of the injury, and inconsistent stories from the parents should always suggest physical abuse. Serious intra-abdominal and head injuries may lead to death from physical abuse.

Once a child has been physically abused he has a 60 per cent chance of being abused again; 10 per cent of abused children die from their injuries.

The siblings of an abused child are also at risk. Children subjected to regular abuse become withdrawn, listless, frightened, wary and untrusting of both adults and their peer group. Some become aggressive and all have low self-esteem and show poor academic achievement.

Management

Once physical abuse has been detected, intervention must be made immediately by both doctors and social workers to prevent further injuries. A child may need to be removed from his home, perhaps by being admitted to a paediatric ward, if necessary under a place of safety order obtained from the magistrates court if the parents object. The degree of risk to the child can then be assessed at a case conference. This should involve all the professionals in contact with the child: doctors, nurses, social workers, teachers and health visitors. The child may need to be put on the 'at risk' register held by the local authority or placed under a care order which allows the local authority to assume parental rights. The child psychiatric team may then become involved in the child's rehabilitation. Sometimes the child may return home under the careful supervision of the social services while attempts are made to help the family both in practical ways and in family therapy. Frequent moves between placements in a foster home or institution and the child's own home should be avoided if possible, as such repeated separations are likely to cause further psychological harm. Older children may benefit from individual psychotherapy to overcome the serious psychological after-effects of abuse or neglect earlier in life.

FURTHER READING

Freud, A. (1980). *Normality and Pathology in Childhood: assessments of development*, 3rd ed. Hogarth, London.

Graham, P.J. (1986). *Child Psychiatry: a developmental approach*. OUP, Oxford.

Rutter, M. (1974). *Helping Troubled Children*. Penguin, Harmondsworth.

Rutter, M. and Hersov, L. (eds) (1985). *Child and Adolescent Psychiatry: modern approaches*, 2nd ed. Blackwell, Oxford.

Wolff, S. (1981). *Children under Stress*, 2nd ed. Penguin, Harmondsworth.

41

Mental Handicap*

Most parents look forward to and greatly enjoy their new baby. How deeply this early expectation is shattered by their realisation that their child is mentally retarded cannot be too strongly emphasised. The emotional impact of such an event is profound; it generates distress, shame and anger and eventually resignation to their child's permanent disability. It touches parental, indeed human, feelings very deeply. In few situations is the doctor so painfully confronted with his own inadequacy; rarely is there a greater need for him to recognise how far his own discomfort affects his management of the child and the family. Nor does the situation really change. Because their expected normal child cannot be restored to them, parents often find explanations of the tragedy and treatment programmes unsatisfying and may seek many diagnostic opinions or pursue various remedies; often the more time-consuming or expensive they are the more they are valued. Such reactions are common defences against understandable anger and sense of loss; they need to be recognised as such and treated appropriately. It is no mean task.

The competent clinical management of the mentally handicapped child demands time and patience in guiding the parents into a realistic view of his disability, which in turn requires an understanding of the parents' own view. Above all, parents need to be asked what they think is wrong with their child, not simply told, however erudite or thorough the explanation may be.

TERMINOLOGY

Several different terms have been used to describe individuals who suffer intellectual impairment from infancy or childhood. These include mental impairment, mental subnormality and mental retardation; the branch of psychiatry concerned with these disorders used, in the past, to be called mental deficiency.

The term *mental subnormality* was adopted in the 1959 Mental Health Act to describe 'a delayed or arrested development of the mind', and the term continued to be used until recently. In the ICD-9 (1978) the term

* Although this chapter is mainly concerned with mental handicap in children, the adult mentally handicapped are also considered.

mental retardation is used. It is defined as 'a condition of arrested or incomplete development of the mind which is especially characterised by subnormality of intelligence'. The ICD-9 divides mental retardation into mild, moderate and severe; mild cases have an IQ between 70 and 50, moderate cases an IQ between 49 and 35 and severe cases an IQ below 35.

Definitions in terms of the IQ alone are unsatisfactory. It is difficult accurately to assess the IQ, especially in mentally retarded children. In addition to the IQ, clinical data must be considered in assessing the degree of intellectual impairment. Further, physical defects are often associated with impaired intelligence, especially in those who are moderately or severely retarded, e.g. impaired sight or hearing, motor disabilities and epilepsy. The individual's total disability or handicap in terms of his personal and social functioning may therefore go well beyond the effects of his impaired intelligence.

Since the 1970s the term *mental handicap* has begun to replace the earlier terms. This change reflects the increasing emphasis on the social consequences of the individual's disabilities, including his impaired intelligence and his psychological and physical deficits. The term mental handicap is therefore used for the title of this chapter, while the terms mental retardation or mental impairment are used in the text to refer more specifically to intellectual impairment. There is some danger that the importance of the medical aspects of mental handicap could be overlooked as a result of this emphasis on the social aspects. This must be avoided because the nature of the pathology responsible for cases of mental handicap, especially those of moderate or severe degree, remains important. This is particularly the case if the condition is preventable or treatable, as for example in hypothyroidism or phenylketonuria.

The important educational aspects of mental handicap have given rise to the term *educationally subnormal* (ESN). A distinction is made between those individuals who are severely educationally subnormal (IQ below 50) and those who are moderately educationally subnormal (IQ between 50 and 70). Here again, clinical observation of the child's learning difficulties is at least as important as psychometric testing.

PREVALENCE

The prevalence of mental handicap is difficult to assess precisely. This applies particularly to mild mental handicap (IQ between 70 and 50) because this grades into the dull normal, whose IQ lies between 70 and 100. The latter represent those normal members of the population who fall within 2 standard deviations (SD) below the mean of 100 in the normal distribution curve of intelligence, with an SD of 15. The distinction between the dull normal and mildly mentally handicapped is particularly difficult to make when a child of low normal intelligence has perceptual or motor disabilities which interfere with the reliable assessment or demonstration of his intelligence. As a result, a child with low normal intelligence may be wrongly classified as mentally retarded.

The mildly retarded group (IQ 70-50), though slow in response or backward in learning, may have no overt neurological abnormality, nor any serious emotional disorder or problems in social adjustment, though all these are more common than in the more intelligent population. Moreover, signs of below normal intelligence in thé mildly retarded group may only become apparent at school age so that the correct diagnosis may at first be overlooked.

The prevalence of moderate and severe mental handicap (IQ below 50) is much easier to determine. The development of such children is likely to be slow from the beginning and neurological or other physical abnormalities are frequently associated with their mental retardation, causing severe mental handicap early in life.

The following figures indicate the prevalence in these different groups. The prevalence of moderate and severe mental handicap (IQ below 50) is 3-4 per 1000 population for children, and 2-3 per 1000 for adults. The prevalence is higher in males than females. The lower figures for adults are due to the fact that a proportion of severely handicapped children will have died from associated physical disorders before they reach adulthood.

The total prevalence of mental handicap, i.e. the mildly retarded (IQ 70-50) and the moderately and severely retarded (IQ below 50), is estimated at 20-30 per 1000 of the population. About 80 per cent of the total number of mentally handicapped belong to the group of mildly retarded and 20 per cent to the moderately and severely retarded. Many of the former can lead more or less independent lives as adults given some family or social support, but they may require assistance when this breaks down, e.g. when a close relative with whom they have lived dies.

About 300,000 severely mentally handicapped children and adults live in the UK at any one time, and the cause is known in only about 35 per cent. Depending on the degree and kind of their disability they need help, either from their families with the assistance of the social and community services, or in small residential homes or hostels. These are now taking the place of the large institutions or hospitals in which the mentally retarded used to be housed; many of these were isolated, over-crowded and poorly staffed, making it difficult to provide an adequate level of personal attention and social stimulation.

TYPES OF DISABILITY

Most of the severely mentally handicapped have a combination of disabilities; the proportion with epilepsy, cerebral palsy, sensory defects, communication disorders or behavioural problems is much higher than in the normal population, so that many retarded patients present their doctor with an array of clinical problems, some of which may be far more disabling than others. All these problems, though often with different priorities, may be thought to merit treatment by the doctor, the family and, if he is able to express it, by the retarded person himself.

In many cases the interaction between these disabilities interferes with the development of learning ability in the handicapped person. In others the underlying pathology retards such development to a far greater extent than would be expected from the individual disabilities it generates. Thus some deaf, supposedly retarded children have a communication disorder far in excess of that expected from the level of their hearing loss, while conversely some children with cerebral palsy are far more spontaneous and skilled in overcoming their disabilities than others with clinically similar, or even worse motor defect. It is also difficult to estimate how much the level of current performance is due to early detection and hence appropriate treatment, or to the degree of pathology, or even to significant personal qualities, since the mentally handicapped child is as much an individual as any other person.

There are complex and as yet poorly understood causal relationships between pathology, if established, and resulting disability and potential. This justifies the treatment efforts, particularly with the young child, so urgently and enthusiastically promoted by many parents and by professional staff. Until we have a clearer understanding of such causal relationships it is important to respect their efforts and, if concerned about their realism, to give careful reasons for one's doubts, however serious they may be. Parents are apt to assume that the connection between diagnosed pathology, symptomatology and prescribed treatment is as clear-cut in mental handicap, with its many medical components, as in acute and curable illnesses. They need to be helped to recognise the limitations of such a medical approach when dealing with the chronic disability of their mentally handicapped child. This must be carefully explained, along with the probable impact of the disability on the child's development and his social function throughout life. At the same time they need to be safeguarded from a conviction that any progress is unlikely or can be obtained only through social or educational efforts.

Mental impairment, disability and handicap

In this context it is useful to distinguish between impairment, disability and handicap. Wood (World Health Organisation 1980) offers the following definitions.

> *Impairment* (Why is my child handicapped?)
> In the context of health experience, an impairment is any loss or abnormality of psychological, physiological or anatomical structure or function.

This is the focus of diagnosis; it indicates, in the family's view, what is 'wrong', what may have been present from birth or acquired subsequently; what may be permanent or temporary, remediable or not. It is with these topics that the family is first concerned.

Disability (How is my child handicapped?)
In the context of health experience, disability is any restriction or lack (resulting from an impairment) of ability to perform an activity, or within the range considered normal for a human being.

These are the subjects of assessment and treatment, such as dysarthria, hearing loss or inability to walk. Parents will view such disabilities as a hindrance to acquiring simple developmental skills and will thus understandably press for active intervention to reduce or correct them. They will often assume that the tactics they imagine elicit such skills in their normal children should be pursued that much more vigorously in their disabled child. Such initiatives and such a sense of purpose are of great value, but the doctor must occasionally help parents to realise how over-simplified, indeed occasionally obstructive, such enthusiasm may be. In particular he will need to protect them from disappointment or self-blame when they feel that in spite of their efforts they have achieved inadequate progress.

Handicap (How normal will my child become?)
In the context of health experience, a handicap is a disadvantage for any given individual, resulting from an impairment or disability that limits or prevents the fulfilment of a role that is normal (depending on age, sex and social and cultural factors) for that individual.

This concerns the direct personal experience of the retarded person and of his family while living with him. It is what really matters to them all. It relates to how much help he needs, how closely he must be supervised, how rewarding or wearying his care may be. It will vary over time, not simply because the level of disability may change, but because the family's expectations and their tolerance of practical difficulties change. These changes may be upward or downward, quite independently of the disability, though often family members when dismayed at deterioration or encouraged by improvement will attribute this to 'treatment', in the broadest sense, or to its lack. Assumed changes in handicap may well be the result of changes in attitudes of family members. This can be a valuable distinction for the doctor to use when assessing the family's insight into their own capacity to cope.

CAUSES OF MENTAL IMPAIRMENT

The array of possible causal factors in mental impairment is very wide. Since each pathological process may occur with varying severity and in varying combinations, it may have varying disabling effects; it is important therefore to be cautious about categories of clinical types. At the same time it must always be remembered that the retarded person has as much an individual personality as anyone else, so that although sufferers from e.g. Down's syndrome may be helpfully regarded as similar to each other and conforming to a clinical type, they will each have personal characteristics which are distinctive to them as individuals. None the less, there are broad groupings of retarded people who can be regarded as having similar features relevant to their behaviour or learning problems, and to the support needed to help their progress and to resolve conflicts they generate within the family.

The more common reasons for impairment will be outlined next, together with examples of the clinical types associated with them. (For further information see the texts listed on p. 533.) Close cooperation with a paediatrician is needed in the diagnosis and management of the physical disorders associated with mental retardation.

One reason for impaired mental development present from birth is that range of biological conditions, regarded as inherited or familial, which distort embryological processes in the growing baby. These include abnormal genes, abnormal chromosomes, and associated biochemical abnormalities. However, it is important to realise, as many parents do not unless they are so advised, that if the baby is abnormal from birth this may not necessarily be the result of defective inheritance. Other conditions due, for example, to maternal infections, or adverse effects of smoking, alcohol or drugs, can occur before birth, but are acquired. Mental impairment may also be acquired during birth (perinatal) or after birth (postnatal).

Table 41.1. Some known causes of mental handicap

Aetiology	Examples of syndromes
Abnormalities of single genes	Phenylketonuria (recessive)
	Gargoylism (Hurler's syndrome) (recessive)
	Hunter's syndrome (sex-linked recessive)
	Tuberous sclerosis (epiloia) (dominant)
Chromosomal abnormalities	
Autosomal	Down's syndrome
	Cri-du-chat syndrome
X-chromosome	Fragile X syndrome
Acquired	
Prenatal	Rubella
	Coxsackie virus
	Toxoplasmosis
	Drugs (e.g. phenytoin, alcohol)
	Cretinism (congenital hypothyroidism)
Perinatal	Prematurity
	Hyperbilirubinaemia (rhesus incompatibility)
	Anoxia
	Birth trauma
Postnatal	Epilepsy, e.g. febrile convulsions
	Infantile spasms (salaam attacks)
	Infections
	Lead intoxication
	Hydrocephalus, microcephaly

Polygenic effects

Intelligence is difficult to define and even more difficult to quantify, though it is recognised that some have more of it than others. It is likely that the largest group of people who could be considered mentally handicapped are those whose cognitive abilities are retarded to a handicapping level by being at the lower end of the range in the distribution of variation of human intelligence. The size of such a group in any given population is difficult to ascertain, because quite apart from grading into the 'unretarded' population (see p. 518), their prevalence will vary from place to place. They tend to be found more often among the socially disadvantaged, and their problems can in part arise from a variety of social and environmental circumstances.

In this group of retarded people the acquisition of developmental skills, although very slow, may be even in its delay. Self-help and domestic skills may also be slower, and antisocial behaviour may arise simply through their vulnerability and their lack of awareness when advantage is taken of them. As children they are found in schools for those with moderate learning difficulties, but in the future may become the earliest candidates for integration into normal schools if that policy is pursued.

In so far as intelligence is definable or quantifiable and can be regarded to some extent as a biological variable like height, it is the result of a continuous gradation due to many factors, genetic and environmental, each of small effect. The genetic component of this gradation is called *polygenic inheritance*. However, the distribution of intelligence within a given population is not symmetrical about a mean IQ of 100 because at the lower end of the distribution curve there are a number of severely affected people in excess of that expected by normal distribution alone. Their severe mental impairment, if inherited, is due either to rare abnormal single genes, inferred from the pattern of inheritance, or to chromosome abnormalities, now demonstrable by miscroscopic techniques. Abnormal genetic markers and their location on specific chromosomes will no doubt be increasingly identified by modern DNA probing techniques and linked with different forms of inherited mental handicap.

Abnormal genes

In clinical practice mental impairment is inferred as being due to an abnormal gene from its pattern of manifestation within a family as well as from associated specific clinical features. The commonest modes of inheritance are of two kinds: dominant or recessive autosomal. Some others are carried on a sex chromosome.

Dominant autosomal conditions present in the heterozygous form; they occur when the affected child has the relevant gene from one parent only. They therefore have a theoretical risk of occurrence of 1 in 2; they have a high mutation rate and their penetrance tends to be very variable. The severity of manifestation in affected family members therefore varies a great deal. An example is *tuberous sclerosis (epiloia)*, a severely disabling condition comprising a triad of epilepsy, mental retardation and various skin abnormalities, particularly adenoma sebaceum with a typical facial distribution. Nodules of neuroglia are present in the brain. It may be evident in the affected parent of a severely disabled child as no more than a minor previously undetected skin abnormality such as an achromic spot.

Recessive autosomal conditions, by contrast, need to be present in the homozygous form for the condition to be fully manifested, so the gene must be present in and contributed by each parent. With such inheritance the risk of occurrence is 1 in 4, and the conditions are more likely to occur if the parents are consanguineous or come from isolated or closely-knit communities in which intermarriage is common. A rare example is gargoylism (Hurler's syndrome), in which deposits of mucopolysaccharides are found in the brain, liver and spleen.

As a very broad generalisation dominant conditions have a tendency to be dysmorphic, i.e. to have a distinctive collection of abnormal physical features, though not all may be present together, as well as mental retardation. Recessive conditions tend to be associated with biochemical disorders and errors of metabolism such as phenylketonuria. As knowledge progresses this distinction is becoming increasingly blurred, but it is helpful to be alert to the possibility of autosomal recessive disorder in the case of a child with severely retarded development who none the less has normal appearance. An awareness of this will indicate the need for biochemical screening of the child, and possibly loading tests to detect a carrier state in his parents. Phenylketonuria may serve as an example of an autosomal recessive cause of mental retardation.

Phenylketonuria

This is one of the best known of the metabolic disorders of genetic origin and is characterised by autosomal recessive transmission. Lack of phenylalanine hydroxylase, responsible for the conversion of phenylalanine to tyrosine, causes an excess of phenylalanine and its metabolite phenylpyruvic acid in the blood; this is responsible for abnormal cerebral development and mental retardation. It is a rare disorder, found on average in 1 in 10,000 births in the UK, with some geographical variations.

The excess of phenylalanine in the blood can now be detected by a heel prick screening test which should be carried out on all newborn babies 5-10 days after birth, when the milk intake is adequate. If the test is positive the baby should at once be put on a diet low in phenylalanine to prevent the development of mental retardation, and this diet must be maintained at least until the early or mid-teens. If an adult phenylketonuric woman plans to have a baby she should go back on a low phenylalanine diet to protect the foetus from high levels of maternal phenylalanine (Lenke and Levy 1980).

Sex-linked transmission

This is associated with abnormal genes on the X-chromosome. Most are recessive and are manifested in only half the males born to a female carrier, who will herself be apparently unaffected. Since she will theoretically pass on her normal x gene to the other half of her male children they will be normal. Similarly 1 in 2 of her daughters will be carriers and the others normal. Such sex-linked conditions are much rarer than those due to abnormal autosomal genes. *Hunter's syndrome* serves as an example. Here the child has stunted growth, coarse facies, stiffening joints and mental retardation, and suffers from a storage disorder associated with mucopolysaccharidosis, affecting the brain, the liver and other organs.

Chromosome abnormalities

Whereas inherited disorders are as yet largely inferred from patterns of inheritance and recognition of associated clinical abnormalities, some inherited conditions with mental defect have recognisable chromosome abnormalities revealed by miscroscopic techniques. The commonest of these is Down's syndrome.

Down's syndrome

This was first described by Langdon Down in 1866. It used to be called mongolism, a term originally coined to describe some of the abnormal facial features characteristic of the syndrome. It constitutes a third of the moderately or severely mentally handicapped population and occurs in about one out of every 600 births. These children have a number of characteristic physical features, including short stature, a small rounded head, downward sloping epicanthic folds, a small mouth, furrowed tongue and high arched palate, broad hands with a curved little finger, and a single transverse palmar crease. There may also be associated congenital heart disease, e.g. septal defects, and duodenal atresia.

The syndrome is associated with an additional chromosome in pair 21 of the 22 pairs of autosomes. Usually the extra chromosome lies free, additional to pair 21, hence the term *trisomy 21*. In about 3 per cent of cases the extra chromosome is fused with another, in a *translocated state*. This may arise as a mutation, in which case the parents' chromosomes will be normal, but it may be present in one parent in a balanced form with a consequent high transmission risk. Chromosome studies should therefore always be undertaken to exclude the balanced translocated form.

In trisomy 21 the risk of giving birth to a child with Down's syndrome increases with maternal age, rising from a risk of 1 per 1000 births if the mother's age is below thirty-five, to 13 per 1000 if she is between forty and forty-five, and to 35 per 1000 if she is over forty-five. If the condition is due to translocation in one of the parents the risk is greatly increased and not related to maternal age.

The diagnosis of Down's syndrome can now be made before birth by amniocentesis followed by chromosome studies. This should therefore be offered to pregnant women in their thirties so that they can consider the possibility of a termination if the foetus is affected.

There is a wide range of mental impairment, from mild to severe, among people with Down's syndrome, and in any individual this is independent of the number of associated physical features characteristic of the syndrome. In many cases the extent of the disability, initially apparently mild, becomes increasingly and sadly obvious as the child grows older and the discrepancy between his and the normal acquisition of developmental skills emerges.

With improvements in the treatment of those medical conditions associated with the syndrome affecting the heart or gastro-intestinal system, patients with Down's syndrome now often survive into middle age. Such patients often develop signs of premature Alzheimer-type dementia. The onset at this age of epileptic attacks, otherwise rare in Down's syndrome, and of ill-coordinated rather than reluctant mobility, with an unsteady gait, adds to the suspicion of a dementing process.

Other chromosome abnormalities

Mental impairment may also be associated not with the addition but with the deletion of chromosome material. An example is the *cri-du-chat syndrome*, in which a part is missing from chromosome 5; this results in a microcephalic hypotonic child with epicanthus, mental retardation and a distinctive mewing cry which gives the syndrome its name.

Although many mentally handicapped individuals with chromosome abnormalities have distinctive dysmorphic features, there are others with recognised chromosome defects who have only mild or few such features. One of these is the *fragile X syndrome*, also known as the Martin-Bell syndrome (Richards *et al.* 1980; Turner 1982). In this condition a fragile or broken site on the X-chromosome can be identified microscopically. It is estimated to be responsible for 6 per cent of cases of severe retardation in males, which may be one of the reasons for the excess of males among the mentally handicapped. The disorder is sometimes associated with large testes, macro-orchidism. An association has also been found between the fragile X syndrome and some cases of autism.

Congenital hypothyroidism (cretinism)

Congenital hypothyroidism is usually due to a defect in development of the thyroid gland and synthesis of thyroxine. In the past iodine deficiency in the mother's diet was a common cause. It does not cause impairment of growth or mental retardation until after birth when both become progressively impaired if untreated. Early detection and thyroid replacement therapy are therefore essential. Blood screening tests for thyroxine (T4) and TSH should therefore be carried out on all newborn babies, and this can now be done at the same time as the heel prick test for phenylketonuria. This is not yet obligatory in the UK, but there is a national screening test in Eire where an incidence of 1 in 4000 births has been reported.

If the condition remains undetected and untreated the baby soon becomes sluggish and sleepy; it fails to feed and becomes constipated. The abdomen becomes prominent, the skin coarse and puffy, and the tongue gets large and begins to protrude. Unduly prolonged physiological jaundice should also arouse suspicion. The detrimental effects on mental development are irreversible. Permanent mental retardation can only be prevented by early and adequate replacement therapy, starting as soon after birth as it is detected and maintained in adequate dosage throughout life.

Acquired impairment

A major practical difficulty not only in the diagnosis of mental handicap but also in offering explanations to parents and planning treatment programmes is the wide array of external factors which can cause mental handicap. It is helpful to divide these conditions according to the timing of their effect, into prenatal, perinatal and postnatal or later causes.

Prenatal causes

Maternal infections which may cause damage to the embryo by affecting the brain can occur in acute or chronic (recurrent) form. Acute infections with this effect include some viruses (coxsackie A and B, echo, measles and mumps) and the group B streptococci. These have a self-limiting, i.e. circumscribed, impact because they are eliminated by the mother's immune defence mechanisms. Other infections are more serious because the conditions, which include rubella, toxoplasmosis, cytomegalovirus (CMV) and herpes simplex, can result in persistent infective damage not only through their recurrent nature but also by their ability to traverse the placenta. Such persistent infection in the child can cause a variety of impairments.

Maternal rubella during the first trimester can cause congenital rubella, characterised by hearing loss, cataract, microcephaly, congenital heart disease and mental retardation. The incidence of congenital rubella can now be much reduced by immunisation in childhood, although in the UK this is not yet taken up as much as it should be. Other infections do not usually result in such recognisable symptoms, but visual loss is common in all children retarded through prenatal infections. For example, toxoplasmosis may cause choroidoretinitis and mental retardation.

As maternal infections may produce few symptoms during the mother's pregnancy, and since many babies, e.g. those with CMV defect, may be symptom-free at birth, an infection may not be suspected. This can be particularly disabling as the infection may be progressive in the young child, who could have been more effectively treated by earlier intervention. It is important to be alert to the significance in a mother's history of being vaguely unwell in her pregnancy when one is confronted with a very slowly developing child; relevant antibody studies should then be carried out. Some infants with CMV infection have microcephaly at birth, and more severely affected children may die of encephalitis. Congenital syphilis is rarely seen since the introduction of serological testing of the mother.

Drug effects in pregnancy are becoming increasingly suspected as a cause of developmental defects. Some, such as thalidomide, cause severe developmental defects without involving the brain. Others, such as phenytoin, affect both the brain and other organs producing distinctive facial and limb features, impaired growth as well as mental retardation. It is estimated that as many as 1 in 10 phenytoin-exposed foetuses have some combination of these features, which are grouped together as the *foetal phenytoin syndrome* (Albengres and Tillement 1983).

High maternal alcohol consumption during pregnancy also carries a risk of producing a malformed infant, the so-called *foetal alcohol syndrome* (Clarren and Smith 1978). These infants have a low birth weight, their intelligence may be slightly impaired or they may be mentally retarded and slow in developing. There may be associated physical deformity, especially microcephaly and abnormal facial appearance. The perinatal mortality is also increased. To what extent these abnormalities are the direct result of the mother's high alcohol consumption or due to associated factors, such as heavy smoking or ill-health due to heavy drinking, is still uncertain.

Perinatal causes

Perinatal *brain damage* is a controversial topic. There is no doubt that a variety of conditions around the period of birth can result in severe brain damage, e.g. cerebral trauma, anoxia and electrolyte imbalance. What is complex and still being studied in obstetrics and neonatal care is the relationship between particular adverse events, the cerebral pathology they produce and the resulting pattern of impaired function in the child. Some broad generalisations can be made relating to the timing of the damaging episode.

Late pregnancy may be complicated by hypertension and toxaemia with widespread capillary disturbance over the cortex and diffuse cortical hypoxaemia in the foetus. Such widespread bilateral damage can be further complicated by delayed onset of labour and can result in substantial intellectual impairment, attention deficit and subsequent hyperactivity. However, this syndrome of 'distractible hyperactivity', sometimes called the 'hyperkinetic syndrome', can be due to many causes other than perinatal factors (see p. 503).

Cerebral trauma during or shortly after birth, particularly in the premature baby, is likely to produce discrete localised lesions in the brain resembling a cerebrovascular accident in adults so that, if severe, the child is both mentally retarded and has *cerebral palsy*.

In the neonatal period, *hypoxaemic damage* is more likely to occur in children who are vulnerable through prematurity or cardiovascular conditions which reduce the oxygen supply to the brain. Such cases are less acute than those due to birth trauma; the low-grade hypoxia may damage parts of the brain which are especially vulnerable to oxygen lack, leading to cortical, striatal or cerebellar symptoms, as in the retarded, athetoid or ataxic child. Multiple handicap, including retardation, epilepsy and cerebral palsy, tends to be associated with severe problems during delivery or neonatal care, though advances in these fields have reduced the frequency and severity of such disabilities. There is evidence that such multiple handicap tends to be associated less with obstetric complications or problems during perinatal care than with risk factors during pregnancy.

Postnatal and later causes

Epilepsy

Severe or frequent fits in infancy or early childhood are often associated with mental handicap. Whether in any given case the fits cause the retardation or whether both are part of an underlying pathology is often unclear. Generalised convulsions with febrile illness are common in young children and are not in themselves associated with retardation, but severe fits, especially if they occur in bouts within the first few months of life, can produce bilateral temporal damage which later results in severe learning defects and mental handicap.

Infantile spasms due to frequent epileptic seizures in the first year of life, often associated with salaam attacks, may be accompanied by gross cortical disorganisation. This is confirmed by a characteristic EEG showing *hypsarrythmia*, i.e. widespread spikes and slow waves of high amplitude (Friedman and Pampiglione 1971). Such children, though motor intact, usually develop extreme learning difficulty, mental retardation and social inaccessibility. Some of them show features of autism. About 25 per cent die before reaching adulthood.

Lead toxicity

Ingestion of lead, e.g. from toys with lead-based paints, or by inhaling industrial or petrol fumes with a high lead content has long been known as a cause of acute lead encephalopathy. More recent surveys have suggested that impaired intelligence, reduced educational attainment and behaviour disorders can be associated with raised blood lead levels even though these are much lower than those producing lead encephalopathy. The evidence has been reviewed by Yule and Rutter (1984). It seems likely that lead can have a graded neurotoxic effect. In many countries legislation has been introduced to reduce environmental exposure to lead.

To what extent the neurotoxic effects of lead can reinforce co-existent defects in the retarded population is still a matter for speculation. For example, some cases of mental retardation and the condition called *pica* (McLoughlin 1987), i.e. the habit of some children of ingesting or sucking a large variety of inedible substances, are both associated with increased blood lead levels. This could be due to the fact that pica, independently caused, has led to the ingestion of lead, resulting in raised blood lead levels, which could then lead to or increase the degree of any co-existent mental impairment. Alternatively, a high blood lead level due to environmental exposure could cause some degree of mental impairment which then results in pica. Such interdependence and mutual reinforcement of environmental neurotoxic hazards, psychosocial disorder and organic cerebral defect is common in the retarded population.

Adverse immunological reactions

These reactions may be very serious. For example, it has been suggested that immunisation against whooping cough could cause an acute encephalopathy and result in permanent mental retardation, but there is no convincing evidence that this is the case.

Allergic reactions to food substances

There is growing interest in and a great deal of controversy about the effects of various food components, including additives and dyestuffs, on behaviour and intelligence. A review by Conners (1980) of various studies using controlled diets suggests that the role of allergic reactions to certain foods or food additives in the aetiology of retardation and behaviour disturbance may at best be significant only in a very small proportion of patients.

PSYCHIATRIC DISORDERS

Psychiatric disorder can of course affect the mentally handicapped just as it does the normal population. The diagnosis of mental illness in the normal population largely depends on eliciting thoughts and feelings through dialogue in the course of interviewing the patient. This is often not possible with the mentally handicapped. Moreover, a major obstacle to diagnosing psychiatric disorder in the mentally handicapped is the extent to which their everyday behaviour in response to stress may in many respects resemble the symptomatology of mental illness. Emotional lability and disinhibited or impulsive reactions or, conversely, withdrawal and sluggish responses to situations all occur in the mentally handicapped population. Nevertheless, psychiatric morbidity is commonly seen among the mentally handicapped and the full spectrum of mental illness, behaviour problems and personality disorder can be found (Corbett 1985).

Alzheimer-type dementia

This occurs in mentally retarded adults and usually presents as a loss of already impaired language skills, deterioration in self-care, disorientation and often loss of continence. The onset is likely to be insidious, and this helps to distinguish it from a similar clinical picture emerging in response to moving into an unfamiliar setting or in response to drastic changes in routine, particularly in a settled or institutionalised retarded person. Changes in affect, e.g. passivity, withdrawal or unpredictable, impulsive aggressive behaviour, may also occur, often with little indication of situational triggers. Such changes due to dementia occur, for example, in a proportion of Down's syndrome patients after the age of thirty-five (see p. 526).

Dementia may be confused with the progressive effects of *hypothyroidism*. Although this is now rare as a cause of mental impairment in children, it may develop in mentally handicapped adults. As with dementia, hypothyroidism may go unrecognised because the onset is insidious and its symptoms may be exaggerations of those already present, e.g. depression and sluggish responses. It should always be kept in mind since treatment with thyroxine has very beneficial effects even in later stages (see also p. 295).

Schizophrenia

The recognition and appropriate treatment of schizophrenia is difficult in the mentally handicapped. This is particularly so in the more severely retarded since, because of their poverty of language, diagnosis depends mainly or entirely on observed behaviour. The abnormal behavioural features due to schizophrenia may well resemble those resulting from the onset of dementia or an adverse reaction to institutional care. Conversely, the behavioural features such as social withdrawal, stereotypies and unpredictable, impulsive outbursts may be the result of stress reactions in a deteriorating handicapped adult and not due to schizophrenia. Mistakes in diagnosis are therefore easily made. As a result mentally handicapped patients are often treated with psychotropic drugs for clinical conditions loosely but often wrongly labelled as psychotic, a practice particularly ill-advised if the medication is long-term, infrequently reviewed and hence unaltered.

In order to make a correct diagnosis of schizophrenia in the severely mentally handicapped it is essential to pay attention to *changes* in the individual's behaviour over longer periods of time. This depends on the presence of consistent staffing in any residential setting so that carers can get to know the individual patients and can be sensitive to such changes, however gradual.

Psychotic disorders, including schizophrenia, when diagnosed correctly probably run a more benign course in the mentally retarded. Paranoid disorders have a later onset than in the non-retarded psychiatric population. Treatment with psychotropic drugs is as appropriate for the retarded psychotic patient as for the non-retarded, provided the safeguards outlined above are respected.

Affective disorders

In the affective disorders, as in schizophrenia, the presentation of relevant symptoms in the mentally handicapped may be obscure. Many retarded people are limited verbally and prone to frustration at their inability to communicate, which can lead either to apathy and withdrawal or to impulsive reactions to being thwarted. They are also less well equipped to adapt to the unfamiliar, or to changes in demands made on them.

In order to recognise significant indicators of affective disorders, especially *depression*, in the mentally handicapped it is again essential to have staff caring for them consistently so that they can observe *changes* in the individual patient's pattern of life. Slowing up, generally reduced mobility, loss of appetite, weight loss and disruption of sleep pattern are all suggestive of depression. So are the development of irritability, increased stubbornness or rigid responses where these were previously absent, or were only a mild component of the patient's earlier range of behaviour. Acts of self-harm not previously seen in the patient are also highly suggestive.

In contrast to the likelihood of over-diagnosis of schizophrenia and unnecessary and prolonged treatment with antipsychotic drugs, affective disorders, especially depression, are likely to be under-diagnosed in the mentally retarded. This leads to the patient's depressive illness remaining unrecognised and untreated. In fact the treatment of depression in the retarded is not significantly different from that in the non-retarded patient.

Secondary mental handicap

Some handicapped people, children or adults, try to protect themselves from what is for them a bewildering and threatening world of non-retarded people by becoming even less able to use their already limited intelligence, so that they become isolated and increasingly less communicative. This secondary mental handicap can be greatly helped, as described by Bicknell (1983, 1988) and by Hollins and Bicknell (1988) (see also p. 566). Counselling and group discussion, sensitively adapted to the more able retarded individual's needs, can also help him to improve his personal and social functioning.

*

In conclusion, major distortions of mood, social response and levels of activity can all too readily be regarded as the product of the handicapping condition itself, though that may not be clearly defined. Conversely, such changes in behaviour, even though they resemble psychiatric disorder, may in fact be a reaction to changes in the environment and life circumstances in the handicapped person. Unequipped as he may be to reveal or cope with his feelings, he is by no means less sensitive than the non-retarded and reacts in ways which are occasionally wrongly labelled as ill and treated accordingly. The diagnosis and effective treatment of psychiatric illness in the mentally handicapped is a taxing professional skill. The practitioner should be able to distinguish disorder from levels of reaction that are typical or understandable for that individual in his particular circumstances, and to treat each appropriately. With the increasing emphasis on community care, there is an even greater need for the clinical sensitivity required to make such distinctions competently, to advise on and initiate appropriate treatment and to supervise its effectiveness.

The more the mentally handicapped enjoy the independence and the opportunities to which they are entitled the more urgent is the recognition of their special needs and a level of care which respects their vulnerability as well as their potential.

FURTHER READING

Detailed textbooks

Penrose, L.S. (1972). *The Biology of Mental Defect*, 4th ed. Sidgwick & Jackson, London.
Clarke, A.M., Clarke, A.D.B. and Berg, J.M. (eds) (1985). *Mental Deficiency: the changing outlook*, 4th ed. Methuen, London.
Kirman, B. and Bicknell, J. (1975). *Mental Handicap*. Churchill Livingstone, London.

Shorter general texts

Russell, O. (1985). *Mental Handicap*. Churchill Livingstone, Edinburgh.
Ricks, D.M. (1983) 'Severe subnormality' in *Handbook of Psychiatry*, vol. 2 (Lader, M.H., ed.), ch. 16. CUP, Cambridge.

Specialised topics

Cooper, B. (ed.) (1981). *Assessing the Handicaps and Needs of Mentally Retarded Children*. Academic Press, London.

Department of Health and Social Security (1971). *Better Services for the Mentally Handicapped*. HMSO, London.

Rutter, M. (ed.) (1984). *Developmental Neuropsychiatry*. Churchill Livingstone, London.

Smith, D.W. (1982). *Recognisable Patterns of Human Malformation: genetic, embryological and clinical aspects*, 3rd ed. Saunders, London.

Wilkins, D. (1979). *Caring for the Mentally Handicapped Child*. Croom Helm, London.

Practical problems

Simon, G.B. (ed.) (1980). *The Modern Management of Mental Handicap: a manual of practice*. MTP Press, Leicester.

Carr, J. (1985). *Helping your Handicapped Child*. Penguin, Harmondsworth

Finnie, N. (1971). *Handling the Young Cerebral Palsied Child at Home*. Heinemann, London

Freeman, P. (1975). *Understanding the Deaf/Blind Child*. Heinemann, London.

42

Infantile Autism

The term autism is used in two senses, either to describe a collection of symptoms found in a variety of disorders, or as the clinical entity called infantile autism.

Autism as a symptom complex refers to marked withdrawal, socially inaccessible behaviour and severe difficulty in relating to others. It is found in a wide range of psychiatric disorders, including schizophrenia, borderline states (see p. 342), and especially in severe mental retardation when the term 'retarded with autistic features' is often used.

In contrast, infantile autism, first described by Kanner (1943), is a clinical entity characterised by

(1) an inability to develop personal, affective and social relationships
(2) a failure or distortion of language acquisition
(3) ritualistic, stereotyped behaviour.

Its prevalence is about 2-4 per 10,000 children, and the condition is seen about three times more often in boys than in girls.

Among all the disabilities related to mental handicap, infantile autism is among the most controversial and emotive. This is due both to the distressing and bizarre nature of the disorder and to the conflicting views about its origin.

CLINICAL FEATURES

The symptoms of infantile autism become apparent within the first 30 months of life. Characteristically autistic children are unable to form attachments to their parents or other people and do not respond either appropriately or predictably to affectionate gestures. Some avoid eye contact; others, when they look at people, visually scan the face in a distant or impersonal manner. Such unresponsive behaviour is very distressing to parents because their efforts to form a close, affectionate relationship with their child seem to be ignored or rejected. Because autistic children give the impression of resisting or being afraid of closeness, they appear to be indifferent to people and withdraw into themselves: hence the term autism, which is derived from the Greek *autos*, meaning 'self'.

Autistic children also avoid and may react with fear to anything strange or unfamiliar. This desire for 'sameness' leads to stereotyped behaviour. They cling rigidly to routine and become distressed when this is changed in any way, e.g. by a change of surroundings, the presence of strangers, or new clothes, food or toys. Their play also tends to be repetitive and rigid, without originality or imagination. Although unable to play representationally, the child may absorb himself with meticulous skill in construction or inset toys or jig-saw puzzles. He may get attached to some particular toy or object, e.g. a solid toy or piece of metal, which he carries with him, firmly clutched in his hand.

Particularly serious is the failure of such children to acquire language. Some are mute, others learn to talk but find it difficult to use language to communicate with others, and the ability to talk may remain severely limited.

Despite these gross deficits, distinctive congnitive assets may be present, including rote memory, visuospatial skills, an acute sense of direction, or awareness of pitch patterns and response to music. Thus a perplexing and uneven pattern of cognitive defects and assets is common in each individual autistic child.

The level of apparent intelligence also varies a great deal from one child to the next. Some show moderate or severe mental retardation, but others have normal and a few even have superior intelligence when assessed by non-verbal performance tests. A similar wide range also applies to the other defects seen in infantile autism. Thus some autistic children have no speech while others may speak reasonably well although communicating badly, if at all, in the sense of meangingfully sharing experience or conveying feelings and needs. They may articulate clearly and employ quite complex sentences, but the way in which they use language is uncommunicative and odd, speaking at you rather than to you. There is no sense of dialogue nor indeed any indication that the autistic child is aware of you as a person similar to himself.

Hobson (1986a, 1986b), in a series of studies comparing the responses of autistic and non-autistic children to the facial expression of emotions by other people, has demonstrated that the autistic child has a specific inability to recognise and to respond to the meaning of facial expression of feelings. This disability is much greater than any difficulty the child may also have in recognising individual inanimate objects and their characteristics.

In general, much of the child's behaviour is marked by a self-contained detachment, lack of emotional contact with people, absence or poverty of speech and preoccupation with order. The autistic child's insistence on maintaining order and routine is so great that he may be regarded as struggling to overcome confusion in his experience of events, settings and people. Attempts to explain how this confusion arises have generated considerable controversy (see below).

COURSE AND PROGNOSIS

This is very variable, but a few indications influence the likely outcome. The most important of these is the degree of cognitive impairment in childhood, as assessed by performance tests which do not depend on the child's verbal ability. Those who are severely retarded and whose ability to speak has not improved by about the age of five are likely to remain severely handicapped throughout life in terms of their intellectual and social function. This applies to about 60 per cent of autistic children. Severely retarded autistic children also run a greatly increased risk of developing epilepsy in adolescence.

Those children whose intelligence is not seriously impaired and whose behaviour and language skills start to improve significantly by the time they reach the age of five have a better prognosis and may later on be able to make a reasonable social adjustment. Indeed there may well be autistic people, so mildly affected that their disability has remained unrecognised other than being odd and introspective with a strange way of speaking, who live isolated lives among the rest of us.

AETIOLOGY

It used to be thought that infantile autism was a form of childhood schizophrenia. However, the absence or rarity of schizophrenia in relatives; the reduction in intelligence, however measured; the higher than normal prevalence of epilepsy; the absence of delusions and hallucinations; and the ineffectiveness of phenothiazines all contrast with schizophrenia, whatever assumptions are made about similar symptomatology. This view has therefore been abandoned.

There has been much debate as to whether the condition is of biological origin, psychologically determined, or due to a combination of both. Those who have studied possible *psychogenic aspects* have suggested that the child becomes autistic as a result of conflicts in relation to his mother (Tustin 1981). Feeling unsafe and in danger of being rejected or hurt by his mother interferes with the way the child perceives his world, preventing him from making the same sort of stable sense out of his experience as would a child without such fears and conflicts. He then becomes frightened and uncomprehending and withdraws into an autistic state.

Several reasons make it difficult to accept such a purely psychogenic hypothesis. First, studies of the behaviour of the mothers of autistic children have not confirmed that they are unresponsive or cold in relation to their babies; further, some of the abnormalities that have been found in retrospective studies could have been due to the effect on the mother of having an autistic child rather than the cause of the disability.

Secondly, a purely psychogenic explanation assumes that the affected child is born with at least potentially normal perceptual, affective and cognitive functions. This conflicts with evidence that autistic children have deficits in all these areas from the start. For example, the studies by Hobson (1986a, 1986b) have demonstrated the autistic child's inability to perceive and respond to the facial expression of emotions of other people, and hence of his mother. As a result the child's response to his mother is distorted so that he reacts to her in abnormal and unpredictable ways. This in turn adversely affects the mother's responses to her child. The inevitable interpersonal difficulties that result when a mother finds that her baby is not responding to her as she had expected, are thus more likely to be a consequence rather than the primary cause of the autistic disability. However, the distressing interaction that is thus set up could in some cases aggravate the disorder.

There is now increasing evidence that *biological abnormalities* causing cerebral dysfunction are present in children with infantile autism. First, there is a high incidence of epilepsy in some autistic children when they reach adolescence. Secondly, an array of biochemical abnormalities, e.g. in the dopamine and tryptophan metabolic pathways, have been found in a consistent proportion of cases. Thirdly, there is some suggestion that there may be an abnormality in cerebral lateralisation, e.g. the more frequent than normal finding of ambidexterity and lack of eye, hand or foot preference. Failure to develop language skills and symbolisation suggests a defect in dominant hemisphere function, while non-dominant hemisphere functions, e.g. visuospatial skills, are intact or even exceptionally well developed. Some studies using CT scans have shown the brains of autistics to be more symmetrical than those of controls, though other studies have shown the reverse; these findings are as yet inconclusive. Minor EEG abnormalities are also common in autistic children, though nothing specific to the syndrome has yet emerged. Lack of adequate data in normal children and of clear agreement on the clinical group studied as autistic, however, make it difficult to assess the significance of these observations.

There is also increasing evidence that *genetic factors* are important. One difficulty in carrying out genetic studies on autism is the fact that very few autistic individuals are able to marry and have children. However, the concordance rate of infantile autism among monozygotic twins is significantly greater than in dizygotic twins (Folstein and Rutter 1977). Furthermore, although the incidence of infantile autism among the siblings of an affected child is low, it is significantly higher than in the general population, and some of the apparently unaffected siblings show a greater than expected incidence of learning difficulties or impairment of speech. To what extent this could be due to environmental factors in a family with an autistic child is uncertain. In some cases autism is associated with the fragile X syndrome (see p. 526); this might account in part for the higher incidence in males than females.

In conclusion, it seems likely that several distinct, probably interrelated, neurophysiological abnormalities are involved in the causation of autism, leading to abnormal cerebral function early in childhood. This would then be responsible for the disruption of the child's perceptual processes and affective responses in relation to his environment. This primary deficit could then lead to disturbed interaction between the child and his mother, resulting in exacerbation of the child's disability.

DIFFERENTIAL DIAGNOSIS

A child with infantile autism must be differentiated from a child who is severely mentally retarded and shows some autistic features, such as withdrawal and stereotyped behaviour. In infantile autism the degree of language impairment and withdrawal from personal relationships is usually more severe than his intellectual impairment would suggest, while in mental retardation these discrepancies are either absent or less marked. The distinction may be difficult to make unless some other cause of mental retardation can be identified.

Infantile autism must also be distinguished from the disintegrative childhood psychoses (see p. 505). Such children, unlike autistic children, at first develop normally but after a few years suffer rapid and progressive deterioration of their speech, intellectual function, behaviour and personal relationships. The disintegrative psychoses are usually of organic origin, e.g. due to measles encephalitis or one of the lipoidoses or leucodystrophies, so that the child either dies or becomes severely and permanently mentally handicapped.

Another related but rare condition is *Asperger's syndrome* (L. Wing 1981). Here impairment of relationships and sterotyped behaviour becomes worryingly evident later in childhood, after the age of three, although language skills and intelligence are usually more or less normal. The abnormalities persist into adult life. The condition resembles and may be mistaken for a severe schizoid personality disorder, whereas it is more likely to be a mild, though socially very disabling, form of infantile autism.

TREATMENT

This has to be considered in relation to both the child and his family. Whatever one's view about the aetiology of autism, there is general agreement on the importance of attempting to help the autistic child to learn how to relate to others and to improve his social functioning. This has to be done by educational measures aimed at stabilising the child's awareness of the world around him and the people within it. This involves a great deal of explanation and support of the parents in order to help them understand their child's perplexing disability and provide the stable, highly structured home environment he needs. Those children who are not too severely retarded (which is difficult to predict) benefit from early education in a structured school environment appropriate to their age, intelligence and verbal ability.

Behaviour programmes, if established after adequate and careful observation, are likely to improve social and self-help skills, language and the child's capacity to relate to others. Psychotropic drugs have been found to have variable effects but may sometimes be helpful in controlling episodic disturbed behaviour or in a crisis; anticonvulsant drugs may be needed in children with epileptic fits or where impulsive behaviour is associated with paroxysmal disturbance in the EEG, if recordable.

An array of other treatments are used, including psychotherapy (see p. 566), holding therapy, dietary control, vitamin supplements and drugs which correct abnormal levels of neurotransmitters or counteract the effects of suspected abnormal endorphin output. Careful and controlled follow-up studies evaluating their effects are, as yet, unfortunately rare. It is however important to keep an open mind in the hope that reliably effective remedies will emerge in the treatment of this very distressing condition.

FURTHER READING

Rutter, M. (1985). 'Infantile autism and other pervasive developmental disorders' in *Child and Adolescent Psychiatry: modern approaches*, 2nd ed. (Rutter, M. and Hersov, L., eds). Blackwell, Oxford.

Tustin, F. (1981). *Autistic States in Children*. Routledge, London.

Wing, L. (ed.) (1976). *Early Childhood Autism: clinical, educational and social aspects*, 2nd ed. Pergamon, Oxford.

Wing, L. (1980). *Autistic Children: a guide for parents*. Constable, London.

43

Child Sexual Abuse

HISTORY

The history of childhood is a nightmare from which we have only just
recently begun to awaken. The further back in history one goes, the lower
the level of childcare, and the more likely children are to be killed,
abandoned, terrorised and sexually abused.

Lloyd de Mause (1976)

Children have been physically, emotionally and sexually abused
throughout history. It is a sign of the progress our society has made that
we find the continuing existence of sexual abuse so disturbing. Indeed, it
is only in the last ten years that we have even reached a position from
which we can begin to comprehend the nature and extent of sexual abuse.

Throughout history great thinkers have drawn attention to this issue,
but society as a whole has been unable or unwilling to take in the
message. In the fourth century BC Aristotle was one of the first to note the
link between abuse and later repetitive sexual behaviour, observing in
his *Politics* that homosexuality often became habitual in those abused
from childhood. The orator Aeschines spoke of Athenian laws that tried to
limit the sexual attacks on boys by their teachers, aided by the teachers'
legal powers to punish physically. In ancient Rome in the first century AD
Quintilian also underlined the child's helplessness against the legal and
physical power of the adult in his *Institutio Oratoria*: 'If inadequate care
is taken in the choice of respectable governors and instructors, I blush to
mention the shameful abuse which scoundrels sometimes make of their
right to administer corporal punishment.' In our own time STOPP, the
Society of Teachers Opposed to Physical Punishment, has made the same
statement, underlining the difficulty the child has in saying no to
intrusions on its body when the law is still largely permissive of such
adult physical attack. STOPP has now made it easier for abuse in the
classroom to be made public more speedily.

Nearly a century ago, Freud (1896), in his work on the aetiology of
hysteria, provided us with an understanding of the sexual abuse of
children and its long-term effects. He expressed the view that in all the
eighteen cases of hysterical illness that he had dealt with by then,

repression of the memory of sexual abuse by an adult or sibling was at the core. He delineated three categories of sexual abuse that are still the most important today:

> In the first group it is a question of assaults – of single, or at any rate, isolated instances of abuse, mostly practised on female children, by adults who were strangers, and who, incidentally, knew how to avoid inflicting gross mechanical injury. In these assaults there was no question of the child's consent and the first effect of the experience was preponderantly one of fright. The second group consists of the much more numerous cases in which some adult looking after the child – a nursery-maid or governess or tutor, or unhappily, all too often, a close relative, has initiated the child into sexual intercourse and has maintained a regular love relationship with it – a love relationship, moreover, with its mental side developed – which has often lasted for years. The third group, finally, contains child-relationships proper – sexual relations between two children of different sexes, mostly a brother and a sister, which are often prolonged beyond puberty and which have the most far-reaching consequences for the pair ... Where there had been a relation between two children I was sometimes able to prove that the boy – who here too played the part of aggressor – had previously been seduced by an adult of the female sex ... In view of this I am inclined to suppose that children cannot find their way to acts of sexual aggression unless they have been seduced previously (Freud 1896, p. 208).

Freud was himself shocked by the facts he had uncovered. The shock that he as a pioneer felt was exacerbated by the fact that none of his colleagues were able to accept his theory of sexual trauma. In a letter to Fliess dated 21 September 1897 he wrote: '...surely such widespread perversions against children are not very probable' (Freud 1897). Current figures would appear to underline some of Freud's doubts. For example, in a general review of published data Tower Hamlets Social Service Information (1984) found that only just over half of juvenile offenders guilty of child sexual abuse gave a history of having been physically or sexually abused themselves.

It is important, however, to appreciate that Freud never withdrew from the fact that his early findings of sexual abuse mattered. He only revised his view that they applied to all hysterical phenomena. In the context of his work on the origins of sexual disorders he laid great emphasis on 'the effects of seduction which treats a child as a sexual object prematurely and teaches him, in highly emotional circumstances, how to obtain satisfaction from his genital zones, a satisfaction which he is then usually obliged to repeat again and again by masturbation. An influence of this kind may originate either from adults or from other children. I cannot admit that in my paper on "The Aetiology of Hysteria" (1896) I exaggerated the frequency or importance of that influence' (Freud 1905, p. 190).

It is not surprising that Freud has often been criticised or even blamed for recognising the importance of sexual abuse (McFarlane and

Waterman 1986; Masson 1986). It seems to be a dynamic of child sexual abuse that someone in the professional team, even today, becomes the recipient of the outrage for the act of abuse that would otherwise go to the abuser (Furniss 1983), and that unusually critical feelings are directed at colleagues (Kraemer 1987). This affects writers on the subject as well as practitioners and needs to be carefully monitored and understood.

PROFESSIONAL RESPONSES

A common response is either to blame the child for bringing the trauma upon himself or to vent hatred on the perpetrator and rush into precipitous action. It is far easier to empathise with a child in an average family who has been suddenly assaulted by a stranger, than to feel empathic with the child who has eroticised his emotions as a result of long-term abuse within the family and has become addicted to it. More frequently, there is a wish not to see what the child is presenting. As Sgroi (1982) has pointed out, 'recognition of sexual molestation in a child is entirely dependent on the individual's inherent willingness to entertain the possibility that the condition may exist'. Freud, in his lone position, was willing to entertain that possibility. Many workers today, with the benefit of long training, are still struggling to do so. Abusers often take care to avoid physical injury so that physical examination only occasionally provides convincing evidence. We can therefore see why, unless there is a clear-cut confession from an adult, this work is so fraught with diagnostic, emotional, ethical, legal and clinical difficulties.

DEFINITION

Many authorities have provided their own definitions of child sexual abuse. There is, however, a core concept that, in the words of Bentovim (1987), is 'the most widely accepted definition of sexual abuse'. That is, 'the involvement of dependent developmentally immature children and young people in sexual activities which they cannot fully comprehend, to which they cannot give informed consent, and which violate the social taboos of the culture *and are against the law* (italics added by DHSS Draft Guidelines 1986).' Additions to this core definition, first formulated by Schechter and Roberge (1976), have been made by many local authorities, including the Tower Hamlets District Review Committee (1986). These include the whole spectrum of inappropriate sexual behaviour from fondling, exhibition of genitals, masturbation of the adult by the child or vice versa, mutual masturbation, oral, anal or genital contact, full vaginal or anal intercourse and the involvement of children in pornographic activities. Various forms of passive sexual abuse have since been added, in which children are made to watch pornographic or horror movies or watch adult sexual activity.

There are two other areas of sexual abuse, one that is defined by law and one that is a disturbingly grey area. First, child prostitution is estimated to include 170 million children, i.e. 3.8 per cent of the world's total population (Defence for Children International 1984). Using children for pornography and prostitution is an international multi-million pound business. The children most vulnerable to this are the poorest (International Children's Rights Monitor 1985).

Secondly, there is the very difficult problem of correct sexual boundaries in everyday life. A small child needs help to dress, undress, wash and go to the toilet. Although these intimate activities are parts of normal family life they can sometimes serve as expressions of disturbed sexuality in the family. Educational videos, such as 'Kids can say no!' by Carolyn Okell-Jones (1985) help to make young children more aware of their rights to their own body, of the difference between a 'good' and a 'bad' touch and the meaning of a secret. However, for many children it is hard to say no to kisses and touches that are satisfying the adult's secret erotic needs. Where a child is not only at the physical mercy of adults but at the same time loves and needs to be loved by them, an inner awareness of 'no' can easily be blunted. A child can find it so unbearable to have the knowledge that it is being betrayed by a parent that the 'no' can even be transformed into a 'yes'.

Some of the *'grey areas'* in ordinary family life are open to controversy. For example, there is some disagreement whether sharing the parents' bedroom and hence watching them having intercourse necessarily has a damaging effect on the sexual and personal development of children. It is important to understand what constitutes normal family life in a particular culture before we can appreciate the conditions in which actual sexual abuse occurs. However, sexual disturbances in everyday life will not be recognised while defences of culture are used. Some societies (Tucker 1987) 'encourage the gentle stroking of a restless or upset infant's genitals as a way of inducing calm and contentment'. The fact that a custom is spread widely does not necessarily make it free of damaging effects; it merely underlines the fact that whole societies or sub-groups can follow a disturbed practice. Forward and Buck (1978) call these grey areas 'pseudo-incest' but say that they can be just as damaging as true incest.

FREQUENCY

Kempe (1979) drew attention to the frequency of child sexual abuse in the 1970s. In 1986 the NSPCC issued figures showing that new cases of sexual abuse, severe enough to be included in a child abuse register, had risen from 500 in 1984 to 2,932 in 1985. In 1986 the number had increased to 6,330 children from infants to sixteen-year-olds, an annual incidence of 0.57 cases per 1000 children under seventeen. Mrazek *et al.* (1981) found an incidence of 3 per 1000 children up to the age of fifteen who came to the notice of professionals. However, many workers have seen these figures as just 'the tip of the iceberg' (Okell-Jones 1987), as many cases are not detected or reported.

Retrospective studies of adults reveal a different story. D. Russell (1983) found that 38 per cent of a group of 930 adult women in San Francisco gave a history of sexual abuse, either intra- or extra-familial, before the age of eighteen, and A. Rosenfeld (1979) found that 33 per cent of a small sample of psychiatric patients gave a history of incest. Finkelhor (1979) found that 19.2 per cent of women and 9 per cent of men in a college population gave a history of sexual abuse in childhood. The marked difference between the figures obtained in childhood and the retrospective figures obtained from adults points to one of the key elements in sexual abuse of children – secrecy and guilt, and children's fear of breaking the secret. This clearly contributes to the difficulty in obtaining reliable figures for the incidence and prevalence of sexual abuse in the community (Markowe 1988). No reliable figures exist so far.

As diagnostic skills have improved, there has also been growing awareness of the early age of onset of abuse. Bentovim *et al.* (1988) report a significant number of under-fives being referred in the UK. Since 1981 in the USA the average reported age of initiation has dropped from nine to seven years (Summit 1983). Overall, in the UK and USA, children referred on account of sexual abuse are over the age of eleven in 60 per cent of cases, 27 per cent are between six and ten and 13 per cent are under six (Tower Hamlets Social Services Research and Information 1984). Abuse within the family affects boys and girls over eleven about equally, while under the age of ten girls are abused more often than boys. A child is three times more likely to be abused by a recognised trusted adult than by a stranger. The perpetrator is known to the child in 75 per cent of cases (Finkelhor 1979; Summit and Kryso 1978). Between 90 and 98 per cent of abusers are men (Elliott 1985), many of them married with children. They come from all social classes and many were abused themselves as children.

SIGNS AND SYMPTOMS

The emotional signs of child sexual abuse can cover a wide range of childhood psychiatric symptoms. Only occasionally are there physical signs which help in diagnosis, for example vaginal or anal lacerations, bleeding, bruising or infections. In small children there may be evidence of regression and sexualisation of behaviour. At school age conduct disorders and low achievement become noticeable. There can be loss of self-esteem and self-care. In adolescence there can be overdosing, truancy, self-mutilation, pregnancy, promiscuity, abuse of younger children, anorexia nervosa and regression.

Very rarely does sexual abuse come to light from medical examination alone, and unless the examination takes place shortly after the abuse spermatozoa will not be found. The examination must be done with a great deal of tact and the minimum of trauma to the child; repeated examinations must be avoided. This means that while the attention of a doctor, including a paediatrician or police surgeon in some cases, is necessary to see if any physical signs of abuse are present, the assessment skills of a multi-disciplinary team, including a doctor, social worker, psychiatrist, psychotherapist and police officer, are all needed. Careful work must always be done with the child and the family before a diagnosis can be made and a decision is reached about the management of the child and the family (Department of Health and Social Security 1988a, 1988b). In the words of Lord Justice Butler-Sloss in her Report on the Cleveland Inquiry (Butler-Sloss 1988): 'There is a danger that in looking to the welfare of children believed to be the victims of sexual abuse the children themselves may be overlooked. The child is a person and not an object of concern.'

DISCLOSURE

Disclosure is very rarely due to the abused child telling someone. The child is terrified of losing parental love or his family, and of a parent going to prison. Sometimes abuse comes to light through other family conflict.

For example, Kevin, a small eight-year-old, evoked concern in his school. He was underachieving, withdrawn and easily bullied. His mother was twenty-eight, divorced and living with a new boyfriend. Sexual abuse had never been suspected. It would have remained a secret within the family had the boyfriend not started an affair with a friend of the mother. In her hurt at his betrayal of her she was able to voice more clearly her compliance in and anger at his betrayal of her child. Only when Kevin's mother firmly and strongly made clear to the multi-disciplinary team that she knew her boyfriend was abusing Kevin but was frightened of losing him, was Kevin able to nod his acceptance of her story.

Sometimes there is incidental discovery by a third party. For example, a neighbour wrote to her local hospital's child psychiatry department saying she was worried about six-year-old Mary who was always publicly masturbating and involved in sexual games with older children. A visit by a social worker revealed that sexual abuse was taking place within the family.

The work of child protection workers and agencies brings in other disclosures. In 1986, after two years of running Kidscape, child psychologist Michele Elliott received disclosures of sexual abuse from over 400 children, amounting to 10 per cent of all the children she had interviewed in schools as part of her prevention programme. The BBC programme Childwatch and subsequently Childline have 'been swamped by thousands of calls from troubled children, many of whom are current victims of sexual abuse' (Okell-Jones 1987). Child psychotherapists in child guidance clinics and child psychiatry departments have also reported an increase of disclosure in the course of psychotherapy, but a child might be in therapy for years before revealing abuse.

DIAGNOSTIC INTERVIEWS

Even after a parent or other person has disclosed abuse or made an allegation about it, it nevertheless remains difficult to prove. Every member of our society has a right not to be convicted of a serious crime without evidence. However, the therapeutic kind of interview that would allow a child the freedom to reveal more is rarely productive of the kind of evidence that would be accepted in a court of law. As Douglas and Willmore (1987) state, 'interviews are conducted by clinicians primarily concerned with aiding the recovery of abused children rather than the forensic needs of the courts'. The child sexual abuse team at Great Ormond Street Hospital, London, has pioneered important diagnostic methods and techniques (Bentovim *et al.* 1988; Vizard and Tranter 1988). These involve a structured interview conducted by trained workers using anatomically correct dolls. There is a free play period, followed by undressing the dolls and naming body parts. Sometimes the secrecy surrounding abuse has deprived the child of the means of expressing himself. By having dolls with sexual parts the interviewer can find out what words, if any, the child uses. With the adult's permission to name what might be unnameable in the home the child feels freer to describe the abuse or re-enact it with the dolls. However, there is still a discrepancy between a therapeutic interview and a forensic one, although the gap is narrowing.

Legal aspects

The use of video-recorded interviews with children now amounts to documentary evidence and is an admissable form of evidence in court. However, judges have not surprisingly expressed concern about the principles involved. Thus Waite (1987) recognised the benefits of using a video-recording but pointed out that some questions would be seen as leading questions in court; e.g. 'When daddy does that, does it ever feel a bit wet down there?' when enquiring about ejaculation. Leading questions are not suitable for a court of law, and Vizard (1987) has changed aspects of her interviewing method to meet these difficulties.

In some areas police officers are working directly with doctors and social workers, and the police are themselves considering filming forensic interviews. Police are trained in questioning and if they were able to undertake the assessment interviews with support from other professionals some of the legal difficulties might be avoided.

Therapeutic assessment

Every adult working in any capacity with a child who they suspect may have been abused needs to hold that possibility in mind. This means there may at times be a change in the more usual structuring of an interview.

> Josie, aged fourteen, had already been in therapy with me (Sinason 1988a) for 1½ years when a teacher reported that she had suddenly 'clammed up' after talking about doing 'funny things' with her brother.

> 'How can you be sexy without being dirty?' she asked suddenly.
> Because of the external information I replied that maybe someone was making her feel sexy and dirty at the moment.
> *Josie*: My boyfriend makes me feel sexy and happy.
> *Therapist*: Maybe someone else has made you feel sexy and dirty.
> *Josie*: (whispering) My brother.
> *Therapist*: Something you do with your brother makes you feel sexy and dirty.
> (Josie was then unable to speak.)
> *Therapist*: Maybe it would be easier to tell me with the dolls. (I brought a teenage girl doll and a bear. I pointed to the doll.) This is Josie coming home. Where is her brother bear?
> *Josie*: (pointing at the bear) Josie is in her bedroom because she is sent to bed at 6 o'clock and her brother comes in to say goodnight.
> *Therapist*: Right, Josie is in her bedroom and now her brother bear comes in. What happens?
> (Josie looks intently at the dolls and then picks them up, miming actions as she speaks.)
> *Josie*: Johnny hits Josie doll around the face and knocks her out onto the bed and says he will kill her if she does not keep the secret. (She bursts into tears)
> *Therapist*: What happens next?
> *Josie*: (miming with the dolls) He puts his willy in. (Loudly) He did it first when I was five and I told my mum and she told me not to be stupid.

After that assessment of the abuse with Josie I told her that what she had told me was very important and could not just stay with me. I needed to tell her social worker. Josie understood but wanted to make sure I realised that her mother's neglect and emotional abuse hurt her more than her brother's actions. A meeting of the whole team, including a police representative, resolved finally to move Josie to a boarding school without taking her brother to court.

Assessment interviews to determine the nature of the abuse where it is already known can run into difficulties if the worker takes the over-simple line: 'You are not to blame. It is daddy's fault.' This fails to deal with the child's feeling of guilt; it also fails to recognise the sexual satisfaction the child may have gained. When undertaking a forensic assessment it may help to say: 'Even if you enjoyed it, that did not make it right for the grown up to have been doing that to you.'

Assessment problems

Where there has been no disclosure but the team feel certain that there has been abuse a very specific training is needed to work with the child. Psychodynamic understanding is necessary as the child, in order to survive, has had to make adjustments which have serious psychological consequences. As Shengold (1979) expresses it:

> If the very parent who abuses and is experienced as bad must be turned to for relief of the distress that the parent has caused then the child must, out of desperate need, register the parent – delusionally – as good. Only the mental image of a good parent can help the child deal with the terrifying intensity of fear and rage which is the effect of tormenting experiences. The alternative – the maintenance of the overwhelming stimulation and the bad parent imago – means annihilation of identity, of the feeling of the self. So the bad has to be registered as good. This is a mind-splitting, fragmenting experience.

The unskilled worker can completely overlook or underestimate this process in a mistaken attempt to 'educate' the child out of its good opinion of its parent or relatives. Conversely, the helping adult can find it intolerable to be seen by the child as a bad person waiting for the right moment to seduce her. An understanding of the processes of projection and splitting is therefore essential (see also pp. 55-6).

EFFECTS ON THE CHILD

Sexualisation of behaviour

One of the main effects of child abuse is the sexualisation of children's behaviour, e.g. compulsive masturbation and the abuse of others. Sexual activity can be felt to be so pleasurable that it is hard to find comparable rewards to reinforce more acceptable behaviour (Yates 1982). The high focus on sexual learning detracts from social and educational learning. The breakdown of differentiation between sexual touch and affectionate touch means that the child can be stimulated by any physical or emotional closeness. Mentioning sexual excitement in a treatment session can itself act as a concrete sign to be excited. This blurring of normal boundaries between socially appropriate and inappropriate behaviour leads to further difficulty and distress.

Foster placements can break down under the duress of this breaking of boundaries, and there are calls for foster-parents to be trained to deal with abused children. The foster-parents first feel they are receiving a tragic victim and their empathy helps them manage the first inappropriate sexualised actions of the child. They next tend to believe that the behaviour has nothing to do with the child but is the terrible effect of previous abuse. When after a year in the new home the child's sexualised behaviour continues and the foster-family are unable to cope with this, the placement may break down, adding to the cycle of rejection and despair.

> Four-year-old Matthew had been sexually abused by both his mother and father. His foster-mother, a woman with three daughters, felt very proud to gain a handsome little son and was full of compassion for the mental and physical abuse he had suffered. After five months she said, 'I can put up with all his violence and his falling over all the time and all the children ringing the door to tell me he has been fighting them even though he's so tiny. But I can't have him rocking up and down all the time playing with his willy in front of my daughters and my neighbours and relatives. I send him upstairs and he carries on, and at night none of us can sleep hearing his bed creaking all the time.' After one year, despite her understanding, she was unable to continue although she was very fond of him. 'I never thought he would stay bad despite what you said. Not this long. I thought a good home would help him by now but when he starts lifting up neighbours' skirts and trying to touch them and playing with himself, I can't take him anywhere or have anyone over. And if I shout at him or hit him it just gets him more excited.'

Learning difficulties

Learning and sexual learning are closely linked in childhood. In the Oedipal period (see p. 73) a normal child playing with the fantasy of marrying his opposite sex parent has to learn that this wish cannot be fulfilled in reality. The fantasy play helps the child prepare for future adulthood. However, the abused boy or girl has *become* the mummy or daddy; symbolic functioning has been destroyed and there is a reduction of intellectual development. Brooks (1985), in a study of 29 adolescents in a secondary school for emotionally disturbed girls, found that 18 had been abused. We are facing the prospect of finding out how many of our disturbed children with special needs have in fact been sexually abused.

Recent studies in America (Cohen and Warren 1987) suggest that various kinds of secondary mental and multiple handicap may be an acquired disability resulting from abuse in childhood. Similarly, psychoanalytical psychotherapy is revealing that secondary mental handicap (see p. 532) sometimes serves as a defence against the past trauma of sexual abuse (Sinason 1986).

The repetitive nature of sexual abuse

As mentioned earlier, children who have been abused may later, or as adolescents or adults, abuse others. It would seem that the only way to deal with an intolerable experience, the memory of which cannot be borne, is to expel it by making someone else experience it instead (Sinason 1988b). For example, during his therapy a boy called Ali looked desperate when it was time for his therapy session to end. He raced around the room sticking his penis in the dolls' mouths and bottoms. 'I can't go until I have made all the dolls sick,' he cried. Only when he had evacuated his experience into the dolls and me could he bear to leave. The compulsive masturbation that is a feature of many sexually abused children's behaviour and the repetitive nature of the abuse may have a similar origin.

Loneliness and isolation

Sexual abuse of a child is usually a crime for which there is no witness except for the abuser and abused. The perpetrator nearly always tells the child that the sexual relationship is a secret. The abuser has often used violence or has threatened the child with the blame for break-up of the family or his imprisonment if the child tells. At the same time the abuser, if one of the parents, is also likely to be one of the people from whom the child expects protection. The consequence of this conflict is that the child has no one to talk to and share the experience with, nor can she bear to comprehend the enormous betrayal of trust. Some children may give up forever the hope that there is any honourable adult authority. This makes future delinquency more likely.

If in addition the child is disbelieved by the non-abusing parent whom she tries to tell, she feels so psychologically orphaned that she may retract the accusation and as a result be branded as a liar. If the child is believed there is a greater chance of psychological recovery (Herman 1982). If an outsider whom the child tells does not believe her there is a similar loss of hope, and this also applies to the disbelieving professional. Skilled work is essential, for the child can rarely stand up against adult authority for long and denials are likely to appear, leaving no proof whatsoever. The growing but often harmful practice of second or even third opinions is often experienced by the child as a further abuse by adults. Sometimes the abuse will never be proved and will never again be spoken of. The team may then have to live with the painful fact that they may never know (Trowell 1987).

TREATMENT

Treatment depends partly on what is available locally. Ideally, an integrated judicial/social/psychotherapeutic intervention is best, but this is rarely available. *Group therapy* for abused children and adolescents can offer relief and social contact to those who feel abnormal and alone: 'It felt good just knowing I wasn't the only person in the world,' said fifteen-year-old Louise. At the actual time of disclosure *family work* can be therapeutic and may avoid the breaking-up of the family. Family work can prove more difficult later on as the family becomes more resistant to change and may have united against the victim or, less frequently, the perpetrator. However, the protection of the child is paramount and, if there is no alternative, it is better for the child to be sadly and properly alone and lonely in care than to be unhealthily 'at home' in a dangerous family.

Individual psychotherapy or psychoanalysis is the only treatment that offers some abused children a chance of lasting internal change and recovery, but provision for such treatment is limited and still largely centred in London. Psychoanalytical psychotherapy is long-term work that experiences painful setbacks at times when circumstances make the individual more vulnerable. For example, Ali, the boy mentioned earlier, who revealed his abuse during therapy, found that whenever he was badly bullied he would be driven to seek out further abuse or to struggle with the temptation of abusing a smaller child himself.

Stages in psychotherapy

At the beginning of therapy the child may be withdrawn, monosyllabic and distant. Conversely, the child may be physically too close, trying to give kisses, and be both repellant and appealing at the same time. After a period of maybe less than a year if the family has admitted the abuse, or several years if there is total family denial, the child will start to show more feelings of a genuine kind, sadness and rage. This can often culminate in a painful re-enactment of the abuse during play therapy with whatever toys are available.

There is often a short productive period in which the child as victim mourns the loss of her trust in adults. At this point the therapist is the witness of the innocent child's helplessness against adult power and need. This is extremely painful but proves to be the easiest part of the therapy.

During the next stage, the child, having mourned for herself as victim, takes on the role of her aggressor and shows the power of her identification with him. The therapist may now come under physical and sexual attack, sometimes standing for the child as victim, sometimes for the abusing parent. It is important for the therapist to allow the child to perceive him in this way and not insist on being seen as a good adult. As a further expression of identification with the aggressor, the child might start becoming abusive to smaller children. Only after this has been worked through is there any chance of future safety and sanity. The child will gradually recognise the incongruity of these feelings and re-evaluate them with the therapist.

FURTHER READING

Bentovim, A. (1987). 'The diagnosis of child sexual abuse'. *Bull. Roy. Coll. Psychiatrists* 11, 295-299.
Bentovim, A., Elton, A., Hildebrand, J., Tranter, M. and Vizard, E. (eds)

(1988). *Sexual Abuse in the Family: assessment and treatment.* John Wright, London.

Ciba Foundation (1984). *Child Sexual Abuse within the Family* (Porter R., ed.). Tavistock, London.

De Mause, L. (ed.) (1976). *The History of Childhood: the evolution of parent-child relationships as a factor in history.* Condor Books, London.

Department of Health and Social Security (1988). *Diagnosis of Child Sexual Abuse: guidance for doctors.* HMSO, London.

Mrazek, P.B. and Kempe, C.H. (eds) (1981). *Sexually Abused Children and their Families.* Pergamon, Oxford.

Sinason V. (1988a) 'Dolls and bears: from symbolic equation to symbol. The significance of different play material for sexually abused children and others'. *Brit J. Psychother.* 4, 349-363.

Sinason, V. (1988b). 'Smiling, swallowing, stupefying and sickening. The effect of sexual abuse on the child'. *Psychoanalytic Psychotherapy* 3, 97-111.

Part VIII

Treatment Methods

The methods used to help psychiatrically and psychologically disturbed patients can be divided into three groups:

(1) *Psychological treatments*, including psychoanalysis and other forms of individual psychotherapy, group, marital and family therapy, and behaviour therapy.
(2) *Physical treatments*, including pharmacotherapy, electroconvulsive therapy and psychosurgery.
(3) *Social treatments*, including the use of the environment, therapeutic communities and rehabilitation.

The choice of method is determined in each case by the diagnosis, the patient's mental state, personality, and any interpersonal and social factors that may be causing or contributing to the disorder. In clinical practice different methods often need to be combined: a patient suffering from a depressive illness may need antidepressant drugs and supportive psychotherapy in the acute phase and benefit from analytical psychotherapy later on, or a patient with agoraphobia may need behaviour therapy as well as marital or family therapy.

44

Psychotherapy

It is difficult to give one concise definition of psychotherapy, as there are many different methods. The term is used here to describe those psychological treatment methods which take place in a professional context and in which the relationship between the patient and therapist plays a central role in helping the patient deal with his difficulties by understanding and working through them at an emotional level.

Behaviour therapy, in which the patient-therapist relationship is not thought to be of central importance and whose theoretical and practical orientation differ from psychotherapy as defined above, is considered separately (see Chapter 46). Some patients may benefit from a combination of psychotherapy and behaviour therapy, just as some patients require treatment with drugs as well as psychotherapy.

The different methods of psychotherapy will be described under the following headings:

(1) psychoanalysis
(2) various forms of individual psychoanalytic psychotherapy, often also referred to as psychodynamic, insight-directed or analytically-oriented psychotherapy
(3) child psychotherapy
(4) group psychotherapy, including group analysis
(5) supportive psychotherapy
(6) counselling.

A few other forms of psychotherapy will also be considered briefly. Marital and family therapy will be considered separately in Chapter 45.

Psychotherapeutic methods differ from each other according to the following criteria:

Treatment setting: this can either be individual, as in psychoanalysis and analytical psychotherapy; joint, as in marital or family therapy; in small groups, as in group therapy or group analysis of six to eight patients; or in large groups.

Frequency of treatment sessions: this ranges from four or five sessions a week in psychoanalysis to one or two sessions a week in individual analytical psychotherapy or group psychotherapy, to less frequent sessions, e.g. at fortnightly intervals, in marital or family therapy, to occasional sessions at varying intervals, as in supportive therapy. The duration of the sessions also varies, e.g. 50 minutes in psychoanalysis and 1½ hours in small group therapy.

Depth of understanding: this ranges from deep and widespread exploration, including work at an unconscious level, in psychoanalysis and analytical psychotherapy or group analysis, to work focussed on more specific problems, mainly at a conscious level, as in counselling and supportive therapy.

Aims: in supportive psychotherapy and counselling the primary aim is to provide symptom relief. In psychoanalysis the main emphasis is placed on bringing about changes in the patient's personality in order to promote psychological maturation, with symptom relief occurring as a result of these changes. The various forms of analytical psychotherapy, group therapy and marital or family therapy occupy an intermediate position. These differences and the degree to which some of these methods overlap will become clearer as the different forms of psychotherapy are described.

Psychotherapy is carried out not only by doctors but increasingly also by other professionals trained in one or more forms of psychotherapy; these include non-medical psychoanalysts and psychotherapists, child psychotherapists, clinical psychologists, psychiatric social workers, nurses and counsellors.

PSYCHOANALYSIS

Although the use of psychoanalysis as a treatment method is limited for economic, social and clinical reasons, its principles form the basis of most of the other analytical or psychodynamic methods of psychotherapy in use today. It will therefore be described first.

Historical background

The origins of psychoanalysis are well described in biographies of Freud by, for example, Jones (1964), Sulloway (1979) and Gay (1988). As described in Chapter 1 (p. 16), Freud became interested in the aetiology and treatment of hysterical symptoms during his work as a neurologist; in this he was influenced by Breuer, a colleague who had treated a patient with multiple hysterical symptoms between 1880 and 1882. In 1885 Freud spent some time with Charcot in Paris and saw him use suggestion under hypnosis to cure patients with hysterical symptoms. Charcot had also been able to demonstrate that hysterical symptoms could be produced by suggestion under hypnosis. This led Freud to explore the role of unconscious mental processes in the origin of hysteria (Breuer and Freud 1895). Freud started to use hypnosis to bring repressed unconscious processes into consciousness, but soon replaced this by *free-association*, i.e. by asking his patients to say aloud whatever entered their minds. This was the beginning of psychoanalysis as a treatment method. Since then Freud himself and many other psychoanalysts have revised and improved the early psychoanalytical theories and practice. Some of these developments and the modern concepts of psychoanalytic theory and personality development have already been described (see Chapters 5 and 7). The following account refers to psychoanalysis as it is practised today.

Present practice

A psychoanalyst usually sees his patient four or five times a week for a 50-minute session. The duration of an analysis has increased greatly since Freud first introduced it and tends to last for between two and five years, sometimes longer (Freud 1937). Several factors are responsible for this. Instead of concentrating on symptom relief, increasing emphasis is nowadays placed on the resolution of long-standing underlying conflicts and on the promotion of personal growth. Moreover, since the development of object-relations theory (see p. 64) analysts have learnt how to help patients whose personal development has been seriously affected by emotional deprivation due to losses or failures in relation to their mother or father at very early developmental stages. They are therefore prepared to treat not only psychoneurotic patients but also those with long-standing personality disorders, borderline states (see p. 342), and some who are suffering from psychotic symptoms (see p. 248). These patients often require much longer treatment than patients with psychoneuroses, whose symptoms are due to unconscious conflicts that were once thought to have their origin at later stages of development.

The patient usually lies on a couch with the analyst sitting behind him. This makes it easier for patients to stay in touch with their own thoughts and feelings without having to maintain conventional social contact with their therapist. It also promotes regression and assists the development of the transference (see below). Some patients, however, especially those with borderline states and impaired reality testing, may be better treated sitting up to maintain contact with reality. The patient is encouraged to talk as freely as possible about whatever comes to his mind. Free-association in the classical sense is less insisted upon nowadays; silences often occur and need to be accepted and their meaning understood, when possible.

The exploration and interpretation of unconscious conflicts, of resistances and defences (see Chapters 5 and 6) remain an important aspect of psychoanalytic work. Dreams in particular may provide insight into the patient's conflicts, both conscious and unconscious (see p. 50). It is, however, recognised nowadays that the nature and analysis of the relationship between patient and analyst constitute the central core of the psychoanalytic process. Both the real relationship and transference and counter-transference phenomena need constant attention. The various clinical concepts of psychoanalysis are discussed by Sandler *et al.* (1973).

The term *transference*, first used by Freud in 1895, is used to describe the process by which the patient transfers on to his analyst past experiences and strong feelings, e.g. of dependency, love, sexual attraction, jealousy, frustration or hatred, which he used to experience in relation to significant persons such as his mother, father or siblings earlier in life. Transference phenomena occur in all psychotherapeutic relationships as well as in everyday life, but in analysis they are particularly pronounced. This is partly due to the fact that in the analytical setting the patient has very little factual knowledge of the analyst's personal life and attitudes. Through the experience of the transference the patient can relive important aspects of his infancy and childhood in the therapeutic situation; interpretation and ultimate resolution of the transference is now regarded as one of the most important tools in psychoanalysis and analytical psychotherapy.

The term *counter-transference* has two different meanings. Originally the term referred to the fact that the analyst may develop strong feelings towards his patient which are at least in part the result of unresolved feelings he himself had experienced in the past in relation to significant figures in his own life and which he is now transferring on to his patient. For example, an analyst or therapist who had a domineering and rejecting mother he often disliked may feel resentful of patients with similar characteristics. It is important for the therapist to be aware of the origin of such counter-transference reactions in order not to let them interfere with the progress of therapy.

A more important modern use of the term counter-transference is to describe the thoughts and feelings the analyst experiences in response to his patient's communications, feelings, wishes, fantasies and behaviour. The patient is often not fully aware of what goes on in his mind and hence unable to express this directly. The analyst's counter-transference can then be a response to what is going on within his patient at an unconscious level and can thus help him to get in touch with unconscious or only partly conscious aspects of his patient's mental functioning. This function of the analyst's counter-transference as an important tool in analysis was described by Heimann (1950).

> For example, an analyst was treating a heavily defended and apparently strong and independent man of forty-five whose resistances made progress slow and difficult. The analyst began to feel that he wanted to take special care of his patient and to protect and mother him as if he were an unhappy little boy. He knew that the patient's mother had been a rather cold, distant person who had given her son little affection when he was little. Taking notice of his desire to protect and mother the patient, made him decide to say to him that he got the feeling that he, the patient, might be feeling

vulnerable like a small child and wished that he, the analyst, could give him the care and affection he had failed to get from his own mother when he was little. In response, the patient for the first time became tearful and said that he sometimes felt he wanted to be mothered and looked after but had never dared to admit this as it went against his determination to appear self-sufficient and independent. This opened up new areas in the patient's inner world, previously heavily defended against, and led to more rapid progress in treatment.

This illustrates how feelings and thoughts experienced by the analyst in his counter-transference may lead to better understanding of the patient's problems, sometimes at a hidden or unconscious level. The example also indicates that in psychoanalysis a great deal of attention is nowadays being paid to the child within the adult, and that the patient's emotional experiences in relation to the analyst are at least as important and probably more so than insight at an intellectual level.

Indications for psychoanalysis

Apart from the obvious practical and economic limitations, it will be evident from the above that for a patient to be suitable for analysis certain clinical criteria are essential. He needs to be sufficiently motivated to undergo such intensive, prolonged treatment; he needs to be intelligent enough and able to use psychological understanding, and sufficiently flexible to undergo at least some changes in his personality. Sufficient internal resources to tolerate painful insights, and an adequate capacity for reality testing and self-observation are further desirable characteristics. Some of these characteristics may be deficient at the beginning but develop in the course of treatment.

In terms of diagnostic considerations, patients with psychoneuroses, personality problems, psychosexual disorders and some psychosomatic symptoms are particularly suitable. Patients with borderline personality disorders (see p. 342) are also increasingly taken on for analysis. Its use for the treatment of patients with manic-depressive psychosis and acute schizophrenia is debatable and by itself does not constitute adequate treatment (see p. 248). A few psychoanalysts specialise in the treatment of psychoses. If such patients are treated analytically this has to be combined with the use of psychotropic drugs, at least during the acute phases of the illness. The outcome of psychoanalysis of patients with psychoses remains uncertain, but a great deal has been learnt about the nature of psychotic mental processes from the use of analysis and such knowledge is of considerable value in the understanding and management of psychotic patients in general (see p. 249) (T. Freeman *et al.* 1965; T. Freeman 1969, 1988; Rosenfeld 1965, 1987).

Much of what has been said about modern concepts and practice of psychoanalysis also applies to Jungian analysis or 'analytical psychology' as practised today. The differences and similarities will be discussed next.

ANALYTICAL PSYCHOLOGY

Analytical psychology is the name given to the form of psychotherapy developed by Carl Gustav Jung (1875-1961). Jung, whose father was a protestant pastor in Switzerland, became a psychiatrist and worked for nine years at the Burghölzli Hospital in Zurich. There he became particularly interested in the inner, subjective experience of schizophrenic patients. He extended this interest in the inner world to his non-psychotic patients and used the language of metaphor, symbolism and imagination to describe their experiences rather than apply an objective, scientific and causal approach. Jung's personal background and main concepts have been described by Storr (1973).

Jung developed the concept of the *collective unconscious*, a deeper layer of unconscious processes common to all mankind, as distinct from each individual's personal unconscious (Jung 1943). He based this view on the finding that the experience of each individual echoed themes common to many different cultures, races and religions, and thought that the collective unconscious was influenced by an innate unconscious *archetypal* patterning. He stressed the creative power of the collective unconscious, which directs each individual towards a sense of wholeness and self-realisation. At the same time he was aware of its potentially destructive power. He considered that its positive influence on personal development and on the outcome of therapy depended on insight and conscious self-awareness.

After reading Freud's *Interpretation of Dreams* (1900) Jung contacted Freud, and the two men corresponded from 1906 and subsequently worked closely together until 1913 (Freud/Jung letters 1974). This period of collaboration and friendship then came to an abrupt end. This was partly the result of personal disagreements following a period of what almost amounted to mutual idealisation, but professional differences also played a prominent part. Freud's emphasis on a scientific and objective approach to the understanding of the mind came increasingly in conflict with Jung's more mystical and subjective approach. In particular, Jung disagreed with the emphasis Freud at that time placed on the role of sexual energy or libido in human development; he also disagreed with Freud's purely causal explanation of neurotic symptoms in terms of early childhood experiences. Jung saw the libido as a life-giving force which included sexuality, power and religion; he also attributed meaning to neurotic experiences in the sense that he thought they opened up potential solutions to problems encountered at critical periods in life.

After this split, followers of Freud and Jung worked separately, and the Jungian school called itself the school of *analytical pyschology*. Over the years both schools have changed and evolved a great deal, and clinical work has demonstrated much common ground between them in spite of their different origins. Both stress the importance of unconscious processes and of dreams. Nowadays Jungians see personal and collective unconscious processes less as separate entities and more as a continuum, while Freudian psychoanalysts tend to lay greater stress on the role of unconscious fantasies and object relationships (see p. 64), concepts which have much in common with innate archetypal images in Jungian terminology. Jungian analysts see the process of psychotherapy as leading to greater integration or individuation, to use Jung's expression, a view very similar to that of many psychoanalysts who speak of healing splits in the patient's personality and of personal growth and the development of the Self. Both schools recognise the central role of transference and counter-transference in analysis and in psychotherapy.

However, quite apart from their different concepts and languages, differences in attitudes and emphasis between Jungian analysts and psychoanalysts do persist. There are some groups of Jungian analysts who still prefer to work more in accordance with Jung's classical concepts. In practice, whether an individual patient chooses to have a psychoanalysis or a Jungian analysis will at least in part be determined by his personal interests, attitudes and beliefs. The practical procedures and indications for a Jungian analysis are essentially the same as for psychoanalysis.

ANALYTICAL PSYCHOTHERAPY

Analytical psychotherapy is also referred to as analytically oriented, psychoanalytic, psychodynamic or insight-directed psychotherapy, a confusing array of terms. It is the commonest method of formal individual psychotherapy used in the UK, in other European countries and in the USA. It differs from psychoanalysis in that treatment sessions are less frequent, usually once or twice a week. As there is now a tendency even in psychoanalysis for the patient sometimes to be seen only three or four instead of five times a week, the exact boundary between psychoanalysis and analytically oriented psychotherapy has become difficult to define, especially as the basic concepts and the method of working are very similar. However, in terms of the patient's experience and the intensity of the interaction and development of transference between patient and therapist, there is a great difference between the two extremes of only one session a week in psychoanalytic psychotherapy on the one hand and five sessions a week in psychoanalysis on the other. The fact that in once weekly analytical psychotherapy patient and therapist usually sit facing each other while in psychoanalysis the patient usually lies on a couch adds further to the difference in the experience.

Another difference between psychoanalysis and analytical psychotherapy lies in the duration and aims of therapy. In general, analytical psychotherapy lasts for a shorter period, varying from a minimum of six months to perhaps one or two years, though it sometimes lasts longer. Nowadays attempts are made in 'brief' psychotherapy of a few months to focus treatment on fairly specific goals, and to set a date for termination at the beginning (Malan 1976a, 1976b; Sifneos 1987). Many patients, however, require wider, open-ended therapy.

An advantage of starting on a once or twice a week basis is that the aims, frequency and duration of therapy can be adjusted to the needs of the individual patient as treatment progresses, some patients requiring longer treatment than was envisaged originally, others perhaps benefiting from a change from individual to group therapy, and a few deciding, after a period of analytical psychotherapy, to undergo psychoanalysis.

The concepts used in analytical psychotherapy are the same as in psychoanalysis. The relationship between patient and therapist is of fundamental importance; initially, as in psychoanalysis, a good relationship needs to be created in order to work together in what is called a *therapeutic alliance*. Careful attention must be paid throughout to transference and counter-transference phenomena. The patient's difficulties need to be understood not only in terms of his present problems and conflicts but also in terms of underlying conscious and unconscious problems dating back to early disruption of his object-relationships and disturbances at later stages of development. As therapy approaches its end, it is particularly important to deal with the patient's reaction to the impending separation from his therapist; this is likely to stir up memories and feelings related to much earlier losses and separations. The same applies to the ending of an analysis, but in briefer forms of analytical psychotherapy where the patient knows from the outset that the duration of therapy is limited these issues of separation need to be faced early on.

The clinical indications for analytical psychotherapy are similar to those for psychoanalysis (see p. 561). The choice is determined partly by the patient's motivation, social circumstances and personal preferences, and partly by the therapist's assessment of the aims, depth and intensity of treatment required and of the number of sessions per week needed to achieve this. There is, however, no general agreement as to the number of sessions per week any particular patient may need. Some borderline patients are thought to do better in two or three times a week therapy, while long-standing character or personality disorders may do better in four or five times a week analysis. Many patients with less severe neurotic disorders may only need therapy once a week. In practice the decision usually has to be made on the basis of the psychotherapeutic facilities available. In the UK and especially in the National Health Service these still fall far short of what is needed for the many patients who require psychotherapy; in some parts of the UK there are hardly any trained and experienced therapists or psychoanalysts.

CHILD PSYCHOTHERAPY

As described in Chapter 40, in many cases psychological disturbance in the child is closely related to problems in the relationship of the child to his parents. In such cases counselling or brief psychotherapy for the parents may be effective in relieving the child's problems without the child being involved directly.

If the child's problems are part of disturbance in the family, family therapy may be more appropriate (see Chapter 45). In other cases educational methods are needed rather than psychotherapy. Behavioural treatments may help some children with specific behaviour problems such as a phobic disorder or enuresis (see Chapter 46).

The choice of treatment is best made after diagnostic interviews with the child and the parents. These should include an assessment of the family dynamics and of the child's own feelings and conflicts. In some cases it will become apparent that intrapsychic problems play a major role in the child's disturbance. In that case individual psychotherapy for the child may be needed. Even when this is the case the parents should be seen separately so that they can be given the counselling and support they need to learn how best to help their child. For example, in child guidance clinics or child psychiatric departments, one member of the treatment team, e.g. a social worker, may see the parents while a child therapist sees the child for individual pyschotherapy.

Individual psychotherapy of children, like adult psychotherapy, depends on the establishment of a therapeutic relationship between the child and his therapist, usually a trained child psychotherapist. The aim is to understand the child's inner world, including his conflicts, feelings and fantasies, and their relation to his parental and family background. With young children it is not possible to do this by means of verbal communication alone, and *play therapy* is therefore an important method in child psychotherapy. The therapist provides a number of small toys, such as dolls, soldiers, cars, trains, houses, animals and so on, and attempts to understand the child's problems from the way he relates to and plays with these toys. Drawing materials or sand and water may also be used to enable the child to express what he feels, including transference feelings towards the therapist. The therapist's main task is to understand the child through the meaning of his play, to make appropriate comments, and to join in his play when appropriate.

Play therapy was first introduced in the 1920s by Melanie Klein in order to treat young children along psychoanalytic lines (Klein 1975). Later Anna Freud (1946) stressed the need to establish a helpful and trusting relationship with the child while combining this with interpretative work, using play therapy depending on the child's age. While child analysts may see the child several times a week, most children are only seen once or twice a week or less often while the parents are seen separately for guidance and support. Winnicott (1977), Reisman (1973) and Axline (1971) have described their psychotherapeutic work with children.

The main indications for child psychotherapy are serious emotional, developmental and conduct disorders (see Chapter 40) and problems in relation to other family members. Children who have been sexually abused may also benefit from psychotherapy (see Chapter 43).

Recently attempts have also been made to help some children with mental handicap and children with infantile autism by means of a flexible psychotherapeutic approach. This use of child psychotherapy remains controversial, but Tustin (1981, 1986) has helped some autistic children as well as children with emotional problems and associated autistic features. Similarly, Sinason (1986) has drawn attention to the serious effects of secondary mental handicap which can be superimposed on and aggravate the degree of primary handicap. Secondary handicap can also serve as a defence in response to severe mental trauma, e.g. sexual abuse (see p. 550). Sinason's psychotherapeutic work with some of these children has led to relief from the secondary handicap. No claim is made that psychotherapy can cure the primary organic disorder present in autism or mental handicap, but the child may learn how to express and come to terms with his sadness, anger and sense of inferiority, and to function better in personal and social relationships. As a result he may also make better use of educational measures and rehabilitation.

While such children are being treated with psychotherapy, the parents need continued support and counselling so that they can reach a better understanding of their handicapped child and their reactions to him. Bicknell (1983) has described the many painful feelings with which both the handicapped child, especially as he gets older, and his family have to struggle, and has emphasised their need for help and understanding. Attempts have also been made to help mentally handicapped adults by means of psychotherapy (Symington 1981).

GROUP PSYCHOTHERAPY

It has long been recognised that people in need of help and support can benefit from meeting together in groups to help each other with common problems. The use of small groups to provide formal psychotherapeutic help for patients with psychiatric problems is a much more recent development. During the Second World War a few psychoanalysts and psychiatrists at Northfield Military Hospital in Birmingham started to apply psychoanalytic concepts to the treatment of six to eight patients with psychoneurotic and other psychological problems, meeting regularly in a group setting. Since then small group psychotherapy has become established as a common method of formal psychotherapy. It is an economic method of treatment, one therapist being able to treat several patients together regularly once a week, and it is now recognised as an effective method of treating patients with neurotic and psychosomatic symptoms, personality disorders and difficulties in social relationships. The most widely used method of group therapy is known as *group-analysis*, developed by Foulkes (1964, 1975). The following account is largely based on the practice of group-analysis and related forms of group therapy. Yalom (1985) has reviewed the practice of group therapy in general.

Six to eight patients meet regularly once or twice a week for 1½ hours in a group led by a group therapist, called the conductor; sometimes the conductor works together with a co-therapist or observer. The patients and the conductor sit in a circle facing each other. In 'closed' groups the composition of the group remains constant throughout, all patients starting and finishing at the same time, usually after two to three years. More often groups are run as 'slow-open' groups, patients who leave because they are ready to go or because they break off therapy being replaced by new group members; such groups can therefore continue indefinitely, and the duration of treatment of individual members will vary depending on their needs and rate of progress.

The group should as far as possible be composed of equal numbers of men and women, and their ages, levels of intelligence and ability to make use of verbal communication should be sufficiently similar for no one to feel a complete outsider. For example, one adolescent should not be in a group whose other members are all between, say, thirty and fifty. He would be better treated in a group for adolescents.

The wide range of the patients' problems helps the members of the group to recognise the shared factors that have contributed to their different disorders. One or two socially isolated and initially inhibited or withdrawn patients may gradually find themselves accepted by the rest of the group; they may learn to overcome their social inhibitions and become active participants. Psychotic patients or antisocial psychopaths should not be mixed with other patients, but special groups either for psychotics or for psychopaths can be used to treat such patients (see p. 340).

When group therapy began some therapists treated each member in the group as an individual, paying little attention to group interaction or what was going on in the group as a whole. Bion (1961) at the Tavistock Clinic, London, instead focused attention mainly, if not entirely, on the group itself, commenting only on how the group as a whole was relating to the conductor, e.g. being dependent on or hostile towards him. He paid little attention to the problems of individual members, who were supposed to benefit from the group being 'treated as a whole'. The results of this procedure were often unsatisfactory and there was a high drop-out rate.

The method used in group-analysis, as developed by Foulkes, is more flexible and assumes an intermediate position. Individual members benefit from actively participating in the group process, talking about their own and other members' problems and thus relating to and interacting with each other and the conductor. One of the group conductor's tasks is to encourage and facilitate the active work done by the members themselves. He does so by remaining relatively inactive without being too detached or distant. He has to be sensitive to the atmosphere and dynamics in the group, called the *group matrix* (Foulkes 1964). He also has to remain aware of the individual members' needs, attitudes and behaviour, including transference manifestations (see p. 560) between each other and towards himself. His comments or interpretations will sometimes be directed towards individual members, e.g. if one of them tries to dominate the group, or to their interaction, and sometimes to what is going on in the group as a whole. The attitude of the group to the conductor needs to be carefully watched and commented upon when necessary; for example the whole group may be dependent on him and try to force him to assume a more active role, or it may be hostile towards him, making him feel useless and angry. His own counter-transference usually helps him recognise and put into words what the group is doing to him or expecting from him, and his interpretation is aimed at bringing about a shift in the attitude of the group and its members.

As the group progresses the members will learn how to share more and more intimate and personal problems with each other; a strong sense of *cohesion* develops, and in a group which functions well each member learns how to help the others to gain understanding of their difficulties and change while deriving similar benefits himself. As treatment approaches its end members share their feelings of loss and separation from each other and the conductor. The aim is to help them outgrow some of their maladaptive, conscious or unconscious attitudes, assumptions and patterns of behaviour, and to leave the group with increased personal resources. One man who was particularly isolated and withdrawn when he first joined a group said sadly when he was ready to leave, 'After all, this is the only family I have ever had and learnt to grow up in.'

SUPPORTIVE PSYCHOTHERAPY

Unlike the various types of formal psychotherapy described so far, supportive psychotherapy does not attempt to uncover hidden and unconscious factors that underlie the patient's difficulties or symptoms. Its main aim is to provide a safe setting in which the patient feels free to talk about his problems and to express what he feels. The doctor or other professional worker – counsellor, social worker, psychologist or nurse – therefore has to listen without being judgmental and to reflect back what the patient is telling him. His comments will be mainly directed towards encouraging the patient to enlarge on what he feels his problems are, and to help explore possible ways of dealing with them but not to impose his own prejudices or solutions. Supportive psychotherapy does not aim to bring about major changes in the patient's personality or inner world, but it may help him function better in his interpersonal relationships at home or at work if they are contributing to his difficulties.

There are three main areas in which supportive psychotherapy is particularly helpful. First, any person asking for help, be it with a physical or psychological problem, is bound to be anxious to some degree. In a general sense a supportive approach should be one aspect of every consultation, whether in general practice (see p. 648), in a hospital, or in a community setting, and alongside whatever other form of investigation or treatment may be needed. Providing support is merely one aspect of good professional care, and it should include explaining to the patient as far as possible what his symptoms, mental or physical, are likely to be due to, and why the various examinations and investigations are being done.

Secondly, there are many patients who are inadequate, dependent people, and others who suffer from long-standing or incurable conditions, physical or psychiatric, who require support either regularly or from time to time. Here the patient may need to be seen and supported at irregular intervals, often over prolonged periods, and the doctor or other professional helper has to accept that the patient's dependence on him is an inevitable and essential part of their relationship.

Thirdly, some people who are otherwise stable and coping well may go through a serious crisis, e.g. after a bereavement or other loss, or illness, or some serious problem in the family. They may need more regular sessions of supportive psychotherapy, sometimes together with another family member – e.g. husband or wife – over a limited period of time. Such *crisis intervention* is aimed at providing temporary support so that the patient can learn to muster his own resources and cope with the crisis that initially undermined his defences.

The doctor or other professional who provides supportive psychotherapy is bound to find that the patient at times stirs up strong feelings in himself. A very dependent, demanding patient is likely to make him feel threatened and angry; a patient who contradicts and denies everything he says may make him fell useless and irritable. Self-awareness and the ability to understand and control such feelings in relation to the patient or client are as essential in supportive as in other forms of psychotherapy.

COUNSELLING

Some counselling methods overlap with supportive or dynamic psychotherapy, while others are more concerned with giving information and practical advice. Counsellors are either non-medical profe sionals, such as social workers, psychologists, teachers or clergymen, or lay people interested in helping others. Most undertake formal training in their particular form of counselling work, e.g. marriage guidance counsellors, student counsellors in university settings or polytechnics, counsellors for people with suicidal tendencies (the Samaritans), counsellors for alcoholics, for the physically disabled, and so on.

As in supportive psychotherapy, counsellors largely rely on their ability to listen and provide information, understanding and support in the hope that this will enable their patients, sometimes referred to as clients, to find their own solutions. Counsellors must be able to recognise when some of their clients need more formal, insight-directed, analytical psychotherapy. They may then refer their clients for formal psychotherapy, but some counsellors themselves become trained as psychotherapists. There is some danger that patients or clients who require more intensive psychotherapy will believe that a few sessions of counselling is all they need, and some doctors collude with this point of view. On the other hand counselling services provide help for many who do not need more intensive therapy.

ALTERNATIVE METHODS

Several other methods of psychotherapy have been introduced over the last few decades, e.g. Rogerian client-centred therapy, transactional analysis, psychodrama, Gestalt therapy, bioenergetics and encounter groups. These will be described briefly below.

Some of these therapies make use of concepts derived from psychoanalysis or group psychotherapy. They may combine these concepts with other approaches and sometimes with more active techniques. Therapies like bioenergetics and encounter groups have gained more popularity among their followers than within the context of psychiatry and are sometimes referred to as 'fringe' therapies. They may be of value to people who are not suffering from psychiatric disorders but are searching for personal growth and greater freedom of self-expression in their personal relationships and creative activities. However, there is considerable overlap between the aims of these and more orthodox therapies. For example, the various forms of analytical psychotherapy described above are also used to help patients outgrow problems in their personal growth and development. However, individuals who enter one or other form of the fringe therapies in their search for growth may be more seriously disturbed than they, and sometimes their therapists realise, and may need psychiatric help.

Rogerian client-centred therapy

This well established form of therapy was introduced by Carl Rogers (1951) in the USA. The therapist uses his relationship to the client to encourage open and frank discussion of his problems. Client-centred therapy stresses the need for 'accurate empathy', 'non-possessive warmth' and 'genuineness' in the therapist's relationship to the client. By being truly empathic the therapist helps the client to feel understood; by means of non-possessive warmth he avoids excessive closeness but provides warmth and accepts without disapproval whatever the client brings to the session; by being genuine he reacts to the client with self-awareness, honesty and openness. In this way the client's feelings and conflicts are brought into the open and accepted without criticism so that his self-acceptance and self-esteem increase. At the same time the therapist, by remaining non-directive, encourages the client to find his own solutions. Deeper and unconscious conflicts, defences and transference phenomena are not usually dealt with. Client-centred therapy can therefore best be looked upon as a more intensive and effective form of counselling or supportive therapy, emphasising the client's positive qualities but ignoring negative feelings and deeper problems in his personality. To some extent the three characteristics of the therapist mentioned above are essential in any form of psychoanalysis or psychotherapy, but by themselves they are often not sufficient to bring about more fundamental changes.

Transactional analysis

This method, developed by Eric Berne (1961) in the USA, is based on the view that in each individual three aspects of the personality can be distinguished. These are the *Parent*, the *Adult* and the *Child* parts of the person, and everyone is liable to relate to others from one or other of these parts of himself at different times. Relatively straightforward, unemotional interactions usually take place between Adult and Adult. For example, when someone asks for simple information like the time of the day he does so from his Adult Self and expects a simple Adult answer from the other person. When a father talks to the headmaster of his son's school he may feel anxious and inferior and talk to him from the Child part of himself, expecting the headmaster to behave like a Parent figure in an authoritarian manner; if the headmaster instead relates to his pupil's father in a factual and friendly manner from his Adult Self, this may help the father to relate to him from his Adult Self after all.

The Parent aspect of each of us is largely determined by what we have internalised from our parents, and to some extent it corresponds to the psychoanalytic concept of the superego (see p. 48), especially if the actual parents were experienced as authoritarian and omniscient. The Child aspect corresponds to all those aspects of ourselves which have survived within us since we actually were children. The Adult aspect corresponds to our more grown-up, reality-oriented and rational Self. There are, of course, many occasions when it is perfectly acceptable for us to function from our Child Self, e.g. when relaxed and playful; or from our Parent Self when we have to keep control over others, e.g. a teacher when confronted with a difficult class.

In transactional analysis the therapist actively explores with his client with what part of himself he is relating to other people, including at times the therapist himself. Many inappropriate and conflicting modes of relating may come to light, and the client may discover the various 'games' he plays in life (Berne 1968). The aim is to help him to relate to others in a more appropriate and direct manner, often as Adult to Adult. Transactional analysis is frequently carried out in a group setting but can be used in individual therapy. It does not usually pay attention to unconscious phenomena, and deeper conflicts are not explored. Its uses are therefore limited, but some of the concepts outlined above are helpful in conjunction with other forms of psychotherapy.

Psychodrama

Unlike client-centred therapy and transactional analysis, psychodrama and other methods to be described below make use of more active techniques. Psychodrama was introduced by Jacob Moreno (1892-1974), first in Vienna and later in the USA. He originally became involved in encouraging spontaneous activity by actors in the theatre, the 'Theatre of Spontaneity', and subsequently applied this to the treatment of patients (Davies 1976). Psychodrama is usually practised in groups and conducted by non-medical staff, including occupational therapists, trained in psychodrama. The aim is to re-enact the patient's conflicts underlying his psychoneurotic or other psychological disturbances in the group setting. The therapist instructs the patient or 'protagonist' to select other members of the group to act as 'auxiliaries' and take on the roles of, say, his father, mother and sibling in relation to himself. In this way he can relive relevant past or present conflict-laden situations. This not only leads to emotional release or 'abreaction', but also to the discovery of more appropriate ways of handling problems. If the patient himself cannot find a better way of responding during psychodrama sessions another group member may be asked to act as his 'alter-ego' and show him an alternative way of reacting. For example, a patient who has always assumed a defeatist and submissive role may be shown by an alter-ego how to stand up to or get angry with the auxiliaries who are acting the role of his parents.

Gestalt therapy

This was promoted by Fritz Perls (1893-1970) in California (Perls 1969). It is based on the psychoanalytic concept that neurotic and other forms of abnormal behaviour result from certain aspects and feelings of the person being split off, denied or repressed and hence not available to the person as a whole. To reconstitute wholeness or 'Gestalt', a term derived from Gestalt psychology, a number of active techniques were devised by Perls and used in therapy, usually in a group. One of these is that each member of the group is made to express here and now what he actually thinks and feels rather than talk about it as something he experienced in the past or might do in the future. Again, instead of talking about another person in the group he has to tell him directly what he thinks of him. Instead of complaining about a bodily sensation like having a pain in the neck he is made to say who in the group is a 'pain in the neck to him'. Active techniques also include hitting a pillow or breaking an object like a chair that is meant to represent someone with whom he is angry. In this way the group members are brought in touch with feelings in the here-and-now which they had not been aware of or acknowledged or expressed before. These strong emotional experiences may help some patients or clients to achieve greater self-awareness and self-expression, but others may find them too disturbing and potentially disruptive. An experienced Gestalt therapist will therefore combine these techniques with a more cautious insight-directed and supportive approach, and the group members should also support and comfort each other. Some of these methods are occasionally used in the course of conventional group therapy to overcome resistances.

Bioenergetics

Freud (1923) pointed out that the ego is 'first and foremost a bodily ego', thus stressing the basic unity of mental and physical processes. One of his followers, Wilhelm Reich (1897-1957), who later left the psychoanalytic movement and formed his own school, formulated the view that the body, especially posture and movements, provide direct expression of underlying attitudes and defences. He called these bodily constellations the 'character armour' and correlated each of them with specific psychological characteristics (Reich 1950). Following Reich's concepts Lowen (1958) and others developed various bioenergetic techniques. The meaning of the patient's posture is pointed out to him, and physical exercises, massage, relaxation and breathing exercises are used to alter his posture and behaviour, and to release muscular tension. The hope is that this will bring about corresponding changes in psychological function and self-expression.

Such bioenergetic methods can be helpful provided they are not used in isolation but integrated with insight-directed forms of therapy. Unfortunately, as in some of the other forms of fringe therapy, bioenergetic therapists tend to ignore the intrapsychic, developmental and transference aspects of psychotherapy. On the other hand, analytical psychotherapists often overlook the importance of non-verbal communication.

Encounter groups

Carl Rogers, who initiated client-centred therapy, later also developed encounter groups (Rogers 1970). The number of participants in encounter groups is usually larger than that in small group psychotherapy and ranges between 8 and 16. These groups are attended by people searching for personal growth who are therefore usually not referred by members of the medical profession.

Attendance at an encounter group may be a one-off experience, usually lasting for several hours or a whole weekend, a so-called marathon group, or clients attend the same group regularly for a whole day once a week as well as for an occasional weekend. The main emphasis is on frank self-expression and honesty. Closeness, interaction and cohesion are encouraged by the encounter group leader, and a strong sense of belonging and mutual concern rapidly develop. The leader may start each group by encouraging relaxed interaction, including movement, exercises and physical contact. This leads on to the sharing of problems and feelings, and the leader takes an active part in fostering open communication. Unfortunately some encounter group leaders do so by behaving in a somewhat aggressive manner that can be dangerous.

Most encounter group leaders make use of methods derived from Gestalt therapy, psychodrama and bioenergetics in order to foster self-revelation and emotional release. Less emphasis is placed on exploration of intrapsychic conflicts or the understanding of problems in terms of past experience, and transference manifestations are usually not recognised or ignored.

Attendance at these groups can provide a powerful personal experience that may assist self-awareness and promote easier communication and self-expression for those who previously felt limited or inhibited. People who function mainly on a cautious, intellectual and rational level are less likely to attend or benefit from encounter groups. Individuals who are more suggestible or emotionally aroused, perhaps because they are passing through an emotional crisis, are more likely to benefit. For people who are seriously disturbed or have a psychiatric disorder the experience may be too overwhelming and cause them to break down. Encounter groups, their functions and hazards have been reviewed by Lieberman *et al.* (1973).

FURTHER READING

Aveline, M.O. (1979). 'Action techniques in psychotherapy.' *Brit. J. Hosp. Med.* 22, 78-84.

Axline, V. (1971). *Dibbs: in search of self.* Penguin, Harmondsworth.

Bloch, S. (ed.) (1986). *An Introduction to the Psychotherapies,* 2nd ed. OUP, Oxford.

Brown, D. and Pedder, J. (1979). *Introduction to Psychotherapy: an outline of psychodynamic principles and practice.* Tavistock, London.

Brown, J.A.C. (1961). *Freud and the Post-Freudians.* Penguin, Harmondsworth.

Casement, P. (1985). *On Learning from the Patient.* Tavistock, London.

Foulkes, S.H. (1975). *Group Analytic Psychotherapy: method and principles.* Gordon & Breach, London.

Malan, D.H. (1979). *Individual Psychotherapy and the Science of Psychodynamics.* Butterworths, London.

Sandler, J., Dare, C. and Holder, A. (1973). *The Patient and the Analyst: the basis of the psychoanalytic process.* Karnac Books, London.

Sifneos, P.E. (1987). *Short-term Dynamic Psychotherapy: evaluation and technique,* 2nd ed. Plenum Press, New York.

Storr, A. (1979). *The Art of Psychotherapy.* Heinemann, London.

Yalom, I.D. (1985). *The Theory and Practice of Group Psychotherapy,* 3rd ed. Basic Books, New York.

45

Marital and Family Therapy

MARITAL THERAPY

Doctors and other members of helping professions should be familiar with the basic skills of interviewing and helping couples. This usually applies to married couples, but the techniques described below also apply to other couples, such as unmarried partners and homosexual pairs.

Formal marital therapy in which both partners are seen together is indicated in three main situations:

(1) When there is a specific marital problem, e.g. sexual difficulties, escalating rows, threats of divorce, marital violence.

(2) When marital problems are thought to be making a major contribution to an illness, e.g. a woman with depression who is unhappily married, or an alcoholic man whose marriage is on the point of breaking up.

(3) In some chronic psychiatric illnesses, e.g. schizophrenia, chronic anxiety states or recurrent depression, the spouse may need to be shown how to understand and support the sick partner and assist in treatment. This may relieve some of the tension associated with looking after a chronically ill partner, and this in turn may benefit the patient, if only by making him feel less guilty.

Marital therapy is often conducted by a pair of co-therapists of opposite sex. This ensures that both male and female points of view are represented. Also, the therapists can act as a 'role-model' for the unhappy couple, showing, for example, that it is possible to disagree without becoming destructively angry with each other. Perhaps the most important task for marital therapists is to integrate the methods described below so as to meet the needs and expectations of a particular couple, and to learn how to avoid getting too identified with one or other partner, focusing instead on the interaction between them.

There are three basic approaches to marital therapy. These will be considered more or less in the order in which they have developed since the 1950s. They are the psychodynamic, behavioural and structural or strategic approaches, the latter being based on systems theory (see p. 578).

Psychodynamic marital therapy

The role that psychodynamic factors, including unconscious processes, play in the choice of marriage partner and in the subsequent relationship between the partners has already been described in Chapter 8 (see pp. 86-7). Such factors also contribute to the threat of marital breakdown, and may interfere with the balance between mutual dependency and respect for one another's individuality and separateness, necessary for a successful marriage (see p. 87).

In Chapter 8 we saw how the experience of intimacy and sexual and emotional closeness in marriage may stir up feelings and conflicts which stem from earlier experiences with parents in infancy and childhood. Such feelings may then be projected or transferred onto the marriage partner, just as in psychotherapy where they are transferred onto the therapist. For example, a husband may unconsciously project onto his wife aspects of himself which his parents found unacceptable when he was a child and which he still perceives as bad; he then blames her for all their problems and sees himself as entirely good and blameless. Or a wife who lost her father when she was a child may still harbour unresolved feelings of loss and sadness which she covers up by appearing bright and cheerful. Her unexpressed sadness may be sensed and experienced by her husband who, as it were, carries her sadness and becomes depressed.

In psychodynamic marital therapy the partners are seen together, usually by two co-therapists who aim to help them acknowledge their own feelings and conflicts by working on these mutual projections. They may thus learn to appreciate and understand each other in a less distorted way and be helped to respect and accept each other as separate people with their own individual assets and deficits. Dynamic marital therapists therefore aim to find out the reasons, often unconscious and dating back to childhood, why one couple avoids intimacy and becomes too separate, while another clings together and becomes too dependent.

Behavioural marital therapy

Behavioural marital therapists try to understand marital interaction, whether normal or pathological, in terms of mutually reinforcing or extinguishing sequences of behaviour. Their therapeutic interventions therefore aim to reinforce those forms of behaviour that are mutually desirable and rewarding, and to free the couple from a vicious circle of mutually destructive behaviour.

The couple are instructed to refrain from complaints about what their spouse has *not* done, and instead to respond positively to what they *have* done. For example, a husband is told not to complain about the mess in the house, and the wife not to nag about how late he comes home; instead he is to comment on how he enjoys her cooking, while she is to tell him how pleased she is when he does come home early. The sex-roles are stereotyped in this example but could easily be reversed. A particular example of behavioural marital therapy is sex therapy, as described by Masters and Johnson (1970) (see p. 352).

Structural and strategic marital therapy

These important, more recent approaches are discussed below under Family Therapy.

FAMILY THERAPY

Medical education teaches students and doctors how to interview individual patients in order to identify one or more clearly defined causes that may have led to their symptoms or illness. But people are not islands; they live in groups and the social context within which a patient lives, his family, social setting and ethnic group, may have a profound effect on the development of symptoms, the nature and course of an illness and the chances of recovery. This applies particularly to psychiatric disorders. The family therapist sees the symptoms or disturbed behaviour of one family member as an expression of how the family functions as a whole; instead of looking for the cause of the symptom in the individual he tries to understand it in terms of the interaction and feed-back between family members. For example, a child's refusal to go to school may be a response to constant friction and quarrels between the parents and reflect a fear that his mother might leave home to get away from his father. As a result the child may avoid going to school in order to stay close to his mother. Thus the child's symptom may be an expression of a problem affecting the family. Rather than focus on the child alone, the doctor or other professional has to pay attention to the child, siblings and parents together.

Family therapy is based on a set of theoretical concepts about how families function, and how family dysfunction can lead to or exacerbate psychiatric illness. It is also a set of practical techniques for engaging families in treatment, for interviewing couples and families together, and for helping families to change. The unit of treatment in family therapy is the family as a whole, not the individual. Family members are considered as sub-units of a larger organisation which has its own rules of functioning, just as the organs of the body are part of an interactive and delicately balanced system.

There is increasing clinical and experimental evidence that family theory and therapy are important dimensions of psychiatry. For example, it has been shown that by reducing high expressed emotion within the family the relapse rate for a schizophrenic member of the family can be reduced (see p. 252). There is some evidence that family therapy may be more effective in treating a girl with anorexia nervosa than individual supportive therapy if the patient is under seventeen and the illness has not yet reached a chronic, relapsing stage (Dare 1986; Russell *et al.* 1988) (see p. 446).

Theoretical concepts

The theoretical basis of much of family therapy is *systems theory*. This has evolved from cybernetics, the study of control, regulation and communication which is applicable both to inanimate objects and to living organisms and social organisations. Systems theory holds that there are a number of features which characterise biological and social systems, all of which need to be intact for optimal function. When these principles are applied to families certain features of family structure and function are found to be particularly important. These will be described next.

Boundaries

The family is separated from the outside world by a boundary which may be more or less permeable, allowing either a great deal or very little communication with the outside world. In most families the boundary is 'semi-permeable', the family communicating well with the outside while preserving a sense of being a coherent family. Families with too rigid boundaries permit little interplay with the outside world. They are called *enmeshed* families as the members cling closely together and any disagreements or marital disharmony remain hidden and covert. Such families may function reasonably well when the children are small, but problems emerge when the children become adolescent and start to form stronger peer relationships outside the home. Enmeshment is a common feature of disturbed families in which one of the members develops anorexia nervosa. By contrast, in *disengaged* families the external boundaries are blurred and ill-defined; each member tends to function as a separate unit and marital disharmony tends to be overt. This pattern is sometimes associated with delinquency in teenagers.

Sub-systems

Within a family there are several sub-systems, e.g. parents and children, males and females, humans and pets. Just as the external boundary of the family needs to be semi-permeable, so too do sub-system boundaries. Families whose infants are in the parental bed every night, thus ruining parental sleep and sex-life, have too permeable sub-system boundaries. Conversely, if the parents are remote and cannot play and communicate with their children, or never snuggle up to them, the sub-system boundaries are too rigid.

Hierarchy

In healthy families the parents, or parent in single-parent families, have the final say in what happens or does not happen in the family, preferably with the agreement and acceptance of other family members. There is thus a hierarchy of power within the family, often challenged by the children as they become older and by the growing independence and natural rebelliouness of adolescents. When parents are unable to exercise control and authority, symptoms may emerge; for example, the mother may feel helpless and become depressed, the father may opt out and spend more and more time in the pub, and the adolescents may become disturbed, neglect their studies, or get into difficulties with the law. If parental authority is inconsistent this can lead to adolescent rebelliousness and destructive behaviour inside or outside the family.

Communication

Communication in families can be divided into two types: instrumental (doing) and affective (feeling). In more traditional families, the male members tended to be more associated with the instrumental aspects, and the female members more with the affective aspects of family life, but this is gradually changing. For families to function effectively there must be a free flow of both sorts of communication. Both partners need to be able to talk about feelings and practical issues for effective decision-making to take place. Where communication is impaired the family is vulnerable to dysfunction. For instance, if parents are unable to express their love for each other they may instead lavish all their love and attention on the child. The child is thus locked or *triangulated* in the parental relationship; he may feel responsible for the parents and may develop symptoms or disturbed behaviour, e.g. excessive dependency and school refusal. As he becomes older he may feel unable to leave home and become more independent. A son who continues to feel responsible for his mother may find it impossible to form relationships with other women.

It is always useful to ask oneself the question, 'Where is the "marriage" in this family?' It may be between, say, mother and daughter, with a step-father excluded; between father and daughter, with a mother who is depressed; between siblings, with an exhausted single parent. These alliances, while sometimes supportive and helpful, can lead to serious difficulties. They are frequently seen in cases of child sexual abuse (see Chapter 43).

An example of faulty communication in families is that of the pathogenic *double bind* (Bateson *et al.* 1956), where a family member, usually a parent, gives two conflicting messages to another family member, usually a child. The parent may offer love verbally but indicate non-verbally that the child is not wanted or disapproved of, e.g. by tone of voice or gesture. The child, who is dependent on the parent and hence cannot escape, may become confused and anxious and lose his sense of identity.

Techniques of family therapy

These are drawn from a variety of sources. In the 1950s *psychoanalytic concepts*, especially the role of past events and interpretation of unconscious conflicts of individual family members, played a central role in family therapy. This has been superseded by a more active approach based on *systems theory*, which deals with present interaction and communication within the family. Techniques derived from *behaviour therapy* are also used. For example, reciprocal positive reinforcement may lead to mutually rewarding behaviour and discourage undesirable behaviour (see p. 576).

In general nowadays a family therapist is a lively and active agent of change, issuing directions and instructions; he does not just reflect back or interpret the feelings and problems the family members express. The family therapist tends to be less interested in the symptoms of the family member who is the 'identified patient', such as the mother who is depressed, than in the effects her symptoms are having on the other members of the family. Thus he will not ask the mother what makes her depressed, or how it feels to be depressed. Instead he may ask the husband, 'What do you do when your wife is depressed?' or 'Which of the children is most upset when their mother gets depressed and has to go into hospital?'

Techniques based on systems theory can be divided into two main approaches: structural therapy and strategic therapy.

Structural therapy

Here the therapist aims to bring about change directly by altering the structure of the family during the interview. For example, if during the session an adolescent anorexic girl sits between her parents and becomes the focus of attention by constantly getting them to argue with her and each other about her disturbed eating behaviour, the therapist may ask her to stop sitting between them, and ask the parents to sit together instead. The parents are then given the joint task of discussing their own marital difficulties while the therapist talks to the girl, perhaps expressing surprise that she is still so heavily involved with her parents instead of leading her own more independent life. In this way boundaries between the girl and her parents can be re-established.

Strategic therapy

Some families are so entrenched in their dysfunction that structural approaches lead to increased resistance rather than change. These families need to be approached more indirectly, and more devious strategies are sometimes used to achieve change. One strategy is to challenge the family by offering them a therapeutic double bind. For example, some anorexic patients believe that if they recover their parents will split up. The anorexic patient may be told to go on sacrificing herself for her parents' sake by remaining anorexic. This is sometimes called 'prescribing the symptom'. Such a surprising intervention may challenge the patient so that she starts eating, and the parents may begin to work on their own problems. By further challenging the family, perhaps by expressing the view that the improvement will not last, the family may again be made to prove the therapist wrong and further improvement will take place. Alternatively, the family implicitly accepts the therapist's original instruction and authority, and the anorexic behaviour continues. This can later be used to therapeutic advantage as the family is more likely at a later stage to follow the therapist's instruction now to change their behaviour so that the girl starts to eat and the parents face their marital problems. In either case the desired therapeutic effect will have been achieved.

Indications for family therapy

Family therapy is a broad-spectrum treatment with wide applications. Unlike individual therapy, questions of intelligence, verbal ability or psychological awareness are not important in selecting families for treatment. In child psychiatry it is a widely used form of treatment, with drug and individual therapy only being offered in selected cases. In adult psychiatry family therapy is indicated if there are thought to be major family dynamics maintaining an illness or symptom. Family therapy can also be used when a patient is unsuitable for or unable to benefit from individual therapy. It can also be effective when intervening in a family crisis. The main limitation of family therapy is that by focusing primarily on family dynamics one or more individual members of the family, even though their symptoms or illness may improve, may be left with unresolved problems in their personality. If this causes them difficulties later on they may then need individual psychotherapy.

FURTHER READING

Barker, P. (1986). *Basic Family Therapy*, 2nd ed. Blackwell, Oxford.

Bentovim, A. (1986). 'Family therapy when the child is the referred patient' in *An Introduction to the Psychotherapies*, 2nd ed. (Bloch, S., ed.). OUP, Oxford.

Holmes, J.A. (1985). 'Family and individual therapy – comparison and contrasts'. *Brit. J. Psychiat.* 147, 668-676.

46

Behaviour Therapy

Behaviour therapy includes a variety of psychological treatment methods which have originated from experimental psychology, especially the principles of learning. These methods are directed at modifying symptoms and abnormal behaviour. The development of behaviour therapy in the 1950s and 1960s arose particularly out of the clinical application of concepts derived from classical Pavlovian conditioning, and out of operant conditioning described by Skinner (1938, 1953). Since then cognitive and social psychology and clinical experience and research on patients have made important contributions to present-day practice of behaviour therapy, which aims not only to alleviate undesirable symptoms and behaviour but also to encourage more desirable forms.

Behaviour therapy was first used mainly in the treatment of simple phobias, agoraphobia and social phobias (Wolpe 1958). It is now also used, sometimes in conjunction with other treatment methods such as counselling or psychotherapy, in generalised anxiety states, obsessive-compulsive neurosis, some sexual and marital problems, nocturnal enuresis and alcoholism; it can also be helpful in the modification of disturbed social behaviour due to chronic psychiatric disorders such as chronic schizophrenia and mental handicap. It has been estimated that its applications are useful in about 10 per cent of psychiatric outpatients. A common factor in these applications is that the patient learns and practises new ways of coping with anxiety and of confronting and changing his abnormal behaviour or symptoms.

ASSESSMENT

Before any decision about treatment is made an assessment is needed to ascertain whether a psychiatric condition, e.g. a depressive illness, is present which might require treatment in its own right. If not, consideration should be given to the possibility of treating the patient's symptoms by behavioural methods. In some cases these may have to be combined with physical treatments or other forms of psychological treatment. For behaviour therapy to be successful it is essential that the abnormal behaviour or symptom to be changed is clearly identified by both patient and therapist, although in the case of some mentally handicapped or chronically institutionalised patients this may not be possible.

Once the decision to use behaviour therapy has been made a detailed analysis of the disturbed behaviour is essential; this *behavioural analysis* aims at establishing under what circumstances the symptoms and undesirable behaviour arise and what increases or decreases their severity. It is sometimes useful to ask the patient to keep detailed diaries in order to obtain a measure of the frequency, duration and severity of the symptoms, and to find out under what circumstances they occur and what relieves them. Carefully kept diaries also help to assess the qualitative and quantitative changes that occur during the course of treatment.

In addition to the behavioural analysis the patient's thoughts, anxieties, expectations and his motivation for treatment need to be explored. Successful treatment requires a well-motivated and cooperative patient. Some patients refuse or find it difficult to cooperate for a variety of reasons. These may be related to problems within the family or be due to more widespread psychopathology. Lack of cooperation may also be due to the patient's fear of what the treatment will involve or preference for a psychodynamic approach.

The patient's physiological response to anxiety must also be assessed. A high level of arousal and of physical manifestations of anxiety may suggest the need for additional relaxation exercises and the use of tranquillisers before the patient is exposed to the anxiety-provoking situation.

When treatment starts the therapist should present the patient with a clear, well-structured and directive treatment plan. In some cases treatment may require the cooperation of a friend or family member. Such an ally may be called upon to act as a surrogate therapist whenever treatment is carried out in the absence of the therapist in between sessions, perhaps in a setting which is more appropriate to the problem. For example, a husband might be instructed to accompany his agoraphobic wife when she goes out, and to follow a treatment programme which has previously been agreed with the therapist; or a friend or close relative might be told how to prevent a patient with compulsive rituals from carrying out his compulsive behaviour.

Relationship between patient and therapist

It is not always clear how much of the effect of treatment is attributable to the specific behavioural technique used and how much to other factors such as suggestion, praise or active encouragement from an enthusiastic therapist. The patient's relationship with the therapist and his own expectations of treatment can influence the results. As in other forms of psychological treatment, the patient may for a while become dependent on the therapist even though he is encouraged to be self-reliant and to carry out much of the treatment programme by himself in between treatment sessions. Sometimes a patient's disappointment with the therapy may lead to difficulties or interruption of treatment. Training and experience should help the therapist to prevent or deal with such negative reactions. Many behaviour therapists now recognise that discussion of other personal problems or of emotional conflicts may be necessary alongside the use of behavioural techniques.

In general there is an increasing tendency to integrate behavioural techniques with counselling or psychodynamic psychotherapy. This is especially important when removal of a symptom leads to the development of difficulties in close relationships. For example, when a woman becomes more independent after treatment of her agoraphobia, her husband may become jealous, depressed and afraid of her leaving him; in that case marital therapy may be needed as well. If a patient needs a combined approach it may be preferable for the behavioural treatment to be carried out by one therapist, and the dynamically orientated therapy by another.

APPLICATIONS

There are many different behavioural techniques, and many different ways of classifying them. They will be described here in relation to the disorders for which they are commonly used. There are also some procedures which are shared by various techniques.

Simple phobias

Simple phobias (see p. 163) respond well to behavioural methods (Marks 1986, 1987) and the following techniques have been used:

Desensitisation in reality
(Real-life confrontation of the phobia; exposure in vivo)

This technique aims to help the patient overcome his avoidance behaviour by introducing him to the feared situation in stages, starting with the least and gradually building up to the most severe anxiety-provoking situation. This is called a *hierarchy*. Either the frightening nature of the situation or the duration of exposure to it are gradually increased. At each stage the patient is taught and encouraged to relax as far as possible to counter his anxiety. For example, a patient with a spider phobia is first exposed to photographs of spiders. This may result in a surge of anxiety, which the patient is taught to tolerate by learning to relax. Once this is achieved the next more difficult step, e.g. seeing a live spider in a glass jar, is confronted. The patient thus learns to endure anxiety and not to avoid the phobic object. After having passed through further successive steps in the hierarchy the patient may eventually be able to touch a spider without anxiety or panic. The desired behaviour is reinforced by virtue of success. This, combined with praise from the therapist, may in itself be helpful and lead to further improvement, as in operant conditioning.

It is essential for the patient to confront the phobic situation himself in between treatment sessions, preferably once or twice a day for about an hour. Too short or too long periods, and exposure to too little or too much anxiety are less effective than repeated, regular exposure to moderate anxiety for an hour at a time.

Desensitisation in reality has now become established as the best form of treatment not only for simple phobias but also for more severe and disabling ones (Mathews *et al.* 1981), as described below. Earlier fears that new symptoms might replace the original phobia, so-called *symptom substitution*, have not been confirmed.

Desensitisation in imagination

This differs from desensitisation in reality in that the patient is asked to face the phobic stimulus by imagining it instead of facing it in reality. Wolpe (1958) pioneered this method of deconditioning in South Africa and later in the United States. It concentrates on the use of graded exposure in imagination. A hierarchy is constructed by identifying and grading the phobia from its least frightening to its most frightening aspects. Then the patient is asked to imagine the least fearful aspects of the phobia. When he becomes anxious he is asked to relax by using previously learned muscle relaxation in order to counteract his fear. Occasionally a tranquilliser may be used as well to reduce anxiety. When the first fear-producing step in the hierarchy has been mastered, the patient is instructed to move up the hierarchy and to imagine the next more anxiety-provoking situation. Relaxation and mastery follow and counteract the anxiety at each stage by reciprocal inhibition. This stepwise coupling of relaxation with the phobic situation leads to eventual mastery of the most fear-arousing situation.

This technique is sometimes more acceptable to patients than exposure in reality, but it is slow and time-consuming and may fail when the patient has to face the real situation. It is rarely effective in conditions other than simple phobias and has largely been replaced by desensitisation in reality.

Flooding (implosion)

In flooding there is no gradual exposure to the feared situation. Instead the patient is asked at once to confront the situation which produces maximum anxiety in reality for as long as possible, usually an hour or longer. This technique is rarely used nowadays because it is extremely stressful and the patient may refuse or break off treatment. It has also been shown that the results are no better then those obtained by gradual desensitisation in reality (Gelder *et al.* 1973).

Agoraphobia

Principles similar to those described above may also be used in the treatment of agoraphobia (Mathews *et al*. 1981). Exposure in reality is the treatment of choice. The patient is instructed gradually to increase the time, distance and frequency of journeys away from home or into crowds or supermarkets. He has to practise this daily, at first with the help of a friend or relative and later on his own, so-called *programmed practice*. Through such regular practice the patient learns that fear and anxiety at each successive stage can be mastered. By repeated performance, each improvement acts as a positive reinforcer of the desired behaviour.

Agoraphobic patients tend to fare less well in behavioural treatments than patients with simple phobias, and in some patients agoraphobia runs a long and fluctuating course in spite of treatment. However, in a follow-up study after behavioural treatment Munby and Johnston (1980) found that the degree of improvement attained after six months was still present 5-9 years later.

Similar behavioural treatment methods can be used for claustrophia and travel phobias.

Social phobias

Treatment of patients with social phobias makes use of similar principles. For example, a patient who is afraid of eating in public places may first be asked to face the real situation by gradually exposing himself to the feared situation in the company of a friend until he is able to do so alone. Alternatively he may be desensitised by role-playing or modelling in a group and then be asked to face the real situation by going to a restaurant on his own, or among strangers.

Many people feel anxious in a variety of social situations, such as talking to strangers, asking someone out, or returning goods to a shop. Here social skills training can help. It includes the use of role-playing, modelling and gradual confrontation with the actual situation, either in a group or individually. When several patients are treated together in a group their mutual support and encouragement acts as an additional curative factor (see also Chapter 60).

General anxiety states

In anxiety states physical symptoms often accompany the psychological distress. The use of relaxation techniques and anxiety management may be helpful for such patients. Regular practice of muscular relaxation leads to enhanced control over muscular tension. In this way the anxiety and some physical symptoms, such as tension headaches, palpitations or hyperventilation can be alleviated. Success depends on the patient's persistence in practising these methods. Tape-recorded relaxation exercises are used occasionally, and biofeedback instruments may help the patient to monitor one or more physiological parameters, e.g. muscle tension and heart rate.

Obsessive-compulsive neurosis

Behavioural methods are used in the treatment of obsessive-compulsive neurosis to control both the compulsions and the obsessional thoughts (Rachman and Hodgson 1980).

Treatment of compulsions is carried out by *response prevention*. The patient is told to resist his compulsive behaviour, e.g. hand-washing, at first with the help of the therapist, perhaps a nurse trained in behaviour therapy, or a relative or friend instructed by the therapist, but later on his own. When this has been achieved the patient is deliberately exposed to the stimulus that provokes his compulsive rituals, e.g. touching dirty objects. This may once more trigger off the compulsion to wash, but he is strongly discouraged from doing so. With the support and encouragement of the therapist he learns that it is possible to resist the hand-washing, his anxiety subsides and he finds that no ill-effects follow. He has to practise this procedure repeatedly and for several hours at home, if necessary with the assistance of a member of the family. As in the other behavioural treatments, persistence and prolonged practice are essential for a successful outcome.

The treatment of obsessional thoughts by behavioural methods is less successful. The technique used is called *thought stopping*. The principle is forcibly to interrupt the patient's obsessional thoughts by distracting his attention. For example, as soon as the patient indicates that his obsessional thoughts are occurring the therapist says 'Stop'. Later the patient has to say 'Stop' to himself, at first aloud and later silently. Alternatively, the patient may divert his attention by thinking of some pleasant subject of his choice, or use an external stimulus, such as snapping an elastic band worn on the wrist, as a distraction. There is no evidence that these methods are successful in the long run.

Marital problems

Behavioural techniques may be useful in the treatment of some marital problems. The couple are usually seen together and a contract is made using the 'give to get' principle in which a bargain is struck. Each partner is asked to behave in a specific manner to please the other so that the couple learn how to fulfil each other's needs. This has been considered in Chapter 45 (p. 576).

Sexual dysfunction

Techniques originally pioneered in the USA by Masters and Johnson (1970) are used in the treatment of sexual dysfunction. They are described in Chapter 28 (p. 352).

Sexual perversions

In the 1960s *aversion therapy*, previously used in the treatment of alcoholism (see below) was introduced in an attempt to stop patients engaging in fetishism, transvestism and sometimes homosexual activity. Aversion therapy is based on the observation that undesirable behaviour can be suppressed by linking it with an unpleasant or painful stimulus. In the treatment of sexual perversions minor electric shocks were used as the aversive stimulus. For obvious humane and ethical reasons aversion therapy was only attempted in patients who had themselves asked to be relieved of some aspects of their sexual behaviour and had agreed to this form of treatment. Aversion therapy has since been largely abandoned, partly for ethical reasons and because it is distressing and may leave the patient without any alternative satisfying sexual outlet; but mainly because it often fails and its effects are at best short-lived. Instead, behavioural methods designed to encourage more desirable sexual behaviour have been introduced (Gelder 1979; Bancroft 1983). The subject is discussed more fully in Chapter 28 (p. 366).

Mental handicap, chronic schizophrenia and institutionalisation

Patients with these disorders often have severe difficulties in everyday activities such as feeding themselves, getting dressed and attending to personal hygiene. Behaviour modification can sometimes be used to improve their skills. Behaviour can be 'shaped' by reinforcing desired behaviour with appropriate rewards. Both social and personal skills can be developed by systematically rewarding the achievement of certain aspects of behaviour which, when strung together, make up the whole of an intended pattern. The reward may take the form of points or tokens which can then be exchanged for goods. This method is known as *token economy*. The earlier method in which patients were punished for undesirable behaviour, e.g. by the withdrawal of privileges, is now rarely used, partly because of the ethical problems involved, and partly because of the distressing effect on the patient. Token-economy methods require careful planning and implementation by trained staff. They can be used either in the setting of a community, say a hospital ward, or in the treatment of families, couples or individuals. Unfortunately even if behaviour modification of, say, a mentally handicapped patient is successful in a ward setting the effects may not be generalised, i.e. the improved behaviour may not be manifested in other situations.

Nocturnal enuresis (bedwetting)

The patient, usually a child, sleeps with a pad under his bottom sheet. The pad consists of two metal plates separated by a cotton sheet; the plates are attached to an electric circuit incorporating a battery and a bell or buzzer. If the child begins to pass urine a circuit is completed as the cotton sheet between the plates gets moist. The sound of the bell then wakes the child who turns it off and completes the act of micturition by going to the toilet. In addition to conditioning, the parents' praise and approval of his success probably play an important role in the child's recovery (see also p. 507).

Alcoholism

Aversion therapy was first introduced in the treatment of alcoholism. The patient was given apomorphine to induce nausea and vomiting and this was linked with the taste and smell of alcohol by classical conditioning. The treatment was very unpleasant and the results usually short-lived, and it has therefore been abandoned. Instead attempts have been made to use cognitive methods (see below) in an attempt to promote greater self-control and to reduce the patient's desire to drink.

Depression

Attempts have been made to treat depression with *cognitive behaviour therapy* (Beck *et al.* 1979). This recent form of behaviour therapy tries to teach the patient to replace his erroneous assumptions, e.g. his self-deprecating, gloomy and despairing thoughts, by alternative positive thoughts about himself (see also p. 205). Cognitive therapy has also been used in the treatment of anxiety and alcoholism. It is not yet known whether the results of cognitive therapy have a lasting effect. If the patient's negative thoughts are due to a severe depressive illness antidepressants will be needed instead; patients with underlying conflicts and personality disorders due to past experiences may require treatment with psychotherapy.

FURTHER READING

Marks, I.M. (1986). *Behavioural Psychotherapy*. Wright, Bristol.
Mathews, A.M., Gelder, M.G. and Johnston, D.W. (1981). *Agoraphobia: nature and treatment*. Tavistock, London.

47

Outcome of Psychotherapy and Behaviour Therapy

As with other treatment methods in psychiatry, and for that matter in medicine as a whole, it is important to study the effectiveness or outcome of psychological treatments. A great deal of research has been done in this field. Here we shall summarise some of the findings, describe the present position and draw attention to the difficulties that face research workers in this field. The subject has been reviewed by Bergin and Lambert (1978), Bloch (1982) and Lambert et al. (1986).

OVERALL REVIEW STUDIES

Most patients treated with dynamic psychotherapy or by behaviour therapy present with psychoneurotic symptoms, behaviour disturbance and personality disorders. One of the many questions asked in outcome research is whether such patients can be shown to improve significantly more when treated with psychotherapy or behaviour therapy than patients who receive no treatment or only minimal support.

A crucial issue, to be discussed below, is what is meant by improvement. Researchers have often concentrated on symptom relief, and sometimes also on social functioning and adjustment. Intrapsychic changes, personal growth, development and maturation are often at least as important and sometimes more so, but they are much more difficult to assess.

Since the early 1930s many studies have tried to answer these and related questions. Several were based on relatively small numbers of patients; the diagnoses were often uncertain and varied; and some studies did not include adequate control groups. Some were even carried out on volunteer subjects without significant complaints so that they in no way resembled actual patients seen in clinical practice. In order to overcome some of these serious limitations, several research workers have extracted and re-evaluated the findings from some of the more reliable earlier studies and then applied statistical methods to the combined and hence larger group of patients treated. Such investigations or review studies, however, cannot compensate for inadequacies in the original studies. In spite of this several important findings have emerged.

Outstanding among these reviews are those by Bergin (1971), Bergin and Lambert (1978) and Lambert *et al.* (1986) which clearly showed that patients who receive psychotherapy or behaviour therapy show significantly greater symptomatic improvement than patients in control groups who receive either no treatment, e.g. by being kept on a waiting list, or only minimal support.

In his 1971 review Bergin also demonstrated that previous claims made by Eysenck (1952) contained several inaccuracies. Eysenck had claimed that two-thirds of neurotic patients improved 'spontaneously', i.e. without treatment, over a two-year period, and that patients treated with dynamic psychotherapy did no better than those who were left untreated. Bergin (1971) and Bergin and Lambert (1978) discussed the reasons which led to Eysenck's mistaken conclusions. They also pointed out that the concept of so-called spontaneous improvement of neurotic symptoms is of doubtful value. This concept is derived from and applicable to some medical disorders of organic origin in which the progress without treatment is well known and predictable; in that case the progress in a group of patients receiving treatment can readily be compared with that of an untreated control group. In contrast, the course of the neuroses, when untreated, is very variable and depends on many factors, some known, some unknown. These include the nature and duration of the symptoms (those of recent onset often clearing up more quickly than those of long standing), the patient's personality, his early development, his present interpersonal relationships, social circumstances and any changes in his life situation. For example, symptoms of neurotic depression caused by the loss of a partner may clear up if the patient finds a new satisfactory relationship, but they may become worse if he experiences further losses and disappointments. This makes the use of untreated control groups very difficult. There is no guarantee that these uncontrollable factors will necessarily be the same in a group of patients treated with formal psychotherapy compared with those in an untreated control group, especially if the number of patients is small. Further research is needed to investigate the influence of the various factors mentioned above on the course of specific psychoneurotic symptoms in the absence of treatment.

The conclusions reached by Bergin and Lambert (1978) from their overall review study are as follows. Eysenck's claim that two-thirds of patients with psychoneurotic symptoms improve in two years without treatment is erroneous. An average figure of 43 per cent, with a wide range from 18 to 67 per cent for improvement in untreated groups, emerges from their review of several papers. Patients treated with psychotherapy showed significantly greater improvement than those in the untreated group; moreover, in the treatment groups patients on average improved significantly faster. Bergin and Lambert summarised their findings by saying that if patients receive psychotherapy this yields 'clearly positive results compared with no treatment, waiting list, and placebo or pseudotherapies'.

Recently a new statistical method, meta-analysis, which measures the 'effect size' of psychotherapy by comparing treated with untreated control groups, has led to similar conclusions (Smith *et al.* 1980). Briefly, they found that on average patients who received psychotherapy did significantly better in terms of symptom relief than 80 per cent of patients in untreated control groups. Their findings have been confirmed by Andrews and Harvey (1981).

While there is therefore strong statistical evidence that patients who receive some form of psychotherapy do better than control groups of untreated patients, it has been much more difficult to demonstrate statistically significant differences between different forms of treatment. Luborsky *et al.* (1975) in a paper entitled 'Comparative studies of psychotherapies. Is it true that "everyone has won and all must have prizes?" ' reviewed 105 controlled studies of different therapies. They were unable to demonstrate any significant differences when they compared the overall figures for individual and group therapies, time-limited and unlimited treatment methods, or client-centred and other forms of psychotherapy. While these findings are often quoted, their other significant findings are referred to less often. They found that all these forms of therapy led to improvements which were significantly greater than in the untreated control groups. Further, when they concentrated on studies of patients with clearly specified disorders they found, perhaps not surprisingly, that, for example, patients with circumscribed phobias did better with behaviour therapy than other forms of therapy, and that patients with psychosomatic symptoms did better with psychodynamic therapy combined with medical treatment than with medical treatment only. This underlines the need for more research on clearly defined symptoms or disorders.

Bergin and Lambert (1978) have drawn attention to the *deterioration effect* of psychotherapy. They pointed out that the psychological treatment methods, psychoanalytic or behavioural, both of which have been shown to be effective and hence to have positive effects, can in some patients have harmful effects, as demonstrated in several studies. It follows that outcome studies based on large numbers of patients with different disorders, and treated by a variety of methods and therapists, will include patients who have improved as well as patients who have deteriorated; it is important therefore to measure the variance as well as the average change in all such studies. To what extent the deterioration effect depends on the patient's particular personality or disorder, on the treatment method used, on the skill or lack of skill of the therapist and on the quality of their relationship, requires further investigation. It is likely that all these factors play a part.

INDIVIDUAL OUTCOME STUDIES

There are many different forms of psychotherapy and behaviour therapy, carried out by many different therapists, and used to treat a large variety of patients with different personalities and different disorders or symptoms. It is therefore necessary to conduct individual outcome studies designed to answer specific questions, such as whether analytical psychotherapy or behaviour therapy is more or less effective in the treatment of a clearly defined symptom or disorder; or how psychoanalysis compares with brief forms of once-weekly analytical psychotherapy, and so on.

One of the best known studies of this kind is that by Sloane *et al.* (1975) carried out in the Temple University Psychiatric Outpatient Clinic in Philadelphia. Ninety-four patients were divided into three groups, those treated with short-term (four months) psychoanalytic psychotherapy, those treated with behaviour therapy and those kept on a waiting list. The latter went through the same detailed initial assessment procedure as those in the two treatment groups. They were, however, kept in regular contact with a research assistant by telephone and were promised treatment after four months; they could therefore better be described as a 'minimal contact' group. The psychotherapists and behaviour therapists were all experienced therapists in their respective fields and the duration of treatment was the same in both therapy groups, i.e. four months. The patients suffered from neurotic symptoms or personality disorders. All patients were assessed in terms of their target symptoms and their social and work adjustment at the initial assessment, after four months and again after a year by independent assessors.

After four months all three groups showed improvement in terms of target symptoms, but it was significantly greater in both the psychotherapy and the behaviour therapy groups than in the waiting list group. There was no significant difference in the degree of improvement between the two treatment groups, a finding in keeping with that obtained in other studies.

Unfortunately the follow-up assessment at one year was made less conclusive by the fact that a significant proportion of patients in all three groups had sought therapy for themselves in the intervening eight months. However, any improvement in target symptoms and social adjustment reached at the end of four months of treatment was maintained or had increased further at one year.

Another important finding was that in both the psychotherapy and the behaviour therapy groups a mutually satisfactory relationship between patient and therapist was a significant factor which correlated with satisfactory outcome of treatment, a finding to which we shall return shortly.

An important criticism of this study is that the patients treated with psychoanalytic psychotherapy only received four months of therapy, a very short period even for brief psychotherapy. This does not detract from the fact that even in this short period the patients derived equal benefit compared with those who received behavioural treatment. Whether significantly greater improvement would have taken place if the psychotherapy patients had been treated for one or two years, as is much more usual in analytical psychotherapy, cannot be determined from this study. This raises a difficult methodological issue. In this study it was decided to treat the patients in both therapy groups for the same length of time; as behaviour therapy hardly ever extends beyond a few months the psychotherapy had to be limited to the same period. Moreover, improvement was only assessed in terms of target symptoms and social and work adjustment. Personality development and intrapsychic changes were not assessed. In clinical practice patients who are severely disturbed and who receive analytical psychotherapy may require many months or longer to establish a working therapeutic relationship before they get fully engaged in therapy and start to derive benefit. A different research project in which all patients received analytical psychotherapy, one group for six months and the other for two years or longer, might answer the question of relative effectiveness of short-term and more long-term analytical psychotherapy, provided changes in personality and intrapsychic structure are assessed as well as target symptoms.

In general, behaviour therapy lends itself more readily to outcome reseach than psychotherapy, not only because of its shorter duration but also because it is more often used to treat circumscribed and readily defined symptoms, e.g. phobic anxiety states. Moreover the main aim of behaviour therapy is symptom relief and social adjustment, and these are more readily assessed in quantitative terms than personality and intrapsychic changes which, alongside symptomatic improvement, constitute important aims in analytical psychotherapy. In one study (Gelder *et al.* 1967) the effect of desensitisation in imagination (see p. 585) in the treatment of patients with phobic anxiety states was compared with the effects of either group psychotherapy or individual psychotherapy. Desensitisation led to more patients with phobic symptoms having improved at the end of treatment than group or individual psychotherapy. At follow-up the psychotherapy patients in whom symptom relief took place more slowly had almost caught up with those treated by desensitisation. Patients with agoraphobia did less well with either treatment than those with simpler phobias. It has since been shown that desensitisation in reality (see p. 584) gives considerably better results in the treatment of agoraphobic patients than desensitisation in imagination (Mathews *et al.* 1981).

Malan (1963, 1973, 1976b) at the Tavistock Clinic, London, has carried out several studies on patients with a variety of psychoneurotic and psychosomatic symptoms in an attempt to identify factors which influence the outcome of brief analytically oriented psychotherapy. In these studies outcome was assessed quantitatively by means of rating scales not only in terms of symptom relief but also in terms of psychodynamic changes defined in depth for each individual patient before treatment began. The following *specific psychotherapeutic factors* correlated with a positive outcome of brief psychoanalytically oriented psychotherapy:

(1) The patient's motivation to obtain insight based on psychodynamic understanding.

(2) The therapist's ability to make use of a focused psychotherapeutic plan based on psychodynamic understanding of each individual patient.

(3) Interpretation and working through of the transference in terms of earlier problems in relation to parents, the so-called 'transference/parent link'.

Malan (1976b) also drew attention to some non-specific factors which emerged from his studies. In nine patients who had been seen once only for a diagnostic interview but who had not entered psychotherapy, follow-up showed that this single diagnostic interview had had a significant and lasting therapeutic effect. In other patients who did receive psychotherapy, maturation in response to helpful life events contributed to a satisfactory outcome in addition to the specific psychotherapeutic factors described above. This study thus provides some quantitative data in support of the view that the capacity for insight and working through the transference are important specific factors leading to a positive outcome of psychoanalytically oriented psychotherapy, but it also shows that non-specific factors can play a significant role. The study was not designed to compare the outcome of brief psychodynamic therapy, conducted once weekly for several months, with psychoanalysis over several years, or with other forms of psychotherapy or behaviour therapy.

NON-SPECIFIC FACTORS

The role that non-specific psychological factors, previously sometimes called placebos, may play in contributing to a satisfactory outcome of psychotherapy has been investigated by many research workers other than Malan, especially by Jerome Frank (Frank 1968, 1973, 1974; Frank *et al.* 1978), and also in the study by Sloane *et al.* (1975) described earlier. The term is used to identify those factors which are not specific to the techniques used in a particular method of therapy, such as transference interpretations in analytical psychotherapy, and desensitisation in behaviour therapy. It has been shown that such non-specific factors as the patient's motivation and a good patient-therapist relationship contribute to a positive outcome in a variety of different treatment procedures, both psychodynamic and behavioural. A better term might therefore be *common therapeutic factors*, i.e. factors common to a variety of therapeutic methods (Bloch 1982; Lambert *et al.* 1986). The following are some of these common factors: the patient's motivation to enter therapy; his hope that the therapy offered will help him; the therapist's liking for the patient and enthusiasm to help him; and a satisfactory match between therapist and patient. Psychotherapists often pay attention to the last factor in clinical practice when selecting a therapist for a particular patient. The therapist's personality and experience in the particular treatment method are also significant. The effects of therapist variables have been reviewed by Beutler *et al.* (1986).

The positive effect of helpful life events has already been noted as a non-specific factor, but it is difficult to keep this factor separate from the specific effects of treatment; for example, a patient may have been helped by dynamic psychotherapy to establish better interpersonal relationships, and this may have made it possible for him to enter into and maintain a lasting relationship he would otherwise have rejected or broken up. Similarly a patient with social phobias may have been helped by behaviour therapy to enter new relationships he would previously have avoided. In either case the new, satisfactory relationship may in turn contribute further to a satisfactory outcome.

In conclusion, the overall superiority of psychological treatment methods over untreated control groups has now been established, as has their superiority over the effect of non-specific factors alone (Lambert 1986). More specific studies are needed to decide which particular therapy of what duration and intensity is needed for what kind of patient with what kind of problem or symptom, and by what kind of therapist. Perhaps the most challenging task is to devise new ways of assessing intrapsychic changes and maturational processes, especially in order to evaluate short-term and long-term psychoanalytic psychotherapy and psychoanalysis.

FURTHER READING

Bergin, A.E. and Lambert, M.J. (1978). 'The evaluation of therapeutic outcomes' in *Handbook of Psychotherapy and Behaviour Change*, 2nd ed. (Garfield, S.L. and Bergin, A.E., eds). John Wiley, New York.

Bloch, S. (1982). 'Psychotherapy' in *Recent Advances in Clinical Psychiatry*, No. 4 (Granville-Grossman, K., ed.). Churchill Livingstone, Edinburgh.

Frank, J.D. Hoehn-Saric, R., Imber, S.D. Liberman, B.L. and Stone, A. (1978). *Effective Ingredients of Successful Psychotherapy*. Brunner/Mazel, New York.

Lambert, M.J. Shapiro, D.A. and Bergin, A.E. (1986). 'The effectiveness of psychotherapy' in *Handbook of Psychotherapy and Behaviour Change*, 3rd ed. (Garfield, S.L. and Bergin, A.E., eds). John Wiley, New York.

48

Psychopharmacology and the Placebo Response

HISTORY

Drugs have been used from earliest times to alter mental functions such as sleep, memory, cognition, perception or mood and, as a consequence, to bring about changes in behaviour. Extracts of such plants as the mandrake, poppy and blue-water lily, known to the ancient Egyptians, all have psychotropic effects. Mandragora, derived from the mandrake plant, is mentioned in the Old Testament, and its production is described in the early Arabic formularies.

Nowadays the active compounds are isolated, purified and subjected to experimental trials. New, precisely delineated chemical compounds are constantly being developed. As a result a large variety of psychotropic drugs, i.e. drugs used to control mental symptoms, have been introduced since the early 1950s. These include drugs to control anxiety, also called anxiolytics or minor tranquillisers, antidepressants, stimulants and antipsychotic drugs, also called neuroleptics or major tranquillisers. In addition anti-parkinsonian drugs are used to control the extrapyramidal side-effects of antipsychotic drugs.

The initial discovery of the psychotropic action of certain drugs was often made by chance. For example, the finding that derivatives of ethylamine protected against histamine was made before the Second World War and later led to the development of more potent and less toxic antihistamines; some of these were then found to have marked sedative but fewer anthistamine properties, and one of them, chlorpromazine, was produced in 1950 by Charpentier in Paris and introduced into anaesthetic practice as a tranquilliser. It was soon found to have marked antipsychotic effects, and a whole range of other antipsychotic drugs and tranquillisers was developed from it. The marked antidepressant effects of imipramine, a drug closely related structurally to chlorpromazine, were first noted in 1957. The monoamine oxidase inhibitor group of antidepressants, on the other hand, owe their origin to the observation that certain antituberculous drugs, including isoniazid, synthesised in 1951, had marked euphoric action. Iproniazid, a closely related compound which acts as an inhibitor of monoamine oxidase, was then shown to have marked antidepressant effects.

Other substances were discovered quite fortuitously. For example, the hallucinogenic properties of lysergic acid diethylamide (LSD) were noted accidentally in 1943. Hofmann, a chemist working with LSD at Sandoz Laboratories, on returning home from the laboratory, experienced a pleasant state of sleepiness during which he had a stream of fantastic and vivid images lasting for about two hours. He suspected that these effects were the result of having worked with LSD earlier in the day, and he confirmed this by deliberately taking a small dose of LSD. Later a chemical relationship between LSD and other hallucinogenic compounds, such as mescaline and psilocybin, was worked out.

The development of psychotropic drugs and of hallucinogens and the treatment of disturbed mental states has therefore grown out of a combination of folk remedies, pharmacological research and clinical observation (Hordern 1968).

EVALUATION

In psychiatry, as in the rest of medicine, a balance has to be struck between the clinical usefulness of a drug and its possible toxicity and side-effects. When drugs are used to relieve subjective distress, such as mood changes and deterioration in the quality of life, their effects are particularly difficult to assess quantitatively. As a result there is often considerable uncertainty and debate about the clinical usefulness of a particular psychotropic drug relative to its possible toxicity and side-effects. For example, such a serious long-term effect of chlorpromazine as tardive dyskinesia (see p. 246), may sometimes outweigh its usefulness as an antipsychotic drug, especially when given in large doses over a long period of time.

Carefully controlled evaluation of drug therapy is essential in assessing the effectiveness of a psychotropic drug. Even when this has been established, it may only become apparent later that the drug has significant toxic effects. When this happens the use of the drug may have to be modified or abandoned, and sometimes it has to be withdrawn.

The effectiveness or otherwise of a particular drug can only be determined by comparison with the effect of another drug or of dummy medication acting as a placebo. Gaddum (1954) proposed that the term 'dummy tablets' be used to describe a pharmacologically inert preparation which can be used as a control in a drug trial and other experimental procedures, reserving the term 'placebo' for preparations known to the doctor to be inert but used in clinical practice to please and help the patient. However, 'placebo' is now generally used for both. The placebo response is considered below.

Drug trials

When a placebo is used in double blind drug trials it is important to ensure that neither the patient nor the observer is aware which drug is being given. The two tablets should look, taste and smell exactly the same, and any side-effects should also be identical. In practice this is often difficult to achieve so that either the patient or observer or both may make a shrewd guess as to which is which.

Another method is to compare a new psychotropic drug with an established remedy without using placebo controls. These trials can be difficult to interpret statistically unless a large number of patients, say 100-200, are studied. When no significant difference is found in a drug trial using a smaller number of patients, this may only indicate that the sample range was insufficient to discriminate between the effectiveness of the two drugs.

THE PLACEBO RESPONSE

The discovery that inert substances, since called placebos, could have as marked an effect on patients as scientifically proven drugs at first caused some embarrassment among those clinicians who were reluctant to acknowledge the importance of the psychological influence of the doctor on his patient. Some even considered it unethical to help a patient by giving him a placebo. The medical profession had reacted similarly to the discovery of the role of suggestion and hypnosis at the beginning of the nineteenth century (see p. 15).

Attempts to estimate the incidence of the placebo response in groups of patients have given very variable results, but an average figure of 35 per cent is often quoted. The fact that a high proportion of patients can react to a placebo makes it a significant tool in treatment and underlines the importance of establishing whether a drug's effectiveness is due to its placebo effect or its pharmacological properties, or a combination of both. This applies especially to psychotropic drugs.

Research on the placebo response has been reviewed by Shapiro and Morris (1978). The age, sex and degree of neuroticism of patients do not play a consistent role in determining whether or not they are placebo reactors. However, the patient's expectations of the treatment, based on his earlier experience and encounters with doctors, are of considerable importance. Previous experience of having benefited from treatment with drugs correlates with a positive response to being given a placebo; previous disappointing experiences tend to lead to the patient either not responding to a placebo or even developing adverse side-effects, a so-called negative placebo reaction.

The doctor's personality plays a very important role. That different practitioners of medicine or psychiatry should have varying powers to alleviate suffering will surprise no one but the most unobservant. Shapiro and Morris (1978) even speak of 'iatroplacebogenesis'. The doctor's personal attitude is of decisive importance in determining how he administers the placebo and hence its therapeutic effectiveness. His personal interest in the patient, his warmth and friendliness all increase the positive response to the placebo, while lack of interest, coldness, rejection or even hostility have the opposite effect. The overt message he gives to the patient, emphasising that the treatment will help him, and the covert influence of his own belief or disbelief in its effectiveness both have a significant influence. This also applies to the administration of drugs of known pharmacological value. For example, a study by Feldman (1956) showed the additional beneficial effect which enthusiastic doctors can have on the results of treatment of schizophrenia with antipsychotic drugs; and similar observations have been made during treatment of patients with antidepressants.

It is the interaction between doctor and patient which is of major importance in determining the effect or otherwise of a placebo. Trust in the doctor and his ability to inspire confidence and hope have a positive influence, while mistrust and a poor doctor-patient relationship have the opposite effect.

The role of the placebo response in psychological treatments has also been investigated, e.g. in relation to the various forms of psychotherapy and behaviour therapy (Shapiro and Morris 1978). It has long been known that the outcome of psychological treatments is influenced by non-specific factors, common to the different methods used, e.g. the patient's expectations and his relationship to the therapist. This is discussed further on p. 595.

FURTHER READING

Iverson, S.D. (1985). *Psychopharmacology: recent advances and future prospects.* OUP, Oxford.

Shapiro, A.K. and Morris, L.A. (1978). 'The placebo effect in medical and psychological therapies' in *Handbook of Psychotherapy and Behaviour Change*, 2nd ed. (Garfield, S. and Bergin, A.E., ed.). John Wiley, New York.

49

Psychotropic Drugs

These will be considered under the following headings:

(1) anxiolytics and hypnotics
(2) antidepressants
(3) drugs used in manic-depressive illness
(4) antipsychotic drugs

ANXIOLYTICS AND HYPNOTICS

Three main groups of drugs have anxiolytic properties: (1) the centrally acting sedatives, such as barbiturates and alcohol, which have widespread effects throughout the central nervous system; (2) the centrally acting sedatives – sometimes known as minor tranquillisers – such as the benzodiazepines, which are relatively specific in their effect on the limbic system; (3) a group whose anxiolytic effects are part of a more widespread pharmacological effect, e.g. peripheral beta-adrenoceptor blockers such as propranolol, and some antidepressant drugs.

Barbiturates are no longer prescribed as anxiolytics in view of their toxicity and propensity to cause dependence. Furthermore their anxiolytic action is poor in comparison to the benzodiazepines. The use of alcohol as a socially acceptable way of coping with anxiety is probably quite common, especially in individuals who experience social anxiety. Unfortunately dependence may result and its use is not usually recommended, but it is sometimes useful as night sedation in the elderly.

Benzodiazepines

The most widely prescribed group of drugs in the treatment of anxiety are the benzodiazepines. They were first noted to have sedative properties in the 1950s, and since then a whole range of compounds, all with somewhat similar actions, have been synthesised even though the justification for marketing so many is limited.

Pharmacology

Most benzodiazepines are variations of the basic 1.4 benzodiazepine structure which is essentially a seven-membered ring of carbon and nitrogen atoms. Recently the 1.5 benzodiazepine structure has also been shown to be pharmacologically active. Benzodiazepines bind to postsynaptic sites at GABAergic synapses. These are found throughout the central nervous system, especially in the limbic system, cerebral cortex and the cerebellum, and also in the spinal cord. Gamma-aminobutyric acid (GABA) is an inhibitory neurotransmitter, and the benzodiazepines potentiate this inhibitory effect by increasing the permeability of the neuron to chloride ions, which makes the cell more difficult to excite. Recently several types of benzodiazepine receptors have been discovered, only some of which appear to be involved in anxiety. This may lead to the development of compounds which have a more specific anxiolytic effect.

Clinicians are particularly concerned with the duration of action of the benzodiazepines, long-acting drugs being used to control anxiety and short-acting drugs to treat insomnia. Many of the benzodiazepines are partially metabolised to desmethyldiazepam, which though less potent is also pharmacologically active and has a very long half-life of between 50-180 hours. This group, which includes medazepam, chlorazepam and diazepam, have a long duration of action. Other long-acting benzodiaze-pines are nitrazepam, flurazepam and chlordiazepoxide. These drugs have the advantage of a continuous anxiolytic effect but may give rise to hangover effects and problems associated with continuing mild sedation. Shorter-acting benzodiazepines, such as temazepam, oxazepam and lorazepam, are often more useful in the treatment of insomnia, i.e. as hypnotics, especially if there is initial sleeplessness such as occurs in anxiety states.

Clinical uses

The benzodiazepines are valuable in helping to alleviate anxiety and insomnia. They also have muscle-relaxant and anti-convulsant proper-ties. For anxiety a short course of a long-acting benzodiazepine is usually prescribed, e.g. chlordiazepoxide or diazepam orally 5 mg three times a day. A flexible dosage regime varying from 2-10 mg is valuable when symptoms wax and wane, but care should be taken that the patient does not exceed the prescribed dose. In insomnia a shorter-acting benzodiaze-pine is usually prescribed, e.g. temazepam 20 mg at night.

The patient should be cautioned against taking night sedation regularly so that it becomes a habit. In many cases insomnia will resolve or recede and the need to prescribe will be short-lived, but some people suffer from chronic insomnia and take benzodiazepines on a regular basis for many years. These patients need to be encouraged to have short periods without any medication, so-called 'drug holidays'. If this is not done the dose of the drug will gradually have to be increased to achieve the desired hypnotic effect as tolerance develops.

In general, because of the serious risk of dependence, benzodiazepines should only be prescribed for a limited period, preferably no longer than a few weeks. Until recently they were often prescribed for much longer, especially in patients with a chronic anxiety state. This should be avoided if at all possible. Instead efforts should be made to control the anxiety with support, psychotherapy and relaxation exercises to minimise reliance on drug treatment.

Benzodiazepines are also used in the treatment of phobic states. Specific phobic states are probably best treated by desensitisation alone and without the use of drugs. The more diffuse phobias, such as agoraphobia and social phobia, are also best treated with desensitisation, but the use of benzodiazepines may be helpful during the treatment, e.g. taking them shortly before exposure to the feared situation to control excessive anxiety. Occasionally claustrophobia or agoraphobia are associated with vestibular dysfunction and care must be taken to ensure that the unsteadiness is not worsened by the benzodiazepines.

Diazepam, 10 mg orally or intravenously, is also used to control the acute symptoms of delirium tremens and in status epilepticus.

Side-effects

The benzodiazepines are relatively free from side-effects and are generally safe even when taken as an overdose. However they can cause confusion in the elderly and lead to ataxia even at low doses. Their sedative effect may make driving dangerous. Their effect is potentiated by alcohol.

As mentioned above, psychological and physical dependence are now recognised as a serious problem in a high proportion of cases, and a withdrawal syndrome may occur after only a few weeks of regular consumption (see p. 393). Lader and Higgitt (1986) have discussed the management of dependence on benzodiazepines.

Other anxiolytic drugs

Beta-blocking drugs such as *propranolol* are effective in reducing somatic symptoms of anxiety such as tremor and palpitations. They probably do this by acting peripherally and so may be combined with a centrally acting anxiolytic drug if anxiety is severe. A low dose is used, such as propranolol orally 40-80 mg daily, and physical dependence does not occur. As they can cause hypotension, heart block and bronchospasm, they should not be prescribed for people with heart disease and asthma.

Some psychiatrists use antipsychotic medication such as thioridazine in the treatment of anxiety. However, even at low doses tardive dyskinesia may develop and so their use in anxiety is best avoided.

ANTIDEPRESSANTS

At present two main classes of drugs are used in the treatment of depression. These are the tricyclic and tetracyclic group of antidepressants, and the monoamine oxidase inhibitors (MAOIs). A variety of other drugs also have antidepressant effects; these are discussed below under the heading 'miscellaneous antidepressants'.

Psychopharmacology of depression

The monoamine hypothesis of depression is discussed in Chapter 18 (see p. 195). In essence it states that depressive illness is associated with a reduction or relative deficiency of noradrenaline or 5-hydroxytryptamine (5HT) at the synapses in as yet unknown areas of the brain. The discovery that drugs such as the tricyclic antidepressants and MAOIs, which increase the amount of noradrenaline and 5HT available in the synapse, have an antidepressant effect seemed to confirm this hypothesis. At present it is not clear which of the monoamines are primarily involved in depressive illness.

Tricyclic and tetracyclic antidepressants

The tricyclic antidepressant drugs block the active re-uptake into cellular stores of noradrenaline and 5HT released into the synaptic cleft. This increases the amount of monoamines at the synapse. Some antidepressants act predominantly on noradrenaline, e.g. maprotiline, protryptiline and desipramine, while others act primarily on the re-uptake of 5HT, e.g. fluvoxamine, clomipramine and trazodone. Some of the newer antidepressants seem to act slightly differently: mianserin, a tetracyclic antidepressant, acts on the presynaptic receptors and has little effect on amine re-uptake.

Clinical uses

The effectiveness of tricyclic and related antidepressants in the treatment of depressive illness has been clearly established. The more closely the clinical picture resembles the classical description of endogenous depression, the more likely is the patient to respond. In clinical practice tricyclic antidepressants can be divided into those that are sedative, e.g. amitryptiline, dothiepin, trimipramine, and those that have more stimulant properties, e.g. desipramine, lofepramine and sometimes imipramine. The *sedative antidepressants* are of greater use in agitated depression, the *stimulant antidepressants* in retarded depression. Patients should be warned that improvement will take time, usually 7-14 days, and that it will be gradual. They should also be informed about the expected and common side-effects. These usually start within a few days, often before any antidepressant effects are noted; this may lead the patient to stop taking the drug prematurely. Moreover the doctor may change the patient's antidepressant medication after too short a trial period or prescribe an inadequate dose. If antidepressants are stopped too early relapse is common. In general, patients who respond to antidepressants should continue to take them for some time after the symptoms cease. The depressive illness should have run its course by the time the drug is gradually withdrawn.

Tricyclic antidepressant drugs have also been used in the treatment of obsessional neurosis, anxiety states and phobic anxiety. The sedative antidepressants such as amitryptiline are effective in anxiety states and phobic anxiety; clomipramine has been claimed to be effective in obsessional illness but there is little evidence for this claim; it is probably only useful in those obsessional patients who also have a depressed mood.

The use of antidepressant drugs in nocturnal enuresis is discussed elsewhere (see p. 507).

Side-effects

In general tetracyclic antidepressants have fewer side-effects than tricyclics. The commonest unwanted effects of antidepressants result from their anticholinergic action and include dry mouth, blurred vision, constipation and urinary retention. The tricyclic antidepressants should be avoided in patients with glaucoma and prostatic enlargement. There may be some risk to patients with cardiac disease as tricyclic antidepressants impair conduction in the Bundle of His and can cause tachycardia, arrhythmia and heart block. Some of the newer preparations such as mianserin and lofepramine have fewer anticholinergic effects and are said to be less cardiotoxic.

Tricyclic antidepressants antagonise adrenergic neuron blockers used in the treatment of hypertension, e.g. bethanidine and guanethidine, and they should not be prescribed together. Excessive doses of tricyclics may lead to hypertension, cardiac arrhythmias, hallucinations, excitement and convulsions.

Individual antidepressants

The following section describes the effects of several tricyclic and tetracyclic antidepressants in common use. Although both patients and their doctors hold strong views as to the best antidepressants, the range of drugs available would indicate that no one preparation is markedly more successful than another. Reasons for the choice of drug may have more to do with conviction and enthusiasm than with particular pharmacological characteristics.

Amitryptiline

This tricyclic antidepressant, in view of its marked sedative properties, is most useful in agitated depression. It has pronounced anticholinergic side-effects and can cause cardiac arrhythmias. The dose is gradually increased from 75 mg up to 200 mg daily and can be given as a single dose taken at night.

Imipramine

This tricyclic antidepressant is less sedative than amitryptiline and is therefore of greater use in retarded depression. It also has marked anticholinergic properties and is cardiotoxic at higher doses. The dose is 75 to 150 mg daily and is usually given in divided doses.

Desipramine

This metabolite of imipramine is thought to have no advantage over it as an antidepressant, although initially it was claimed that it acted more quickly. It acts selectively on noradrenaline re-uptake and has similar toxicity to imipramine. Dosage is 75-200 mg daily.

Clomipramine

This drug is similar to imipramine. It acts on the re-uptake of 5HT. Some patients find it sedative, others more alerting. It is used in obsessional and phobic disorders where there is a marked anxiety or depressive component. The dose is 50-150 mg daily and it can be taken in a single dose at night.

Dothiepin

This drug is very similar to amitryptiline but has fewer anticholinergic side-effects and is less cardiotoxic. The dose is 75-150 mg daily.

Lofepramine

This relatively new antidepressant drug has fewer anticholinergic effects than imipramine or amitryptiline. It is not particularly sedative in its action and is not as cardiotoxic as many other tricyclic antidepressants. If further study and use confirm its potency and effectiveness as an antidepressant, it should make a useful addition to the range of drugs available. The dose is 70-210 mg daily in divided doses.

Maprotiline

This tetracyclic antidepressant seems to act mainly on the re-uptake of noradrenaline. It is less sedative than amitryptiline, has a long half-life and can be used in a once daily dosage. The dose is 50-150 mg daily.

Mianserin

This tetracyclic antidepressant has very few anticholinergic side-effects and is said to have little cardiotoxicity. Recently there have been reports of bone marrow suppression, and it is now recommended that a full blood count is done every month during the first three months of treatment. Patients should be warned to report the onset of any fever or sore throat. After the first three months of treatment blood counts should be done periodically. The dose is 30-120 mg daily, although higher doses can be used.

Nortriptyline

This is the only tricyclic antidepressant in which there is good evidence that the plasma level correlates with the antidepressant effect. Too low or too high a plasma level is ineffective, and the drug is most effective at a mid-range level. The therapeutic range of nortriptyline plasma concentration is 50-140 ng/ml. The dose is 30-75 mg daily in divided doses three times a day.

Trimipramine

This is similar to imipramine but slightly more sedative. It is sometimes therefore combined with imipramine; imipramine is given during the day and trimipramine at night. It is useful in depressive illnesses with marked insomnia. The dose is usually 50-100 mg taken at night.

Monoamine oxidase inhibitors (MAOIs)

MAOIs are potent antidepressant drugs, but their usefulness is limited both by their side-effects and by their interaction with sympathomimetics. MAOIs were originally thought to inhibit the enzyme which removes noradrenaline, serotonin and dopamine from the synaptic cleft, hence increasing the availability of these substances at the synapse. However, the pharmacological explanation for their activity is probably more complex. Some drugs that inhibit monoamine oxidase are nevertheless ineffective in depression.

Clinical uses

The role of MAOIs in clinical practice is controversial. In endogenous or psychotic depressive illness there is no doubt that the drugs of first choice are the tricyclic or tetracyclic group of antidepressants. If these fail after a therapeutic trial at an adequate dosage most clinicians would then use ECT and not the MAOI group of drugs. The MAOIs tend to be effective in depressive illnesses characterised by neurotic features, particularly anxiety, especially if endogenous features are absent. These are sometimes referred to as the atypical depressions and tend to be unresponsive to tricyclic antidepressants. MAOIs are also used to treat agoraphobia and social phobias.

Side-effects and interactions

MAOIs sometimes produce insomnia, dizziness due to postural hypotension, excitement, tremulousness and ankle oedema due to fluid retention. Anticholinergic side-effects are common, and in men delayed ejaculation sometimes occurs. The hydrazine group, which includes all the MAOIs currently in use other than tranylcypromine, may cause hepatocellular damage with jaundice. This is rare except in patients with alcoholism. Dependence occurs with tranylcypromine perhaps less than would be expected from its amphetamine-like structure.

When taken in conjunction with sympathomimetics, MAOIs may cause a hypertensive crisis. Any food subject to bacterial decomposition may contain pressor amines, as do many cough medicines and other remedies for colds. Foods to be avoided are those that contain tyramine, including cheese, pickled herring, seasoned game, Bovril, Oxo, Marmite and broad beans. Chianti wine also contains tyramine as do some Canadian beers. Before these dietary restrictions were imposed many patients ate these foods but only a few seemed to develop disastrous hypertensive crises. Patients must be given detailed instructions about their diet and always carry a card explaining that they are taking MAOIs. This enables other doctors and dentists to avoid prescribing drugs which may cause dangerous interactions. Such drugs include other antidepressants, narcotic analgesics such as pethidine, and CNS depressants such as the barbiturates and anti-parkinsonian drugs. Some psychiatrists have claimed that it is safe to combine MAOIs and tricyclic antidepressants in the treatment of severe depression. This is not recommended. In fact a gap of two weeks is advised when changing a patient from a tricyclic antidepressant to an MAOI or vice versa.

Individual MAOIs

The drugs described below are the most commonly used MAOIs.

Phenelzine

This is a hydrazine MAOI. The interactions and side-effects noted above do occur, but in normal doses a hypertensive reaction with food is rare. Phenelzine has a sedative action and is therefore useful in the treatment of anxiety associated with atypical depression. The dose is 30-60 mg daily in divided doses.

Isocarboxazid

This appears to be less potent than phenelzine and less likely to produce unwanted side-effects. The dose is 20-30 mg daily in divided doses.

Tranylcypromine

This is a non-hydrazine MAOI structurally related to amphetamines. It has a stimulant and euphoriant effect and seems to act quickly, sometimes quite dramatically. It is prone to produce dependence. The clinicial impression is that it is more potent than other MAOIs but also more likely to lead to a hypertensive crisis if taken with foods containing tyramine. The dose is 10-30 mg daily in divided doses.

A preparation containing both tranylcypromine and trifluoperazine is available. Some patients seem to do well on this mixture of antidepressant and sedative, but the evidence for its usefulness is limited.

Other antidepressants

A variety of other drugs are used in the treatment of depression. These include L-tryptophan, lithium, both the minor and major tranquillisers and the psychostimulants.

L-tryptophan

L-tryptophan is a precursor of serotonin. There is some evidence that it has an antidepressant action in its own right, but it is usually used as an adjunct to another antidepressant drug, such as an MAOI or the tricyclic clomipramine. The usual dose is 1 gram three times a day.

Lithium

The use of lithium in affective disorders is discussed in detail below, but there is evidence that it has antidepressant properties as well as protecting against recurrent affective swings. It is therefore occasionally useful in those patients who do not appear to respond to other antidepressants.

Tranquillisers

Both minor tranquillisers, such as diazepam and chlordiazepoxide, and major tranquillisers, such as chlorpromazine, are sometimes used in the treatment of depression. Overall they are probably more effective in decreasing anxiety and agitation than relieving depressed mood, but there is some evidence that chlorpromazine and flupenthixol in low doses have antidepressant properties. In most cases a sedative antidepressant, such as amitriptyline, is probably as effective as the minor tranquillisers in relieving anxiety.

Psychostimulant drugs

Amphetamine, dextroamphetamine and methylamphetamine have all been used to relieve depression, but they are hardly ever prescribed for this condition now because of the danger of psychological dependence. Their rapid action also makes them popular drugs of misuse, and this aspect is discussed further on p. 394. They are occasionally used in the treatment of narcolepsy and the hyperkinetic sydrome in children.

DRUGS USED IN MANIC-DEPRESSIVE ILLNESS

The drugs used in the treatment of the depressive episodes of a manic-depressive psychosis have been described above. In the manic episodes antipsychotic drugs such as chlorpromazine, haloperidol and pimozide are used to control the acute symptoms and calm the patient. They are discussed on p. 613. Two further drugs, lithium and carbamazepine, require further mention.

Lithium

One of the most significant psychopharmacological advances in the treatment of manic-depressive illness over recent years has been the introduction of lithium therapy. Its actions and clinical use have been reviewed by Johnson (1980).

Lithium has widespread effects in the body. Many of its actions depend on its concentration. Fortunately its psychological effects are achieved at relatively low plasma levels. High plasma levels result in severe toxic effects, so all patients on lithium must have their plasma levels regularly monitored. It is unclear which action of lithium is important for its psychological effects. It replaces sodium and potassium in the cells, acts on cyclic adenosine monophosphate (cAMP), interferes with carbohydrate metabolism and alters endocrine function. It is excreted by the kidney.

Clinical uses

Lithium carbonate is used in the prevention of recurrent attacks of mania, unipolar depression, and bipolar manic-depressive illness. Occasionally it is useful in the control of acute mania and aggressive outbursts in patients with mental handicap. About two-thirds of patients with manic or manic-depressive illness will improve considerably with lithium. Lithium is of most use in the prevention of bipolar manic-depressive illness.

There are no absolute indications for starting lithium therapy in manic-depressive illness. Most psychiatrists agree that before it is used the patient should have had at least two clear episodes of the illness within a period of two years.

Before lithium treatment is begun, an initial screening should be made of electrolyte levels, creatinine clearance and thyroid function. This is because lithium can cause renal impairment and decreased thyroid function. Lithium should be avoided in early pregnancy because of the increased incidence of congenital malformations in the foetus; if possible it should also be avoided in late pregnancy and the puerperium because it can produce a hypotonic infant and is excreted in the breast milk.

The plasma level of lithium required for effective prophylaxis is uncertain and probably varies from patient to patient. A level between 0.4 to 1.0 mmol/l is usually recommended. The blood level at which toxic symptoms occur also varies from patient to patient, but early signs of toxicity may occur at levels above 1.4 mmol/l. A typical initial dosage, giving an appropriate plasma level, is lithium carbonate orally 800 mg at night, but this may have to be increased. To start with the blood level should be checked once a week, but once the level is stabilised, this need be done only once every two to three months. Blood should be taken at a regular time after the ingestion of lithium, shortly before the next dose is due. This is because lithium is rapidly absorbed, its level rising quickly initially and then falling equally rapidly before decreasing more slowly to a basal level. It is this basal level, just before the next dose, that is most useful in deciding the appropriate dosage.

Side-effects and interactions

Early and transient side-effects include nausea, diarrhoea and fine tremor. These do not contraindicate the continued use of lithium as they tend to diminish after a week or so or only occur as a result of a transient high level following a single dose. Other side-effects only occur after taking lithium for a few months on a regular basis. These include tremor, polyuria and polydypsia, and considerable weight gain. The excessive thirst results from the kidney becoming insensitive to antidiuretic hormone. This is reversible. The cause of the weight gain is less certain but may be a result of the patient drinking high calorific fluids in order to quench his thirst. Hypothyroidism occurs in a small percentage of patients taking lithium for long periods. This either requires the cessation of lithium treatment or the administration of thyroxine. Occasionally the hypothyroidism recovers spontaneously. Psoriasis can be markedly exacerbated by lithium.

It is essential to warn patients of the signs of lithium toxicity. These are the onset of a fine tremor, almost like an intention tremor, pronounced somnolence, vertigo and dysarthria, nausea, diarrhoea and vomiting. Epileptic fits and coma may also occur, in which case lithium should be stopped at once and a plasma lithium estimation obtained urgently.

As lithium is excreted by the kidney, it should not be used in patients with impaired renal function. Furthermore urinary tract infection or diuretics, both of which interfere with renal function, will markedly elevate the plasma lithium level and result in toxicity. Caution must therefore be exercised if the patient is likely to become dehydrated, either as a result of diuretic therapy or as a result of extreme sweating in hot climates.

Lithium therapy requires a cooperative patient and adequate resources for rapid and efficient monitoring of his clinical and biochemical state. Given this, the successful prophylaxis of such a severe psychiatric illness as recurrent affective disorder is gratifying.

Carbamazepine

Recently carbamazepine has been tried in the prophylaxis of manic-depressive illness (Nolen 1983). In general it is only used in those patients who fail to respond to lithium and as an adjunct to lithium therapy. Patients with a rapidly cycling illness, i.e. four significant mood changes in one year, may respond best. The dose is gradually increased from 200 mg daily to give a plasma level of 4-12 mg/l. Neurotoxic effects such as confusion, disorientation and ataxia may occur, especially in patients treated with both drugs simultaneously.

Other anti-epileptic drugs such as sodium valproate have also been tried in the treatment of manic-depressive illness but with limited success.

ANTIPSYCHOTIC DRUGS

As described in Chapter 48, the discovery of the antipsychotic effects of chlorpromazine in the 1950s led to the development of a variety of drugs capable of controlling psychotic symptoms, especially schizophrenia and mania. These antipsychotic drugs are also called neuroleptics or major tranquillisers. They can be classified, according to their chemical structure, in three main groups: the *phenothiazines*, the *thioxanthenes* and the *butyrophenones*. All these drugs block the dopamine receptors at the synapses in the brain, especially in the mesolimbic, nigrostriatal, medullary and hypothalamic-pituitary pathways. As discussed in Chapter 20 (p. 238), the discovery that all the drugs which control the acute symptoms of schizophrenia are dopamine antagonists has given rise to the hypothesis that schizophrenia might be due to increased dopamine activity in one or more of the dopaminergic pathways in the brain – the dopamine hypothesis. There is so far insufficient evidence to confirm this theory, but there is no doubt that the antipsychotic action of the drugs used in the treatment of schizophrenia is closely correlated with their ability to block dopamine receptors.

The action of the various drugs in the *phenothiazine* group at each of the dopaminergic sites varies according to modifications in the side-chain on the phenothiazine nucleus. Those with an aliphatic side-chain, e.g. chlorpromazine and promazine, have strong hypnotic properties. Those with a piperazine side-chain, e.g. trifluoperazine and fluphenazine, are less sedative and have fewer autonomic side-effects but are more prone to produce extrapyramidal side-effects. Those with a piperidine side-chain, e.g. thioridazine, have fewer side-effects but can cause pigmentary retinopathy when used in high doses.

Other dopaminergic sites, such as the medullary pathways, account for the anti-emetic effect of the phenothiazines. They also block the inhibition of prolactin release in the hypothalamic-pituitary pathway, and hence produce hyperprolactinaemia. Measurement of the serum prolactin has been used in an attempt to assess the degree of dopamine blockade. While it may correlate with the plasma levels of the phenothiazine drugs it does not reflect the symptom response in schizophrenia.

The *thioxanthenes*, e.g. flupenthixol and clopenthixol, are chemically related to the phenothiazines but extrapyramidal side-effects are less common.

The *butyrophenones* differ from the phenothiazines in their chemical structure although their clinical effects are similar. Haloperidol is most commonly used. Overall the butyrophenones have strong antipsychotic but fewer sedative effects. Extrapyramidal side-effects are common.

Individual drugs

Chlorpromazine

This was the original drug used to control psychotic symptoms, and it is still widely used especially in the treatment of schizophrenia. It is more sedative than some other phenothiazines and is therefore particularly useful in the treatment of excited schizophrenic patients. The drug can be given as a syrup, tablet or intramuscular preparation. The initial dosage varies between 100-200 mg three times a day, although in acute schizophrenia the dose may be built up to 1,000 or even, exceptionally, 2,000 mg a day to control the symtoms. The side-effects, including extrapyramidal effects, are described in Chapter 20 (p. 245).

Trifluoperazine

This is related to chlorpromazine but is less sedative and has fewer anticholinergic effects. However, it has a greater tendency to produce extrapyramidal side-effects than chlorpromazine. It is particularly useful in the treatment of paranoid symptoms. The dose is 5-20 mg three times daily for control of psychotic symptoms. It is used for oral maintenance therapy in schizophrenia, especially as a slow release preparation once daily by mouth, e.g. trifluoperazine spansule 15 mg at night.

Thioridazine

This resembles chlorpromazine but has more sedative properties and anticholinergic effects. It is therefore also used as a sedative. In doses above 500 mg a day pigmentary retinopathy with loss of vision may occur. The usual dose for control of psychotic symptoms is 100-150 mg three times daily.

Promazine

In clinical practice promazine appears to have limited antipsychotic activity, but its sedative properties make it valuable in controlling agitation, especially in the elderly. The dose is 25-100 mg daily.

Sulpiride

This drug has only recently been used in the UK, although it has been used elsewhere for several years as both an antidepressant and an antipsychotic. It is effective in treating the acute symptoms of schizophrenia. It also has a stimulant effect, and may therefore be useful in the treatment of withdrawn, apathetic patients with negative symptoms of chronic schizophrenia. Occasionally it can precipitate excitement, insomnia and restlessness. The usual dose is 400-800 mg daily.

Pimozide

This is an antipsychotic of the diphenyl butyl-piperidine series. It is occasionally used in the treatment of acute and chronic schizophrenia but is thought to be particularly useful in monosymptomatic delusional states and mania. The dose is 2-20 mg once daily.

Haloperidol

This drug, a butyrophenone, is useful in the management of acutely disturbed schizophrenic and manic patients. It is also used in the treatment of the Gilles de la Tourette syndrome (see p. 480). Its rapid action, which results from the speed with which the drug is absorbed from the gastrointestinal tract, is particularly useful. Extrapyramidal side-effects are common, and can occur soon after starting treatment. It can also produce drowsiness and anticholinergic side-effects, and tends to produce depressive symptoms if continued for long periods as maintenance therapy. The dose is usually 3-30 mg daily in divided doses. For control of acute symptoms in mania 5-10 mg can be given intramuscularly.

Benperidol

This is a butyrophenone related to haloperidol. It has been used to reduce excessive sexual drive.

Depot preparations

There is no doubt that the use of long-acting injectable drugs in schizophrenia is useful in the management of many patients, especially those whose illness makes it difficult for them to cooperate fully with oral medication. Injections are usually given once a fortnight either in the patient's home or in an outpatient clinic. This provides an opportunity to monitor each patient's progress and to involve medical, social or other help when necessary. Pharmacotherapy can thus be combined with psychological support.

The commonly used long-acting injectable preparations are fluphenazine decanoate, flupenthixol decanoate and zuclopenthixol decanoate.

Fluphenazine decanoate

An initial test dose of 12.5 mg intramuscularly is given to ensure that the patient is not unduly sensitive, particularly to the extrapyramidal effects of the drug. Thereafter, 25 mg fortnightly is usually the lowest dose to prevent re-emergence of psychotic symptoms. The dose may be increased gradually to 100 mg fortnightly if psychotic symptoms persist. Side-effects are similar to those of the phenothiazines.

Flupenthixol decanoate

This drug is useful as an antidepressant in low doses (see p. 609) as it has an activating effect. In higher doses it is effective against psychotic symptoms. As a result of these two actions it is useful in the treatment of schizophrenic patients who are depressed, retarded, apathetic and withdrawn. An initial test dose of 20 mg intramuscularly is commonly followed by a maintenance dose of 40 mg fortnightly. Higher doses of 100-200 mg are occasionally necessary. Side-effects are similar to those of the phenothiazines.

Zuclopenthixol decanoate

This injectable long-acting preparation resembles flupenthixol but it is more sedative and therefore of greater use in overactive, aggressive schizophrenic patients. 200-400 mg may be given intramuscularly every fortnight, following a test dose of 100 mg.

*

It may well be asked why so many different drugs, all somewhat similar, are used in the treatment of schizophrenia. In the long-term management of a patient, however, a change of medication is often necessary, not only because of pharmacological indications and side-effects caused by one or other drug but also because the patient may periodically become disenchanted with a particular preparation and request a change.

Side-effects

We have referred frequently to the side-effects of antipsychotic drugs. Those of the phenothiazines have been described in detail in Chapter 20 (pp. 245-7). The side-effects of other antipsychotic drugs are very similar, so only a few general comments need be made here.

The most important side-effects of the antipsychotic drugs are their extrapyramidal effects. Those that can occur early in treatment are *Parkinsonian symptoms, acute dystonia* and *akathisia*. Their clinical features and treatment are described on p. 246. *Tardive dyskinesia* develops considerably later, usually during long-term maintenance therapy. It is described more fully on p. 246. Tardive dyskinesia is particularly serious as it may not clear up even when the drug is discontinued so that this distressing disorder may persist in about half the cases. It must therefore be stressed that long-term treatment with antipsychotic drugs, especially in high dosage, should only be undertaken if essential.

The neuroleptic malignant syndrome

This is a very rare but potentially fatal syndrome which can occur during treatment with neuroleptic drugs, usually during the course of a schizophrenic illness. The condition has been reviewed by Kellam (1987). The annual incidence among patients who have been treated with neuroleptics is still unclear as figures from different studies vary widely. Clinical descriptions of fulminating illnesses resembling this syndrome were recorded in schizophrenia, especially of the catatonic variety, and in mania long before the advent of neuroleptic medication. None the less the association between psychotropic drug therapy and the syndrome seems to be established. The syndrome consists of diffuse rigidity of the muscles with cogwheeling and waxy flexibility. Consciousness is often impaired but most significantly there is pyrexia, sweating, tachycardia and a fall in blood pressure. Fatalities are usually due to hyperpyrexia, unless they follow bronchopneumonia or some other complication. Treatment needs to be urgently instituted with the cessation of neuroleptic medication and the use of bromocriptine and dantrolene, a muscle relaxant, as described by Abbott and Loizou (1986). Benzodiazepines may be of use occasionally.

FURTHER READING

Crammer, J., Barraclough, B. and Heine, B. (1982). *The Use of Drugs in Psychiatry*, 2nd ed. Gaskell, London.

Iverson, S.D. (1985). *Psychopharmacology: recent advances and future prospects.* OUP, Oxford.

Silverstone, T. and Turner, P. (1982). *Drug Treatment in Psychiatry*, 3rd ed. Routledge & Kegan Paul, London.

Tyrer, P.J. (1982). *Drugs in Psychiatric Practice*. Butterworths, London.

50

Electroconvulsive Therapy

The concept of convulsive therapy owes a great deal to von Meduna (1937) of Budapest. In 1933, in the belief that schizophrenia and epilepsy were mutually antagonistic, he induced fits artificially in his patients by injecting camphor preparations. Some success led him to do the same with depressives, who did better. It is now known that schizophrenia and epilepsy are not in fact antagonistic; the belief was based on a statistical artefact: both conditions are rare, so the occurrence of both in one patient is even rarer. Further, although the results in depression were good, the camphor method was risky and impractical and soon superseded by the electrical method of inducing fits.

Electroconvulsive therapy (ECT) was introduced by Cerletti and Bini (1938); they designed a machine with electrodes that were placed on either side of the head in the posterior frontal regions; the passage of the current between them evoked a major convulsion. This could be distressing and dangerous; fractures, for example, were not uncommon. Nowadays, an anaesthetist gives a short-acting anaesthetic and a muscle relaxant before treatment. Oxygen is required while the subsequent respiratory paralysis lasts. The patient recovers consciousness in a few minutes but may be confused and forgetful for several hours afterwards. Mild memory deficits may persist for three or four weeks after a course of ECT, but it is extremely rare for memory impairment to last for longer than this. An average course of ECT consists of 6-12 treatments given twice weekly. It is now given unilaterally, i.e. with both electrodes placed over the non-dominant hemisphere. Unilateral ECT is as effective as bilateral ECT in the treatment of depression, and there are fewer adverse effects on memory.

ECT is of proven value in depressive illness, and its risks are now negligible with the above procedures. It is still occasionally used to treat catatonic schizophrenia, but this is rare since the advent of psychotropic drugs. Though normally used for inpatients, ECT is occasionally given on an outpatient basis; this is sometimes difficult to arrange unless relatives or friends are available. Many people are afraid of the treatment and it is therefore used only where other treatments such as antidepressant drugs have failed, or where a rapid response is required. For example, if a patient is severely psychotic or at risk of suicide or serious self-neglect,

ECT may be effective after two treatments whereas antidepressant drugs often take two weeks before an effect is seen.

The mode of action of ECT is still uncertain, but it is believed that, as with antidepressant drugs (p. 604), it acts on the central amine transmission system, probably in the diencephalon. ECT may increase the sensitivity of post-synaptic amine receptors.

FURTHER READING

Fink, M. (1979). *Convulsive Therapy: theory and practice*. Raven Press, New York.

Fraser, M. (1982). *ECT: a clinical guide*, John Wiley, Chichester.

Kendell, R.E. (1982). 'The present status of electroconvulsive therapy'. *Brit. J. Psychiat.* 139, 265-283.

Pippard, J. and Ellam, L. (1981). *Electroconvulsive treatment in Great Britain, 1980*. A report to the Royal College of Psychiatrists. Gaskell, London.

51

Psychosurgery

The surgical treatment of psychiatric illness developed from the observation in 1935 that bilateral ablation of the frontal association areas of chimpanzees led to a reduction in their experimentally induced 'temper tantrums'. The Portuguese neuropsychiatrist Egas Moniz (1936) then performed over a hundred similar operations on people suffering from psychiatric illness, most of whom had schizophrenia. The operation became known as *frontal leucotomy*. Since then it has been refined and no longer severs large areas of the frontal lobe from its connections with the rest of the brain. Stereotactic procedures give greater accuracy and minimise destruction of brain tissue; these procedures either destroy small areas of the orbito-frontal region (*stereotactic subcordate tractotomy*), or ablate part of the cingulum and the ventro-medial quadrant of the frontal lobe (*stereotactic limbic leucotomy*). The lesions are made either by heat coagulation or, more usually, by radioactive yttrium implants.

The indications for psychosurgery are said to be intractable depressive illness, refractory obsessional illness, severe anxiety states and some forms of chronic schizophrenia with increased tension (Mitchell-Heggs *et al.* 1976). However, only those patients who have failed to respond to persistent treatment with drugs, ECT, rehabilitation and other therapies are nowadays considered for such irreversible procedures. Adverse effects such as apathy, weight-gain, epilepsy and personality changes such as disinhibition and fatuous affect occur, but these are less common since the stereotactic procedures were introduced.

Before the 1970s there were no reliable figures as to the number of psychosurgical operations carried out in the UK. During the three-year period 1974 to 1976, 431 neurosurgical operations for psychological disorder were performed in England and Wales (Barraclough and Mitchell-Heggs 1978). The number has probably diminished considerably since. Now that psychosurgery is limited by the terms of the Mental Health Act 1983 (see p. 707), the number performed is likely to become fewer and fewer.

FURTHER READING

Bartlett, J., Bridges, P. and Kelly, D. (1981) 'Contemporary indications for psychosurgery'. *Brit. J. Psychiat.* 138, 507-511.

52

Social Therapy

We have described the various methods of psychotherapy conducted in an individual, marital, family or small group setting. Each individual is, however, also influenced by the wider social network to which he belongs, for example, the institution in which he works. Sociologists, systems theorists, psychoanalysts and psychologists have all contributed to our understanding of the structure and function of such institutions, how they affect the individuals within them, and how in turn the individual members influence the institution as a whole.

Here we are concerned only with the social setting in which psychiatrically ill and psychologically disturbed patients are treated. This may be a specialised hospital for, say, psychopaths or offenders, a psychiatric unit in a district general hospital, a mental hospital, an inpatient ward, a day hospital, a hostel or a sheltered workshop for psychiatric patients in the community.

TERMINOLOGY

It is important to distinguish between three terms often used when considering the treatment of psychiatric patients in one or other of these social settings: social therapy, therapeutic milieu and therapeutic community. The term *social therapy* or sociotherapy is applied in a wide sense to all forms of therapy that specifically rely on the use of the social setting in which the patients are being treated: 'the use of the environment as a means of promoting desired change in clients' (Clark 1977). The term *therapeutic milieu* refers to the atmosphere and conditions that are needed in the social environment for it to have a therapeutic effect on the people within it. The term *therapeutic community* is best reserved for those usually relatively small psychiatric inpatient facilities or hostels specially set up and designed to provide social therapy for a selected group of patients. The concept of a therapeutic community was described by Main (1946) when considering the conditions necessary for effective treatment of psychoneurotic patients in an inpatient setting at the Cassel hospital in Richmond, London. It was later developed further by Maxwell Jones (1968) at the Belmont, since re-named the Henderson hospital for the treatment of antisocial psychopaths.

To some extent the concepts of social therapy, therapeutic milieu and therapeutic community have arisen out of the growing awareness that many of the traditional methods of treating psychiatric patients in mental hospitals could be anti-therapeutic (Goffman 1961). These included locked wards and a strict hierarchical demarcation between staff who were in authority and patients who were expected to do what they were told. The passive role of the patients often led to apathy and 'institutionalisation'. The introduction of open wards and a more egalitarian relationship between staff and patients, and especially the emphasis placed on open communication and shared responsibility, have all contributed to the concepts of social therapy and the use of therapeutic communities (see also p. 41).

MODERN PRACTICE

Since the 1950s, when therapeutic communities had many enthusiastic followers, their advantages and limitations have become clearer. Extremes of permissiveness and equality between staff and patients are now usually recognised as being as disadvantageous as the previous opposite extremes of authoritarianism and a strictly hierarchical structure. A therapeutic milieu is hard to establish and maintain in large psychiatric institutions with a rapidly changing population, and has been made more difficult by the present policy of early discharge of patients into the community. The presence of patients with very different needs also makes the methods of social therapy difficult to maintain in general psychiatric units. The methods described below are more appropriate to small therapeutic communities with a relatively slow turnover of patients and designed for selected groups, especially psychopaths and patients with other severe personality disorders, adolescents, drug addicts, alcoholics, offenders and some severely disturbed psychoneurotic patients requiring inpatient treatment.

Open communication and the sharing of responsibility between patients and staff are crucial. Large community meetings, held daily or several times a week, regular large and small groups all play an important role. The use of large groups, e.g. of all the patients and staff, has been described by Kreeger (1975). Crisis meetings are called in some units when an acute problem arises so that staff and patients can all take part in discovering the reasons for what has happened and deciding how to deal with it. In some therapeutic communities, such as the Henderson hospital, the selection of patients for admission is carried out by the newly referred patients being assessed in a group which includes not only a consultant psychiatrist and other members of staff but patients who have been in the unit for a few months. These 'senior' patients are thus given responsibility in decision-making, while new patients are given the opportunity to decide whether they wish to be treated in the unit. Separate meetings for the staff are needed to help them understand their own attitudes and reactions in what are often very stressful circumstances. Whiteley (1986) has described how at the Henderson hospital patients with personality disorders can be helped by an intensive inpatient treatment programme in which a personal psychotherapeutic experience is combined with the 'sociotherapeutic' experience of living in a highly structured social environment.

Attention must be paid to the boundaries between different professionals, between patients and staff and between the unit and the outside world. In order not to over-emphasise these distinctions, in most units the professional staff no longer wear uniforms. It is now recognised, however, that to deny all the differences between various professionals – doctors, nursing staff, social workers, psychologists, occupational therapists, etc. – and between patients and staff is unrealistic and unhelpful. Their different roles and expertise, the need to collaborate and not to put professional pride or envy before the needs of the community must be acknowledged. For example, if a patient suddenly becomes violent due to an acute psychotic episode it may be necessary for the medical and nursing staff to take responsibility. Problems caused by hierarchical differences, e.g. between senior and junior medical or nursing staff, must all be discussed at community meetings. At such meetings the chairman may be sometimes a senior patient, sometimes a member of the professional staff, so that responsibility can be shared. However, unrealistic egalitarianism and denial of real differences is counter-productive. In these and all other respects reality testing remains essential for the community to function and the patients to benefit.

It is equally important to be aware of interactions at the boundary between the unit itself and outside organisations, such as a larger hospital of which the unit may be a part, or the unit and its administration or the National Health Service. Problems within the unit are often blamed on some outside influence or vice versa; such issues need to be clearly faced by all concerned and dealt with as realistically as possible.

Social therapy continues to change. There is little doubt that it can be of considerable value in small specialised therapeutic communities. For example, recent follow-up studies of 28 inpatients at the Cassel hospital treated for severe psychoneurotic disorders have thrown light on the value of combining individual analytically oriented psychotherapy with an intensive inpatient therapeutic community regime (Denford *et al.* 1983; Rosser *et al.* 1986, 1987). The results showed that at the initial assessment interview the following characteristics could serve as predictors of a favourable outcome at discharge after nine months to two years, and at follow-up after five years: neurotic psychopathology, considerable depression, superior intelligence and minimal previous outpatient treatment. An adequate duration of therapy, up to two years, was another significant factor in determining a successful outcome at follow-up. Chronically depressed patients with borderline personality organisation (see p. 342) and of lesser intelligence responded less well to this inpatient regime.

Some of the concepts and methods included under the term therapeutic milieu have helped to create a better and more beneficial atmosphere in larger, less specialised psychiatric institutions, day hospitals and inpatient units. In any of these settings such methods can, of course, be used in conjunction with small group or individual psychotherapy.

FURTHER READING

Clark, D. (1977). 'The therapeutic community – review article.' *Brit. J. Psychiat.* 131, 553-564.

Jones, M. (1968). *Social Psychiatry in Practice: the idea of the therapeutic community*. Penguin, Harmondsworth.

Main, T.F. (1946). 'The hospital as a therapeutic institution'. *Bulletin, Menninger Clinic* 10, 66-70.

Whiteley, J.S. (1986). 'Sociotherapy and psychotherapy in the treatment of personality disorder: discussion paper'. *J. Roy. Soc. Med.* 79, 721-725.

53

Psychiatric Rehabilitation

DEFINITION AND SCOPE

No single word adequately sums up the endeavour to minimise the impairments of function resulting from mental illness, the social handicap which results from stigma and isolation, and the adverse personal reactions to disability such as low self-esteem, passivity and helplessness. Psychiatric *rehabilitation*, a term borrowed from physical medicine, is the most widely applicable; *treatment* sounds too specifically medical and interventionist: *care* too static and patronising. Terms such as *enablement* and *habilitation* are sometimes advocated, since they acknowledge that the patient may need to acquire skills that had not been developed even before the onset of illness. The more questionable *normalisation*, a term taken from a particular approach to mental handicap, has been adopted by some non-medical staff eager to avoid medical terminology.

At its worst, rehabilitation can be a euphemism for the inactivity or mechanical routine of neglected hospital back wards, or the inhumane turfing-out of unprepared long-term patients into inadequate 'community care'. At its most positive, however, it embraces a wide range of activities in a cooperative venture between hospital services (both in special units and more generally) and local community services concerned with minimising disability and promoting maximum independence and well-being of people with longer-term or relapsing mental disorders. These aims are pursued, if possible, in patients' own homes or in domestic-scale accommodation which provides the necessary minimum of personal support and as full as possible a range of opportunities for interesting and rewarding work, recreation and social intercourse. A central feature should be a clear and enduring commitment to people and families to help them articulate their wishes and achieve the best quality of life they can. The general practitioner, psychiatrist and other professionals involved in rehabilitation must be concerned with the total psychological, social and physical welfare of patients on an indefinite time-scale.

In about half the adult population under the age of sixty-five with such needs, the diagnosis is schizophrenia. Others suffer from affective psychoses and severe neurotic and personality disorders. A minority have organic brain disorders, problems of alcohol and drug dependence or minor degrees of mental handicap. The adverse effects of psychiatric illness are often complicated by multiple difficulties and social disadvantages.

There is very much more to a rehabilitation service than a lot of grand-sounding jargon and declarations of intent. Experience built up in progressive mental hospitals over recent decades, the pioneering example of a small number of innovative psychiatrists, and the research studies particularly of John Wing and his associates (Wing 1978) have enabled several essential principles and practices to be identified. These are summarised in a series of recommendations prepared by the Royal College of Psychiatrists in 1980 and described in greater detail in two more recent books (Wing and Morris 1981: Watts and Bennett 1983). In the USA an outline of aims and good practices is exemplified by the Community Support Programme (Tessler and Goldman 1982).

KEY COMPONENTS

Good rehabilitation practice should include the following:

(1) Methods of assessment, goal-setting, monitoring and evaluation.

(2) Techniques of treatment and therapy designed to enlist the patient's interest, promote his independence and autonomy and improve his level of social functioning.

(3) The provision of social and physical environments in which to promote these techniques and provide appropriately supportive accommodation, occupation and recreation.

(4) Systems of staff deployment, coordination and multidisciplinary management which can effectively knit together the skills of staff of many disciplines, services and community agencies, and direct them to meet the needs of patients, their families and the community.

The overall aim is to help the patient function at the best level of which he is capable. To achieve this it will be necessary to seek changes in the patient or the environment, or usually in both. The governing principles of the exercise, as Babiker (1987) succinctly puts it, are those of common sense and sound psychiatric practice.

ASSESSMENT

As a prelude to rehabilitation, clinical assessment needs to be wider in scope than the standard psychiatric history and mental state. It should comprise a detailed practical review of the patient's social functioning throughout the 24-hour day, in the context of a comprehensive picture of his past life, achievements and social environment. Aspects of present function can be noted under such headings as capacity for self-care and independence, communication and interaction with others, occupational ability and motivation, use of leisure time, ability to handle money or use public amenities, such as transport or the telephone, and physical health.

It is especially important to identify personal preferences and positive strengths as well as lost or undeveloped potential interests and abilities. The standard psychiatric history and formulation tends too often to be a catalogue of negative features, unduly weighted towards morbidity rather than the positive elements upon which progress can be built. Simple observations that Mr A, for example, is kind to very handicapped people and is good with his hands, Mrs B enjoys activities in the open air and likes bus journeys, Miss C enjoys singing and has a sister who would like to see more of her if travel was easier, and Mr D likes helping in the kitchen and is popular with staff, can all be important in the assessment.

Problem areas can be noted as *psychological*, such as enduring or intermittent symptoms and signs of illness, difficulties with motivation or cooperation, disabilities in learning or acquiring new skills; *social*, such as antisocial elements of behaviour, lack of good family relationships and other social adversity such as unemployment; and *physical*, including not only physical illness, but other aspects of physical health such as adverse effects of medication, excessive drinking or smoking, poor dentition, deficits of eyesight and hearing, inadequate nutrition, etc. A variety of more or less systematic methods of recording and scoring these observations have been used in rehabilitation units and community teams, and there are also standardised scales such as Baker and Hall's REHAB (1983).

Two points liable to be overlooked require special emphasis. First, a person's functioning in one situation is commonly not accurately predictive of his functioning in another. If an assessment is to be made, say, of a patient's likely capacity to live outside hospital, it should be done in an environment which resembles most closely the new one rather than the old. Secondly, people with long-term mental illness are much less static in their functioning than is commonly believed. Major fluctuations of well-being and mental state are common and need to be allowed for as far as possible in the planning and provision of services: someone who is capable and independent one day may be severely disordered and in need of protective care the next, and vice versa. The word 'chronic' is therefore often best avoided, since it may carry negative connotations of permanence and stasis which are quite misleading, particularly as most long-term mental disorders, unlike most chronic physical impairments, are not necessarily associated with irreversible tissue damage. The limits of possible change for the better are therefore often not known. In practice it may be difficult to distinguish between limitations of function that are an intrinsic product of the illness, the adverse effects of 'institutionalisation' (often today wrongly blamed as the sole cause of problems) and personality vulnerabilities predating the onset of illness or admission to hospital. A realistic approach which takes things as they are and looks for achievable steps forward is likely to be more beneficial than one based on theories about causes or on unproven predictions.

Goal-setting

The initial assessment of problems and positive strengths enables *targets* or *goals* for rehabilitative work with the patient to be identified. These vary from the short term, e.g. to help the patient get up for breakfast rather than lie in bed, to the long term, e.g. to leave hospital or to work in open employment or live independently in a flat. The active cooperation of the patient and his family should be sought and enlisted in identifying and working towards these goals.

The process of assessment is continuing and open-ended, aiming towards increasing depth of understanding of the patient's history, disabilities, needs, qualities and potential, and the formulation and review of an evolving series of goals and objectives. Methods of record-keeping should aim to provide a continuity of cumulative knowledge which can survive frequent changes in staff personnel.

Monitoring and evaluation

These are two essential aspects of assessment over time. They apply not only to work with the individual patient and his family but also to the assessment of the work of the rehabilitation services as a whole.

Monitoring is an assessment of the extent to which identified goals for the individual and the service are being met. For the individual patient, the task requires good coordination of multidisciplinary team effort and a clear identification of roles and responsibilities for each member of the staff team and for associated agencies who may need to be involved. Services as a whole still have a long way to go in developing methods of keeping track of patients living outside hospital, many of whom slip through the large gaps in the usually very incomplete network of services, so that contact is broken, therapeutic efforts are interrupted and their benefits quickly lost. Computerised case registers have provided valuable statistical information for research purposes. There is a need now for new sorts of registers to provide a continuing practical system of monitoring and review of individual patients, with a capacity to prompt the services to action when contact is interrupted. Low-cost systems of this kind are now feasible.

Evaluation is the task of assessing the effectiveness of services in terms of their discernible benefit in relation to improved functioning, satisfaction to users and their families, the health-care needs of the community and the expenditure incurred. It tends to be much easier to demand than to measure. The vulnerability of mentally ill people to being made the object of other peoples' fanciful notions of what should be done with them and the high cost of providing the facilities and staff to enable them to function as independently as possible make it essential to assess outcome, value and cost-effectiveness.

METHODS OF REHABILITATION

There is a very wide range of therapeutic methods.

Individual psychological therapies

These range from personal guidance, education and support in dealing with practical aspects of daily living to more intensive kinds of psychotherapeutic work aimed at helping patients resolve conflicts and develop positive aspects of their personality in relationships with other people. A common practice is the identification of a *keyworker* among the staff team who will offer a consistent focus of personal support to the individual patient and his family over an appropriate period.

Group methods

These mobilise the capacities of patients to work towards shared goals and to provide mutual support. They include discussion groups, programmes for improving social skills, outings and other activities. Fostering a sense of group identity can be an important part of the preparatory work needed for patients moving out of hospital to, say, a shared hostel or group home.

Family therapy

This may help to reduce relapses, especially in schizophrenic patients living at home (see p. 250).

Structured behavioural programmes

These programmes, often designed and monitored by psychologists, use techniques of providing rewards, extra privileges and approval in a systematic and measurable way. They can be particularly helpful in the earlier phases of trying to improve patients' activity and motivation and in reducing the incidence of difficult and unacceptable behaviours. The *token economy* approach (see p. 588) whereby patients showing desirable behaviour earn tokens which can be exchanged for privileges or comforts such as sweets or cigarettes, has tended to give way to more individually-designed methods better able to achieve results which can be sustained in the world outside the institution. Overall, it is vital to achieve a flexible balance between directive and non-directive techniques which can adapt to changing circumstances.

Use of drugs

Drug therapy, providing (1) optimal control of symptoms, (2) protection where possible from relapse and (3) minimal occurrence of side-effects, is likely to be a crucial part of many therapeutic plans. Drug response and dosage must be very carefully assessed and intensive efforts made to gain the patient's cooperation. The importance of this aspect of the total therapy may be underestimated by non-medical staff who, in the mistaken belief that drugs are the cause of the patient's problems, may press for discontinuation; this may eventually precipitate a relapse and may even lead to the patient being rejected when a florid psychosis ensues. Good medicinal treatment should be seen as just one necessary but minimally obtrusive factor in helping the patient to attain an improved quality of life.

Occupational and work therapies

It has been said that even if nobody had to work to earn a living, work would still be valuable as a treatment for schizophrenia and other enduring mental disorders. Such hyperbole acknowledges the immense value of structured and rewarding activity to counter the apathy, social withdrawal and personal disorganisation which are among the most damaging consequences of severe mental illness. Work provides a purposeful structure for pacing daytime activity, a sense of self-respect, usefulness and normality as well as tangible reward. This still applies even though widespread unemployment and the increasing emphasis on self-fulfilment and rights to leisure-time have combined to diminish regard for the work ethic.

Industrial therapy has had a particularly important role in the development of rehabilitation practice in progressive mental hospitals. Their workshops and gardens, linking in with imaginative schemes and opportunities developed outside hospital, such as in the Industrial Therapy Organisation developed by Early in Bristol, became an essential avenue of return to greater independence. Now that the chances of people finding open employment after discharge from hospital have greatly diminished, the hospital workshops still have a valuable role in providing sheltered work opportunities for those who are well enough to attend for the day from accommodation outside the hospital, especially when local alternatives are not yet available.

Other forms of *occupational therapy* (see Chapter 60) have gained increasing importance and now include a wide range of techniques to improve domestic and social skills, and capacities for leisure activities. Special techniques of art, music and drama therapy may be valuable for some patients. Education to improve literacy, knowledge of welfare benefits and entitlements, civil rights, and community services and amenities can be helpful.

ACCOMMODATION AND DAY ACTIVITIES

None of these therapeutic endeavours can flourish without the provision of appropriate settings and social environments. The emphasis today is on:

(1) Small-scale domestic settings as similar as possible to an ordinary house.
(2) Ready access to family members and ordinary community services, to minimise geographical isolation and stigma.

As the move to close mental hospitals has gathered momentum, expectations in some areas have rapidly risen, with increasing reluctance by social services and health authority planners to provide anything that smacks of institutional care. Much debate continues about how far this process can be taken if the most disabled and disordered patients are to live outside hospital without a return to destitution or exploitation by private landlords. The problem is particularly acute in metropolitan areas where suitably spacious sites which allow patients the benefits of ordinary domestic living and access to community facilities, as well as adequate amounts of personal space apart from each other, can be hard to find. Earlier developments such as the provision of small housing projects in the hospital grounds, as illustrated by the pioneering 'hospital-hostel' at the Maudsley hospital (Wykes 1982), may now be seen as too institutional and hospital-orientated a model for future planning. If expectations become too high, however, there is a risk of rejecting the more difficult and disabled patient. The cynic may then remark that only a normal person will last any length of time in some of the new mental health facilities, whose staff may be looking for the untroublesome users best able to meet their own needs.

It is easier to acknowledge than to ensure that a wide variety of different settings is available to provide for different needs and preferences; these range from independent accommodation with mobile support staff from a community resource centre available in a crisis, through group homes, supported housing schemes in small hostels, supervised adult foster-care with families, to more staff-intensive settings and even specialised hospital units capable of providing for the most disabled or for more difficult patients whose behaviour is socially disruptive. Residents should be able to move between different levels of care as their needs alter over time.

The need for flexible and interlinked options is just as necessary in the provision of day-care; many different attractive models and facilities now exist but provisions are still often inadequate and patchy, with better facilities for the physically handicapped than for people with a background of mental illness. With regard to settings for promoting work opportunities outside hospital, for instance, the Royal College of Psychiatrists Working Party (1980) listed the following existing services in addition to facilities provided by voluntary organisations or non-profit-making companies:

Local authority day centres
Local authority rehabilitation and
  assessment centres
Industrial therapy organisations
Community-based industrial units
Sheltered industrial groups

Employment rehabilitation centres
Skill centres
Residential training colleges
Colleges of further education
Sheltered workshops including
  Remploy factories

The local authority's Disablement Resettlement Officer (DRO) can provide advice and introduction to local opportunities. Job Clubs and Community Programmes may provide support in job-hunting or work experience for those not too disabled.

ORGANISATION OF SERVICES

The organisation of rehabilitation services is crucial to good management. It includes making optimum provisions for the individual patient and his family, the coordination of many professional disciplines and service agencies, and an overall responsiveness to community needs and opportunities. A flexible range of residential, daytime and 'out-of-hours' facilities is required to encourage the patient to progress at his own optimum pace towards greater independence. Staff must be ready to intervene actively at times of crisis or relapse, as well as providing continuing supervision and review. No formula, however, can substitute for the essential requirements of strong team leadership and cohesion backed by high-level interest from senior administrators and resource allocators in the relevant services; these include the National Health Service, social services, other government agencies such as the Manpower Services Commission and voluntary organisations. Equally important is the ability to attract and retain enthusiastic and well-trained staff who are eager to learn.

FURTHER READING

Babiker, I.E. (1987). 'Rehabilitation in psychiatry'. *Brit. J. Hosp. Med.* 38, 112-114.
Baker, R. and Hall, J. (1983). *REHAB*. Vine Publications, Aberdeen.
Watts, F.N. and Bennett, D.H. (eds) (1983). *Theory and Practice of Psychiatric Rehabilitation*. John Wiley, Chichester.
Wing, J.K. and Morris, B. (eds) (1981). *Handbook of Psychiatric Rehabilitation Practice*. OUP, Oxford.

54

Psychiatric Emergencies

Some patients suffer from behavioural and mental state changes severe enough to constitute a psychiatric emergency:

(1) The suicidal patient.
(2) The violent patient.
(3) The intoxicated patient.
(4) The acutely anxious patient.

As a general rule it is the behaviour of the patient which requires emergency management. Only then can the mental changes underlying the behavioural change be fully assessed and treated.

THE SUICIDAL PATIENT

All patients who are depressed, threaten suicide or have committed an act of self-harm must be assessed for suicide risk. (See Table 54.1)

Table 54.1. Factors associated with high suicide risk

Age: 45 years or older	Alcoholism
Male	Preparation for suicide,
Unemployed	e.g. a suicide note or recent will
Social isolation	Previous attempts
Poor physical health	Violent method
Depression	

The interview should cover three vital areas:

(1) Assessment of pre-morbid factors.
(2) Circumstances surrounding an act of self-harm, if committed.
(3) Assessment of the patient's mental state and current problems.

A quiet room should be set aside and the interview conducted in a sympathetic unhurried manner, encouraging a good rapport between patient and interviewer. Whenever possible, an informant should also be interviewed.

Pre-morbid factors

A full history should be taken, paying special attention to previous harmful acts, past psychiatric history, pre-morbid personality and relevant family, personal and social details. In particular, emotional instability, frequent changes of work and accommodation, and severe breakdowns in personal relationships should be looked for. An excessive emotional outburst in a previously stable personality should also act as a danger signal.

Act of self-harm

If an act of self-harm has been committed it is important to obtain a picture of the patient's beliefs and feelings beforehand and at the time of the act. His expectations are more important than the doctor's knowledge of the effects of that act. Thus an elderly lady who believes that five benzodiazepine sleeping tablets will put her to sleep forever may be a suicide risk even though the doctor knows the tablets are relatively harmless in such a dose.

Carefully planned acts committed in a calm, calculated way are more worrying than unplanned impulsive acts. The winding-up of outstanding debts and bills, the writing of a suicide note, making a will, and efforts to avoid discovery all suggest high risk. Conversely patients who commit their acts at a time when they know discovery is likely are probably at lower risk.

Mental state and current problems

Doctors are often frightened to broach the topic of suicide, but suicidal patients may be relieved that the subject can be talked about openly and frankly. Direct questions about suicidal thoughts should always be asked. There is no evidence that talking about suicide increases the risk of its enactment. A fleeting thought about suicide or a passing wish to be dead are quite common and may be of little significance. Persistent suicidal thoughts should be taken seriously and the details of the intent obtained. For example, a patient who has experienced suicidal thoughts for some weeks may have formulated a plan. He should be asked about the plan and any activities undertaken to put it into practice. Thus one patient who had considered hanging himself was clearly at high risk as he had tested out the strength of the joists in his house by swinging on them and had bought a rope.

Special attention should be paid to the presence of depressive features such as depressed mood, hopelessness, inability to see a future and guilt feelings; somatic symptoms such as appetite change, weight loss, poor concentration and sleep disturbance all suggest the presence of a depressive illness requiring urgent treatment.

Psychotic patients are extremely difficult to assess, as suicidal features may be masked by delusions and hallucinations. Patients who have begun to act on delusional beliefs may be particularly at risk. For example, a patient suffering from schizophrenia became frightened by paranoid delusions. Finding no safe place to hide from his persecutors, he felt life was not worth living and jumped out of the window.

Current problems may be either physical or social or both. Chronic physical illness and persistent pain, especially in the elderly, are high risk factors and may be difficult to alleviate. Covert alcohol abuse should always be considered. Social problems such as social isolation, poor accommodation, absence of a supportive network, vagrancy and recurrent or intractable life problems increase suicidal risk and may be difficult to alleviate.

Action after assessment

In the UK the Department of Health no longer recommends that all patients who have taken an overdose should see a psychiatrist, and the trend over the last few years has been to involve non-medical personnel. A multi-disciplinary approach is now used and treatment decisions should, if possible, only be taken after discussion between doctors, social workers, nurses, and other personnel. Usually the nearest relative should also be involved in the decision-making process and the general practitioner informed about the patient's difficulties. Of course, some patients clearly require hospital admission and the doctor often makes this decision unilaterally and then alerts the multi-disciplinary team later.

THE VIOLENT PATIENT

Patients may become violent towards others for many reasons. Some people live within a violent sub-culture and if they become violent in hospital this may be a continuation of their behaviour elsewhere. Serious violence in hospital to members of staff should always be reported to the police in case an enquiry is needed (see also p. 698).

However, violent outbursts by mentally ill patients are often secondary to mental state changes. Common causes include severe personality disorder, psychotic states, and alcohol and drug abuse.

Personality and violence

The patient's underlying personality is probably an important factor in many cases of violence, even if they are mentally ill. For example, a tendency for a psychotic patient to become violent may arise from pre-morbid personality traits rather than the psychosis itself. However, this inter-relationship between personality and violence is unclear and some patients may become violent only when suffering from delusional beliefs or other psychotic symptoms. The personality type most commonly linked to violence is the psychopathic personality disorder, which is discussed in Chapter 26 (p. 336).

Psychotic states

The commonest psychotic state associated with violence to others is schizophrenia. However, only a small percentage of schizophrenic patients are violent; this small sub-group is made up for the most part of male patients suffering from paranoid schizophrenia. People in close contact with the patient, such as relatives, nurses or doctors, tend to be the victims of any violent outburst. Acts of aggression may be a result of psychiatric symptoms such as paranoid delusions or hallucinations (Planansky and Johnston 1977), but in a study by Virkkunen (1974) 60 per cent of the acts of violence committed by schizophrenic patients took place outside the acute phase of the illness (see also p. 697).

Psychotic depression may result in violence. For example, some cases of infanticide result from the mother becoming depressed in the puerperium (see Chapter 33). In these cases delusions of guilt and belief in the necessity of death to atone for evil, or hallucinations may be the motivating force. Suicide results if the violence becomes directed towards the self.

Alcohol and drug abuse

Alcohol is often associated with violence. Approximately 50 per cent of murderers have been drinking before their violent act, and violence clusters in and around public houses (Sheard 1977). Drunken individuals cause difficulties in casualty departments and may threaten staff and patients. It is difficult to decide whether to treat them for their alcohol abuse by admitting them or have them removed by security staff or the police. Of course a patient suffering from withdrawal symptoms or other associated physical and psychiatric problems should be admitted.

Drug abuse may lead to violence either as a result of the direct effects of the drug or because of the criminal lifestyle associated with obtaining supplies. Intoxication with any drug can lead to violence, but the underlying personality characteristics are an important contributory factor. Heroin and amphetamine intoxication can lead to paranoid beliefs which result in attacks on innocent people.

Management

Handling a potentially violent patient is a skilled task, whatever the causes of the aggression. A patient who threatens violence is invariably frightened and the psychiatrist must discover the basis of these fears if a volatile situation is to be defused. Under these circumstances the behaviour and feelings of the psychiatrist are critical. The psychiatrist may rightly be frightened himself, but he should take measures to protect himself without communicating his fear to the patient. A calm and firm attitude combined with subtle protective measures are mandatory in dealing with a threatening patient. For example, the psychiatrist, when quietly introducing himself to the patient, may pick up a chair and sit down with the back of the chair facing the patient; he should always remain nearer to the door than the patient so that he can leave rapidly if necessary, protecting himself with the legs of the chair.

The psychiatrist may be called after several members of staff or police have tried to subdue a patient. The fears of paranoid patients are increased by confrontation and it is often useful for the psychiatrist to ask everyone to leave the room after making careful arrangements for help to be out of sight but close at hand. This action will allow a paranoid patient to feel some trust in the psychiatrist as he has 'saved the day' by removing all the persecutors and should reduce tension in both the patient and the staff. The psychiatrist may then talk to the patient in a firm confident manner; there should be no hint of anger or threats of punishment. Eye contact should be maintained. This will reassure the patient that his destructive impulses are not as powerful as he fears as they do not frighten the doctor. On no account should the psychiatrist make any physical contact with the patient as this will increase the danger of an attack.

Sometimes one may be forewarned that a patient may become violent. Warning signs include increasing agitation, verbal threats and the breaking of objects.

Occasionally a patient is so disturbed, for example in casualty, that the interventions described above are impossible. The psychiatrist should then discuss the situation with the staff, listen carefully to their opinions and consider all the available information about the patient. Informants should be interviewed whenever possible. Initially the patient may be offered medication 'to help reduce tension and to stay in control'. This may be refused; if so, sedation will still be necessary if the patient's disturbance has arisen from mental state changes. Once this decision has been made, action must be rapid. Uncertainty and vacillation on the part of the psychiatrist will increase the danger to both staff and patient. Enough staff should be available to restrain the patient while an intramuscular injection of either chlorpromazine or haloperidol is given. It often happens that the patient quietens down soon after restraint even though the drugs have not had time to take effect, because he is relieved that his own fears of uncontrollable violence have not terrified everyone around him and that he is no longer at the mercy of his own violent impulses.

Once the danger is over the patient, if still in casualty, should be admitted. The acute episode and further management should then be discussed with all the staff. Once in hospital the patient can be carefully assessed while his behaviour is safely controlled with sedation.

THE INTOXICATED PATIENT

Drug intoxication and alcohol withdrawal are a medical and psychiatric emergency, requiring close cooperation between psychiatrist and physician. Often the physical effects of drug and alcohol are best treated by the physician and the psychiatrist takes over once physical complications have been dealt with. The symptoms of alcohol withdrawal and delirium tremens are discussed in Chapter 30 (see p. 380). Patients presenting to casualty departments should be sedated rapidly. Chlordiazepoxide 20 mg orally four times a day, or chlormethiazole 192 mg three times daily are the drugs of choice. They not only act as sedatives but also reduce the likelihood of epileptic fits. Chlordiazepoxide is the safer drug to use in view of the side-effects of chlormethiazole. The dose should be reduced gradually during the next few days. A vitamin supplement such as parentrovite may also be given.

The behavioural, physical and psychological consequences of drug intoxication and withdrawal are diverse and dependent on the drug taken. Their treatment is discussed in Chapter 31.

THE ACUTELY ANXIOUS PATIENT

Patients experiencing panic, perhaps in fear of imminent collapse or death, may require immediate help. They should be reassured and helped to relax as quickly as possible; only then will it be possible to explore the precipitants of the panic. Reassurance alone may not diminish a patient's anxiety and a benzodiazepine, e.g. diazepam 5 mg orally, may be required.

GENERAL GUIDELINES

Obtain an adequate history

It is tempting to act immediately in a psychiatric emergency, but the psychiatrist should make every effort to establish the course of events leading up to the crisis. Inadequate information may lead to inappropriate treatment, so as much information as possible should be obtained from the staff, patient and other informants. If the picture remains unclear only measures which are absolutely necessary should be taken. The judicious use of tranquillisers may help, but their excessive use may mask symptoms and make diagnosis more difficult.

Admit the patient to hospital

Disturbed patients often refuse an offer of hospital admission. The patient may drop his protestations and accept informal admission if the psychiatrist is clear and firm about his intentions, but if admission is still refused, compulsory admission under Section 4 of the Mental Health Act will be required (see p. 705). This should be fully explained to the patient and an approved social worker called for a further opinion.

Sedate the patient if necessary

Major tranquillisers should be used with care. Their side-effects may be severe (see p. 245) and over-sedation will mask important clinical signs. Intramuscular haloperidol 5-20 mg, or chlorpromazine 100-200 mg are the drugs of choice. Haloperidol has the advantage of not inducing a hypotensive crisis and may be used safely in high doses. Sedation may be done under common law in an emergency.

No heroics

Discuss the management of the patient with all the staff involved and be open and frank with worried relatives. In an emergency the doctor should never act alone.

Exclude any organic factors

A full physical examination and any necessary physical investigations should be performed as soon as practically possible. A drug screen is essential.

FURTHER READING

McGrath, G. and Bowker, M.L. (1987). *Common Psychiatric Emergencies*. Wright, Bristol.

Part IX

Psychiatric Services

55

The General Practitioner

In the UK the general practitioner is usually the doctor to whom members of the public first turn when in need of medical or psychiatric help. Even if a person with psychiatric or psychosomatic symptoms or emotional problems first contacts a physician, psychiatrist or psychotherapist directy, the GP will almost certainly be informed and is likely to get involved in his management. In this chapter we shall consider first the number and kind of psychiatric patients seen in general practice, and then the role of the general practitioner in providing help for such patients.

EPIDEMIOLOGY AND DIAGNOSIS

We shall attempt to answer two related questions in this section: (1) On average, what proportion of patients registered with a GP will consult him on account of psychiatric or emotional disorders? (2) What proportion of all patients actually seen by the GP suffer from such disorders?

Different GPs are known to give widely different figures concerning the number of patients with psychiatric complaints in their practices. Some give figures as low as 10 per cent, others as high as 60 per cent. Such wide differences are partly determined by the individual GP's personal level of interest in psychiatric and psychosomatic illness and emotional problems. If it is known that a particular GP is interested in and willing to help patients with psychological problems, he will attract such patients and be more likely to recognise emotional problems in his patients. If, on the contrary, a GP is known to be disinterested or even antagonistic to patients with psychological problems, such patients will either conceal these problems, or consult him complaining of physical symptoms instead, or register with a different practice. Moreover, a GP who is uninterested in the psychological aspects of medicine is likely to miss a psychiatric diagnosis or emotional problem unless the patient is suffering from major psychiatric symptoms due to serious psychiatric illness, e.g. a severe affective illness or schizophrenia.

In order to discover what proportion of patients registered in general practice on average consult their GP on account of psychiatric problems, Shepherd *et al.* (1966) studied 46 general practices in the Greater London area over a survey period of one year. They found that out of a 1 in 8 sample of all patients over the age of fifteen registered in these practices, i.e. a sample of 14,697 patients, 139.4 per 1000 or 14 per cent consulted their GP at least once during the survey period of one year with a disorder either wholly or partly of psychiatric or emotional origin (see Table 55.1). To put it more simply, if a GP has a list of 2,500 patients he is likely to see 350 of them at least once a year on account of problems of psychiatric or emotional origin. The study also showed that patients with psychiatric and emotionally determined illnesses consulted their GP more often and made significantly greater demands on his time and energy than patients with physical illnesses. It is interesting to note that compared with the figure of 14 per cent for psychiatric morbidity the corresponding figures for respiratory or gastrointestinal disorders at the time of the study were 25 per cent and 9 per cent respectively.

The study by Shepherd *et al.* (1966) has also provided useful information on the frequency of different psychiatric disorders seen in general practice (Table 55.1). The table shows that 88.5 per 1000 (just under 9 per cent) of patients were suffering from neuroses and 29.9 per 1000 (3 per cent) from psychosomatic conditions, i.e. physical symptoms or illnesses which the GP considered to be wholly or in part of psychological origin (see Chapter 37). The next highest rate was 15 per 1000 for organic illnesses with psychiatric overlay. None of the other conditions exceeded 7.5 per 1000 or 0.75 per cent. Between them the neuroses and psychosomatic conditions accounted for over 80 per cent of the total psychiatric morbidity.

The table also shows that in almost all the diagnostic categories, the neuroses and psychosomatic conditions included, the number of female exceeded the number of male patients. In the neuroses the ratio of female to male was 2.1:1.

The low figure of 5.9 per 1000 for the psychoses compared with 88.5 for the neuroses is of interest. In terms of percentages of the total for psychiatric disorders in general practice this corresponds to a figure of 4.2 per cent for psychoses compared with 63.4 per cent for neuroses. Corresponding figures for first admission to mental hospitals in 1957, close to the time of Shepherd's study, were 72.3 per cent for psychoses and 18.1 per cent for neuroses. The marked difference reflects the fact that only very few patients with neuroses but a much higher proportion of patients with psychoses required hospital admission. This still applies today, although the present policy of discharging patients with psychoses and other major psychiatric disorders from mental or district general hospitals into the community means that the number of psychotic patients being seen and cared for in general practice is increasing.

Table 55.1 does not provide figures for alcoholism and drug dependence although these play an important part in general practice, and patients with drug dependence are on the increase (see Chapters 30 and 31). Nor does it give separate figures for eating disorders, another group of patients often seen in general practice. Disorders of childhood and early adolescence are not included either as patients under fifteen were excluded

Table 55.1. Patient consulting rates per 1000 registered, i.e. at risk for
psychiatric morbidity, in general practice
(at least one consultation during the survey year)

Diagnostic categories	Male	Female	Both sexes
Neuroses	55.7	116.6	88.5
Psychoses	2.7	8.6	5.9
Personality disorders	7.2	4.0	5.5
Mental subnormality	1.6	2.9	2.3
Dementia	1.2	1.6	1.4
Formal psychiatric illness*	67.2	131.9	102.1
Psychosomatic conditions	24.5	34.5	29.9
Organic illness with psychiatric overlay	13.1	16.6	15.0
Psychosocial problems	4.6	10.0	7.5
Psychiatric 'associated' conditions*	38.6	57.2	48.6
Total psychiatric morbidity*	97.9	175.0	139.4 (14%)

* These totals cannot be obtained by adding the rates for the relevant diagnostic
groups because while a patient may be included in more than one diagnostic group
he will be included only once in the total.

Adapted from Shepherd *et al.* 1966.

from the study. The developmental, behavioural, educational, psychiatric
and psychosomatic problems of children and adolescents in fact play an
important part in the work of general practitioners. About 20 per cent of
children and adolescents suffer from such disorders. The prevalence is
higher in large cities than in small towns (Rutter *et al.* 1975b).

Lastly, Table 55.1 does not give any details concerning the kind of
emotional problems encountered in the patients seen in general practice.
Many of these problems are concerned with difficulties in interpersonal
relationships within the family, with marital and sexual problems, or
with more long-standing emotional difficulties, sometimes dating back to
childhood.

We now turn to the second question concerning psychiatric morbidity
in general practice, i.e. what proportion of all patients actually seen by
the GP, as opposed to those registered, suffer from psychiatric problems?
There is now wide agreement that about a third of the patients a GP sees
suffer wholly or in part from either psychiatric disorders, psychosomatic
symptoms or emotional problems. Watts (1958) on behalf of the Royal

College of General Practitioners arrived at an average figure of 34 per cent.

Goldberg and Blackwell (1970), using interviews and the General Health Questionnaire, studied the prevalence of psychiatric patients in one general practice run by a GP who had previously trained as a psychiatrist. They arrived at a very similar figure: 30 per cent of 553 consecutive attenders were found to have psychiatric or emotionally determined symptoms or disorders. This study is of special interest because Goldberg and Blackwell also investigated the degree to which the GP was able to identify the patients with psychiatric or emotional disorders. All the 553 patients were seen by the GP, but a sample of 200 of the patients he saw were also seen by a psychiatrist. The GP, who only had about ten minutes in which to see each patient and who had to attend to their physical complaints as well, identified psychiatric disorders in only 20 per cent of the patients he saw; but the psychiatrist, who had half to one hour in which to interview each patient, identified an additional 10 per cent, thus arriving at the figure of 30 per cent. Goldberg and Blackwell therefore made a distinction between the *conspicuous psychiatric morbidity* of 20 per cent and a 'hidden' psychiatric morbidity of 10 per cent. However, it has since been shown (Skuse and Williams 1984) that GPs differ considerably in their ability to identify psychiatric and emotional problems in their patients. The hidden psychiatric morbidity may therefore vary in different practices.

Although psychiatrists may be better at diagnosing major psychiatric disturbances, they are not necessarily better than GPs at discovering less obvious emotional problems. The GP may have known the patient for a long while, be familiar with his personal and social problems, and aware of problems within the family which may help him to make the diagnosis (see p. 647)

It is important to note that GPs only refer about 5 per ent of the psychiatric or emotionally disturbed patients they see to the psychiatric services. This means that they themselves accept the responsibility for treating 95 per cent of these patients, sometimes in conjunction with a social worker, community psychiatric nurse, psychologist or counsellor attached to the practice (see p. 648).

A great deal of epidemiological research on general practice continues to be done. This has been helped greatly by the use of standardised questionnaire methods, especially the General Health Questionnaire (Goldberg 1972), and standardised interviews, including the Clinical Psychiatric Interview (Goldberg *et al.* 1970). These more recent studies have shown that the psychiatric morbidity among patients registered in general practice is somewhat higher than 14 per cent, on average nearer 20 per cent, women again being affected twice as often as men. An association between physical illness, especially cardiovascular and respiratory disorders, and psychiatric illness has also been demonstrated. Some of the more recent findings have been described by Shepherd and Clare in Shepherd *et al.* (1981) and by Goldberg and Huxley (1980).

ACCESS TO PSYCHIATRIC CARE

Goldberg and Huxley have investigated the process by which psychiatrically and emotionally disturbed people in the community can gain access to psychiatric care, including help from GPs. They discussed this process in terms of five 'levels' and a series of four 'filters' through which patients have to pass (see Table 55.2). The first filter between level 1 and 2, i.e. the factors that determine the proportion of patients with psychiatric problems in the community who consult the GP, includes the severity of their symptoms, their reactions to the symptoms – so-called illness behaviour (Mechanic 1977, 1986), the attitude of their relatives, and the availability of medical services. In the UK most patients in the community, over 90 per cent, pass through the first filter.

Passage through the second filter, i.e. recognition by the GP of the patients he sees as psychiatrically ill, depends on the GP's attitude to psychiatric illness and on his interviewing and diagnostic skills, the nature and severity of the patient's symptoms and the way in which they are presented; for example, recognition is more difficult if the patient complains of physical rather than of psychological symptoms. Patients with symptoms of anxiety and depression are among those most commonly diagnosed as psychiatrically ill.

The third filter, i.e. the GP's decision to refer the patient to the psychiatric services, will be determined by the severity and nature of the symptoms, the GP's interest and his degree of confidence in being able to manage the patient in the general practice setting, the patient's family and social circumstances and the availability of suitable psychiatric

Table 55.2. Pathway to psychiatric care

Level 1	Psychiatric morbidity in the community ↓
Filter 1	The decision to consult the GP ↓
Level 2	Total psychiatric morbidity in general practice ↓
Filter 2	Recognition by the GP as psychiatrically ill or emotionally disturbed ↓
Level 3	Conspicuous (detected) psychiatric morbidity in general practice ↓
Filter 3	Decision to refer to the psychiatric services ↓
Level 4	Patients seen in the psychiatric services ↓
Filter 4	Decision to admit ↓
Level 5	Psychiatric inpatients

services. As mentioned earlier, only about 5 per cent of patients diagnosed by the GP as psychiatrically disturbed are referred by him to a psychiatrist. This, incidentally, shows that the patients seen by psychiatrists belong to a highly selected group.

The fourth filter, i.e. the psychiatrist's decision to admit the patient, will largely depend on the nature and severity of the disorder, the attitude of the patient and his family, and the availability of inpatient beds or adequate community services. A few patients are admitted directly as an emergency, say from the casualty department, bypassing levels 2, 3 and 4.

THE DOCTOR-PATIENT RELATIONSHIP

How can the GP best help his patients to start talking about their emotional problems and identify their psychiatric or psychosomatic disorders in the short time of about ten minutes he usually has available when a patient comes to see him? Much attention has rightly been paid to the *interviewing skills* needed in general practice, but it must be stressed that interviewing is not just a matter of technique. The GP's personality, attitudes and experience are at least equally and probably more important as they largely determine how he relates to his patients.

The doctor-patient relationship has always been known to play an important role in general practice. In the 1950s Michael Balint, working at the Tavistock Clinic in London, started to work with GPs in small weekly groups, in which the GPs reported on patients they were seeing in their practices. This led to the development of *Balint groups* whose main aim was to study the doctor-patient relationship in detail and to modify the GPs' attitudes in order to improve and develop their ability to relate to their patients. These groups met weekly for two to three years or longer and often provided an important personal and educational experience for the doctors who had applied to join and been accepted by the group leader. Balint subsequently described his findings in *The Doctor, his Patient and the Illness* (Balint 1957, 1964). Although Balint was a psychoanalyst, the groups were not run along psychoanalytic lines. Instead, attention was paid throughout to the doctor-patient relationship, to the way in which the doctor's personality influenced this relationship, and to the GP's ability to uncover and handle the patient's emotional problems. The influence of Balint groups has been reviewed by Hopkins (1979). Bloomfield (1983) has described a group led by Balint at University College Hospital, London.

Much of what was learnt from Balint groups has since been incorporated in general practice and in post-graduate training seminars for GPs. Only a few GPs in the UK nowadays attend Balint groups for further training; they are now more popular in several other European countries, especially Germany (Bräutigam 1983), Switzerland and Holland, and also in the USA.

More recently psychiatrists have studied interviewing techniques in general practice from a more descriptive and technical point of view (Goldberg 1979; Davenport *et al.* 1987), and have explored the use of videotape feedback in training GPs (Gask *et al.* 1987). The following comments are based on a combination of psychodynamic findings derived from Balint-type sensitivity groups, and the study of teaching interviewing techniques and the use of videotape feedback.

General interest in the patient as a person is the first priority. Most doctors who choose to become general practitioners do so because of their interest in the individual person, seen in the context of his family and social relationships.

Next in importance is the GP's sensitivity to the patient's emotional problems. This is largely determined by his ability to empathise with the patient and convey to him that he understands what troubles him. Sometimes the patient may openly tell the GP how he feels, e.g. unhappy or depressed, anxious or frightened. He may even tell the GP what he thinks is making him feel as he does. Other patients hide their feelings and may present with physical symptoms instead (Bridges and Goldberg 1985). Often the GP has to respond to indirect cues, e.g. a complaint of insomnia may lead him to ask what is keeping the patient awake or what is on his mind while he tries to get off to sleep. Or a patient may be complaining of some physical symptom, say backache, that he has had for a long time; the GP may then ask what made him decide to come and see him with this symptom just now? A sensitive GP may often pick up non-verbal cues: if the patient looks tense or anxious he may comment on his appearance and say that this makes him wonder what it might be that is making him feel so tense.

Once the patient has begun to open up it is important for the GP to *listen* and not to interrupt unnecessarily. Empathic listening is perhaps the GP's most important task, along with his ability to reflect back the meaning of what the patient is telling him.

A few specific aspects of the consultation are worth considering. At the beginning it is essential for the GP to be relaxed and unhurried in order to make the patient feel at ease. It is helpful to look at the patient in a relaxed manner, while looking at notes may make the patient feel that the doctor is not really interested in him. It is usually best to start the consultation with an open-ended question, such as 'What is it that brings you to see me?' More direct or closed questions, such as 'Are you sleeping better?' or 'Are you still feeling depressed?' can be answered by a simple yes or no, thus preventing the patient from talking about what is on his mind. Throughout the consultation open-ended rather than closed questions tend to be more effective in helping the patient express how he feels. Sometimes it is while the GP is examining him physically that the patient begins to say what is on his mind.

Equally important is the end of the consultation. If the patient appears to hesitate as he is about to leave, the GP should pick this up and perhaps comment on the fact that the patient seems to have something more he wants to say. Some crucial information may then be revealed, or the patient may start to cry having so far concealed how depressed he really feels.

Of course, there are occasions when the GP has to ask more direct questions. For example, once the GP has realised that the patient is depressed he needs to enquire whether the patient has suicidal thoughts or plans, and whether he has such biological symptoms as sleep disturbance, anorexia or weight loss. A full examination of the mental state cannot be carried out during a brief consultation in general practice, but an experienced GP will ask a few relevant questions to obtain enough information about the patient's history and mental state to make a preliminary diagnosis. Alternatively he may ask the patient to make an appointment for a longer consultation in a day or two. This is particularly important on those frequent occasions when it appears that the patient has some troublesome emotional problems, not necessarily amounting to a formal psychiatric disorder. By seeing him again soon for a longer interview the patient's problems can be explored more fully.

Methods of consultation have recently been discussed in detail by Neighbour (1987) and Pendleton *et al.* (1984).

MANAGEMENT

As we have seen, 95 per cent of patients with emotional problems and psychiatric or psychosomatic disorders will be treated within the general practice without referral elsewhere. Some psychiatrically ill patients will require treatment with psychotropic drugs (see Chapter 49.) The majority of patients, however, present with emotional problems which do not amount to a major psychiatric illness, or with psychoneurotic or psychosomatic symptoms; some kind of psychotherapeutic approach is therefore often needed, either on its own or occasionally in combination with drugs. In the past many GPs worked single-handed, but nowadays most work in group practices or in primary care teams which may include a number of non-medical workers, such as a social worker, health visitor, community psychiatric nurse, counsellor, or clinical psychologist, often on a part-time basis. This makes it easier to arrange appropriate psychotherapeutic and social support than in the days of single-handed practices. It must, however, be remembered that the ultimate clinical and legal responsibility rests with the GP. Many GPs will, of course, take their own share in providing psychotherapeutic help.

PSYCHOTHERAPY

What then are the characteristics and types of psychotherapy used in general practice?

First, GPs differ widely in their interest in and ability to use a psychotherapeutic approach. This will be determined largely by their personality, training and experience. Some GPs will not wish to undertake psychotherapy and those who do will vary in the kind of psychotherapy they are prepared to provide.

It is helpful to think in terms of simple and more formal types of psychotherapy in general practice. Simple therapy correponds roughly to supportive psychotherapy (see p. 568), and formal therapy to brief and modified forms of individual psychodynamic psychotherapy (see p. 563). In many cases the distinction is not clear-cut and the two types of therapy may overlap.

Supportive psychotherapy is needed particularly by patients with long-standing and often incurable emotional, physical or psychiatric disorders who may need to be supported for long periods. Other patients who are relatively stable emotionally but are passing through a crisis following, say, a bereavement or marital breakdown, may need supportive therapy for a short period until their own resources have recovered sufficiently for them to cope on their own.

More formal types of psychotherapy may be needed by some patients with psychoneurotic or psychosomatic symptoms, and by patients with sexual, marital, family or other emotional problems. GPs with an interest and some training in psychotherapy may decide to treat a few such patients themselves for short periods, recognising the limits of what can be achieved in the general practice setting. Other patients may be treated within the practice team by, say, a social worker, counsellor, clinical psychologist or psychiatric nurse attached to the practice, provided he has had training in the form of psychotherapy required. For example, a couple with marital or sexual problems may be taken on for marital therapy by a marriage guidance counsellor or by a psychologist trained in marital or sex therapy. Or a patient with a phobic anxiety state may receive treatment from a psychologist or a psychiatric nurse trained in behaviour therapy (Marks and Horder 1987).

If these facilities are not available in the practice team the patient may have to be referred for therapy to the psychiatric services. However, in many districts there is still a great shortage of consultant psychotherapists and psychotherapeutic facilities in the NHS, and there are long waiting lists. GPs are therefore understandably reluctant to refer such patients and may prefer to treat them themselves. Moreover, many patients find the practice setting more acceptable than a hospital psychiatric outpatient department. They feel less stigmatised, the practice is familiar to them, often nearer to their home, and the hours may be more flexible. Other patients may prefer to be referred for psychotherapy in the private sector.

Psychotherapeutic skills

In some respects these do not differ fundamentally from the GP's interviewing skills outlined earlier. In essence they consist of a genuine interest in and sensitivity to the patient's psychological problems, and the ability to listen with empathy and reflect back to the patient what he has been saying. For example, if a depressed woman whose husband has died recently is talking about the fact that her only daughter is about to leave home, a GP who can empathise with her might say 'This must be very hard for you, especially now!' This will show her that her doctor understands and accepts how she is feeling and enable her to enlarge on how she feels.

A GP who carries out more formal psychotherapy should be able to recognise transference phenomena (see p. 560). Some aspects of the patient's relationship to him may mirror experiences the patient has had as a child in relation to, for example, his parents, or more recently to someone close to him, perhaps in his present family. It is often helpful to point this out. For example, if a patient is being submissive to the GP and afraid that he will disapprove of what he is telling him, the GP, who may already know that the patient had a rather authoritarian, frightening father, may comment that the patient seems to think that he, the GP, will, like his father, behave in a superior and disapproving manner. The patient may then not only learn to trust his GP more and hence talk to him more freely, but he may recognise that he tends to react to other people as if they were authority figures.

It will be clear that the acquisition of psychotherapeutic skills in general practice requires both training and experience. The benefit derived from attending a Balint group has already been mentioned (p. 646). GPs may attend postgraduate courses in individual or more specialised forms of psychotherapy, e.g. sex therapy, marital therapy or behaviour therapy. Many GPs may during their training have held a post in psychiatry which provided experience in supervised dynamic psychotherapy. The teaching of basic psychotherapeutic skills to medical students in a voluntary training scheme at University College Hospital will be described later (see p. 715). Such training can serve as a useful preparation for future general practitioners.

Practical issues

A GP who undertakes psychotherapy has several decisions to make with regard to the timing and frequency of sessions for each individual patient.

For some patients the initial consultation may provide an opportunity to give some psychotherapeutic help. Even if the consultation only lasts fifteen minutes, the fact that the patient has felt understood and perhaps has gained some new understanding of his problems may have a psychotherapeutic effect. One or two further similar interviews during surgery hours may then be all that is required, at least for the time being, especially as the patient knows he can return for further talks.

To other patients, especially those who appear in need of a brief period of more intensive therapy, the GP may decide to offer regular sessions, perhaps once every week or two, for a longer period. He may decide to see these patients at pre-arranged times outside surgery hours, for, say, half an hour. Patients who need long-term support may only need to be seen at monthly intervals. In general, the practical arrangements for psychotherapy in general practice tend to be much more flexible than in specialist psychotherapy.

Limitations and aims

The aims of psychotherapy carried out by the GP are bound to be limited and it is essential to be aware of this from the outset. Even those GPs who select a few patients for modified, brief psychodynamic psychotherapy have to recognise that at best they can only bring about limited changes in the patient's personality. Any insight gained usually takes place at a more or less conscious level; interpretations of unconscious conflicts and of the consequences of early emotional deprivation are rarely used. Most of the work will be done in terms of the patient's present problems. The use of transference interpretations has been mentioned above.

In spite of these limitations the patient can derive considerable benefit. Symptoms may clear up or diminish in intensity or duration, and the number of days off work may decrease. The frequency of consultations and requests for tranquillisers or other psychotropic drugs may diminish. In general, the time spent on providing some time for psychotherapeutic intervention may lead to the patient making far fewer demands on the GP's time and energy later on (Balint 1964).

It must, however, be recognised that some patients may fail to respond or get worse. This applies particularly to patients who are very demanding, perhaps as a result of emotional deprivation early in childhood. Their frustration and resentment may lead to the development of a strong negative transference, manifested by constant criticism and ever-increasing demands on the GP. He, in turn, may react to this by feeling useless and a failure, or angry and resentful. A great deal of psychotherapeutic skill and self-awareness is needed to handle these difficult situations, and the GP may need help, especially in coping with his own feelings. This is when being a member of a practice team is particularly valuable, enabling the GP to discuss his patient with one of his partners or in practice meetings. Occasionally referral to or discussion with a specialist psychotherapist may be necessary, either to get his support and advice while continuing to treat the patient, or in order to transfer the patient for specialist psychotherapy by someone else. Other difficult patients may not be suitable for psychotherapy; their management in general practice has been discussed by Gerrard and Riddell (1988).

Attachment of a psychiatrist

The growing tendency to have a psychiatrist or a psychotherapist attached to the practice team for one or two regular weekly sessions is very helpful in the management of psychological problems and of patients with psychiatric disorders. Horder (1988) has described the advantages of such collaboration between general practitioners and psychiatrists.

About 20 per cent of psychiatrists now spend one or two sessions a week working in a general practice (Brook 1978). This has considerable advantages over the more usual method of consultation, whereby the GP refers one of his patients for a psychiatric opinion or advice on psychotherapy to the psychiatrist or psychotherapist in a psychiatric outpatient department. Contact between the GP and psychiatrist is often confined to a referral letter and the consultant's written reply. Such lack of personal contact often leaves both parties dissatisfied, the psychiatrist not knowing exactly what kind of help the GP is hoping for, and the GP feeling disappointed if he receives a reply that does not meet his needs.

If the hospital consultant instead regularly spends one or two sessions a week in the general practice, he and the GPs and other members of the practice team can get to know each other better and discuss problems as they arise. It is probably best for the consultant to adopt a flexible approach. For example, he may see a patient for assessment, diagnosis and advice on treatment, including psychotherapy, followed by discussion with the GP concerned; or he may see a patient himself for a few psychotherapy sessions before, perhaps, handing him back to the GP. Alternatively the consultant may make himself available for discussion with the GP of patients the GP finds it difficult to handle, e.g. very demanding or aggressive patients, or patients the GP has taken on for psychotherapy but who have caused problems in the doctor-patient relationship. Here the help the psychiatrist can provide often consists of helping the GP to understand better and tolerate the feelings the patient has engendered in him, and supporting the GP from time to time while he continues to treat the patient.

Psychotropic drugs

Patients with major psychiatric illnesses, such as a depressive illness or schizophrenia, will require antidepressant or antipsychotic drugs prescribed by their GP.

In other patients, especially those wih psychoneurotic or psychosomatic symptoms or emotional problems, the use of drugs is much more debatable and often not required. Since the early 1960s there has been a great increase in the use of minor tranquillisers, mostly benzodiazepines, and to a lesser extent of antidepressants. The growing awareness of the risk of dependency is now leading to greater caution in the use of tranquillisers and hypnotics, except for brief periods or during a crisis. Many patients do not actually take the tablets that have been prescribed, and there is always a danger that they may build up a large supply that could be used for an overdose. Other patients do not even take the prescription to the chemist, but the GP may remain under the impression that his patient is taking what he has prescribed.

There is always a temptation to give in too readily to a patient's request for drugs in order not to disappoint and upset him, or simply to save time, often by giving repeat prescriptions without even seeing the patient. Instead the GP should discuss with the patient why he wants the tablets and spend some time, if possible, finding out what emotional problems may be responsible for his symptoms. The hope is that by adopting a more psychotherapeutic approach the need for tranquillisers or sedatives will be reduced and ultimately overcome. As Balint (1964) put it, the GP can often offer his patients the drug 'doctor' rather than another prescription.

FURTHER READING

Balint, M. (1964). *The Doctor, His Patient and the Illness*, 2nd enlarged ed. Pitman, London.

Elder, A. and Samuel, O. (eds.) (1987). *While I'm Here Doctor: a study of the doctor-patient relationship*. Tavistock, London.

Goldberg, D. and Huxley, P. (1980). *Mental Illness in the Community: the pathway to psychiatric care*. Tavistock, London.

Horder, J. (1988). 'Working with general practitioners'. *Brit. J. Psychiat.* 153, 513-520.

Neighbour, R. (1987). *The Inner Consultation: how to develop an effective and intuitive consulting style*. MTP Press, Lancaster.

Pendleton, D., Schofield, T., Tate, P. and Havelock, P. (1984). *The Consultation: an approach to learning and teaching*. Oxford General Practice Series 6. OUP, Oxford.

Shepherd, M., Cooper, B., Brown, A.C. and Kalton, G.W. (1981). *Psychiatric Illness in General Practice*, 2nd ed. with new material by Shepherd, M. and Clare, A. OUP, London.

56

Hospital and Community Services

An optimist describing services for mental health in Britain today can report a growing recognition that mental disorder deserves high quality treatment and care from staff of many disciplines working together to help sufferers and their families. He can point to major advances in treatment methods and research into the causes of mental illness and social breakdown, a widespread trend towards intgegration of mental health services into ordinary hospitals, community services and family homes, and diminishing reliance on mental asylums.

A pessimist, by contrast, might find a poorly funded service, fragmented into a dispersed and inconsistent patchwork of provisions, lurching from the dehumanising era of the asylum into the no less inhumane never-never land of 'community care'. He might protest at the growing evidence on city streets of homeless vagrants with mental illness, now disowned by mental hospitals and local authorities, the increase of mental illness among the prison population and the discrepancy between the thousands of patients discharged from mental hospitals and the tiny number of alternative residential services now provided for them.

STRUCTURE OF SERVICES

The present services for mental health in the UK have three main components which function independently in various kinds of liaison. The two statutory services are the *National Health Service* or NHS (incorporating the health authorities at Regional and District level and the primary care services separately administered by Family Practitioner Committees) and the *Social Services* of the Local County and Borough Authorities whose commitment to mental health concerns is highly variable. The third arm is the growing *voluntary sector* of charitable organisations, commonly now employing a variety of paid staff and offering many valuable services in the field of residential aftercare, day provisions, counselling and other supportive help.

Each service has its own geographical range, and the territories may not coincide. Mutual cooperation between the three arms varies greatly and relies largely on local interests and personalities rather than on clear policies. Funding arrangements such as Joint Finance or Care in the Community are available to support cooperative ventures.

Comprehensive district services

The NHS, following major administrative restructuring in 1974 and 1982 and again more recently with the introduction of Griffiths General Management methods, is now committed to the principle of *comprehensive local District services* for mental health, enabling patients as far as possible to be treated in their own homes with recourse to hospital only if it cannot be avoided. These aims are also incorporated in the Mental Health Act of 1983 (see Chapter 62).

The intention is to make each Health District (with a population averaging about 200,000) self-contained, with only some specialist services, e.g. for adolescents, drug dependency and Medium Secure provision, offered on a Regional or sub-Regional scale shared by more than one District. At present the mental hospitals or mental handicap hospitals still commonly cater for more than one District, often at such a distance as to prevent easy visiting by relatives and friends. Some Districts are divided into smaller units so that all specialised mental health services relate to one sector team based on one or more District General Hospital units, perhaps in conjunction with a mental hospital. The gain of increased commitment to a defined population may be offset by limited consumer choice.

SPECIALISED SERVICE SETTINGS

Health services

Most of the NHS's specialist resources for mental health are in hospitals, but the present trend is to try to shift this balance more towards services outside hospital, which are still limited and patchy.

The national policy to make the *psychiatric unit of the District General Hospital* (DGH) the main focus of hospital services for mental illness has not yet been fully implemented; nearly a quarter of England's 190 Districts still lack such a unit. The units provide inpatient beds and outpatient clinics as well as liaison services to the casualty department and other medical and surgical specialities in the hospital. They offer easy access to a variety of medical services, are less associated with the stigma of the mental hospital and are near the patient's home. Against these important advantages have to be set the difficulties such units have commonly found in providing for the needs of patients with severe behavioural disturbance and for those needing longer-term rehabilitation. Despite its title, the DGH unit may not actually be in the main hospital complex, but set apart at a secondary site, housed in less modern or attractive buildings or in a former workhouse vacated by other services.

The *large mental hospitals*, of which there are more than 100 in England and Wales, still provide two-thirds of psychiatric hospital beds and often serve more than one Health District. Their progressive rundown is now to be accelerated by plans to close about half of them. The buildings are often in a dilapidated condition after years of under-funding, the farms which helped feed their residents long since closed. They provide admission units and most of the beds for longer-term care and rehabilitation, together with beds for the elderly demented and a variety of specialist units, e.g. for intensive care or Medium Secure provisions. Many of the residents have lived there for the greater part of their adult lives, the more capable having been discharged leaving behind an increasingly disabled and difficult core of people whose numbers now decline more by death than by discharge.

Though many of he better mental hospitals have provided the first initiatives for a more community-oriented service and staffing levels and facilities have been greatly improved, they have come to be widely regarded as he dinosaurs of psychiatric pratice, overdue for extinction. As elements of a national resource for very disadvantaged people, however, they still provide a flexible back-up to DGH units, with their spacious grounds, economies of scale and opportunities for varied approaches to treatment and occupation which may be expensive and difficult to replicate in local Districts. Questions have still to be answered about what alternative provisions can best be made to provide for their more disturbed and longer-term residents. The asylum offers a sense of home and community not easily replaced in the less accepting world outside.

Day hospitals, provided in the DGH unit or mental hospital, at independent sites, or sometimes in rural areas as a mobile service, offer a full range of medical, nursing and other services for patients able to attend daily from home. They can provide an alternative to hospital admission for people suffering from acute illness or help to shorten the stay in hospital. In addition they provide an extension to the outpatient service by offering more intensive opportunities for treatment.

The newest development is the *community resource centre*, which can take various forms based on a house or day centre offering a variety of multidisciplinary services to people who attend the centre or are visited in their homes.

Social services

Social service departments provide community social workers to help patients and their families in their homes, and hospital-based social workers to assist in services for both inpatients and outpatients (see Chapter 57). The authorities can provide, on their own or now increasingly wih the cooperation of the voluntary agencies and initial health service funding, a wide range of residential services outside hospitals in the form of hostels, adult foster-care placements with families, other supported lodging schemes and day centres (see below).

Many other services, more or less specifically directed at mental health problems can also be offered, such as drop-in centres, relatives' support groups, and bereavement counselling as well as home-help services, meals-on-wheels, community centres and holidays.

Day centres

Day centres are run by non-medical staff and offer a variety of more or less structured occupational and recreational activities and group discussions, sometimes for special needs. They aim to provide a period of supportive help on a medium- or longer-term basis, for people with more enduring or relapsing disorders. In practice much overlap with the function of day hospitals is found, with a tendency in both to accumulate people with indefinitely continuing need for daytime support.

Voluntary organisations

Charitable organiations play an increasingly important part in mental health services; their earlier role of filling gaps in provisions by the statutory agencies is being greatly extended, in some places providing central coordination for major elements of the service in housing, day centres, workshops and many other enterprises. The variety is enormous. Some such as the Richmond Fellowship, the Mental Aftercare Association, Mind, Mencap, the Samaritans, the National Schizophrenia Fellowship and Age Concern are nationally organised with local foci, while others, such as housing associations, serve particular localities. Self-help groups have developed to focus on particular kinds of problems, such as Alcoholics Anonymous and Accept (alcoholism), Narcotics Anonymous, Tranx (drug dependence), Overeaters Anonymous and Anorexic Aid (eating disorders).

Work opportunities are discussed in Chapter 53.

SERVICE PROVIDERS

Relatives and families, often with little or no support from professional agencies, provide the major bulk of care and support for people with mental disorders, even of the most severe and disabling kind. The degree of emotional stress experienced by these relatives is often not sufficiently appreciated (Fadden *et al.* 1987).

The quality of any service depends primarily on those who provide it and, for professional staff, on the training and support that helps them to function most effectively. As services evolve outside hospital without the strong traditions and structure of big institutions, problems in defining roles and responsibilities can repeatedly arise as staff come and go, successively building and dismantling different styles of interaction and management.

The major professional service providers for the mentally ill include general practitioners, psychiatrists, psychiatric nurses, social workers, various social service personnel employed as residential care assistants, day centre supervisors, clinical psychologists and occupational therapists. These professionals may work on their own, but there is an increasing tendency for *multidisciplinary teams* to play a central role in providing services for the mentally ill either in the community or in hospital. Such teams are often led by a consultant psychiatrist or, though less often, by one of the other team members. They usually include nurses (a role taken in the community by community psychiatric nurses), a social worker and perhaps a clinical psychologist and occupational therapist. Such teams can work well together by combining a wide range of skills and perspectives. In some cases, however, conflicts and uncertainties about leadership, treatment approach or the roles of individual team-members can lead to a confused and troubled team lacking consensus or clear purpose. It is increasingly common to designate a *keyworker* as the person most directly in contact with the patient and responsible for providing his continuing personal support and overall coordination of services.

Besides providing teams for general psychiatric services, Districts commonly aim to develop sub-specialist teams concerned with problems of rehabilitation and longer-term illness, elderly patients, children and adolescents, mental handicap and drug dependency.

ACCESS TO PSYCHIATRIC CARE

This has been discussed by Goldberg and Huxley (1980) and is described in Chapter 55 (see p. 645). Once a patient has decided to seek help or has been persuaded to do so by friends or relatives he will usually consult his GP who may provide physical or psychological treatment himself or within the practice setting. If the patient is not well enough to attend the surgery the GP may arrange a domiciliary visit by a psychiatrist or a *crisis intervention team*, including a psychiatrist, social worker and community psychiatric nurse (CPN). Or the general practitioner may refer the patient to a local psychiatric outpatient department, or for admission to an inpatient unit.

In some cases local authority social workers may be the first to be alerted to the need for psychiatric assessment, e.g. by friends or neighbours. Occasionally an approved social worker (see p. 668) may be asked to arrange compulsory admission to a psychiatric unit under the powers granted by the Mental Health Act (1983) (see Chapter 62).

Other routes include attendance at a drop-in centre or emergency clinic available in some centres, or at a casualty department with direct access to a psychiatrist. Some patients may be referred to liaison psychiatrists from the medical or surgical services in a general hospital. Services such as hostels, old people's homes, day centres and prisons usually have special arrangements for calling upon a psychiatrist for assistance. Some patients are referred to the psychiatric services from the Courts; a disturbed patient found in a public place may be taken to a 'place of safety' such as a casualty department under section 136 of the Mental Health Act, or a police surgeon may seek to arrange admission from the police station.

REQUIREMENTS AFTER DISCHARGE

All too often patients are discharged from hospital too early or to an unsupportive environment, with no support to prevent relapse and ultimately readmission. At the very least there should be a continuation of outpatient supervision and follow-up until the patient's state has stabilised. Only then should the patient be transferred back to the care of his GP for continuing support and maintenance drug treatment, if required. The community psychiatric nurse may administer neuroleptics by injection, perhaps in a special 'depot clinic' which can also offer an opportunity for social contact and support. Other special outpatient clinics may be provided, e.g. to supervise lithium treatment or for continued behaviour therapy. Patients in need of formal psychotherapy may attend the outpatient department for individual, group, marital or family therapy.

The need for residential accommodation with or without supervision may delay discharge, especially as the existing facilities in the community are far from adequate. The necessary arrangements are usually made by the hospital-based social worker who should be familiar with the various forms of accommodation in the local community, such as group homes, mental health after-care hostels, or some kind of adult foster care (see Chapter 57).

Similarly, residential arrangements may have to be made for elderly people, e.g. in some kind of sheltered accommodation, or the more intensive provision of part III accommodation, so-called after part III of the National Assistance Act 1948, in old people's homes. These are run by local authorities and have care assistants rather than nurses so that the patient may have to be readmitted if he becomes incontinent or deteriorates mentally or physically.

We have already mentioned the role of day hospitals and day centres, and the support given to patients discharged home by regular visits from social workers or CPNs.

Lastly, it must not be forgotten that the more disabled or itinerant patient, e.g. a chronic schizophrenic discharged into the community, may easily become detached from supportive services and may progressively slide into self-neglect if there is no relative or agency to motivate the services to re-establish and retain contact. The itinerant patient without a fixed address often also loses contact with the general practitioner services. Gains made during periods of active treatment and contact with community services may all too quickly be lost if efforts at maintaining support are not sustained.

COST AND OTHER STATISTICS

NHS spending on hospital mental health services accounts for about 13 per cent of total spending on hospital and community provisions (excluding primary care). Of this total, only about 10 per cent is spent on day-patients and outpatients. Social service departments provide very much less than this for the mentally ill, perhaps 10 per cent of the NHS total, with under 2 per cent of the total budget or Personal Social Services directed towards them. Plans to direct a greater share of funding towards services outside hospital have a very long way to go before the rhetoric of community care becomes a reality.

Over the past 25 years the number of patients in psychiatric hospitals in England and Wales has fallen from 145,000 to under 70,000; the total continues to decline, partly through discharge but mainly through death of long-stay patients. The great majority, over 55,000, are in over 100 mental hospitals. Services outside hospital now offer over 16,000 day hospital places and about 9,000 places in day centres The fall in hospital beds is not matched by the growth of alternative residential accommodation, for which only some 6,000 places have been provided.

Staffing

There are now over 1,000 consultant psychiatrists and some 60 times that number of nurses in psychiatric units. CPNs have increased at least three-fold in the last ten years to over 2,000. Clinical psychologists number about 1,500. In some areas the introduction of Griffiths Management has been associated with disproportionate increases in non-clinical administrative staff. In mental handicap hospitals numbers of residents have also been falling, to about 40,000 in 1983, of whom 1,250 are children. The number of consultant psychiatrists in mental handicap is about 150 with, again, about 60 times as many nurses.

Estimating requirements

In 1975, the White Paper 'Better services for the mentally ill' (DHSS 1975) gave details of our 'norms' of requirements per head of population for mental illness services. A 1971 White Paper had undertaken a similar task for mental handicap services (DHSS 1971).

Though offered as guidelines, the 'norms' were widely adopted more rigidly by health authorities because they offered an attractively concrete approach to planning service requirements; when abused in this way the 'norms' have proved misleading. Additional account must be taken of local factors, such as indices of social deprivation, associated with greatly increased needs for services.

Administrative battles between those who want to dictate what the needs ought to be and those confronted by the actual scale of need are all too common. Particular uncertainty has surrounded the question of how many places will be required for long-stay patients, whose numbers are expected to reach a plateau when the continuing decline of the *old long-stay* is matched by the steady accumulation of *new long-stay* patients who cannot easily be discharged. A 1981 DHSS calculation suggested that by 1991 an average health district would have 140 inpatients per 100,000 of population, 80 of whom would be long-stay; 34 of these would be over the age of sixty-five.

PROBLEMS

The lack of a unified Mental Health Service in Britain militates against ease of coordination of services when more than one agency is needed by the patient and his family. Development plans for the various types of service required differ widely in different parts of the country. Competing demands on scarce resources are made by plans to close mental hospitals, by the needs of special groups such as the behaviourally disturbed, drug abusers, ethnic minorities and the rising tide of the very elderly infirm. Services for people with neurotic and other problems of adjustment have very limited manpower and the scale of need is much greater than can be met within general practice. Often administrators look for savings in mental health budgets to meet the increasing cost of acute medical services and new technologies.

The present upheavals in the delivery of services for mental health pose many challenges for doctors, including the task of clarifying the proper scope for medical and psychiatric intervention in an immense range of human problems which vary from the mainly physical to the entirely social. Continuing improvements in the psychosocial awareness of general practitioners and in the quality of entrants to psychiatry offer the greatest cause for hope.

ILLUSTRATIVE CASE HISTORY*

Henry Holt, aged 46, first turned up at odd intervals in the casualty department of a District General Hospital in a dirty and dishevelled state, smelling of alcohol, and sometimes noisily abusive when his requests for Valium were refused. On several occasions the hospital security staff had to be called to eject him. The psychiatrist who was called to see him could not make much sense of his muttered speech which sounded grossly thought-disordered and probably deluded. He was unshaven and dressed in a filthy Army overcoat, and his feet were wrapped in what looked like off-cuts from a furrier's. So far as could be gathered he was living in the streets and eating scraps of food from restaurant dustbins. The consultant psychiatrist gave him a small number of Valium tablets and asked him to come back sober for a longer interview, but he failed to keep his appointment. After

* The names in this case history are fictitious.

several weeks, the consultant saw him again and this time offered him a bed in the mental hospital admission unit, which he promptly accepted.

In hospital he was cleaned up and quickly settled gratefully into the ward routine. His speech became more intelligible though still grossly thought-disordered. He seemed to have multiple delusions of a fantastic kind. He conveyed the impression that he believed that his penis had been replaced by the IRA with a second-hand one. It emerged that before he became a vagrant he had worked as a porter for many years in a hospital and had been treated for severe anxiety symptoms by a psychiatrist who, when contacted, remembered him well; there had been no hint of psychosis.

In hospital his mental state greatly improved with antipsychotic medication and he became a regular attender at the hospital industrial workshops. The psychologist was able to assess his cognitive abilities, which showed some acquired performance deficit over and above a modest intelligence, and advised a programme of rehabilitation. The social worker had a particularly important role in preparing the liaison with the local authority adult fostering scheme, by whom he was found residential accommodation with a family who were paid for his upkeep and care. Placement in an aftercare hostel or group home had been considered but it was thought he would benefit from the more personal support of a family home. He was registered with a GP in a Health Centre, who prescribed continuing antipsychotic injections. These were administered by a community psychiatric nurse based at the Health Centre, who was able to persuade him to attend the depot injection clinic at the local hospital. If he did not attend she visited him at home. For daytime occupation he initially attended the hospital workshops as an outpatient and then transferred to the local day centre run by the local branch of Mind. Here he was able to take part in a variety of activities and to attend social evenings with other disabled patients.

One thing had been particularly unusual about Mr Holt. An EEG in hospital revealed temporal lobe epileptic activity, which was thought possibly to account for the development of his schizophrenic symptoms (see p. 317) and the extreme social decline associated with them. Anticonvulsant medication was prescribed. He is currently doing well, is always smartly dressed, friendly and cheerful, though rather shy, retiring and nervous. The thought disorder and delusions are no longer evident.

Henry's story illustrates the use of some of the services available in or outside hospital to provide continuing support and assistance in the four major areas of service provision needed by psychiatric patients. Complicated and diverse as services for the mentally ill may at first appear, they can be seen as varying realisations of four main elements:

(1) A place to stay with an appropriately supportive social and phy. environment, e.g. a home, hospital or hostel.

(2) Services to go out to during the day, e.g. for treatment, shelterec work and recreation.

(3) Services that can when necessary come to the patient at his place of residence, e.g. community nurses, doctors, other visiting professionals and support services.

(4) A special person or people to relate to, who make it their responsibility to help the patient achieve the best possible level of functioning, e.g. a GP, keyworker or therapist.

Pared down to the barest essentials, this outline can serve as a basic framework for organising services to help and support people with mental illness; it can also be used to formulate a series of questions as to how each element of care can best be provided to meet the needs and wishes of any particular patient and his relatives.

FURTHER READING

Fadden, G., Bebbington, R. and Kuipers, L. (1987). 'The burden of care: the impact of functional psychiatric illness on the patient's family'. *Brit. J. Psychiat.* 150, 285-292.

Martin, F.M. (1984). *Between the Acts: community mental health services 1959-83.* Nuffield Provincial Hospitals Trust.

Report of the Richmond Fellowship Enquiry (1983). *Mental Health and the Community.* Richmond Fellowship Press.

Social Services Select Committee Second Report (1985). *Community Care with special reference to adult mentally ill and mentally handicapped people*, vols 1-3. HMSO, London.

Wilkinson, G., and Freeman, H. (eds). (1986). *The Provision of Mental Health Services in Britain: the way ahead.* Royal College of Psychiatrists. Gaskell, London.

Wing, J.K. (ed.) (1982). 'Long-term community care: experience in a London borough'. *Psychol. Med. Monograph Supplement* no.2.

57

The Hospital Social Worker

In 1974 the Social Services in the UK were reorganised following the recommendations of the Seebohm Report, and provision of a social work service to hospitals became the responsibility of local authorities. Before reorganisation social workers worked in several separate departments: there were Child Care Officers, Mental Health Social Workers and Welfare Workers employed by the local authority dealing with the elderly and disabled, and Medical and Psychiatric Social Workers working in hospitals employed by the Health Service. This arrangement led to narrow definitions of the social work role and to some families being visited by more than one worker.

After reorganisation the local authorities created departments which provided the full range of social services, including residential, day and domiciliary care. These services were organised by Social Services departments and divided into local area offices. There was also an expansion of training courses leading to the Certificate of Qualification in Social Work (CQSW), which was designed to equip students with the basic skills required to start practising social work in these new 'generic' departments. As a result specialisation became unfashionable. Training remains generic, although students choose fieldwork placements which reflect their special interest. Opportunities for post-qualification training also continue to be provided but these are often limited by the financial constraints on local authorities.

Before the reorganisation the term Psychiatric Social Worker (PSW) referred to a social worker who had specialised training in the mental health field. Nowadays PSW is used to describe a social worker who works primarily in the mental health field, usually in a psychiatric setting, but who has not necessarily had such specialised training although he may have had additional experience in clinical psychiatry, and sometimes in psychotherapy. It is in this sense that the term PSW is used here.

Critics of this less specialised service and training regret the demise of the old system in which the PSW had a more extensive, specialised knowledge of clinical psychiatry, some psychodynamic training, greater familiarity with multi-disciplinary teamwork and a stronger identification with the hospital setting. On the other hand, many social workers in psychiatric settings such as inpatient wards, outpatient departments, day hospitals, child and adolescent departments and drug dependency clinics now have experience of working in area teams and voluntary agencies. They will be familiar with the whole local authority system, all aspects of social services and a wide range of community resources. Communication with area-based colleagues is therefore easier and they are more likely to see admission to hospital as part of a continuum of community care.

ROLE IN THE HOSPITAL TEAM

The PSW, though an integral part of the clinical team, is an employee of the local authority and therefore independent of the hospital hierarchy. He therefore stands at the interface between the health service and community provision and is well placed to ease communication and increase understanding between professionals. Liaison with agencies outside the hospital is an important part of the work; the PSW builds links with local area offices, day care centres, residential homes, housing departments and community centres. Community workers who are encouraged to come into the hospital and to participate in decision-making may be willing to do so only if they feel that their contribution is valued. The presence of a social worker in the hospital team may do just that. Sometimes differences between the medical and social work approaches to patients may lead to a gap in understanding and reinforcement of mutual suspicions. For example, area social workers may be seen as being 'anti-psychiatry', while psychiatrists may be regarded as paternalistic or authoritarian, seeking to control unwanted behaviour with 'damaging' drugs. Each may feel that the other does not live in the 'real world'. Since most contacts between these different groups take place in hospital, area social workers will be on unfamiliar ground. The hospital social worker, used to moving between the two systems, can facilitate communication, counteract these misconceptions and promote mutual understanding and collaboration. It is equally useful for hospital staff to go out to meet community workers on their territory.

Patient care is organised in various ways depending on the setting. The starting point is an assessment. This is followed by treatment, discharge and aftercare. Close cooperation between the social worker and other members of staff is essential. The social worker's particular role in assessment is to gain an understanding of the patient's social network and circumstances, and to ensure that this is communicated to the team and given due consideration alongside other clinical factors. In interviewing people from the family or other supporting networks at this stage, the social worker's task is not only to ask for information, which is often obtained by other members of the team, but also to offer emotional and practical support. It is always useful to ask why an admission occurs at any particular time. It is often due as much to changes in the supporting environment, such as the departure of a familiar GP or community nurse, as to a deterioration in the patient's clinical condition. Admission to hospital or any referral to a psychiatric agency often follows a period of stress for the family as well as the patient. Offering support to families of patients from the start of an admission can lead to an earlier discharge. If patients return to an unchanged stressful environment, the improvement achieved through treatment is unlikely to be maintained. Often family and friends have fears and misconceptions about psychiatric treatment and find the hospital system intimidating. This is especially likely among ethnic minorities, and the social worker can help by identifying and mobilising those services which help such minority groups.

The treatment phase of admission overlaps with assessment and plans for discharge. Often all three proceed simultaneously. Many PSWs, in common with psychiatrists, psychotherapists and other professionals, undertake psychotherapeutic work with patients individually, in families and in groups. Social workers also use a method known as *social casework* which tries to effect change within a trusting relationship. This can be useful with individuals for whom formal psychotherapy would not be considered suitable. Caseworkers deal with both the internal and external worlds, offering emotional support together with practical help when appropriate. Casework values include respect for the individuality and autonomy of the client and acceptance of his right to make decisions about his life.

Social work begins with the problem that is presented to the social worker, e.g. social security or other money matters, accommodation problems, or anxieties to do with a spouse or children. Some parents may be particularly worried that, once children are received into the care of the local authority because they are temporarily unable to look after them, they will be prevented from resuming parental care. This may lead them to view the offer of social work help with suspicion. In recent times there has been a move away from a more exploratory approach towards brief problem-solving or task-centred therapy which identifies small but well-defined goals for the patient. Casework is usually grounded in psychodynamic theory, but some methods from behaviour therapy are being used as well.

FAMILY AND GROUP WORK

Although much of their work is with individual clients, social workers also see patients in groups and work with families. *Group work* ranges from psychotherapeutic groups (see p. 566), treating a small number of outpatients over a long period, to large groups of acutely disturbed patients, where the composition of the group changes rapidly. Social workers may also organise support groups and social activity groups for discharged patients and relatives; these fulfil an important function for patients, who are often isolated people, anxious at leaving the security of the hospital and facing the outside world.

Family therapy (see p. 577) is a growing area of interest for professional mental health workers. Social workers have always sought to understand behaviour in terms of relationships; they have long appreciated the value of seeing the individual's problems in the context of the family and wider social network, and of working with couples and families. Family therapy is therefore increasingly being used as a method of intervention by clinical teams including social workers.

AFTERCARE AND REHABILITATION

After a period of inpatient treatment many patients will return to their former way of life, perhaps supported by outpatient appointments and their GP, and may only need minimal help on leaving hospital. Others may need to attend a psychiatric day hospital or day centre as a continuation of treatment. For a sizeable proportion of inpatients, especially in inner-city areas, once acute symptoms have subsided, social factors may prevent discharge. One of the tasks of the PSW is to look at the options available in terms of accommodation, employment and other social support, and to discuss these with the patient and his family. The local authority, whose duty it is to house those who are vulnerable through ill-health, can often only offer suitable accommodation after a long period of waiting in depressing bed-and-breakfast hotels. Hostel places are also in short supply, in spite of the efforts of voluntary organisations such as the Richmond Fellowship to provide half-way houses. Some local authorities have adult care or fostering schemes which provide family care or lodging in sympathetic households. In group homes ex-patients share a house, sometimes with a caretaker living in and with support from social workers and community psychiatric nurses. There are also specialist hostels dealing with the rehabilitation of patients with a history of alcohol or drug abuse.

Finding the resources to fit the needs of each individual is a time-consuming process. The ideal is often not available, and then a compromise has to be negotiated. Although it may seem to the clinical team, who are concerned with freeing beds, that the process of placement is unnecessarily protracted, the PSW has to allow time for patients to make important choices about their future and must resist pressure to achieve discharge deadlines. It is encouraging to see patients, who had previously drifted or stayed in large impersonal hostels where they felt isolated, become part of a group home where they feel they have a right to be and where they can both receive and give support. Often the PSW responsible for a placement will continue to give support to the patient over a long period.

In London, as in other inner city areas, many of the people sleeping rough in night shelters or homeless hostels are suffering from psychiatric disability. With the threatened closure of large mental hospitals before adequate community care is established, this problem is likely to become considerably worse.

Clinical example

Since coming to London from Scotland four years ago, Mr Smith had had frequent episodes of schizophrenic breakdown requiring hospitalisation. Between admissions he had returned to live in a vast Victorian lodging house where his strange manner made him unpopular and liable to verbal and physical abuse. He in turn became afraid and suspicious of help. He did not attend the outpatient clinic or continue the prescribed medication and within a short time had to be readmitted. His PSW then found a group home for him. He shares this with three other discharged patients, attends a day centre, takes his medication and enjoys shopping, cooking and watching television at home. He still feels depressed at times and talks to himself, but this is not frightening for the other residents, who tolerate his occasional odd behaviour.

COMPULSORY ADMISSION

In the past PSWs based in hospitals rarely undertook the duties of what used to be called a 'Mental Welfare Officer' auhorised to make applications for compulsory admissions under the old Mental Health Act (1959). The arguments against such involvement were first that the PSW would have difficulty in maintaining professional independence in the face of medical recommendations from close colleagues; and secondly that to exercise such authority would damage the therapeutic relationship. Both arguments have some validity. Mind (The National Association for Mental Health) does not consider it good practice for a hospital social worker to make an application for admission or a change of status of an existing patient if this is based on the medical recommendation of a member of the same clinical team. However, many social workers, e.g. probation officers and child-care workers, have to reconcile social control with a therapeutic role. The use of authority may sometimes be an effective demonstration of the worker's caring attitude.

PSWs with their particular expertise and experience in the field of mental health work can in fact bring much of value to the role of what is now called an *Approved Social Worker* (ASW) under the new Mental Health Act 1983. This Act (see p. 704) requires that both medical and social work professionals assess the needs and situation of the patient, weighing social and psychiatric factors in deciding whether to use statutory powers to compel admission to hospital. The Mental Health Act 1983 makes it a positive duty for the ASW to make sure that hospital admission is essential and that no less restrictive alternative course of action is available. PSWs, with their experience in the field of mental illness, are increasingly choosing to take on this role, confident that professional independence can be maintained. The PSW also plays an important part in ensuring that detained patients receive assistance in exercising their rights of appeal and in preparing social reports for

Mental Health Tribunals. Local authorities, together with District Health Authorities, have a duty to provide aftercare for many detained patients on discharge, and this requires close cooperation between hospital and local social workers.

OTHER RESPONSIBILITIES

PSWs, together with psychiatrists and other professionals, need to monitor gaps in the services for the mentally ill and bring collective pressure to bear on the authorities responsible for the provision of care both in hospital and the community. A further and important reason for the continuation of the PSW's hospital-based role lies in the opportunity to teach the understanding of the social aspects of patient care to junior social work staff and students undertaking placements in psychiatric settings.

FURTHER READING

Blestock, F. (1961). *The Case Work Relationship.* Allen & Unwin, London.

Fisher, M., Newton, C. and Sainsbury, E. (1983). *Mental Health Social Work Observed.* Allen & Unwin, London.

Madones, C. (1980). 'The prevention of re-hospitalisation of adolescents and young adults'. *Family Process* 19, 179-191.

Pringle, N. and Thomson, P. (1986). *Social Work, Psychiatry and the Law.* Heinemann, London.

58

The Psychiatric Nurse

The nursing staff provide the largest professional resource in caring for people with mental illness, yet their skills and expertise are still under-rewarded and often unrecognised. Psychiatric nurses meet patients in a great many settings: casualty departments, outpatient departments, inpatient units, day hospitals, health centres and the patient's own home. All have received specialised training and have experience of working in a multidisciplinary team.

When nurses first became involved in caring for the mentally ill, they were primarily responsible for the patients' physical well-being. They would make sure patients were clean and properly dressed, help them to organise their day and administer any medication prescribed by the psychiatrist. They would also supervise special treatments such as ECT. While responsibility for these duties remains important today, psychiatric nurses have become much more personally involved with their patients, and more skilled in developing therapeutic relationships with them. Of all the members of the treatment team, the psychiatric nurse has the greatest opportunity to spend time with patients. The nursing staff can thus observe and assist distressed patients when their need is greatest, and convey information about them to the treatment team which will influence any decisions that have to be made.

Good psychiatric nursing is dependent on the nurse maintaining an attitude of hope and encouragement towards his patients in order to show them that, no matter how depressed or disturbed, they have the capacity for change and recovery. Some patients will at times become uncooperative, manipulative and aggressive. It is important for nurses to try to understand why this is happening and look for ways of helping them. Even patients whose illness is chronic and whose mental functioning has deteriorated can sometimes be helped to function at a better level by a psychiatric nurse who is willing to search for any remaining strength to build on.

This type of nursing makes great demands on personal resources. Relating to patients whose behaviour may be offensive, frightening, bizarre or socially inappropriate demands great professional skill. The task is made easier if the nurse has acquired some psychological understanding of patients' disturbed behaviour and of his own reactions

670

to them.

The many roles of the psychiatric nurse include the following:

(1) To assess the patient's needs, circumstances and difficulties, and to administer and coordinate patient care and treatment.

(2) To plan with the patient and help to implement treatment programmes, coping strategies and methods of self-care.

(3) To share with other members of the team the responsibility for creating and maintaining a supportive and therapeutic environment, be it in a ward, day hospital or the community.

(4) To observe and assess the patient's relationship to other patients and to liaise with relatives, friends and any other health professionals involved.

(5) To assess the patient's own perception of the source of his problems and his response to psychiatric intervention.

Nurses should formulate a *nursing care plan* which takes account of the views of all concerned with the patient's illness and treatment. The care plan is developed from observing the patient, identifying his needs and setting priorities for nursing intervention and goals. For example, a patient who is depressed, socially isolated and withdrawn may be allocated a key-worker nurse (see below) and encouraged to develop a relationship with him. The key-worker will then accompany the patient to other activities, such as group and occupational therapy sessions. As the patient improves and becomes more confident in his own ability to relate to other people, the nurse may gradually encourage him to become more independent and self-reliant.

Evaluation depends on continually assessing the patient's progress and the effect of interventions by other members of the team. This process enables the nursing intervention to be modified and is viewed as a continuing process for both the patient and the psychiatric nurse.

Some nurses have received training in and developed special techniques of treatment and rehabilitation, including behaviour therapy, group therapy and counselling, and can use these on psychiatric wards and in other treatment settings.

A psychiatric nurse is often assigned to an individual patient as a *key-worker*, taking special interest in the treatment and management of that patient and acting as co-ordinator for the various resources within the multidisciplinary team. The key-worker may also act as a *nurse therapist* for a specific treatment programme, e.g. desensitisation in the case of an agoraphobic patient, or he may accompany the patient to his home in order to assess how he is functioning there.

When the patient leaves hospital, a *community psychiatric nurse* (CPN) may become involved in further management, visiting the patient at home, perhaps supervising medication and acting as a link between the patient and his GP and other psychiatric services. As the psychiatric services become more community orientated, the role of the CPN is bound to become even more important in ensuring the continuing support and well-being of psychiatric patients.

FURTHER READING

Dexter, G. and Wash, M. (1986). *Psychiatric Nursing Skills*. Croom Helm, London.

Lyttle, J. (1986). *Mental Disorder: its care and treatment*. Bailliere & Tindall, London.

Martin, P. (1987). *Psychiatric Nursing: a therapeutic approach*. Macmillan, London.

59

The Clinical Psychologist

There is often some confusion in the lay person's mind about the difference between psychologists and psychiatrists. Broadly speaking, psychiatrists treat patients with mental illness and emotional disorders by both physical and psychological means. They must have a detailed knowledge of the interaction between physical and mental function and need to be medically qualified. Psychologists, on the other hand, have a degree in psychology and are specially concerned with the scientific study of psychological processes and behaviour, both in health and in illness. There are several different specialities within the discipline, including developmental psychology, educational psychology, neuropsychology and social psychology. Some psychologists, after their basic training, decide to follow a course of postgraduate studies in order to become clinical psychologists. They can then contribute special skills and expertise to the psychological assessment and treatment of people with mental illnesses or emotional disorders.

In the past clinical psychologists mainly carried out routine tests, e.g. of intelligence or personality, and treated patients with behaviour therapy. Nowadays their work covers a much wider field. The work of individual clinical psychologists is largely determined by their particular interest and specialised postgraduate training. For example, they may carry out cognitive therapy, behaviour therapy, analytical psycho-therapy, group, family, marital or sex therapy; many are also engaged in research and teaching.

Developments in patient care, particularly the growth of community psychiatric services, have also changed the role of psychologists and led to the broader application of their skills. Whereas they tended to be based mainly in departments of adult and child psychiatry and mental handicap, nowadays they also work with psychogeriatric patients, patients with physical handicap, in rehabilitation, day hospitals and general practice. Increasingly they also treat patients directly referred to them without prior referral to a psychiatrist.

The contribution of clinical psychology to psychiatry will be considered under the following headings: psychological assessment; psychological treatments; research and evaluation.

PSYCHOLOGICAL ASSESSMENT

This is concerned with obtaining accurate, often quantitative, information about a patient's symptoms, psychological functioning and behaviour, including learning ability, memory, thought processes, affective state, personality characteristics and social interactions. Psychologists decide on which assessment methods to use in the light of the nature of the patient's problem, usually after discussion with the psychiatrist and other members of the treatment team. Psychological assessment includes an interview, observation of the patient's behaviour, and sometimes psychological tests. The clinical psychologist will then acquaint his colleagues with his findings and discuss how these affect diagnosis and treatment.

Psychological testing

Psychiatrists frequently refer patients for assessment of some specific aspect of their psychological functioning such as intelligence or memory. The psychiatrist will have made some assessment during his clinical interview, but psychological testing can often provide more detailed information and the results can be expressed quantitatively. Clinical psychologists use standardised tests whose reliability and validity have been established. An important function of psychologists is to decide which tests to use and how to administer them accurately. This can be difficult, particularly if the patient is confused, unable to concentrate, overanxious or uncooperative. The patient's mental state at the time of testing must always be taken into account when interpreting the results.

There are many different tests, e.g. of memory, intelligence and personality; some also provide information about the presence of organic brain damage. A few of the most commonly used are described in the appendix at the end of this chapter (p. 676).

Sometimes a psychologist will design a special test for a particular patient if there is no standardised test available to investigate his problem. For example, a partially sighted child of normal intelligence may have difficulties with some day-to-day tasks requiring certain spatial abilities. A test may be constructed by the psychologist, based on the components of such tasks, to determine whether and with what help the child will be able to learn the necessary skills.

Tests repeated at intervals are used to assess the course of a patient's disorder or his response to treatment. For example, in a patient with dementia further intellectual deterioration may become apparent when an intelligence or memory test is repeated after six months or a year. After a patient has completed a treatment programme, changes in his responses to tests of personality function or symptomatology may give quantitative information, sometimes based on rating scales, about the effectiveness of the treatment received.

PSYCHOLOGICAL TREATMENTS

An important task of clinical psychologists is the treatment of patients either individually or in couples, families or groups, using the different psychological treatment methods described in Chapters 44-6.

Psychologists who work with the physically or mentally handicapped, or with brain-damaged or chronic psychotic patients, often organise rehabilitation programmes to teach communication and social skills. For example, many long-stay patients with chronic schizophrenia are withdrawn and socially isolated, and have lost socially desirable behaviour. Clinical psychologists have helped to organise wards on an operant conditioning model, where the staff regularly reward socially desirable behaviour (see also p. 588). Rewards are either tokens which can be used to obtain further privileges or praise and permission to do what the patient enjoys. It seems likely that the social interaction between patients and staff also plays a part in modifying the patients' behaviour.

Psychologists can help patients with other types of problems by means of *social skills training*. For example, people who have difficulty asserting themselves may meet with a psychologist in a group and attempt to identify common experiences. They are then asked to role-play specific situations which they have found difficult to cope with in reality, such as being unfairly criticised by a superior at work. The group strongly encourages the person to assert himself instead of accepting this situation. Such newly learnt behaviour may need rehearsing again and again. Finally, the group sets practical tasks for its members, e.g. returning a shop-soiled article or saying 'No' in a specific situation when they would normally avoid confrontation, with individuals reporting back at the next meeting.

Clinical psychologists may also teach other members of the treatment team, e.g. nurses in hospital or in the community, how to use behavioural or other treatment methods such as anxiety management.

RESEARCH AND EVALUATION

Research often requires collaboration between colleagues from several disciplines, e.g. psychiatrists, psychologists, social workers and sociologists. As the training of psychologists places great emphasis on research and scientific methodology, their participation in such joint ventures is particularly helpful. They may, for example, help to evaluate the results of a drug trial, or methods of reducing violent behaviour on a psychiatric ward. A great deal of research is being done by psychologists on the evaluation of psychological treatment methods. This is discussed in Chapter 47.

Psychological studies are also carried out to assess psychological reactions to medical and surgical conditions and procedures, e.g. the psychological sequelae of coronary artery bypass surgery, psychological reactions to AIDS, and coping strategies for cancer sufferers. In some larger research units, programmes of a more ambitious nature are undertaken, e.g. to study the consequences of unemployment, the relationship between life events and mental illness, or the epidemiology of mental disorders. Psychologists may also teach other professionals the scientific basis of their discipline, especially in relation to research methodology and its applications to psychiatry.

APPENDIX: PSYCHOLOGICAL TESTS

Intelligence tests

These are among the best known psychological tests. The one most widely used nowadays is the *Wechsler Adult Intelligence Scale* (WAIS). It is divided into a verbal scale to measure verbal abilities and a performance scale to test practical abilities. The verbal scale is divided into six sub-tests: information, comprehension, arithmetic, similarities, digit span, vocabulary. The performance scale is divided into five sub-tests: digit symbol, picture completion, block design, picture arrangement, object assembly. Separate scores are obtained for each of the sub-tests of the verbal and the performance scales. The test also provides a full-scale IQ and separate verbal and performance IQs. One advantage of the WAIS is that, in addition to providing a measure of general intelligence – a broad concept, not easy to define – the scores of the various sub-tests provide information on specific abilities and help to distinguish particular areas of dysfunction which can then be tested in greater detail.

In general terms, a full scale IQ between 90 and 109 indicates that the person falls into the average range of intelligence (50 per cent of the population); an IQ of between 110 and 129 indicates above average intelligence (17.8 per cent); and an IQ of above 130 superior intelligence (2.2 per cent). People scoring between 70 and 89 are of below average intelligence (17.8 per cent of the population); those with an IQ below 70 are mentally retarded (2.2 per cent). Individuals with an IQ below 50 are moderately or severely retarded. This is usually the result of brain disease, and their number therefore exceeds that to be expected at the bottom end of the normal distribution curve (see also p. 523).

Discrepancies between the verbal IQ and the performance IQ may provide information about possible brain damage. For example, if the performance IQ is significantly lower than the verbal IQ this may suggest deterioration due to generalised brain damage. If, on the other hand, the verbal IQ is significantly lower than the performance IQ, this may suggest a focal lesion in the dominant hemisphere affecting verbal skills, unless it is due to poor education or lack of verbal stimulation. Modern neurological investigations such as a CT scan may provide more accurate information about a possible organic cause.

There are many other intelligence tests. Two which are commonly used are the *Ravens Progressive Matrices*, which assess non-verbal visuo-spatial abstraction abilities, and the *Mill Hill Vocabulary Scale*, which measures verbal ability.

Several criticisms have been made of the use and interpretation of intelligence tests. Each test is based on the results obtained when the test was first standardised in relation to a particular population. For example, the WAIS was standardised on a sample of 1,700 people aged between sixteen and sixty-four in the USA (Wechsler 1958). It cannot be taken for granted that the results are equally applicable to a different population, culture or age group. Personality factors such as motivation and persistence will also affect the result. In the individual patient inability or refusal to concentrate, fear of failure, confusion, anxiety or depression will all affect the result, and psychologists are used to taking this into account when administering the test.

In spite of these limitations intelligence tests are of value, if interpreted with caution, especially for the following purposes:

(1) To assess the degree of intellectual impairment in children or adults suspected of having below normal intelligence. This is especially important in relation to mental handicap (see Chapter 41).

(2) To identify specific learning deficits or assets, especially in relation to educational or vocational assessment.

(3) To investigate the presence of organic brain lesions affecting intellectual function and behaviour. There are many neuropsychological tests specially designed to investigate the presence of cerebral lesions.

(4) To follow the progress of intellectual deterioration due to organic brain disease by repeating tests over a period of time, e.g. in patients with Alzheimer's disease, Korsakoff's psychosis or multiple sclerosis.

(5) In research, e.g. to investigate the influence of environmental factors like lead or nutrition on intelligence.

Memory tests

One of the earliest effects of organic brain disease is impairment of memory, especially of recent memory and new learning ability (see p. 268). If some evidence of impairment of recent and remote memory has been found during clinical examination, there are many standardised memory tests which can provide more detailed and quantitative information. The psychologist will advise which memory test to use for a particular patient.

As in intelligence testing, the patient's mental state at the time of the test must be taken into account; e.g. a patient with early dementia may feel afraid of not being able to answer the questions and become acutely anxious or unwilling to cooperate.

A commonly used test is the *Wechsler Memory Scale*. The result is expressed as the 'memory quotient', which allows for the patient's age and can be compared with his IQ. It is useful in detecting diffuse brain damage, as in dementia. Memory tests will not be described in detail here.

Personality tests

Personality is usually defined as a consistent collection of characteristics or personality traits, but it may also be considered in terms of recurrent behaviour patterns or intrapsychic, psychodynamic relationships. The method of assessment chosen is thus bound to be influenced by one's concept of personality structure. There are many personality tests, but they can be divided into two major types:

Structured self-report measures

In these tests the patient has to answer a series of questions. He must either choose between two or more alternative answers, or decide where his answer falls on a rating scale. Some tests focus on a specific personality variable, e.g. assertiveness, while others aim at a broader picture of the individual's personality. A common test of this type is the *Minnesota Multiphasic Personality Inventory* (MMPI), which consists of 550 printed statements describing behaviour, attitudes, beliefs, symptoms, traits and feelings, to which the patient responds 'True', 'False' or 'Cannot say'. The answers are computed on several scales which describe various dimensions of personality and psychopathology, e.g. 'hypochondriasis', 'hysteria', 'masculinity-femininity', 'paranoia', and so on.

Projective tests

These consist of ambiguous stimuli to which the patient is asked to give his personal responses. Well-known examples include the *Rorschach Test* and the *Thematic Apperception Test* (TAT). Projective tests are based on psychodynamic concepts and aim to provide an understanding of conscious and unconscious mechanisms and dynamics of the patient's personality. In the Rorschach Test the patient is shown inkblots of various shapes and asked to say what they bring to mind. In the TAT he is shown a series of pictures and asked to invent a story about each one. The patient projects his own fantasies, feelings, thoughts, desires and conflicts onto the inkblot or picture. For example if he responds to a particular inkblot by seeing it as representing an aggressive and devouring object, this is taken to indicate destructive and aggressive fantasies within his personality. In this way it is possible to obtain some understanding of the patient's inner world and psychopathology.

The interpretation of projective tests relies heavily on the psychologist's experience and inferences. Such tests rarely provide more information than a psychodynamic interview conducted by an experienced dynamic psychotherapist, and are used less often nowadays than they once were.

FURTHER READING

Carr, A.C. (1985). 'Psychological testing of personality' in *Comprehensive Textbook of Psychiatry* (Kaplan, H.I. and Sadock, B.J., eds), 4th ed., vol. 1, pp. 514-535, Williams & Wilkins, Baltimore and London.

Matarazzo, J.D. (1985). 'Psychological assessment of intelligence', also in *Comprehensive Textbook of Psychiatry*.

Shackleton, V. and Fletcher, C. (1984). *Individual Differences: Theories and applications*, Methuen, London.

Weinman, J. (1987). *An Outline of Psychology as Applied to Medicine,* 2nd ed. Wright, Bristol.

60

The Occupational Therapist

Occupational therapists (OTs) play an important part in patient care, but their precise role is often unclear and frequently misunderstood. They work in hospitals, outpatient departments, Social Service departments, day hospitals, general practice settings and the patient's home. They work with many different groups of patients ranging from children to the elderly, and including both the physically and the mentally ill. Occupational therapy is part of the overall treatment and management of patients, and special skills and treatment techniques are used by OTs in their work with psychiatric patients.

To qualify as an OT a three-year diploma course must be completed. It includes the study of both psychiatric and physical illness and disability. The OT is trained to consider patients in the context of their social, domestic, psychological and physical difficulties. The course includes one year of clinical placements in a variety of rehabilitation settings, and most colleges teach the students various practical skills, e.g. woodwork, printing, art, pottery and more recently the use of computers.

ROLE IN PSYCHIATRY

The most significant distinction between the work of the OT and the intervention of other disciplines within psychiatry is that occupational therapy is based on the use of practical activities, both manual and social. The skill of OTs lies in their ability to select and grade activities appropriate to the needs of individual patients. A patient's programme may include many different basic aspects of existence, e.g. managing personal hygiene and nutrition, performing work tasks, mixing with and tolerating the company of friends, family and strangers, and pursuing various enjoyable or creative interests. Occupational therapy aims to help patients to perform skills, tasks and roles which are part of their everyday life and necessary for independent living. Where full independence cannot be achieved, the aim of treatment is to help the individual to attain the highest possible level of functioning. Using everyday domestic, work, social and creative activities, including cooking, shopping, craftwork and social groups, the OT assesses the patient's level of functioning within these areas. By engaging in activities the patient is required to step out of the more passive, dependent 'sick role' which he may have adopted, especially if he is in hospital. The OT has a unique opportunity to observe, assess and define the patient's skills and level of ability, and to identify his social and behavioural deficits.

Having made an assessment, the OT will develop a graded and sequential programme of activities. These will vary widely among the patient population, such as a midde-aged woman resuming a full-time job and returning to manage her home with her husband and children; a young single man preparing to live alone and facing the possibility of unemployment; an elderly bereaved widow moving into residential Part III accommodation where domestic independence will be discouraged but where independence in personal care, dressing and feeding may be essential. The nature of the OT's intervention will be determined by the patient's clinical condition and personal circumstances.

Occupational therapy programmes may include both individual and group methods; the programme is usually formulated in discussion with both the patient and the treatment team. In order to be effective the patient's active involvement and cooperation is essential. He must be clear about the purpose of occupational therapy and what it may help him to achieve. Initial lack of motivation can often be improved if the psychiatric treatment team encourages and supports the patient's involvement in occupational therapy.

Assessment

The OT first interviews the patient in order to obtain some basic information about his home, work and social situation. He must explain how occupational therapy may be able to help the patient and try to establish a working relationship with him. The patient is then encouraged to attend selected activity groups so that the OT can assess how he is functioning in the following areas: general behaviour, including reality orientation; task performance, including cognitive and motor skills; and interpersonal behaviour.

Treatment aims

Once the areas of dysfunction have been defined, short-term and long-term aims can be drawn up. Short-term aims have to be achieved in preparation for more long-term aims; the short-term aim may be to increase concentration before the long-term aim of returning to work can be considered.

Treatment plans

A graded programme of activities is then formulated. The programme is designed to match as closely as possible the patient's highest level of present functioning, taking into account his personal needs and interests.

Pressure is then applied gradually through increasing expectations, complexity of tasks and goal-setting.

Evaluation

It is essential to evaluate the patient's progress throughout and to modify the programme accordingly. The OT will be involved in team discussions of resettlement and discharge, with special emphasis on social, domestic, work and leisure activities.

TECHNIQUES

The following is a brief account of some of the more specialised techniques used by OTs. Several are carried out in conjunction with other members of the psychiatric team, such as psychologists, psychiatrists, nurses and social workers.

Social skills training

The aim of social skills training (see also p. 675) is to teach the patient to overcome his social anxieties and become more confident in social situations, such as meeting people and making friends, asking for goods in a shop, attending interviews and facing up to authority figures. Methods include the use of role-play, modelling, positive reinforcement and facing anxiety-rousing situations by undertaking practical assignments. Social skills training programmes are either run in a closed group as a course of, say, ten sessions, or as a continuing weekly session on the OT programme.

Anxiety management

This includes teaching patients to recognise the source of their anxiety and to understand the non-threatening nature of any accompanying physiological manifestations, and helping them acquire methods of coping with their anxiety, mainly through relaxation techniques. This is followed by gradual exposure to anxiety-provoking situations.

Relaxation training

Anxiety management is appropriate for only some patients suffering from anxiety; others may not be sufficiently motivated to cooperate. For these patients relaxation training may be more useful. Patients are taught to practise various relaxation techniques, but the cognitive component and graded exposure used in anxiety management are not included. Relaxation sessions are often available in occupational therapy departments to a wide range of patients, not only those suffering from anxiety.

Physical exercise

Physical exercise increases bodily awareness and physical coordination, and may produce a sense of well-being and reduce tension. Occupational therapy departments therefore often include physical exercise in their activity programme, perhaps running keep-fit or yoga classes in the department, or using hospital or local sports facilities. Team games give an opportunity for social interaction, cooperation and enjoyment. In general, physical activities may help to counteract the inactivity and passivity so often found on psychiatric wards.

Reminiscence therapy

Reminiscence therapy is used in an attempt to help elderly and confused patients with impairment of memory to increase their social interaction with others. Sessions are conducted in a group usually once a week, and discussion of past events, both personal and historical, is encouraged by the use of audio-visual presentations, music, photographs and newspaper articles.

Reality orientation

Reality orientation helps some patients with impairment of memory to become better orientated in their environment and fosters social interaction. Reality orientation programmes are best run on a 24-hour basis in residential and hospital settings and require the cooperation of all members of staff. Large clocks and visual display boards giving the date, time, place, weather and next meal are placed around the ward. This information is continually reinforced by the staff and also through more structured group sessions run by the OT.

Creative therapies

Creative therapy includes the use of art, music, drama, dance and movement. Therapists usually have a qualification in one of these areas. Some hospitals and day facilities employ workers who are not OTs but are qualified art, drama, music or dance therapists. Creative therapists should be familiar with the basic principles of psychotherapy and group dynamics. Creative therapies are based on the principle that patients can benefit from being helped to overcome their inhibitions and express themselves as freely as possible. For example, the dance therapist may encourage each person in the group to express himself through dance and body movement, while the art therapist aims to create an atmosphere in which people can express themselves through the use of paint or other art materials. Group members are encouraged to share their experience, thus increasing their awareness of others.

The type of patients selected for these groups varies. Some therapists choose to work with patients who have a potential for insight and a desire to change, sometimes using what the patient expresses in the creative medium to promote self-understanding. Other therapists work with more severely disturbed patients, mainly to increase social interaction.

Home management skills

OTs traditionally undertake the assessment of domestic skills and provide an opportunity for patients to practise them, both within the occupational therapy department and at home. Some departments run cookery sessions, others include cookery in a home management course which covers a wider range of domestic skills, including budgeting, planning and preparing meals, personal care, safety and first aid in the home.

Work

Some occupational therapy departments provide work-type activities, usually light industrial or clerical jobs, all of which are carried out within the department. Some larger psychiatric institutions have separate workshops which function independently. Some of these pay the workers weekly in cash or goods. Sheltered workshops have also been set up in the community for psychiatric and physically disabled clients. Their work is often of a high standard, and contracts from outside firms can be obtained to provide a steady flow of work.

OTs may also carry out a work assessment of individual patients; the patient's manual skills, including the use of tools, motivation to work, and ability to concentrate and to relate to supervisors and colleagues at work are all evaluated.

Leisure activities

As the likelihood of unemployment increases, the need to find stimulating and rewarding activities for psychiatric patients outside work becomes paramount. Most occupational therapy programmes include group sessions which focus on exploring and discovering the resources available in the local community. These include museums, theatres and parks, libraries, sports centres, Citizens Advice Bureaux, adult education classes, neighbourhood centres and social clubs, as well as voluntary organisations and town hall information centres. Members of the group discuss their ideas and share their knowledge of local resources, often taking responsibility for planning outings and visits for the whole group. Teachers may be employed to teach specific skills and activities like pottery, art or woodwork. These teachers often also run adult education classes in the community, so that they can assist patients in the transition from hospital to join classes or other training facilities outside.

FURTHER READING

Mosey, A.C. (1973). *Activities Therapy*. Raven Press, New York.

Wilkinson, J. and Canter, S. (1983). *Social Skills Training Manual*. John Wiley, London.

Wilson, M. (1983). *Occupational Therapy in Long-term Psychiatry*. Churchill Livingstone, London.

Wilson, M. (1984). *Occupational Therapy in Short-term Psychiatry*. Churchill Livingstone, London.

Part X

Forensic Psychiatry

The legal provisions described in this part apply to England and Wales only. Separate provisions apply in Scotland and Northern Ireland.

see also thiamine; nicotinic
    acid; pyridoxine; cyanocobalamin
    (B12); folic acid
voyeurism, 355, 360

Wernicke's encephalopathy, 381, 382
    see also Wernicke-Korsakoff
    syndrome
Wernicke-Korsakoff syndrome, 381-2
Weschler adult intelligence scale, 676
Weschler memory scale, 677
Willis, F., 10
Willis, T., 9
Winnicott, D. W., contributions of
    child psychotherapy, 500, 565
    false self, concept of, 65
    good enough mother, concept of, 95

mother-infant relationship,
    studies of, 64-6
and object relations theory, 18, 64
play, views on role of, 75
stage of concern, concept of, 70, 197
transitional objects, studies on, 67
witchcraft, 7
Woolf, V., suicide of, 201
word salad, 120
work, meaning of, 90-1
writer's cramp, 478

yoga, 5

zuclopenthixol decanoate, 615
    depot preparation for maintenance
    therapy in schizophrenia, 615